Failed Fracture Fixation

Peter V. Giannoudis • Paul Tornetta III
Editors

Failed Fracture Fixation

Revision Surgery Made Easy

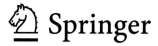

Editors
Peter V. Giannoudis, MD, PhD, FACS, FRCS, MBE
School of Medicine, Trauma and Orthopaedic Surgery
University of Leeds
Leeds, UK

Paul Tornetta III, MD, PhD
Boston University Medical Center
85 East Concord St
Boston, MA, USA

ISBN 978-3-031-39691-5   ISBN 978-3-031-39692-2 (eBook)
https://doi.org/10.1007/978-3-031-39692-2

© The Editor(s) (if applicable) and The Author(s), under exclusive license to Springer Nature Switzerland AG 2024

This work is subject to copyright. All rights are solely and exclusively licensed by the Publisher, whether the whole or part of the material is concerned, specifically the rights of translation, reprinting, reuse of illustrations, recitation, broadcasting, reproduction on microfilms or in any other physical way, and transmission or information storage and retrieval, electronic adaptation, computer software, or by similar or dissimilar methodology now known or hereafter developed. The use of general descriptive names, registered names, trademarks, service marks, etc. in this publication does not imply, even in the absence of a specific statement, that such names are exempt from the relevant protective laws and regulations and therefore free for general use.

The publisher, the authors, and the editors are safe to assume that the advice and information in this book are believed to be true and accurate at the date of publication. Neither the publisher nor the authors or the editors give a warranty, expressed or implied, with respect to the material contained herein or for any errors or omissions that may have been made. The publisher remains neutral with regard to jurisdictional claims in published maps and institutional affiliations.

This Springer imprint is published by the registered company Springer Nature Switzerland AG
The registered company address is: Gewerbestrasse 11, 6330 Cham, Switzerland

Paper in this product is recyclable.

Peter V Giannoudis
Dedicated to my wife Rania and my children Marilena and Vasilis for their love, patience, and support throughout my career.

Paul Tornetta III
To my mother, Phyllis, who found the best in people, had compassion for all, and whose insight, guidance, and love have always made me believe that anything is possible.

Preface

Bone fractures continue to be a global public health issue. The global burden of disease study 2019 (CGD 2019-https://ghdx.healthdata.org/gbd-2019/data-input-sources) reported that in 2019 the prevalence of fractures in all age groups was 455 million worldwide. These primarily affected the appendicular skeleton.

While many fractures can be managed non-operatively, others require fixation to prevent malunion, allow early range of motion, prevent the so-called fracture disease and facilitate early hospital discharge.

Operative fixation includes external fixation, intramedullary nailing, plates and screws, and combinations of these. Each of these options is considered based on the fracture type, anatomical location of the fracture, and patient characteristics (profile).

Despite every surgeon's best intention to achieve optimum fracture fixation and an uneventful healing outcome, failed fixation can occur. While the true incidence of failed fracture fixation is unknown, it varies between different anatomical locations, and its incidence is thought to range between 0% and 15% of operated cases. When a surgeon designs the fracture construct and applies it in the operating room, the race begins between union and fixation failure. The surgeon essentially decides what the mode of fixation failure will be based on the construct applied.

Failed fixation requires revision and that brings additional risks for the patient. In addition, planning and executing revision surgery is more challenging than the initial surgery. It requires an understanding of the failure mode, the mechanics of the injury, and biology of the region.

In this textbook, every chapter describes how to successfully address failed fixation in different anatomical sites with different implants. From the conception of this project, the aim was to help clinicians get experience in this thought process by real examples.

Each chapter provides the reader with the aetiology of failure (why the fixation failed), what kind of investigations would be necessary to formulate an appropriate pre-operative plan, what instruments are needed for removal of the failed implant, what new implant should be used, how the revision surgery should be carried out successfully, and whether any type of bone grafting would be needed.

We hope the book will help in the decision-making process and in the selection of the appropriate implant and surgical technique not just surgeons in training but also qualified orthopaedic surgeons in their busy practice.

We are grateful to all the contributors to make this project possible, and we hope this textbook will be another reference book in the practice of surgeons to improve patient care and clinical outcomes.

Leeds, UK   Peter V. Giannoudis
Boston, MA, USA   Paul Tornetta III
January 2024

Contents

1 Epidemiology of Fracture Fixation Failure 1
Paul L. Rodham, Vasileios Giannoudis, Paul Tornetta III,
and Peter V. Giannoudis

2 Common Causes of Aseptic Fracture Fixation Failure 23
Mark Johnson, Grayson Norris, Jake Checketts,
and Brent L. Norris

**3 General Considerations: Analysis of Failure of Fixation:
A Stepwise Approach** 37
Volker Alt, Markus Rupp, and Siegmund Lang

4 Acromioclavicular Joint Dislocation Failed Fixation 55
Paul Cowling

5 Failed Fixation of Clavicle Fracture 65
Brian J. Page and William M. Ricci

6 Failed Fixation of Proximal Humerus Fracture 77
David Limb

7 Failed Fixation of the Humeral Neck Fracture 87
Carol A. Lin and Milton T. M. Little

**8 Humeral Shaft Fracture: Failed Intramedullary
Nail Fixation** 97
Ashley Lamb, Ian Hasegawa, and Joshua L. Gary

9 Failure of Plate Fixation of Humeral Shaft Fractures 109
Emmanuele Santolini and Peter V. Giannoudis

10 Distal Humerus Failed Plate Fracture Fixation 117
Chang-Wug Oh and Peter V. Giannoudis

11 Failed Fixation of Olecranon Fractures 131
Hüseyin Bilgehan Çevik and Peter V. Giannoudis

12 Failed Fixation of Capitellum Fractures 137
Paul L. Rodham, Vasileios Giannoudis,
and Peter V. Giannoudis

ix

13 Failed Fixation of Radial Head Fractures 145
Charalampos G. Zalavras and John M. Itamura

14 Forearm Fracture Failed Fixation 151
John A. Scolaro

15 Distal Radius K-Wiring Failed Fracture Fixation 157
Michael G. Kontakis and Peter V. Giannoudis

16 Distal Radius Plate Failed Fixation 163
Mitch Rohrback, Erik Slette, Austin Hill, and David Ring

17 Perilunate Dislocation Failed Fixation 173
Chrishan Mariathas

18 Pelvic Fracture Failed Fixation 181
Nathan Olszewski and Reza Firoozabadi

19 Acetabulum Posterior Wall Fracture Failed Fixation 193
Amit A. Davidson, George D. Chloros,
Nikolaos K. Kanakaris, and Peter V. Giannoudis

20 Intracapsular Proximal Femoral Fracture Failed Fixation 201
Paul L. Rodham, Vasileios Giannoudis,
and Peter V. Giannoudis

**21 Extracapsular Proximal Femoral Fracture Intramedullary
Nailing Failed Fixation** 211
Paul L. Rodham, Vasileios Giannoudis,
and Peter V. Giannoudis

22 Susbtrochanteric Femoral Fracture Failed Fixation 219
Vasileios P. Giannoudis, Paul L Rodham,
Nikolaos K. Kanakaris, and Peter V. Giannoudis

23 Midshaft Femoral Plate Failed Fixation 227
Vasileios Giannoudis, Paul L. Rodham,
and Peter V. Giannoudis

24 Distal Femur Plate Failed Fixation 237
Andrea Attenasio, Erick Heiman, Richard S. Yoon,
and Frank A. Liporace

25 Distal Femur Periprosthetic Fracture Failed Fixation 249
Martin Gathen, Koroush Kabir, and Christof Burger

26 Quadriceps Tendon Repair Failed Fixation 259
Patrick M. N. Joslin, Kristian Efremov, Robert L. Parisien,
and Xinning Li

27 Patella Tendon Repair Reconstruction for Failed Fixation 271
Patrick M. N. Joslin, Kristian Efremov, Robert L. Parisien,
and Xinning Li

28 Patella Fracture Failed Fixation 281
Daniel Scott Horwitz and Taikhoom M. Dahodwala

Contents

29 Tibial Plateau Plating Failed Fixation 289
Chang-Wug Oh and Peter V. Giannoudis

30 Proximal Tibial Intramedullary Nailing Failed Fixation 305
Sushrut Babhulkar, Sunil Kulkarni, and Sangeet Gawhale

31 Proximal Tibia Plating Failed Fixation 311
Heather A. Vallier

32 Extra-Articular Tibial Shaft Ilizarov Failed Fixation 325
Paul Nesbitt, Chris West, Waseem Bhat, Martin Taylor,
Patrick Foster, and Paul Harwood

**33 Distal Tibial Extra-Articular Intramedullary
Nail Failed Fixation** 335
Michael J. Price and Peter V. Giannoudis

34 Distal Tibia Extra-Articular Plating Failed Fixation 345
Zoe B. Cheung and Philip R. Wolinsky

35 Distal Tibial Intra-Articular Ilizarov Failed Fixation 357
Paul Nesbitt and Paul Harwood

36 Distal Tibial Intra-Articular Plating Failed Fixation 369
Vincenzo Giordano, Robinson Esteves Pires,
Felipe Serrão de Souza, Franco L. De Cicco,
Mario Herrera-Perez, and Alexandre Godoy-Santos

37 Lateral Malleolus Ankle Failed Fixation 379
Georgios Kotsarinis and Peter V. Giannoudis

38 Bimalleolar Ankle Failed Fixation 391
Jodi Siegel

39 Ankle Syndesmosis Injury Failed Fixation 401
George D. Chloros, Emmanuele Santolini, Amit E. Davidson,
Anastasia Vasilopoulou, and Peter V. Giannoudis

40 Posterior Malleolar Ankle Failed Fixation 417
Scott P. Ryan and Nicholas R. Pagani

41 Talar Fracture Failed Fixation 435
Xinbao Wu, Xiaofeng Gong, and Peter V. Giannoudis

42 Fifth Metatarsal Fracture Failed Fixation 445
George D. Chloros, Adam Lomax, and Peter V. Giannoudis

43 Calcaneus Fracture Failed Fixation 455
Mandeep S. Dhillon and Ankit Khurana

44 Lisfranc Fracture Failed Fixation 467
Mark Yakavonis and Gregory Wayresz

Index 473

Epidemiology of Fracture Fixation Failure

1

Paul L. Rodham, Vasileios Giannoudis, Paul Tornetta III, and Peter V. Giannoudis

Introduction

Since the 1950s and following the introduction of fracture fixation techniques by the AO group in Switzerland, there has been a revolution of implant designs to allow fixation/reconstruction of fractures of all different anatomical areas of the human body [1]. Both internal and external fixation implants with or without specific anatomical profiles are currently being used in the clinical setting [1].

The objective is that the implant selected to stabilise the injured limb will provide adequate fracture stability to obtain bony union, and restore the affected limb axis, rotation, length and joint congruence [2]. It is anticipated that the implant will provide the appropriate biomechanical environment to allow fracture healing and then no longer be needed for physiologic loading. While implants have been divided to load sharing (Intramedullary nailing) and load bearing (plating systems; locking and non-locking) devices, both are at risk of failure prior to the fracture uniting.

The aetiology of metal work failure is multifactorial including selection of wrong implant, sub-optimal fixation technique, non-compliant patient, fragile bone, non-union and infection amongst others [3–5].

Although metal work failure post fracture fixation is infrequent, the overall incidence of this phenomenon is not well reported in the literature. Herein, we report the incidence of fixation failure prior to fracture union in different anatomical sites of the human body.

P. L. Rodham · V. Giannoudis
Academic Department of Trauma and Orthopaedics, School of Medicine, University of Leeds, Leeds, UK
e-mail: p.rodham@nhs.net;
vasileios.giannoudis@nhs.net

P. Tornetta III
Boston University Medical Center, 85 East Concord St, Boston, MA, USA

P. V. Giannoudis (✉)
Academic Department of Trauma and Orthopaedics, School of Medicine, University of Leeds, Leeds, UK

NIHR Leeds Biomedical Research Center, Chapel Allerton Hospital, Leeds, UK

Proximal Humerus

Proximal humeral fractures are the third most common non-axial osteoporotic fracture, affecting 63/100,000 persons [6]. They most commonly affect elderly females sustaining these injuries from low-energy falls [7]. The majority of humeral fractures are low energy with low rates of non-union and can be managed non-operatively [8]. When operative treatment is planned, this can be either in the form of fixation or arthroplasty.

© The Author(s), under exclusive license to Springer Nature Switzerland AG 2024
P. V. Giannoudis, P. Tornetta III (eds.), *Failed Fracture Fixation*,
https://doi.org/10.1007/978-3-031-39692-2_1

The use of locking plates has expanded the role of fixation of proximal humerus fractures, gaining better purchase and fixation in osteoporotic bone. Despite this the failure of these devices continues to be reported in between 7 and 14% of cases [9–13]. Factors associated with the loss of reduction when using locking plates include increasing patient age, presence of osteoporosis, initial varus displacement, degree of reduction achieved, residual varus following fixation and medial comminution [10, 11]. The reported rate for fixation failure in a recent systematic review examining the role of intramedullary nails in the management of proximal humerus fractures suggests a failure rate of up to 24%, with risk factors for failure including the use of this device in three and four-part fractures in addition to the aforementioned risk factors [14].

Humeral Shaft

Humeral shaft factors account for between 1 and 5% of all fractures, with an incidence between 13 and 20/100,000 patients [15]. They have a bimodal distribution with an initial peak in young men between the age of 21 and 30 years, often as a result of high-energy trauma; and a second peak in elderly females between 61 and 80 years, more commonly in the setting of low-energy injuries [15]. Operative management can consist of either plate fixation or fixation with an intramedullary nail, and is utilised in up to 60% of cases [16].

Failure of plate fixation is rarely reported, with small series reporting fixation failure in 4–6% of cases, most commonly associated with osteoporotic bone, short plate span and an early return to weight-bearing activities [17–19]. Similarly low rates of fixation failure are quoted for intramedullary nailing [19].

Distal Humerus

Distal humeral fractures represent one-third of all humeral fractures with an incidence of 6/100,000 patients [20]. As with humeral shaft fractures they have a bimodal distribution with young men sustaining high-energy fractures, and older women sustaining low-energy injuries [20]. Operative treatment is associated with good clinical outcomes, and therefore the role of non-operative management is reducing, generally restricted to undisplaced fractures or those who are not medically fit enough to undergo anaesthesia [21].

When fixation of distal humeral fractures is selected over arthroplasty options, dual plate fixation, either in a parallel or a perpendicular configuration, is generally undertaken. Fixation failure is reported to occur in between 0 and 27% of these cases [22]. Osteoporosis represents a significant risk factor for failure of fixation, and in its presence consideration should be given to the use of arthroplasty [23]. Other risk factors for failure include the use of perpendicular plating, metaphyseal comminution, inadequate volume of screws in the distal segment, usage of short screws in the distal segment [22, 24, 25].

Olecranon

Olecranon fractures are common injuries sustained in the elderly population, with an incidence of 15/100,000 patients [26]. As intra-articular fractures, an operative approach is generally recommended unless the fracture is undisplaced. In those <65 years, an operative approach is taken in 79% of cases, with this tactic reducing in the over 65 s at 65% [27]. Popular techniques for fixation of these fractures include the use of plate fixation, and tension band wiring [27].

Tension band wiring of olecranon fractures is appropriate with simple fracture patterns in the absence of comminution [28–30]. Failure of this technique is reported in between 4 and 16% of cases. Factors that appear to be most associated with failure include the placement of intramedullary wires as opposed to bicortical hold, the use of single knot constructs as opposed to dual knot techniques and failure to adequately secure the proximal end of the K-wire [31–33].

Plate fixation is often utilised in the context of increasing patient age, and increasing com-

1 Epidemiology of Fracture Fixation Failure

plexity of fracture pattern. When utilising plates, current failure rates are quoted to be between 3% and 17% [29, 34, 35]. Prior to locking plate technology the majority of plate fixation would be with the limited contact dynamic compression plate (LCDCP), with failure occurring through screw pull-out [36]. The advent of locking systems specifically for the olecranon has reduced this occurrence, though these constructs may still fail in severely osteoporotic bone, and in highly comminuted fractures [37].

Radial Head

Radial head fractures affect 11/100,000 persons, most commonly females in their 60s [38]. Trends towards operative treatment of these fractures are increasing from 69% in 2007, to 85% in 2016 [38]. This is most commonly performed using screw fixation, although plate fixation and radial head replacement remain options for more comminuted fractures.

Screw fixation is rarely associated with failure, reported in between 0 and 15% of cases [39–42]. Reported risk factors for fixation failure include the presence of osteoporosis, development of non-union, multifragmentary fractures and the use of convergent screw orientations [41, 43]. Plate fixation is less commonly utilised when compared to screw fixation, and as a result there are no clear data available reporting the rates of fixation failure in this cohort.

Forearm

Whilst the highest rates of forearm fractures occur in children, there is a significant increase in these injuries in women aged over 45, and men aged over 70 [44]. The true incidence is poorly defined, but thought to be between 1 and 10/100,000 persons [45]. An operative approach to management is generally advocated due to the

risk of non-union, mal-union and subsequent difficulties with forearm rotation [46]. This is most commonly achieved with plate fixation in the adult population.

Failure of fixation is rare in this cohort, reported in just 2–4% of cases [47, 48]. As with many fracture types, the presence of comminution poses a risk of fixation failure. Additional risk factors include failure to provide compression to the fracture, and the use of short plates which has been demonstrated to be of a higher importance than the number of screws utilised in each segment [48].

Distal Radius

Distal radius fractures represent the most commonly sustained fracture seen by orthopaedic surgeons with an incidence of up to 195/100,000 persons in the United Kingdom [6]. They are increasingly frequently seen in female patients over the age of 60 as a result of a fall from standing height [49]. Extraarticular distal radius fractures that maintain an acceptable alignment can be reliable managed non-operatively; however, displaced fractures or those that extend into the joint surface require fixation. Currently between 14 and 16% of distal radius fractures are managed operatively, most commonly by plate fixation (62%) followed by K-wire fixation (30%) [50, 51].

Modern distal radial plate designs have expanded the scope of fixation including more reliable use in osteoporotic bone and distally based fractures. Within the current literature, the failure rates are noted to be between 1 and 13% [52–54]. Failure rates are reported to be higher in the setting of early return to weight-bearing, close proximity of the fracture to the volar rim with little plate coverage of the unstable fragment, multifragmentary volar rim fractures (AO23-B3), smaller width of the lunate fragment piece, greater ulnar variance on the pre-operative imaging and failure to achieve adequate articular reduction (Fig. 1.1) [54–57].

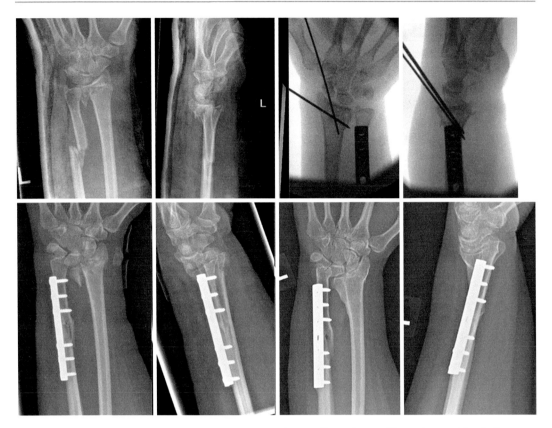

Fig. 1.1 A 42-year-old lady was involved in a rollover RTC sustaining an isolated closed distal radius and ulna fracture. She was taken to theatre on the morning following admission where following bridge plating of the ulna, her swelling did not allow for a second approach to the radius which was, therefore, managed with K-wires with a good intraoperative result. Unfortunately, she did not attend her early follow-up and returned at 6 weeks with a pin site infection, and a significant loss of reduction of the intermediate column of her wrist, resulting in incongruency of both her radiolunate and distal radioulnar joints. Given the concerns surrounding infection, she was treated with 4 weeks of antibiotics in order to suppress the infection until radiological union was achieved. She subsequently underwent removal of metalwork from the ulna accompanied by wrist denervation; however, she subsequently never returned for her planned ulna shortening and corrective radial osteotomy

Distal Ulna

Distal ulna fractures frequently occur in conjunction with distal radius fractures, with an incidence of 3.8/100,000 persons [58]. The majority of distal ulna fractures can be managed nonoperatively, particularly when screened to be stable following the fixation of a distal radius; however, when fixation is pursued, this is most commonly in the form of a plate [59].

Outcome of distal ulna fixation is significantly less frequently reported when compared to the distal radius. In those small series, assessing the outcome of fixation of the distal ulna the reported failure rate is 0%. These studies frequently don't examine the ulna in isolation, having been fixed in conjunction with fixation of the distal radius [60–63]. Whilst clinical data do not currently exist, finite element analysis would suggest that the fixation is under the lowest stress when placed on the dorsal surface of the ulna, with three points of distal fixation [64].

Pelvic Ring

Pelvic ring fractures have an incidence of 23/100,000 persons, with a bimodal distribution affecting young males with high-energy mechanisms, and elderly females with low-energy falls [65]. Operative fixation of pelvic ring injuries is infrequently performed, selected in just over 8% of cases [66]. When operative management is selected, this is frequently a combination of percutaneous screw fixation with open reduction and internal fixation with plates, or use of anterior external fixation [66].

Failure of plate fixation is commonly reported, although frequently asymptomatic. Rates of failure are reported in between 5 and 46% of patients; however, less than 10% of these are symptomatic and require reoperation [67–71]. Risk factors for failure of anterior plate fixation include the use of the technique in osteoporotic bone, the use of a single implant as opposed to dual implant and the use of fewer than 3 holes per segment when spanning the symphysis (Fig. 1.2) [66, 68].

Similarly high rates of fixation failure when employing the technique of anterior external fixation are also reported, in between 23 and 57% of cases [72, 73]. Risk factors for failure of this technique include initial fracture displacement, inadequate reduction particularly in the setting of vertical shear injuries, fixator loosening and the use of this technique in lateral compression type injuries [72, 73].

Fixation of the posterior pelvic ring, typically achieved with percutaneous sacro-iliac (SI) screws, has much lower reported failure rates, occurring in between 4 and 16% of cases [74, 75]. Risk factors for failure of this technique include non-union, intraoperative malpositioning due to either surgeon error or inadequate fluoroscopy, use of a single screw as opposed to two SI screws and patient non-compliance with postoperative weight-bearing instructions [74, 75].

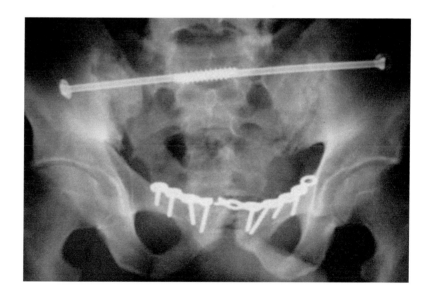

Fig. 1.2 Anteroposterior (AP) pelvic radiograph demonstrating a broken 3.5 mm matta plate. As a plate that spans the symphysis, this construct is continually exposed to bending stresses that lead to plate failure by fatigue (in this case the residual pubis diastasis that developed after failure of the plate did not require any further intervention as the patient was asymptomatic)

Acetabulum

Acetabular fractures are less commonly seen when compared to pelvic ring fractures, with an incidence of only 3/100,000 [76]. In contrast to pelvic ring injuries, they are more frequently observed in males, often as a result of a high-energy injury [77]. As an articular injury, an operative approach is more readily pursued when compared to the pelvic ring, across both the elderly and the non-elderly population [78]. Where fixation is performed, this is most commonly a combination of screw and plate fixation [78].

Failure of fixation is variably reported in the literature with many studies not directly commenting of fixation failure and instead reporting on rates of conversion to total hip arthroplasty (THA). Within the literature, the reported failure rate varies from 10 to 57% [79–82]. Risk factors for fixation failure in this population include increasing age, development of non-union, fracture comminution, initial articular displacement, inability to attain an anatomic articular reduction, fracture classification as an associated type particularly T-type with posterior wall involvement, obesity and surgeon error in siting the fixation device [83–85].

Proximal Femur

Proximal femoral fractures represent the second most commonly sustained osteoporotic fracture with an incidence of 129/100,000 persons [6]. The majority of these fractures affect the intertrochanteric region (60%), with 32% affecting the femoral neck, and 8% affecting the subtrochanteric region [86]. Management is almost exclusively operative unless the patient is unable to undergo an anaesthetic. Fixation is dependent on the location of the fracture and the degree of comminution, how-

ever, frequently involves the use of cannulated screws, a sliding hip screw, or a cephalomedullary nail [87].

Failure of fixation should generally be divided between those implant systems utilised in the management of intracapsular and extracapsular fractures. With regard to intracapsular fractures, the three most commonly utilised systems include the femoral neck system, cannulated screws and the dynamic hip screw with a derotation screw. The failure rates of the femoral neck system is currently reported in between 4 and 6% of cases; however, there is little literature examining this relatively novel implant [88, 89]. Failure rates of cannulated screw fixation are reported in between 13 and 39% cases, compared to failure rates between 0 and 20% when using a dynamic hip screw [90–96]. Risk factors for failure when managing intracapsular neck of femur fractures include increasing age, initial displacement, technical error in siting the implant, inadequate reduction, inferior cannulated screw distance >3 mm from the calcar, cannulated screw configuration (inverted triangle reduces in lowest failure rate) and a delay to fixation of greater than 24 h [88, 90, 97].

When considering extracapsular neck of femur fractures, the most commonly utilised fixation systems include the dynamic hip screw, and cephalomedullary nails. The rate of fixation failure utilising the dynamic hip screw is reported in between 4 and 28% of cases, whilst the rates of failure with an intramedullary nail are reported in between 0 and 13% of cases [98–105]. Risk factors for failure of fixation in extracapsular neck of femur fractures include increasing age, initial displacement, comminution, inadequate reduction, surgeon error, unstable fracture patterns (A2 or A3 compared with A1), comminution of the lateral cortex, calcar tip apex distance, notching of the screw aperture and reduction in a varus alignment (Fig. 1.3) [98–101, 106, 107].

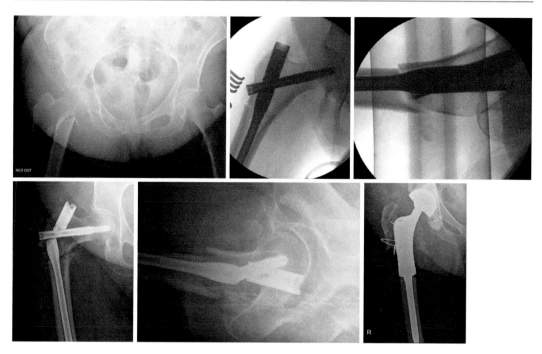

Fig. 1.3 Initial AP pelvic radiograph demonstrating a subtrochanteric proximal femoral fracture in a 74-year-old male that was managed with a cephalomedullary nail. As can be seen, the reduction was not anatomic with residual translation in the sagittal plane, and a degree of malalignment of the medial calcar. The patient represented at 2 months with varus collapse and failure of the nail through the lag screw aperture. This was successfully managed with a proximal femoral replacement to facilitate early patient mobilisation and rehabilitation

Femoral Shaft

The worldwide incidence of femoral shaft fractures ranges between 10 and 21 per 100,000 per year [108, 109]. They have a bimodal distribution affecting young males with high-energy mechanisms, and elderly females with low-energy falls [108]. These fractures are almost exclusively managed operatively. Operative fixation with intramedullary nailing is the gold standard of treatment; however, in transverse fracture patterns use of plate fixation is also observed [110].

The incidence of nail failure is low, reported in between 0.5 and 10% of cases [111, 112]. This is lower than those failure rates seen with plate fixation, which is reported in 1 and 14% of cases [113–115]. Risk factors for failure of femoral shaft fixation include undersising of the nail diameter, failure to lock nail, malreduction, comminution, degree of initial displacement, soft tissue stripping, development of delayed union, sagittal plane malalignment and the use of a short fixation working length when utilising a plate (Fig. 1.4) [114, 116].

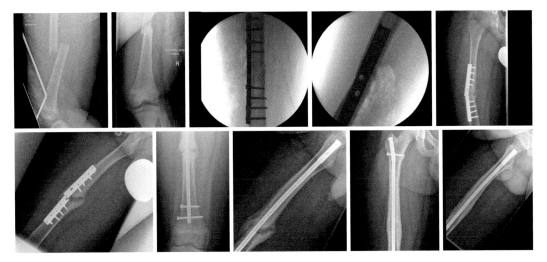

Fig. 1.4 Initial AP and lateral radiograph demonstrating a transverse midshaft femoral fracture in a 12-year-old boy. This was managed with compression plating performed via a lateral approach, as can be seen from the operative films the plate was not pre-contoured, and whilst a good reduction was achieved, there is still some residual gapping on the medial surface. The patient represented at 6 months post-operative with increased pain and swelling of the mid-thigh. Radiographs taken at the time demonstrated evidence of a hypertrophic non-union and breakage of the plate through fatigue. The fixation was removed and an antegrade trochanteric entry nail performed which went onto uneventful union

Distal Femur

Fractures of the distal femur are rare with a reported prevalence of 0.5% of all fractures; they have been slowly increasing in incidence over the past decade with most reported incidence of 8.7/100,000 person per annum [117]. These have been reported traditionally as fragility fractures and the increasing incidence is likely due to a shift towards an aging population worldwide. Distal femur fractures have a bimodal distribution, with patients either being young adults involved in high-energy trauma or elderly osteoporotic individuals who experience a fall from standing.

The most common fracture types are the 33-A1 or 33-A2. Type 33-C (complex articular fracture) is less common. Management is dependent on stability of the fracture pattern, involvement of the knee joint as well as patient-related factors. Where operations are deemed necessary, fixation is dependent on the location of the fracture and the degree of comminution. This normally involves the use of plate fixation (fixed angle blade plate vs. buttress plate vs. locking plate) or intramedullary nailing (antegrade vs. retrograde) [118–120].

The use of locking plates expanded the role of fixation within the distal femur, gaining better purchase and fixation in osteoporotic bone. Despite this, the failure of these devices has been reported in between 6 and 20% of cases [121, 122]. Factors associated with the loss of reduction when using locking plates include increasing patient age, presence of osteoporosis, initial varus displacement, poor initial reduction achieved, residual varus following fixation and medial or posteromedial comminution [121].

Proximal Tibia

Tibial plateau fractures account for 1% of all fractures and are typically sustained with high-energy mechanisms. The incidence of tibial plateau fractures is 10.3 per 100,000 people annually

[123]. They have a bimodal distribution with an initial peak in men younger than 50, often as a result of high-energy trauma; and a second peak in elderly females between years, more commonly in the setting of low-energy injuries leading to tibial plateau insufficiency fractures [123]. In intra-articular fractures, an operative approach is generally recommended unless the fracture is undisplaced. This can be either through the use of plates and screws, external fixator devices or alternatively arthroplasty [124, 125].

Failure of plate fixation has been reported, with small series reporting fixation failure in 30% of cases, most commonly associated with osteoporotic bone, fracture fragmentation and an early return to weight-bearing activities [126]. Failure of fixation elements when utilising a circular fixator is reported in 14% of cases [124].

Tibial Shaft

Tibial shaft fractures are common long bone injuries accounting for 2% of all adult fractures [127]. They have an incidence of 2/100,000 population with a bimodal distribution of peaks at ages 20 and 50 [128]. These injuries may be managed non-operatively if minimally displaced, alternatively they can be treated with Intramedullary nail fixation, external fixator devices or plate osteosynthesis [129]. A cross-sectional survey performed showed that 80% of surgeons treat these Injury patterns with operative intervention [130].

Intramedullary nail fixation failure has been listed as approximately 7.3% [131]. These patients have a higher percentage of open injuries with a higher degree of comminution and had been treated with smaller diameter nails when compared with the group of patients, who had no implant failure. Failure occurred most frequently at the transverse proximal locking screw when a single screw was used [131]. Failure of circular frames is infrequently reported, with most 'failures' constituting broken wires which do not necessarily require intervention in 0–5% of cases [132–134].

Distal Tibia

The incidence of distal tibia fractures is estimated to be 9.1/100,000 persons per annum [135]. Women appear to have an increasing incidence of distal tibia fractures when stratified by age whilst males have a fairly constant incidence [135]. Distal tibia fracture can be treated with a variety of operative treatment methods including external fixators, intramedullary nailing and internal plate fixation [136–138]. Of these fractures there is a reported incidence of 6.9/100,000 distal tibia fractures which are subsequently operated on [139].

Pilon fractures often pose challenging fracture configurations to adequately reduce. There is limited literature assessing failures of differing treatment modalities. Studies suggest a rates of fixation failure between 2 and 10% when utilising plate fixation, and 3% when utilising a circular frame [136, 140–143]. Most commonly cited issues include malreduction of the fracture site and there has been reported to be an association between the use of anteromedial plates and non-unions [140]. Further risk factors include the presence of comminution and periosteal stripping, often seen in open injuries (Fig. 1.5) [141, 142].

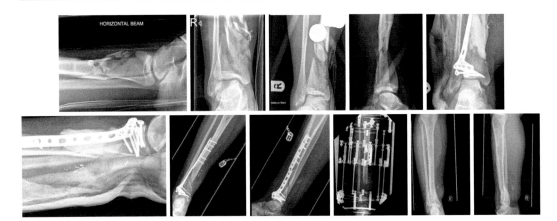

Fig. 1.5 A 34-year-old pregnant lady presented having been crushed between a van and a car. Her injuries included a lateral compression pelvic fracture, a left distal femur fracture and a right open tibial fracture. Following resuscitation, she was taken to theatre for caesarean section, pelvic fixation and debridement of her open tibial fracture with application of an ankle spanning external fixator. Two days following admission, she was returned to theatre for anterolateral plating of her distal tibial fracture and insertion of an antibiotics impregnated cement spacer with plans to reconstruct her bone defect via the Masquelet technique. She had her second stage Masquelet treatment at 6 weeks post first stage. Unfortunately, her graft failed to fully incorporate resulting in a distal tibial non-union and her plate failed via fatigue at 8 months post second stage. This was successfully managed with bone transport

Ankle

Ankle fractures, accounting for 3.9–10.2% of adult fractures, are the most common type of fracture of the lower extremity [144]. They have an incidence rate of 100/100,000 people per year, with the majority occurring secondary to low-energy falls (55%) [6, 145]. Operative management is dependent on the fracture configuration as well as patient-related factors. It may consist of either plate fixation or fixation with an intramedullary nail (Fibular nails/Hind foot nails).

The use of locking plates has significantly expanded the role of fixation within the ankle, gaining better purchase and fixation in osteoporotic bone, leading to a change in treatment paradigm in geriatric ankle fractures with few fixation failures reported. Surgical re-intervention has been reported to range between 1 and 2% [146]. The most common indication for surgical reintervention was syndesmotic malreduction (59%) in a cases series published. This is often secondary to fibula shortening leading to lateral translation with a potential rotational malalignment of the syndesmosis [146]. Furthermore, the importance in reduction of the posterior malleolus has also been shown in biomechanical studies to affect the syndesmosis. Other risk factors for failure fixation include obesity, inability to follow post-operative weight-bearing instructions and the presence of open fractures (Fig. 1.6) [147].

1 Epidemiology of Fracture Fixation Failure

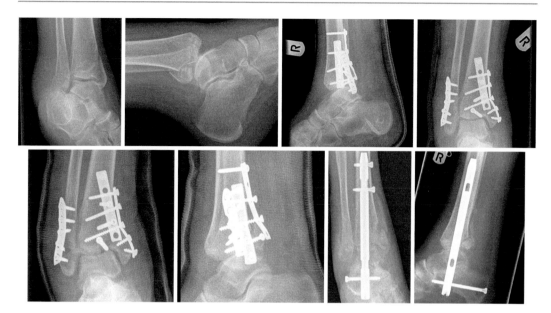

Fig. 1.6 AP and lateral radiograph of a trimalleolar ankle fracture in a frail 53-year-old female that was managed with open reduction and internal fixation with a fibula locking plate, and fragment specific fixation using 1/3 tubular plates for the posteromedial malleolus and the medial malleolar shear fragment. Due to frailty, the patient was not able to comply with post-operative instructions to non-weight-bearing and represented with increased pain and swelling 1 month post-operatively with repeated radiographs demonstrating proximal translation of the medial malleolus, loss of reduction and of joint congruence. Due to the patient's frailty, it was elected to revise this construct to a hindfoot nail which allowed the patient to weight bear without restrictions

Calcaneus

Calcaneal fractures are the most commonly fractured tarsal bone. The annual incidence of calcaneal fractures are 11.5/100,000 people, with a male to female ratio of 2.4:1, most common sustained following falls from height (70%) [148]. The fractures can be broadly classified into extra-articular injuries (25%) often secondary to Achilles avulsion type injuries or intra-articular fractures (75%) [149]. Operative fixation is often recommended when significant disruption to the 'angle of Gissane' or 'Bohlers angle' is present. This can be achieved through percutaneous screw fixation, plate fixation, primary subtalar arthrodesis or C-nails [150–154].

Failure of plate fixation has been documented to be between 0 and 40% and has been most commonly associated with osteoporotic bone [151, 154, 155]. The increasing use of locking plates has attempted to overcome this. There is paucity in literature detailing rates of fixation failures and the rationale behind this. One case series showed that screw fixation had a 24% probability of failure, plates showed a 36% failure and the most unstable seem to be the C-nails with 42% probability of failure. The authors do suggest fixation failure is often linked to patient factors such as smoking status and non-compliance with post-operative weight-bearing status.

Lisfranc

Lisfranc fractures have an incidence of 16/100,000 persons per year [156]. However, there actual incidence may well be higher due to up to 24% of these injuries being missed on their original radiographs [157]. These injuries are more common in males (4 males: 1 female) and most commonly occur in the third decade of life [158].

If true disruption of the ligamentous Lisfranc complex is present, then surgical management is often recommended. Operative intervention can consist of either open reduction internal fixation (ORIF) or primary arthrodesis [158]. The fixation method has been contentious with some surgeons advocating arthrodesis given the decreased need to return at a later date for removal of metalwork and subsequent fusion. Failure of fixation associated with ORIF can often be linked to over compression during the fixation, malreduction of the fracture site when the plates are applied or plantar trajectory of the 'home run screw' [159]. With respect to primary arthrodesis underprepared joints prior to fusion have been implicated with fixation failure, as has an early return to weight-bearing due to poor compliance [159].

Whilst failure of fixation is nor frequently reported, unplanned re-operation rates are similar between ORIF and primary arthrodesis (29.5 vs. 29.6%), most commonly due to post-traumatic arthritis in patients treated with ORIF and non-union in those treated with primary arthrodesis [160].

Discussion

Metal work failure remains a rare complication of fracture fixation, though the overall incidence is poorly defined within the literature. A summary of the current reported rates of fixation failure defined by anatomic site is summarised in Table 1.1.

Table 1.1 Incidence and rates of fixation failure alongside risk factors for fixation failure separated by body site

Site	Incidence	Rate of fixation failure	Risk factors for fixation failure
Proximal humerus	63/100,000 [6]	Plate: 7–14% [9–13] IM nail: 24% [14]	Older age Osteoporosis Varus displacement Varus reduction Medial comminution
Humeral shaft	13–20/100,000 [15]	Plate: 4–6% [17–19] IM nail: 6% [19]	Osteoporosis Short plate span Early return to weight-bearing
Distal humerus	6/100,000 [20]	Plate: 0–27% [22]	Osteoporosis Perpendicular plates Inadequate fixation in distal segment Use of short screws distally
Olecranon	15/100,000 [26]	TBW: 4–16% [28–30] Plate: 3–17% [29, 34], [35]	Osteoporosis Intramedullary wire placement Single wire knot Comminution
Radial head	11/100,000 [38]	Screws: 0–15% [39–42]	Comminution Convergent screws Non-union
Forearm	1–10/100,000 [45]	Plate: 2–4% [47, 48]	Comminution Short fixation span Inability to apply compression
Distal radius	195/100,000 [6]	Plate: 1–13% [52–54]	Early weight-bearing Fracture proximity to volar rim + low size of rim piece AO 23-B3 type Small width of lunate facet fragment Greater ulna variance on pre-op radiographs Residual articular displacement

1 Epidemiology of Fracture Fixation Failure

Table 1.1 (continued)

Site	Incidence	Rate of fixation failure	Risk factors for fixation failure
Distal ulna	3.8/100,000 [58]	Plate: 0% [60–63]	None reported
Pelvic ring	23/100,000 [65]	Plate: 5–46% [67–71] Anterior ex-fix: 23–57% [72, 73] SI screw: 4–16% [74, 75]	Osteoporosis Single symphyseal plate >2 screws per segment Initial displacement Inadequate reduction LC type injuries Fixator loosening Non-compliance Delayed union Inadequate fluoroscopy Second SI screw
Acetabulum	3/100,000 [76]	ORIF: 10–57% [79–82]	Increasing age Non-union Comminution Fracture reduction Associated fracture pattern Initial articular displacement Obesity Surgeon error
Proximal femur	129/100,000 [6]	Intracapsular: FNS: 4–6% [88, 89] Cannulated screw: 13–39% [90–94] DHS: 0–20% [92, 94–96] Extracapsular: DHS: 4–28% [98, 99, 102–104] IM nail: 0–13% [100, 101, 105]	Increasing age Technical error Inadequate reduction Initial displacement Non-inverted triangle configuration of CS Inferior screws distance >3 mm from calcar Delay to fixation >24 h Comminution Reverse obliquity in EC (A2 or A3 vs. A1) Tip apex distance >25 mm CalTAD Lateral cortex comminution Notching of the screw aperture Varus reduction
Femoral shaft	10–21/100,000 [108]	IM nail: 0.5–10% [111, 112] Plate: 1–14% [113–115]	Small nail size Failure to lock nail Malreduction Comminution Initial displacement Soft tissue stripping Delayed union Sagittal plane malalignment Short plate working length
Distal femur	8.7/100,000 [117]	ORIF: 6–20% [121, 122]	Increasing patient age osteoporosis Initial varus displacement, poor reduction Residual varus following fixation Medial or posteromedial comminution
Proximal tibia	10.3/100,000 [123]	Plate: Up to 30% [126] Frame: Up to 14% [124]	Osteoporosis Comminution Early return to weight-bearing

(continued)

Table 1.1 (continued)

Site	Incidence	Rate of fixation failure	Risk factors for fixation failure
Tibial shaft	2/100,000 [6]	IM nail: 0–7% [131] Circular frame: 0–5% [132–134]	Open fractures Comminution Smaller diameter nails
Distal tibia	9.1/100,000 [135]	Plate: 2–10% [136, 140, 141] Circular frame: 3% [143]	Comminution Periosteal stripping Malreduction Anteromedial plate
Ankle	100/100,000 [6]	ORIF: 1–2% [146]	Obesity Open fractures Syndesmotic malreduction
Calcaneus	11.5/100,000 [148]	ORIF: 0–40% [151, 154, 155]	Comminution Non-compliance Technical failures Smoking
Lisfranc	16/100,000 [156]	ORIF: 29.5% [160] Arthrodesis: 29.6% [160]	Over compression Malreduction Plantar trajectory of the home run screw Poor compliance with weight-bearing Inadequate joint preparation

Rates are currently extrapolated from small retrospective series and secondary outcomes of larger trials, varying from 0 to 57% depending on the location of the fracture and the technical application of the technique. Fixation failure is significantly higher in the lower limb where issues with ambulation introduce the risk of early weight-bearing and increased forces to which the fixation construct is exposed to.

Failure was reportedly highest when utilising techniques to stabilise the anterior pelvic ring, be that in the form of an external fixator or a plate. Fixation fails here at a much higher rate as the implant is spanning the symphysis, a joint that whilst stiff will never produce the same strain environment as a healed bone segment. Whilst pelvic 'fixation failure' is commonly reported, severe clinical symptoms are infrequently encountered nor is the requirement for removal of symptomatic hardware [67, 69].

Failure was similarly high in areas where high force transmission and poor vascularity predispose to slow healing, such as the femoral neck; in poor quality cancellous bone where fixation constructs struggle to gain adequate hold, such as the calcaneus; and in the pelvis where cancellous bone combined with an inability to prevent high stress due to its core position place significant stress in the implants utilised in the management of fractures here.

Reports regarding fixation failure are sparse, and often reported as secondary outcomes within larger studies. Whilst an extensive database search was conducted to examine its frequency, this report may still miss some studies which were not identifiable on a standard search. Similarly, the definition of fixation failure is not standardised across all studies, with some reporting on all cases where the integrity of the fixation construct was lost, and others simply reporting when a re-operation was required.

Reporting all cases of fixation failure will often identify metalwork complications that have no bearing on the clinical picture, such as the asymptomatic breakage of syndesmosis screws or loss of tension of an olive wire in a healing fracture segment [161]. Nonetheless reporting only those complications that require revision fixation will miss a number of patients that are symptomatic from their metalwork failure, who may need to alter their post-operative course through adjustment of weight-bearing or splint-

Conclusion

The overall incidence of fixation failure is poorly defined within the literature. Moving forward the true incidence of fixation failure does need to be more accurately defined, ideally via larger cohort studies, with a stricter definition that identifies those patients whose clinical course and outcome are altered by the construct failure.

References

1. Hodgson S. AO principles of fracture management. Ann R Coll Surg Engl. 2009;91(5):448–9. https://doi.org/10.1308/003588409X432419f.
2. Taljanovic MS, Jones MD, Ruth JT, Benjamin JB, Sheppard JE, Hunter TB. Fracture fixation. Radiographics. 2003;23(6):1569–90. https://doi.org/10.1148/rg.236035159.
3. Sharma AK, Kumar A, Joshi GR, John JT. Retrospective study of implant failure in orthopaedic surgery. Med J Armed Forces India. 2006;62(1):70–2. https://doi.org/10.1016/S0377-1237(06)80164-4.
4. Harris LJ, Tarr RR. Implant failures in orthopaedic surgery. Biomater Med Devices Artif Organs. 1979;7(2):243–55. https://doi.org/10.3109/10731197909117579.
5. Nunamaker DM. Orthopedic implant failure. Equine fracture repair; 2019:831–834. https://doi.org/10.1002/9781119108757.ch46.
6. Court-Brown CM, Caesar B. Epidemiology of adult fractures: a review. Injury. 2006;37(8):691–7. https://doi.org/10.1016/j.injury.2006.04.130.
7. Launonen AP, Lepola V, Saranko A, Flinkkilä T, Laitinen M, Mattila VM. Epidemiology of proximal humerus fractures. Arch Osteoporos. 2015;10:209. https://doi.org/10.1007/s11657-015-0209-4.
8. Jo MJ, Gardner MJ. Proximal humerus fractures. Curr Rev Musculoskelet Med. 2012;5(3):192–8. https://doi.org/10.1007/s12178-012-9130-2.
9. Dauwe J, Walters G, Holzer LA, Vanhaecht K, Nijs S. Failure after proximal humeral fracture osteosynthesis: a one year analysis of hospital-related healthcare cost. Int Orthop. 2020;44(6):1217–21. https://doi.org/10.1007/s00264-020-04577-y.
10. Lee C-W, Shin S-J. Prognostic factors for unstable proximal humeral fractures treated with locking-plate fixation. J Shoulder Elb Surg. 2009;18(1):83–8. https://doi.org/10.1016/j.jse.2008.06.014.
11. Jung S-W, Shim S-B, Kim H-M, Lee J-H, Lim H-S. Factors that influence reduction loss in proximal humerus fracture surgery. J Orthop Trauma. 2015;29(6):276–82. https://doi.org/10.1097/BOT.0000000000000252.
12. Agudelo J, Schürmann M, Stahel P, et al. Analysis of efficacy and failure in proximal humerus fractures treated with locking plates. J Orthop Trauma. 2007;21(10):676–81. https://doi.org/10.1097/BOT.0b013e31815bb09d.
13. Brunner F, Sommer C, Bahrs C, et al. Open reduction and internal fixation of proximal humerus fractures using a proximal humeral locked plate: a prospective multicenter analysis. J Orthop Trauma. 2009;23(3):163–72. https://doi.org/10.1097/BOT.0b013e3181920e5b.
14. Wong J, Newman JM, Gruson KI. Outcomes of intramedullary nailing for acute proximal humerus fractures: a systematic review. J Orthop Traumatol. 2016;17(2):113–22. https://doi.org/10.1007/s10195-015-0384-5.
15. Gallusser N, Barimani B, Vauclair F. Humeral shaft fractures. EFORT Open Rev. 2021;6(1):24–34. https://doi.org/10.1302/2058-5241.6.200033.
16. Schoch BS, Padegimas EM, Maltenfort M, Krieg J, Namdari S. Humeral shaft fractures: national trends in management. J Orthop Traumatol. 2017;18(3):259–63. https://doi.org/10.1007/s10195-017-0459-6.
17. Heim D, Herkert F, Hess P, Regazzoni P. Surgical treatment of humeral shaft fractures--the Basel experience. J Trauma. 1993;35(2):226–32.
18. Raghavendra S, Bhalodiya HP. Internal fixation of fractures of the shaft of the humerus by dynamic compression plate or intramedullary nail: a prospective study. Indian J Orthop. 2007;41(3):214–8. https://doi.org/10.4103/0019-5413.33685.
19. Putti AB, Uppin RB, Putti BB. Locked intramedullary nailing versus dynamic compression plating for humeral shaft fractures. J Orthop Surg (Hong Kong). 2009;17(2):139–41. https://doi.org/10.1177/230949900901700202.
20. Amir S, Jannis S, Daniel R. Distal humerus fractures: a review of current therapy concepts. Curr Rev Musculoskelet Med. 2016;9(2):199–206. https://doi.org/10.1007/s12178-016-9341-z.
21. Nauth A, McKee MD, Ristevski B, Hall J, Schemitsch EH. Distal humeral fractures in adults. J Bone Joint Surg Am. 2011;93(7):686–700. https://doi.org/10.2106/JBJS.J.00845.
22. Savvidou OD, Zampeli F, Koutsouradis P, et al. Complications of open reduction and internal fixation of distal humerus fractures. EFORT Open Rev. 2018;3(10):558–67. https://doi.org/10.1302/2058-5241.3.180009.
23. Obert L, Ferrier M, Jacquot A, et al. Distal humerus fractures in patients over 65: complications. Orthop

Traumatol Surg Res. 2013;99(8):909–13. https://doi.org/10.1016/j.otsr.2013.10.002.

24. Yetter TR, Weatherby PJ, Somerson JS. Complications of articular distal humeral fracture fixation: a systematic review and meta-analysis. J Shoulder Elb Surg. 2021;30(8):1957–67. https://doi.org/10.1016/j.jse.2021.02.017.

25. O'Driscoll SW. Optimizing stability in distal humeral fracture fixation. J Shoulder Elb Surg. 2005;14(1 Suppl S):186S–94S. https://doi.org/10.1016/j.jse.2004.09.033.

26. Duckworth AD, Clement ND, Aitken SA, Court-Brown CM, McQueen MM. The epidemiology of fractures of the proximal ulna. Injury. 2012;43(3):343–6. https://doi.org/10.1016/j.injury.2011.10.017.

27. Brüggemann A, Mukka S, Wolf O. Epidemiology, classification and treatment of olecranon fractures in adults: an observational study on 2462 fractures from the Swedish fracture register. Eur J Trauma Emerg Surg. 2022;48(3):2255–63. https://doi.org/10.1007/s00068-021-01765-2.

28. Romero JM, Miran A, Jensen CH. Complications and re-operation rate after tension-band wiring of olecranon fractures. J Orthop Sci. 2000;5(4):318–20. https://doi.org/10.1007/s007760070036.

29. Rantalaiho IK, Laaksonen IE, Ryösä AJ, Perkonoja K, Isotalo KJ, Äärimaa VO. Complications and reoperations related to tension band wiring and plate osteosynthesis of olecranon fractures. J Shoulder Elb Surg. 2021;30(10):2412–7. https://doi.org/10.1016/j.jse.2021.03.138.

30. Macko D, Szabo RM. Complications of tension-band wiring of olecranon fractures. J Bone Joint Surg Am. 1985;67(9):1396–401.

31. Mauffrey CPC, Krikler S. Surgical techniques: how I do it? Open reduction and tension band wiring of olecranon fractures. Injury. 2009;40(4):461–5. https://doi.org/10.1016/j.injury.2008.09.026.

32. Wu C-C, Tai C-L, Shih C-H. Biomechanical comparison for different configurations of tension band wiring techniques in treating an olecranon fracture. J Trauma Acute Care Surg. 2000;48(6):1063.

33. van der Linden SC, van Kampen A, Jaarsma RL. K-wire position in tension-band wiring technique affects stability of wires and long-term outcome in surgical treatment of olecranon fractures. J Shoulder Elb Surg. 2012;21(3):405–11. https://doi.org/10.1016/j.jse.2011.07.022.

34. Wise KL, Peck S, Smith L, Myeroff C. Locked plating of geriatric olecranon fractures leads to low fixation failure and acceptable complication rates. JSES Int. 2021;5(4):809–15. https://doi.org/10.1016/j.jseint.2021.02.013.

35. Campbell ST, DeBaun MR, Goodnough LH, Bishop JA, Gardner MJ. Geriatric olecranon fractures treated with plate fixation have low complication rates. Curr Orthop Pract. 2019;30(4):353–5.

36. Boden AL, Daly CA, Dalwadi PP, et al. Biomechanical evaluation of standard versus extended proximal fixation olecranon plates for fixation of olecranon fractures. Hand. 2019;14(4):554–9. https://doi.org/10.1177/1558944717753206.

37. Siebenlist S, Buchholz A, Braun KF. Fractures of the proximal ulna: current concepts in surgical management. EFORT Open Rev. 2019;4(1):1–9. https://doi.org/10.1302/2058-5241.4.180022.

38. Klug A, Gramlich Y, Wincheringer D, Hoffmann R, Schmidt-Horlohé K. Epidemiology and treatment of radial head fractures: A database analysis of over 70,000 inpatient cases. J Hand Surg Am. 2021;46(1):27–35. https://doi.org/10.1016/j.jhsa.2020.05.029.

39. Swensen SJ, Tyagi V, Uquillas C, Shakked RJ, Yoon RS, Liporace FA. Maximizing outcomes in the treatment of radial head fractures. J Orthop Traumatol. 2019;20(1):15. https://doi.org/10.1186/s10195-019-0523-5.

40. Lindenhovius ALC, Felsch Q, Doornberg JN, Ring D, Kloen P. Open reduction and internal fixation compared with excision for unstable displaced fractures of the radial head. J Hand Surg Am. 2007;32(5):630–6. https://doi.org/10.1016/j.jhsa.2007.02.016.

41. Ring D, Quintero J, Jupiter JB. Open reduction and internal fixation of fractures of the radial head. JBJS. 2002;84(10):1811.

42. Özkan Y, Öztürk A, Özdemir RM, Aykut S, Yalçın N. Open reduction and internal fixation of radial head fractures. Turkish J Trauma Emerg Surg. 2009;15(3):249–55.

43. Shi X, Pan T, Wu D, et al. Effect of different orientations of screw fixation for radial head fractures: a biomechanical comparison. J Orthop Surg Res. 2017;12(1):143. https://doi.org/10.1186/s13018-017-0641-9.

44. Abrahamsen B, Jørgensen NR, Schwarz P. Epidemiology of forearm fractures in adults in Denmark: national age- and gender-specific incidence rates, ratio of forearm to hip fractures, and extent of surgical fracture repair in inpatients and outpatients. Osteoporos Int. 2015;26(1):67–76. https://doi.org/10.1007/s00198-014-2831-1.

45. How HM, Khoo BLJ, Ayeop MAS, Ahmad AR, Bahaudin N, Ahmad AA. Application of WALANT in diaphyseal plating of forearm fractures: an observational study. J Hand Surg Glob Online. 2022;4(6):399–407. https://doi.org/10.1016/j.jhsg.2022.02.004.

46. Schulte LM, Meals CG, Neviaser RJ. Management of adult diaphyseal both-bone forearm fractures. J Am Acad Orthop Surg. 2014;22(7):437–46. https://doi.org/10.5435/JAAOS-22-07-437.

47. Stern PJ, Drury WJ. Complications of plate fixation of forearm fractures. Clin Orthop Relat Res. 1983;175:25–9.

48. Herscovici DJ, Scaduto JM. Failures in fixation of the forearm. Tech Orthop. 2002;17(4):409–16.

49. Stirling ERB, Johnson NA, Dias JJ. Epidemiology of distal radius fractures in a geographi-

cally defined adult population. J Hand Surg Eur Vol. 2018;43(9):974–82. https://doi.org/10.1177/1753193418786378.

50. Armstrong KA, von Schroeder HP, Baxter NN, Zhong T, Huang A, McCabe SJ. Stable rates of operative treatment of distal radius fractures in Ontario, Canada: a population-based retrospective cohort study (2004–2013). Can J Surg. 2019;62(6):386–92. https://doi.org/10.1503/cjs.016218.

51. Mc Colgan R, Dalton DM, Cassar-Gheiti AJ, Fox CM, O'Sullivan ME. Trends in the management of fractures of the distal radius in Ireland: did the distal radius acute fracture fixation trial (DRAFFT) change practice? Bone Joint J. 2019;101-B(12):1550–6. https://doi.org/10.1302/0301-620X.101B12.BJJ-2018-1615.R3.

52. Satake H, Hanaka N, Honma R, et al. Complications of distal radius fractures treated by volar locking plate fixation. Orthopedics. 2016;39(5):e893–6. https://doi.org/10.3928/01477447-20160517-05.

53. Foo T-L, Gan AWT, Soh T, Chew WYC. Mechanical failure of the distal radius volar locking plate. J Orthop Surg (Hong Kong). 2013;21(3):332–6. https://doi.org/10.1177/230949901302100314.

54. Beck JD, Harness NG, Spencer HT. Volar plate fixation failure for volar shearing distal radius fractures with small lunate facet fragments. J Hand Surg Am. 2014;39(4):670–8. https://doi.org/10.1016/j.jhsa.2014.01.006.

55. Cao J, Ozer K. Failure of volar locking plate fixation of an extraarticular distal radius fracture: a case report. Patient Saf Surg. 2010;4(1):19. https://doi.org/10.1186/1754-9493-4-19.

56. Izawa Y, Tsuchida Y, Futamura K, Ochi H, Baba T. Plate coverage predicts failure for volarly unstable distal radius fractures with volar lunate facet fragments. SICOT J. 2020;6:29. https://doi.org/10.1051/sicotj/2020026.

57. Lee DJ, Ghodasra J, Mitchell S. Failure of fixation of volar locked plating of distal radius fractures: level 3 evidence. J Hand Surg Am. 2015;40(9, Supplement):e17. https://doi.org/10.1016/j.jhsa.2015.06.033.

58. Soerensen S, Larsen P, Korup LR, et al. Epidemiology of distal forearm fracture: a population-based study of 5426 fractures. Hand (N Y). 2022:15589447221109968. https://doi.org/10.1177/15589447221109967.

59. Fish MJ, Palazzo M. Distal ulnar fractures. In: StatPearls [Internet]; 2022.

60. Stock K, Benedikt S, Kastenberger T, et al. Outcomes of distal ulna locking plate in management of unstable distal ulna fractures: a prospective case series. Arch Orthop Trauma Surg. 2022;143:3137–44. https://doi.org/10.1007/s00402-022-04549-4.

61. Lee SK, Kim KJ, Park JS, Choy WS. Distal ulna hook plate fixation for unstable distal ulna fracture associated with distal radius fracture. Orthopedics. 2012;35(9):e1358–64. https://doi.org/10.3928/01477447-20120822-22.

62. Nunez FAJ, Li Z, Campbell D, Nunez FAS. Distal ulna hook plate: angular stable implant for fixation of distal ulna. J Wrist Surg. 2013;2(1):87–92. https://doi.org/10.1055/s-0032-1333427.

63. Bakouri MAM, El-Soufy MAA, El-Hewala TA, Fahmy FS. Fixation of distal ulna fractures by distal ulnar locked hook plate. Egypt J Hosp Med. 2021;82(3):506–13. https://doi.org/10.21608/ejhm.2021.147000.

64. Zhang Y, Shao Q, Yang C, et al. Finite element analysis of different locking plate fixation methods for the treatment of ulnar head fracture. J Orthop Surg Res. 2021;16(1):191. https://doi.org/10.1186/s13018-021-02334-4.

65. Balogh Z, King KL, Mackay P, et al. The epidemiology of pelvic ring fractures: a population-based study. J Trauma. 2007;63(5):1063–6. https://doi.org/10.1097/TA.0b013e3181589fa4.

66. Buller LT, Best MJ, Quinnan SM. A nationwide analysis of pelvic ring fractures: incidence and trends in treatment, length of stay, and mortality. Geriatr Orthop Surg Rehabil. 2015;7(1):9–17. https://doi.org/10.1177/2151458515616250.

67. Morris SAC, Loveridge J, Smart DKA, Ward AJ, Chesser TJS. Is fixation failure after plate fixation of the symphysis pubis clinically important? Clin Orthop Relat Res. 2012;470(8):2154–60. https://doi.org/10.1007/s11999-012-2427-z.

68. Herteleer M, Boudissa M, Hofmann A, Wagner D, Rommens PM. Plate fixation of the anterior pelvic ring in patients with fragility fractures of the pelvis. Eur J Trauma Emerg Surg. 2022;48(5):3711–9. https://doi.org/10.1007/s00068-021-01625-z.

69. Giannoudis PV, Chalidis BE, Roberts CS. Internal fixation of traumatic diastasis of pubic symphysis: is plate removal essential? Arch Orthop Trauma Surg. 2008;128(3):325–31. https://doi.org/10.1007/s00402-007-0429-1.

70. Putnis SE, Pearce R, Wali UJ, Bircher MD, Rickman MS. Open reduction and internal fixation of a traumatic diastasis of the pubic symphysis: one-year radiological and functional outcomes. J Bone Joint Surg Br. 2011;93(1):78–84. https://doi.org/10.1302/0301-620X.93B1.23941.

71. Sagi HC, Papp S. Comparative radiographic and clinical outcome of two-hole and multi-hole symphyseal plating. J Orthop Trauma. 2008;22(6):373–8. https://journals.lww.com/jorthotrauma/Fulltext/2008/07000/Comparative_Radiographic_and_Clinical_Outcome_of.1.aspx

72. Lindahl J, Hirvensalo E, Böstman O, Santavirta S. Failure of reduction with an external fixator in the management of injuries of the pelvic ring. Long-term evaluation of 110 patients. J Bone Joint Surg Br. 1999;81(6):955–62. https://doi.org/10.1302/0301-620x.81b6.8571.

73. Bi C, Wang Q, Wu J, et al. Modified pedicle screw-rod fixation versus anterior pelvic external fixation for the management of anterior pelvic ring fractures: a comparative study. J Orthop Surg Res. 2017;12(1):185. https://doi.org/10.1186/s13018-017-0688-7.

74. Routt MLJ, Simonian PT, Mills WJ. Iliosacral screw fixation: early complications of the percutaneous technique. J Orthop Trauma. 1997;11(8):584–9. https://doi.org/10.1097/00005131-199711000-00007.

75. Deng H-L, Li D-Y, Cong Y-X, et al. Clinical analysis of single and double sacroiliac screws in the treatment of tile C1 pelvic fracture. Ye C, ed. Biomed Res Int. 2022;2022:6426977. https://doi.org/10.1155/2022/6426977.

76. Singh A, Lim ASM, Lau BPH, O'Neill G. Epidemiology of pelvic and acetabular fractures in a tertiary hospital in Singapore. Singap Med J. 2022;63(7):388. https://journals.lww.com/SMJ/Fulltext/2022/07000/Epidemiology_of_pelvic_and_acetabular_fractures_in.8.aspx

77. Mauffrey C, Hao J, Cuellar DO 3rd, et al. The epidemiology and injury patterns of acetabular fractures: are the USA and China comparable? Clin Orthop Relat Res. 2014;472(11):3332–7. https://doi.org/10.1007/s11999-014-3462-8.

78. Antell NB, Switzer JA, Schmidt AH. Management of acetabular fractures in the elderly. J Am Acad Orthop Surg. 2017;25(8):577–85. https://journals.lww.com/jaaos/Fulltext/2017/08000/Management_of_Acetabular_Fractures_in_the_Elderly.4.aspx

79. Lehmann W, Spering C, Jäckle K, Acharya MR. Solutions for failed osteosynthesis of the acetabulum. J Clin Orthop Trauma. 2020;11(6):1039–44. https://doi.org/10.1016/j.jcot.2020.09.024.

80. Schnaser E, Scarcella NR, Vallier HA. Acetabular fractures converted to total hip arthroplasties in the elderly: How does function compare to primary total hip arthroplasty? J Orthop Trauma. 2014;28(12):694–9. https://journals.lww.com/jorthotrauma/Fulltext/2014/12000/Acetabular_Fractures_Converted_to_Total_Hip.5.aspx

81. O'Toole RV, Hui E, Chandra A, Nascone JW. How often does open reduction and internal fixation of geriatric acetabular fractures lead to hip arthroplasty? J Orthop Trauma. 2014;28(3):148–53. https://doi.org/10.1097/BOT.0b013e31829c739a.

82. Tannast M, Najibi S, Matta JM. Two to twenty-year survivorship of the hip in 810 patients with operatively treated acetabular fractures. J Bone Joint Surg Am. 2012;94(17):1559–67. https://doi.org/10.2106/JBJS.K.00444.

83. Ziran N, Soles GLS, Matta JM. Outcomes after surgical treatment of acetabular fractures: a review. Patient Saf Surg. 2019;13(1):16. https://doi.org/10.1186/s13037-019-0196-2.

84. Henstenburg JM, Larwa JA, Williams CS, Shah MP, Harding SP. Risk factors for complications following pelvic ring and acetabular fractures: A retrospective analysis at an urban level 1 trauma center. J Orthop Trauma Rehabil. 2021;28:22104917211006890. https://doi.org/10.1177/22104917211006890.

85. Lundin N, Berg HE, Enocson A. Complications after surgical treatment of acetabular fractures: a 5-year follow-up of 229 patients. Eur J Orthop Surg Traumatol. 2022;33:1245–53. https://doi.org/10.1007/s00590-022-03284-1.

86. Yaradılmış YU, Okkaoğlu MC, Ateş A, Kılıç A, Demirkale İ, Altay M. Proximal femur fracture, analysis of epidemiology, complications, and mortality: a cohort with 380 patients. J Surg Med. 2021;5(1):75–9. https://doi.org/10.28982/josam.787253.

87. Mittal R, Banerjee S. Proximal femoral fractures: principles of management and review of literature. J Clin Orthop Trauma. 2012;3(1):15–23. https://doi.org/10.1016/j.jcot.2012.04.001.

88. Davidson A, Blum S, Harats E, et al. Neck of femur fractures treated with the femoral neck system: outcomes of one hundred and two patients and literature review. Int Orthop. 2022;46(9):2105–15. https://doi.org/10.1007/s00264-022-05414-0.

89. Tang Y, Zhang Z, Wang L, Xiong W, Fang Q, Wang G. Femoral neck system versus inverted cannulated cancellous screw for the treatment of femoral neck fractures in adults: a preliminary comparative study. J Orthop Surg Res. 2021;16(1):504. https://doi.org/10.1186/s13018-021-02659-0.

90. Duckworth AD, Bennet SJ, Aderinto J, Keating JF. Fixation of intracapsular fractures of the femoral neck in young patients: risk factors for failure. J Bone Joint Surg Br. 2011;93(6):811–6. https://doi.org/10.1302/0301-620X.93B6.26432.

91. Wang C-T, Chen J-W, Wu K, et al. Suboptimal outcomes after closed reduction and internal fixation of displaced femoral neck fractures in middle-aged patients: is internal fixation adequate in this age group? BMC Musculoskelet Disord. 2018;19(1):190. https://doi.org/10.1186/s12891-018-2120-9.

92. Fixation using Alternative Implants for the Treatment of Hip fractures (FAITH) Investigators. Fracture fixation in the operative management of hip fractures (FAITH): an international, multicentre, randomised controlled trial. Lancet (London, England). 2017;389(10078):1519–27. https://doi.org/10.1016/S0140-6736(17)30066-1.

93. Dolatowski FC, Frihagen F, Bartels S, et al. Screw fixation versus hemiarthroplasty for nondisplaced femoral neck fractures in elderly patients: a multicenter randomized controlled trial. J Bone Joint Surg Am. 2019;101(2):136–44. https://doi.org/10.2106/JBJS.18.00316.

94. Li L, Zhao X, Yang X, Tang X, Liu M. Dynamic hip screws versus cannulated screws for femoral neck fractures: a systematic review and meta-analysis. J Orthop Surg Res. 2020;15(1):352. https://doi.org/10.1186/s13018-020-01842-z.

95. Schwartsmann CR, Jacobus LS, LDF S, et al. Dynamic hip screw for the treatment of femoral neck fractures: a prospective study with 96 patients. ISRN Orthop. 2014;2014:257871. https://doi.org/10.1155/2014/257871.

96. Schwartsmann CR, Lammerhirt HM, Spinelli LD, Ungaretti Neto AD. Treatment of displaced femoral neck fractures in young patients with DHS and its association to osteonecrosis. Rev Bras Ortop. 2018;53(1):82–7. https://doi.org/10.1016/j.rboe.2017.03.003.

97. Yang J-J, Lin L-C, Chao K-H, et al. Risk factors for nonunion in patients with intracapsular femoral neck fractures treated with three cannulated screws placed in either a triangle or an inverted triangle configuration. J Bone Joint Surg Am. 2013;95(1):61–9. https://doi.org/10.2106/JBJS.K.01081.

98. Kim WY, Han CH, Park JI, Kim JY. Failure of intertrochanteric fracture fixation with a dynamic hip screw in relation to pre-operative fracture stability and osteoporosis. Int Orthop. 2001;25(6):360–2. https://doi.org/10.1007/s002640100287.

99. van der Sijp MPL, de Groot M, Meylaerts SA, et al. High risks of failure observed for A1 trochanteric femoral fractures treated with a DHS compared to the PFNA in a prospective observational cohort study. Arch Orthop Trauma Surg. 2022;142(7):1459–67. https://doi.org/10.1007/s00402-021-03824-0.

100. Kashigar A, Vincent A, Gunton MJ, Backstein D, Safir O, Kuzyk PRT. Predictors of failure for cephalomedullary nailing of proximal femoral fractures. Bone Joint J. 2014;96-B(8):1029–34. https://doi.org/10.1302/0301-620X.96B8.33644.

101. Bovbjerg PE, Larsen MS, Madsen CF, Schønnemann J. Failure of short versus long cephalomedullary nail after intertrochanteric fractures. J Orthop. 2020;18:209–12. https://doi.org/10.1016/j.jor.2019.10.018.

102. Jasudason E, Jeyem M. Failure of dynamic hip screw (DHS) fixation for intertrochanteric fracture. Experience of a single district general hospital. Orthop Proc. 2018;88(B)

103. Lin JC-F, Liang W-M. Mortality, readmission, and reoperation after hip fracture in nonagenarians. BMC Musculoskelet Disord. 2017;18(1):144. https://doi.org/10.1186/s12891-017-1493-5.

104. Puram C, Pradhan C, Patil A, Sodhai V, Sancheti P, Shyam A. Outcomes of dynamic hip screw augmented with trochanteric wiring for treatment of unstable type A2 intertrochanteric femur fractures. Injury. 2017;48(Suppl 2):S72–7. https://doi.org/10.1016/S0020-1383(17)30498-9.

105. Pang Y, He Q-F, Zhu L-L, Bian Z-Y, Li M-Q. Loss of reduction after cephalomedullary nail fixation of intertrochanteric femoral fracture: a brief report. Orthop Surg. 2020;12(6):1998–2003. https://doi.org/10.1111/os.12828.

106. Taheriazam A, Saeidinia A. Salvage of failed dynamic hip screw fixation of intertrochanteric frac-

tures. Orthop Res Rev. 2019;11:93–8. https://doi.org/10.2147/ORR.S215240.

107. Petfield JL, Visscher LE, Gueorguiev B, Stoffel K, Pape H-C. Tips and tricks to avoid implant failure in proximal femur fractures treated with cephalomedullary nails: a review of the literature. OTA Int. 2022;5(2S):e191. https://journals.lww.com/otainternational/Fulltext/2022/04001/Tips_and_tricks_to_avoid_implant_failure_in.1.aspx

108. Weiss RJ, Montgomery SM, Al Dabbagh Z, Jansson K-A. National data of 6409 Swedish inpatients with femoral shaft fractures: stable incidence between 1998 and 2004. Injury. 2009;40(3):304–8. https://doi.org/10.1016/j.injury.2008.07.017.

109. Enninghorst N, McDougall D, Evans JA, Sisak K, Balogh ZJ. Population-based epidemiology of femur shaft fractures. J Trauma Acute Care Surg. 2013;74(6):1516–20. https://doi.org/10.1097/TA.0b013e31828c3dc9.

110. Rudloff MI, Smith WR. Intramedullary nailing of the femur: current concepts concerning reaming. J Orthop Trauma. 2009;23(5 Suppl):S12–7. https://doi.org/10.1097/BOT.0b013e31819f258a.

111. Aggerwal S, Gahlot N, Saini UC, Bali K. Failure of intramedullary femoral nail with segmental breakage of distal locking bolts: a case report and review of the literature. Chin J Traumatol (English Ed). 2011;14(3):188–92. https://doi.org/10.3760/cma.j.issn.1008-1275.2011.01.013.

112. Harrington P, Sharif I, Smyth H. Failure of femoral nailing in the elderly. Arch Orthop Trauma Surg. 1997;116(4):244–5. https://doi.org/10.1007/BF00393721.

113. May C, Yen Y-M, Nasreddine AY, Hedequist D, Hresko MT, Heyworth BE. Complications of plate fixation of femoral shaft fractures in children and adolescents. J Child Orthop. 2013;7(3):235–43. https://doi.org/10.1007/s11832-013-0496-5.

114. Hsu C-L, Yang J-J, Yeh T-T, Shen H-C, Pan R-Y, Wu C-C. Early fixation failure of locked plating in complex distal femoral fractures: root causes analysis. J Formos Med Assoc. 2021;120(1, Part 2):395–403. https://doi.org/10.1016/j.jfma.2020.06.017.

115. Min B-W, Lee K-J, Cho C-H, Lee I-G, Kim B-S. High failure rates of locking compression plate Osteosynthesis with transverse fracture around a well-fixed stem tip for periprosthetic femoral fracture. J Clin Med. 2020;9(11):3758. https://doi.org/10.3390/jcm9113758.

116. Said GZ, Said HG, el-Sharkawi MM. Failed intramedullary nailing of femur: open reduction and plate augmentation with the nail in situ. Int Orthop. 2011;35(7):1089–92. https://doi.org/10.1007/s00264-010-1192-4.

117. Elsoe R, Ceccotti AA, Larsen P. Population-based epidemiology and incidence of distal femur fractures. Int Orthop. 2018;42(1):191–6. https://doi.org/10.1007/s00264-017-3665-1.

118. Kolb K, Grützner P, Koller H, Windisch C, Marx F, Kolb W. The condylar plate for treatment of dis-

118. tal femoral fractures: a long-term follow-up study. Injury. 2009;40(4):440–8. https://doi.org/10.1016/j.injury.2008.08.046.

119. Higgins TF, Pittman G, Hines J, Bachus KN. Biomechanical analysis of distal femur fracture fixation: fixed-angle screw-plate construct versus condylar blade plate. J Orthop Trauma. 2007;21(1):43–6. https://doi.org/10.1097/BOT.0b013e31802bb372.

120. Leung KS, Shen WY, So WS, Mui LT, Grosse A. Interlocking intramedullary nailing for supracondylar and intercondylar fractures of the distal part of the femur. J Bone Joint Surg Am. 1991;73(3):332–40.

121. Siddiqui YS, Mohd J, Abbas M, Gupta K, Khan MJ, Istiyak M. Technical difficulties and mechanical failure of distal femoral locking compression plate (DFLCP) in management of unstable distal femoral fractures. Int J Burns Trauma. 2021;11(1):9–19.

122. Collinge CA, Reeb AF, Rodriguez-Buitrago AF, et al. Analysis of 101 mechanical failures in distal femur fractures treated with 3 generations of precontoured locking plates. J Orthop Trauma. 2023;37(1):8–13. https://doi.org/10.1097/BOT.0000000000002460.

123. Elsoe R, Larsen P, Nielsen NPH, Swenne J, Rasmussen S, Ostgaard SE. Population-based epidemiology of tibial plateau fractures. Orthopedics. 2015;38(9):e780–6. https://doi.org/10.3928/01477447-20150902-55.

124. Canadian Orthopaedic Trauma Society. Open reduction and internal fixation compared with circular fixator application for bicondylar tibial plateau fractures. Results of a multicenter, prospective, randomized clinical trial. J Bone Joint Surg Am. 2006;88(12):2613–23. https://doi.org/10.2106/JBJS.E.01416.

125. Scott CEH, Davidson E, MacDonald DJ, White TO, Keating JF. Total knee arthroplasty following tibial plateau fracture: a matched cohort study. Bone Joint J. 2015;97-B(4):532–8. https://doi.org/10.1302/0301-620X.97B4.34789.

126. Ali AM, El-Shafie M, Willett KM. Failure of fixation of tibial plateau fractures. J Orthop Trauma. 2002;16(5):323–9. https://doi.org/10.1097/00005131-200205000-00006.

127. Laurila J, Huttunen TT, Kannus P, Kääriäinen M, Mattila VM. Tibial shaft fractures in Finland between 1997 and 2014. Injury. 2019;50(4):973–7. https://doi.org/10.1016/j.injury.2019.03.034.

128. Anandasivam NS, Russo GS, Swallow MS, et al. Tibial shaft fracture: a large-scale study defining the injured population and associated injuries. J Clin Orthop Trauma. 2017;8(3):225–31. https://doi.org/10.1016/j.jcot.2017.07.012.

129. Tay W-H, de Steiger R, Richardson M, Gruen R, Balogh ZJ. Health outcomes of delayed union and nonunion of femoral and tibial shaft fractures. Injury. 2014;45(10):1653–8. https://doi.org/10.1016/j.injury.2014.06.025.

130. Busse JW, Morton E, Lacchetti C, Guyatt GH, Bhandari M. Current management of tibial shaft fractures: a survey of 450 Canadian orthopedic trauma surgeons. Acta Orthop. 2008;79(5):689–94. https://doi.org/10.1080/17453670810016722.

131. Ruiz AL, Kealey WD, McCoy GF. Implant failure in tibial nailing. Injury. 2000;31(5):359–62. https://doi.org/10.1016/s0020-1383(00)00002-4.

132. Foster PAL, Barton SB, Jones SCE, Morrison RJM, Britten S. The treatment of complex tibial shaft fractures by the Ilizarov method. J Bone Joint Surg Br. 2012;94(12):1678–83. https://doi.org/10.1302/0301-620X.94B12.29266.

133. Dickson DR, Moulder E, Hadland Y, Giannoudis PV, Sharma HK. Grade 3 open tibial shaft fractures treated with a circular frame, functional outcome and systematic review of literature. Injury. 2015;46(4):751–8. https://doi.org/10.1016/j.injury.2015.01.025.

134. Giotakis N, Panchani SK, Narayan B, Larkin JJ, Al Maskari S, Nayagam S. Segmental fractures of the tibia treated by circular external fixation. J Bone Joint Surg Br. 2010;92(5):687–92. https://doi.org/10.1302/0301-620X.92B5.22514.

135. Wennergren D, Bergdahl C, Ekelund J, Juto H, Sundfeldt M, Möller M. Epidemiology and incidence of tibia fractures in the Swedish fracture register. Injury. 2018;49(11):2068–74. https://doi.org/10.1016/j.injury.2018.09.008.

136. Borg T, Larsson S, Lindsjö U. Percutaneous plating of distal tibial fractures. Preliminary results in 21 patients. Injury. 2004;35(6):608–14. https://doi.org/10.1016/j.injury.2003.08.015.

137. Tyllianakis M, Megas P, Giannikas D, Lambiris E. Interlocking intramedullary nailing in distal tibial fractures. Orthopedics. 2000;23(8):805–8. https://doi.org/10.3928/0147-7447-20000801-13.

138. Leung F, Kwok HY, Pun TS, Chow SP. Limited open reduction and Ilizarov external fixation in the treatment of distal tibial fractures. Injury. 2004;35(3):278–83. https://doi.org/10.1016/s0020-1383(03)00172-4.

139. Ylitalo AAJ, Dahl KA, Reito A, Ekman E. Changes in operative treatment of tibia fractures in Finland between 2000 and 2018: a nationwide study. Scand J Surg. 2022;111(3):65–71. https://doi.org/10.1177/14574969221111612.

140. Queipo-de-Llano A, Jimenez-Garrido C, FDB D-R, Mariscal-Lara J, Rodriguez-Delourme I. Complications after plating of articular pilon fractures: a comparison of anteromedial, anterolateral and medial plating. Acta Orthop Belg. 2020;86(3):102–13.

141. Lomax A, Singh A, Jane Madeley N, Senthil KC. Complications and early results after operative fixation of 68 pilon fractures of the distal tibia. Scott Med J. 2015;60(2):79–84. https://doi.org/10.1177/0036933015569159.

142. Ene R, Panti Z, Nica M, et al. Mechanical failure of angle locking plates in distal comminuted Tibial fractures. Key Eng Mater. 2016;695:118–

22. https://doi.org/10.4028/www.scientific.net/KEM.695.118.

143. Lovisetti G, Agus MA, Pace F, Capitani D, Sala F. Management of distal tibial intra-articular fractures with circular external fixation. Strateg Trauma Limb Reconstr. 2009;4(1):1–6. https://doi.org/10.1007/s11751-009-0050-7.

144. Koval KJ, Lurie J, Zhou W, et al. Ankle fractures in the elderly: what you get depends on where you live and who you see. J Orthop Trauma. 2005;19(9):635–9. https://doi.org/10.1097/01.bot.0000177105.53708.a9.

145. Scheer RC, Newman JM, Zhou JJ, et al. Ankle fracture epidemiology in the United States: patient-related trends and mechanisms of injury. J Foot Ankle Surg. 2020;59(3):479–83. https://doi.org/10.1053/j.jfas.2019.09.016.

146. Ovaska MT, Mäkinen TJ, Madanat R, Kiljunen V, Lindahl J. A comprehensive analysis of patients with malreduced ankle fractures undergoing re-operation. Int Orthop. 2014;38(1):83–8. https://doi.org/10.1007/s00264-013-2168-y.

147. Prediger B, Tjardes T, Probst C, et al. Factors predicting failure of internal fixations of fractures of the lower limbs: a prospective cohort study. BMC Musculoskelet Disord. 2021;22(1):798. https://doi.org/10.1186/s12891-021-04688-6.

148. Mitchell MJ, McKinley JC, Robinson CM. The epidemiology of calcaneal fractures. Foot (Edinb). 2009;19(4):197–200. https://doi.org/10.1016/j.foot.2009.05.001.

149. Jiménez-Almonte JH, King JD, Luo TD, Aneja A, Moghadamian E. Classifications in brief: sanders classification of intraarticular fractures of the calcaneus. Clin Orthop Relat Res. 2019;477(2):467–71. https://doi.org/10.1097/CORR.0000000000000539.

150. Weber M, Lehmann O, Sägesser D, Krause F. Limited open reduction and internal fixation of displaced intra-articular fractures of the calcaneum. J Bone Joint Surg Br. 2008;90(12):1608–16. https://doi.org/10.1302/0301-620X.90B12.20638.

151. Jain S, Jain AK, Kumar I. Outcome of open reduction and internal fixation of intraarticular calcaneal fracture fixed with locking calcaneal plate. Chin J Traumatol. 2013;16(6):355–60.

152. Bèzes H, Massart P, Delvaux D, Fourquet JP, Tazi F. The operative treatment of intraarticular calcaneal fractures. Indications, technique, and results in 257 cases. Clin Orthop Relat Res. 1993;290:55–9.

153. Schepers T. The primary arthrodesis for severely comminuted intra-articular fractures of the calcaneus: a systematic review. Foot Ankle Surg. 2012;18(2):84–8. https://doi.org/10.1016/j.fas.2011.04.004.

154. Pompach M, Carda M, Amlang M, Zwipp H. Treatment of calcaneal fractures with a locking nail (C-nail). Oper Orthop Traumatol. 2016;28(3):218–30. https://doi.org/10.1007/s00064-016-0441-0.

155. Yu HH, Ardavanis KS, Durso JT, Garries MP, Erard UE. Novel technique for osteosynthesis of tongue-type calcaneus fractures in osteoporotic bone: a case report. JBJS Case Connect. 2020;10(4):e20.00476. https://doi.org/10.2106/JBJS.CC.20.00476.

156. Hardcastle PH, Reschauer R, Kutscha-Lissberg E, Schoffmann W. Injuries to the tarsometatarsal joint. Incidence, classification and treatment. J Bone Joint Surg Br. 1982;64(3):349–56. https://doi.org/10.1302/0301-620X.64B3.7096403.

157. Haapamaki VV, Kiuru MJ, Koskinen SK. Ankle and foot injuries: analysis of MDCT findings. AJR Am J Roentgenol. 2004;183(3):615–22. https://doi.org/10.2214/ajr.183.3.1830615.

158. Moracia-Ochagavía I, Rodríguez-Merchán EC. Lisfranc fracture-dislocations: current management. EFORT Open Rev. 2019;4(7):430–44. https://doi.org/10.1302/2058-5241.4.180076.

159. Lewis JSJ, Anderson RB. Lisfranc injuries in the athlete. Foot Ankle Int. 2016;37(12):1374–80. https://doi.org/10.1177/1071100716675293.

160. Buda M, Kink S, Stavenuiter R, et al. Reoperation rate differences between open reduction internal fixation and primary arthrodesis of Lisfranc injuries. Foot Ankle Int. 2018;39(9):1089–96. https://doi.org/10.1177/1071100718774005.

161. Khurana A, Kumar A, Katekar S, et al. Is routine removal of syndesmotic screw justified? A meta-analysis. Foot. 2021;49:101776. https://doi.org/10.1016/j.foot.2021.101776.

Common Causes of Aseptic Fracture Fixation Failure

2

Mark Johnson, Grayson Norris, Jake Checketts, and Brent L. Norris

Introduction

Millions of fractures occur annually across the globe. Treating these injuries to union with maintenance of limb alignment and function is the ultimate goal. Surgical and nonsurgical management are used to treat these injuries and are often based on a multitude of factors including, but not limited to, fracture type, fracture displacement and associated injuries. When surgery is chosen, physicians must know the most likely outcome and certainly the possible complications that may occur, including nonunion of the fracture. It is estimated that up to 8–10% of all fractures will go onto nonunion [1]. When a fracture is treated surgically with internal fixation and a nonunion occurs, it is very likely the internal fixation will fail. Failed fixation in a delayed fashion is practically pathognomonic for a nonunion. When this occurs, the root cause of the nonunion must be identified. The following chapter is meant to help guide surgeons in the management of aseptic fracture fixation failure and the associated nonunion. It will reflect on the normal bone healing process, review how the biomechanics of the different surgical devices affect healing and finally, review the types of nonunions and the biomechanical and metabolic causes for nonunion.

Bone Healing Process

The physiologic processes governing bone healing are multifaceted and complex.

However, the general principles behind the various types of fracture healing are well described. It is commonly held that there are two major pathways by which bones can heal, either through the primary (direct) or secondary (indirect) pathway. The direct pathway generally follows an intramembranous physiologic course whereas the indirect pathway involves aspects of both intramembranous and endochondral ossification. The understanding of both physiologic pathways is critical in the management of various fractures so that complications such as delayed union, nonunion and malunion can be avoided [2].

Indirect fracture healing is the most common form of fracture healing, and it is most notably associated with nonoperative treatment but is also associated with relatively stable (nonrigid) surgical fixation of a fracture (external fixators and intramedullary nails) [3, 4]. Indirect healing

M. Johnson
Department of Orthopaedic Surgery, Creighton University, Omaha, NE, USA

G. Norris
University of Oklahoma College of Medicine, Oklahoma City, OK, USA

J. Checketts · B. L. Norris (✉)
Department of Orthopaedic Surgery, Oklahoma State University College of Medicine, Tulsa, OK, USA
e-mail: brent.norris@otsok.com

© The Author(s), under exclusive license to Springer Nature Switzerland AG 2024
P. V. Giannoudis, P. Tornetta III (eds.), *Failed Fracture Fixation*,
https://doi.org/10.1007/978-3-031-39692-2_2

occurs over the span of weeks to months and is a complex process involving many physiologic components. Indirect healing begins with the acute inflammatory phase, which involves the formation of a hematoma surrounding the fractured ends. This hematoma contains blood from both the periphery and medullary canals as well as bone marrow cells. Upon the formation of the hematoma, an inflammatory response mediated by macrophage release of tumour necrosis factor (TNF) promotes hematoma coagulation, angiogenesis and osteogenic differentiation of mesenchymal stem cells (MSCs). Other inflammatory mediators that aid in this process include interleukin-1 (IL-1), IL-6, IL-11 and IL-18 [5]. Following this inflammatory response, granulation tissue forms at the fracture site, which allows structure for endochondral activity to take place [6]. This initial endochondral activity forms what is commonly referred to as the soft callus, a collagenous medium that provides a semi-stable structure. Simultaneous to the formation of the soft callus, intramembranous ossification occurs at each end of the fracture creating what is referred to as the periosteal hard callus [3]. It has been previously described that the TGF superfamily plays an essential role in the signalling process of endochondral ossification, whereas bone morphogenetic protein-5 (BMP-5) and −6 have been shown to be predominant signalling molecules for intramembranous ossification [7].

Following the formation of the cartilaginous callus, angiogenesis and revascularization occur through the actions of vascular endothelial growth factor (VEGF), in combination with chondrocyte apoptosis, so that blood vessels may penetrate the callus. Once the soft callus has been constructed and revascularized, new bone formation begins. This process involves the simultaneous central movement of the periosteal hard callus, combined with the mineralization and resorption of chondrocytes within the soft callus. Soft callus hypertrophic chondrocytes undergo calcification of the extracellular matrix via calcium and phosphate precipitation. These precipitates will later undergo homogeneous nucleation in the process of apatite crystal formation [8]. The combination of both endochondral and intramembranous ossification creates a hard callus

structure that ultimately undergoes TNF-/IL-1-mediated osteoclastic/osteoblastic transformation into woven bone via the formation of Howship's lacunae [3].

Direct fracture healing occurs over the span of a few months to years and requires an anatomic reduction of the fracture and rigid internal fixation (often associated with open reduction and internal fixation with plates and screws). The direct healing process can occur through two different physiologic pathways depending on the size of the fracture gap, contact healing and gap healing. When the fragments are less than 0.01 mm apart and there is an interfragmentary strain of less than 2%, the direct process known as contact healing can take place [6, 9]. When the fragments are around 1 mm apart, the bone can still heal via direct bone healing through a process known as gap healing.

Contact healing begins with the formation of cutting cones on both fragments closest to the fracture site. The front ends of the cutting cones contain osteoclasts, which can cross the fracture line and generate longitudinal canals between the two fragments. Following the formation of these canals, osteoblasts located on the rear ends of the cutting cones lay down new bone and establish a union between fragments [10]. Additionally, the formation of this union restores the Haversian system allowing for angiogenesis and migration of osteoblastic precursors. These precursor cells subsequently remodel the bridged osteons into lamellar bone, eliminating the need for periosteal callus formation [11].

Gap healing differs from contact healing due to additional steps at the beginning of the healing process. Due to the larger fracture gap, the remodelling of the Haversian system and formation of bridging osteons do not occur synchronously [10]. Instead, lamellar bone is initially laid down perpendicular to the long axis of the bone to lessen the size of the gap. This initial structure of lamellar bone is subsequently replaced by correctly orientated vascularized osteons that deliver osteoblastic progenitor cells, which produce a structure that then allows for a secondary remodelling process comparable to contact healing to take place. The additional bone forming steps prior to secondary remodelling observed in gap healing are believed to take anywhere from 3 to 8 weeks [9].

Influence of Mechanics on Fracture Healing

Though there are many challenges to managing fracture healing, advances in treatment methods have progressed rapidly over the last century. Management options include casting, pins, plates/screws, intramedullary devices, uni−/biplanar external fixators, ringed external fixators and arthroplasty [12]. Overall, the aims of these treatment methods are to provide mechanical stability to the fracture and support/direct the biological factors associated with fracture healing. Despite these advances, fracture nonunions continue to occur. Furthermore, hardware failure due to nonunion or poor construct mechanics and new fractures around previously placed orthopaedic hardware are becoming increasingly common as the population ages [13, 14]. Both of these conditions present additional challenges to the treating surgeon from both a practical and a biological standpoint.

Stability and Strain Theory

Fracture healing has been thoughtfully described by Norris et al. as a spectrum of stability. At one end of the spectrum is absolute stability which will induce primary bone healing. At the other end of the spectrum is instability which will likely result in nonunion of the fracture site. In the middle of the spectrum is relative stability which will result in secondary bone healing. If blood supply and soft tissue coverage are adequate, fracture healing will be greatly influenced by the type of mechanical environment induced by the chosen fixation method. Thus, when managing fractures operatively, great care and thought must be placed regarding the environment one is aiming to produce at the fracture site through internal or external fixation. Understanding the fracture healing environment cannot be done without first understanding the strain theory postulated by Perren et al. [15]. This theory summarizes the concept of fracture strain as the degree of deformity or motion that is present at the fracture gap as a consequence of the fixation construct's inherent stability. Strain is measured by comparing the original fracture gap to the size of the gap when it is stressed. If the strain is calculated to be $\leq 2\%$, it can be determined an environment for absolute stability, and thus primary bone healing has been created. However, if the strain is measured between 2% and 10%, a relative stability construct has been obtained and fracture healing will occur in a secondary fashion through a cartilage medium. Understandably, if the strain is measured over 10%, the healing will be through a fibrous tissue intermediate and likely result in nonunion of the fracture site.

Intraoperatively an environment of absolute stability can be obtained through proper technique and fixation of the fracture being managed. This is primarily performed with simple fracture patterns (transverse, oblique and spiral). It is additionally employed in fractures involving the articular surfaces. Absolute stability is primarily accomplished by creating compression at the fracture site utilizing lag screws or compression plates, buttress plates and tension band constructs [12] The goal in treatment using these methods is to approximate the fracture to a point where there is no gapping present to allow cutting cones and appositional bone growth to occur.

Conversely, an environment of relative stability can be obtained where some interfragmentary motion between the fracture fragments occurs. This can be advantageous for several fracture types, including metaphyseal or diaphyseal fractures with comminution in which the conditions of absolute stability would likely not be met. Examples of constructs aimed at relative stability include casting, external fixation, bridge plating or intramedullary nail devices.

Proper preoperative planning and construct selection is essential to increase the odds of fracture healing; however, proper execution of the plan is also of the utmost importance. For example, if the goal is to treat a fracture using an absolute stability construct but fracture gapping is present, a delayed union or nonunion may occur. On the other hand, if one's goal is to treat a fracture with a relative stability construct, but their construct allows too little motion (<2% strain), the construct will be too stiff and a nonunion may occur. An example of this would be attempting to treat a comminuted fracture with bridge plating but placing screws too close to the fracture site, thus creating a short working length and a stiff construct. Conversely, if too much motion is allowed at the fracture site due to inadequate fixation of the fracture fragments (>10% strain), callus formation may occur, but consolidation or bridging may not occur resulting in a nonunion. A classic example of this is seen when treating a proximal tibia and distal femur fractures with intramedullary nailing where too much motion is allowed at the fracture site, and thus delayed or nonunion may occur. Knowledge of fracture healing types, strain theory and construct stability and selection is essential to managing fractures effectively. As stated by Norris et al. [12]' All the preoperative planning based on biomechanics will not overcome severe shortcomings in the biological environment of the fracture. Maintaining and maximizing the healing capacity of a fracture must always be considered when formulating a preoperative plan.'

Plate Fixation Mechanics

Depending on the goals of the treatment, plate constructs have a myriad of possibilities and functions resulting in either primary or secondary fracture healing. These included compression, bridging, neutralization, buttress and tension band constructs. It should be noted that these functions are carried out through the surgical technique applied, not the specific plate selected [16]. When treating fractures with plating, the surgeon is directing and determining the extent of the forces the fracture fragments endure during the healing process. These forces are bending, torsional and axial forces, and for the fixation to endure and fracture healing to occur the construct must provide the stability necessary for either primary or secondary healing. In addition to the forces endured by the fracture, the construct selected affects the biomechanical principles present at the fracture. Other biomechanical properties that must be factored into fracture

management are affected by the bone density, geometry of the fracture, plate thickness (which is directly proportional to the construct stiffness) and bone–plate interface friction. When a construct has load applied to it, the interface between the cortex and hardware utilized is where the forces are directed and the stability of the construct during this load is dependent on friction (non-locking screws) and interlocking mechanical forces (locking screws).

Nonlocking plates (such as compression and buttress plates) classically rely on interlocking mechanical forces (screw torque) and bone–plate friction for their construct stability. Higher screw torque and frictional forces are seen when bone density increases, indicating increased stability of the construct when placed in quality bone. Due to this principle, a different type of plate construct was created for better fixation in poor quality or osteoporotic bone. Locking plates work through different principles, as they primarily serve as internal fixators. They do this by creating a fixed angle construct and a more stable bone–plate unit by using threaded screw heads that interdigitate with the threaded holes of the plate. Thus, stability is determined by the interlocking mechanical forces of the screw to the plate allowing a stiffer construct in less dense bone. However, the biomechanics of the bone–plate construct rely on several factors outside of whether it is locking or nonlocking. The distribution and variety of screws as well as the length of the plate also play a large role in the mechanics of the construct [17]. The resistance to pull out forces is directly proportional to the length of the plate on each side of the fracture as well as the spread of the screws in the plate. The distance between the screws closest to the fracture on each side is defined as the working length, and the closer this distance, the stiffer the construct will be. Conversely, the screws subject to the highest degree of pullout forces are those that are closest to the fracture on each side as they bear the greatest proportion of load. Furthermore, increasing the distance between the proximal and distal screws on each side of the fracture increases the stability of that segment and adding additional screws on each segment increases the torsional rigidity. Finally, the material of the plate used can be a factor in regard to fracture healing. Traditionally, stainless steel plates have been used with great success. However, in recent years the use of titanium plates has been met with enthusiasm as titanium's modulus of elasticity is much closer to bone than stainless steel (less stiff) thus potentially promoting greater osseointegration and healing.

Intramedullary Device Mechanics

Diaphyseal and metadiaphyseal fractures of long bones are common, and to restore length, alignment and rotation, operative intervention is usually necessary. Over the last century, intramedullary fixation has evolved and advanced to become the most prevalent means of stabilizing diaphyseal and metadiaphyseal fractures of the long bones. From a biological perspective, intramedullary nails have advantages that are not seen with plates and screw constructs. When placing an intramedullary device, the incision and access to the long bone is generally at the proximal or distal end of the bone, likely some degree of distance away from the fracture site. Because of this, the biology of fracture healing is maintained and undisturbed as it often is with the direct access necessitated for plate and screw constructs. Furthermore, because the nail is intramedullary in nature, there is less periosteal injury that is associated with a bone–plate construct. The biomechanics of the nail and its relationship with bone can have a direct effect on fracture stability and healing. One of the ways intramedullary nails affect fracture healing is through their flexibility, which is a result of nail material, size and geometry. As such, modern intramedullary nails are largely composed of titanium alloy metals as they have a better modulus of elasticity compared to stainless steel and more closely resemble that of bone. These characteristics promote a relatively stable construct and promote callus formation/fracture healing. Because long bones are exposed to bending and torsional forces to a high degree, intramedullary implants must be able to resist these stresses during fracture healing while still allowing the natural elasticity of bone. At baseline, intramedullary fixation will provide a high degree of bending stability in the sagittal and coronal planes; however, to overcome torsional forces, proximal and distal interlocking screws are introduced on each side of the fracture creating a construct that provides the necessary stability to both bending and torsional forces [18]. When a fracture is treated with intramedullary nailing, there is inherent flexibility as it acts as an internal fixator, and as a result micromovements of the fracture are expected. Because of this, fractures treated with intramedullary devices will heal with secondary healing and callus formation. Furthermore, because locked intramedullary nails provide stability in all planes, early weight-bearing is often encouraged for the patient and this likely also positively influences secondary bone healing.

External Fixators Mechanics

There are two types of external fixation, and they have both evolved significantly over the past few decades. Uniplanar external fixation is predominantly used to provisionally stabilize open fractures or fractures that are too swollen to be treated in an open fashion acutely. Ring fixation has now become associated with a form of definitive fixation for not just complex problems like bone transport, infected nonunions with poor soft tissues and also complex periarticular fractures. For the most part, external fixators are a form of relative stability and behave much like bridge plating or intramedullary nailing. They can however be modified to become very rigid and act like plates placed for absolute stability. In some ways, external fixation, especially ringed fixators, is the ideal surgical treatment as you can dial in the necessary level of stability needed for any given situation. Having said this, the use of the ringed fixator has a steep learning curve and is probably the least well-tolerated device by most patients.

Definition of Nonunion

Every fracture treated with surgical fixation becomes a race of achieving osseous union versus a nonunion with ensuing fixation failure. If osseous union has not been achieved within

9 months or a fracture has failed to show progressive healing over 3 consecutive months on radiographs, a nonunion can be declared [19, 20]. When this occurs the internal fixation present continues to endure cyclical stress and motion. Eventually, the hardware will reach its breaking/endpoint leading to a hardware failure. Failure can be simply loosening of the fixation or catastrophic failure (breakage of the implant).

Types of Nonunion (Septic)

A primary consideration in nonunion revision surgery is understanding the type of nonunion present. The primary factor that must be ruled out first and foremost is whether the fracture failed to unite because of an infectious process (septic nonunion). Septic nonunions are probably the most common type of nonunion. One of the most critical steps in a nonunion workup is to rule out infection. An infection at the nonunion site changes the goals of any revision surgery from achieving union to first eradicating infection. Nonunions with an unknown infection present at the time of definitive treatment have demonstrated an increased need of further surgeries and decreased chance of achieving union when compared to true aseptic nonunions [21–23].

Ruling out an infection begins with taking a thorough history, including mechanism and type of the initial injury, medical comorbidities, social habits, surgical procedures performed and any complications. Details such as history of an open fracture, the environment in which the open fracture occurred, the degree of initial contamination, the Gustilo-Anderson type of open fracture, length of time to soft tissue coverage/closure, extended period in external fixators before conversion to intramedullary nail, history of smoking, persistent wound drainage and prior number of surgeries for nonunions have all been associated with infection and should be clues to the surgeon for further investigation.

Clinical signs of infected nonunions can be obvious or subtle, local or systemic, associated with or without abnormal laboratory findings and associated with or without radiographic abnormalities. Obvious signs of a fracture-related infection are a sinus tract or wound breakdown with purulent drainage. Subtle signs of infection include systemic signs like night sweats, fever or malaise. Local signs like swelling, pain, can also suggest local infection.

In addition to these findings, elevated laboratory values are often seen with septic nonunions [24]. Common inflammatory markers used to examine for infection are white blood cell count (WBC), erythrocyte sedimentation rate (ESR) and C-reactive protein (CRP) [24]. Recently, IL-6, D-Dimer and other inflammatory markers have been examined to see whether they can further aid in the diagnosis of a fracture-related infection, but much more data will need to be obtained before they can be recommended to be part of the screening process [25, 26].

Signs of infection are not always present and when they are not, it can make the process of diagnosing a septic nonunion extremely difficult. If the systemic, local and radiographic signs do not indicate an infection, surgeons rely on inflammatory markers to help rule out infection. However, inflammatory markers remain within normal limits with low virulent organisms [27–29].

Finally, radiographs (plain film, computed tomography [CT] and even magnetic resonance imaging [MRI]) are not diagnostic of infection. They can certainly suggest it with signs like sclerosis, erosive changes to the bone/fracture or even hardware loosening [24]. MRI can also show signs suggestive of infection. Typical findings of osteomyelitis seen on MRI are decreased T1 signal and increased T2 signal due to marrow oedema. However, these can also be seen in the setting of stress reaction, reactive marrow and neuropathic arthropathy.

This places the gold standard for diagnosing fracture/nonunion-related infections intraoperatively. This occurs by having at least two positive cultures from separate deep tissue/implant specimens and/or the presence of microorganisms in deep tissue specimens confirmed by histopathological examination [24]. Ultimately, this makes preoperatively diagnosing an indolent septic nonunion very difficult and places an importance of obtaining intraoperative cultures. Therefore, any revision surgery must include gram stain and cultures to rule out infection (Fig. 2.1). This has led

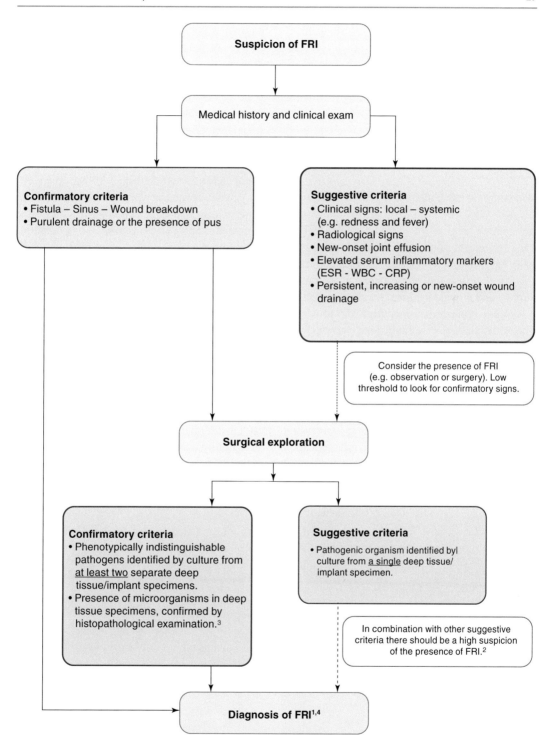

Fig. 2.1 Algorithm for fracture/nonunion-related infection. From WJ Metsemakersa, SM Morgenstern, MA McNally, TF Moriarty, I McFadyen, M Scarborough, NA Athanasou, PE Ochsner, R Kuehl, M Raschke, O Borens, Z Xie, S Velkes, S Hungerer, SL Kates, C Zalavras, PV Giannoudis, RG Richards, MHJ Verhofstad. "Fracture-related infection: A consensus on definition from an international expert group." *Injury*, vol. 49, 2108, pp. 505–510

a lot of surgeons performing staged treatment of the nonunion with first ruling in or out infection followed by definitive treatment if negative cultures are obtained. This is especially important if you are planning on placing an autogenous bone graft.

Types of Nonunion (Aseptic)

Assuming we have ruled out sepsis as the cause of the nonunion, we must then work up and identify any shortcomings of the mechanical and biological requirements that were not met during the prior intervention. Identifying and then correcting these will help optimize the outcome in revision surgery and provide the best chance for union.

Aseptic nonunions are divided into four categories: hypertrophic, oligotrophic, atrophic and pseudoarthrosis. Hypertrophic nonunions are viable and possess adequate blood supply for union but lack fracture stability required to complete union. This results in an abundance of callus present at the fracture with an interfragmentary gap consisting of fibrocartilage persisting (Fig. 2.2). If stability is provided, mineralization of fibrocartilage can occur, which will eventually lead to the formation of mature bone [30]. Hypertrophic nonunions are most frequently seen in internal fixation with inadequate strength such as undersized intramedullary nails and external fixators used for definitive treatment and in nonoperative treatment.

Atrophic nonunions are nonviable and lack any purposeful biological activity. This leads to a lack of callus formation (Fig. 2.3). The nonviability is demonstrated at the fracture edges where sclerotic avascular bone is seen. This can be due to traumatic or systemic causes. Large displacement of the fracture at the time of injury can lead to significant periosteal and soft tissue stripping, potentially devitalizing the fracture. Aggressive surgical dissection and endosteal reaming can also devitalize the bone, limiting the biological response at the fracture site. Systemic causes such as smoking and diabetes can decrease microvascular blood flow to the fracture, limiting the ability to create a biological response.

Oligotrophic nonunions are likely also viable and possess an adequate blood supply, but they result in minimal to no callus formation (Fig. 2.4). The viability can be demonstrated at the fracture

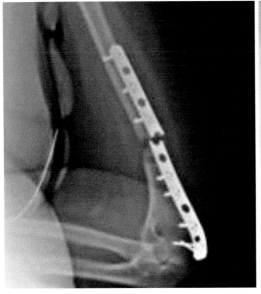
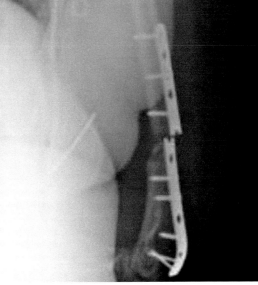

Fig. 2.2 AP and lateral radiographs of left humeral atrophic nonunion

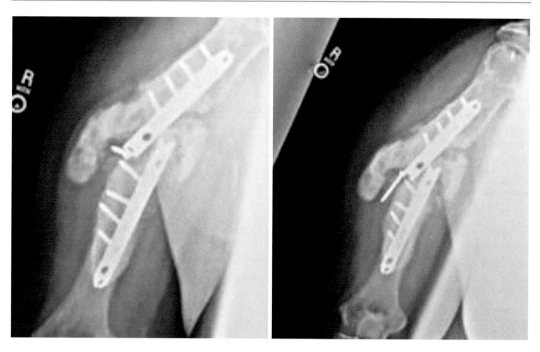

Fig. 2.3 AP and lateral radiographs of left humeral hypertrophic nonunion

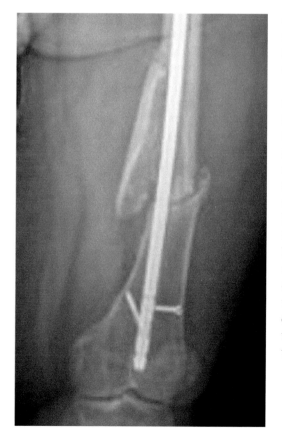

edges with a lack of sclerosis and bleeding present. They are most often caused by inadequate reduction that results in little to no contact at the displaced osseous surfaces.

Pseudoarthrosis is an unusual type of nonunion that can occur for many reasons but commonly occurs when there is excessive motion at a fracture site. There is some thought that this condition might have a genetic predisposition. It can occur from surgical and nonsurgical treatment of the fracture. When it occurs from operative treatment, the surgical stabilization will have failed leading to excessive motion at the fracture. Secondary to the excessive motion, the tissue between the fragments is fibrocartilaginous and/or granulation tissue in nature. This tissue seals off the medullary canal and forms a cavity that will often be lined in synovial-type cells. This cavity bathes the nonunion in fluid giving this type of nonunion its namesake. This type of nonunion is common in the femur, tibia and humerus.

Fig. 2.4 AP radiograph of the left femur showing oligotrophic nonunion

Radiographic and Mechanical Workup for Nonunion

Radiographs from all stages of the injury and treatment should be obtained. Injury films can help determine the initial displacement of the injury and the type of fracture pattern. Fractures with a large displacement can have extensive periosteal stripping, limiting the biological capacity of the fracture after the index surgery. Postoperative imaging allows for assessment of the reduction, fixation technique and the overall hardware construct. Follow-up films will provide a sequential glance of the fracture to see if any healing of comminuted, butterfly or segmental pieces occurred. Follow-up films also help determine if deformity occurred and if it did whether it was a gradual process or if it was a sudden event with hardware failure. Radiographs obtained should include:

- Full length anteroposterior (AP) and lateral of the bone involved.
- AP, lateral and oblique views of the nonunion site.
- Bilateral AP and lateral 51-inch alignment radiographs for lower extremity nonunions to assess length discrepancies and malalignment.
- Flexion and extension lateral radiographs to determine the arc of motion of the adjacent joint to the nonunion site [30].

Even with this extensive amount of radiographs, it may be difficult to determine whether a fracture has healed. A CT scan can be used to help determine this even in the presence of metallic artifact. Healing or healed fractures display greater than 25% of the cross-sectional area while nonunions demonstrate bridging callus over less than 5% of the cross-sectional area [33]. CTs can also be used to determine whether any rotational deformities are present that need to be corrected in the following surgery.

Collecting all this radiographic information allows the surgeon to determine the type of nonunion, if deformity is present, type and status of the hardware implanted and how/when hardware failure occurred. If the wrong fixation technique was paired with a specific fracture, the bone could have been forced down a healing pathway that did not lead to union. This is important when creating a revision operative plan to maximize the hardware construct but also to prevent from using the wrong technique.

This can be seen when surgeons attempt primary bone healing and do not achieve an anatomic reduction and when attempting secondary bone healing and incorrectly place too rigid of a surgical construct around comminuted fractures. In both of these situations the fracture gap is too large to allow primary bone healing, but the fracture is placed in too rigid of an environment to allow secondary bone healing.

If an anatomic reduction cannot be achieved, there are multiple ways to increase motion at the fracture site. Increasing motion can help drive fracture strain to 2–10% where relative stability and secondary bone healing occur [15]. Relative stability is best used to treat comminuted fractures, osteoporotic fractures, paediatric fractures and fractures of the long bones in the lower extremity. Common relative stability treatment methods include casting, intramedullary nails, bridge plating and external fixators.

Creating and maintaining an environment of relative stability during fracture healing is dependent on the surgeon. Surgeons can decrease the construct's rigidity to increase motion at the fracture site with factors including plate design, plate length, plate size, plate material, screw length, screw type, screw density and working length. The working length of a plate construct is defined as the distance between the first screw on either side of the fracture [31]. In the setting of a simple fracture pattern anatomically reduced, a short working length can be advantageous by decreasing the strain at the fracture pushing the bone towards primary bone healing. However, in the setting of comminuted fractures, a shorter working length will create a low strain environment and drive the bone to attempt primary bone healing. If the fracture gap is too large, healing will not occur and an oligotrophic nonunion will likely occur.

2 Common Causes of Aseptic Fracture Fixation Failure

Shorter working lengths can also have undesirable effects on the hardware as well. Shorter plates have shown to be a risk factor for hardware failure on distal femur fractures [32]. A short plate limits the amount of working length that can be obtained. Shorter working lengths create a high-stress environment at the fracture that is transferred to the hardware leading to hardware failure if bony union cannot occur prior to the breaking point of the hardware. A longer working length decreases the stress seen by the hardware decreasing the risk or hardware failure. Increasing the working length in fractures treated with relative stability has shown to increase flexibility, increase strain and in theory promote secondary bone healing, callus formation and fracture healing [33].

Fixation constructs are one of the few things surgeons can control when treating fractures. It is extremely important to critically analyse any hardware failure on how the construct could have prevented failure and promoted union. An ignorance of failed constructs can lead to repeating the same surgical misadventures that previously failed all while expecting a different result to occur. Placing the fracture or nonunion in the optimal mechanical environment will provide the best chance possible for union.

Metabolic Workup for Nonunion

Creating the ideal fracture construct and environment still may not overcome severe shortcomings in the healing capacity of a patient. A variety of contributing factors have been described that deter the biological environment of fracture healing and these must be corrected to place the fracture in the optimal healing environment.

This can start with an assessment of medications the patient uses. Bisphosphonates, systemic corticosteroids, nonsteroidal anti-inflammatory drugs (NSAIDs) and quinolones have all shown to have negative effects on bone healing [34]. The offending medications should be changed or discontinued if possible prior to revision surgery.

Social habits such as smoking and alcohol consumption should be examined. Smoking has not only been shown to slow and inhibit fracture healing but also be a risk factor for osteomyelitis, infection and complications in healing fractures [35–39]. Chronic alcoholism can result in an osteopenic skeleton by suppressing osteoblastic differentiation of bone marrow and promoting adipogenesis [40]. Excessive alcohol in the postinjury period interferes with the fracture healing process by creating bone with decreased strength, density and mineral content [41, 42].

Excessive alcohol use not only changes the biology and healing response of the bone, but also causes falls and noncompliance with postoperative precautions leading to potential hardware failure. Alcohol use of greater than 15 drinks a week has been shown to be a cause for multiple reoperations in clavicle fractures treated operatively [43]. Patients with these habits should be offered assistance in quitting the addiction. Cessation of the habit would be most ideal; however, it may be unrealistic to expect this to occur.

A thorough workup for potential metabolic or endocrine aetiologies of nonunion should be performed prior to any operation. Brinker et al. demonstrated that 84% of patients who failed to heal a simple fracture demonstrated correctable endocrine or metabolic abnormalities [44]. This should be performed by obtaining serum levels of calcium, vitamin D, parathyroid hormone, thyroid panel and an haemoglobin A1c. Brinker et al. even recommend patients with nonunions to be evaluated by an endocrinologist if they fall into one of these criteria: (1) persistent nonunion despite adequate treatment without any obvious technical errors; (2) a history of multiple low-energy fractures with at least one progressing to a nonunion or (3) a nonunion of a nondisplaced pubic rami of sacral ala fracture (Fig. 2.5). This protocol allows endocrine processes such as central hypogonadism to be diagnosed and treated.

Vitamin D, calcium and parathyroid hormone (PTH) have the most direct effect on bone metabolism during fracture healing. Irregularities in their values can be present in up to 50% of people

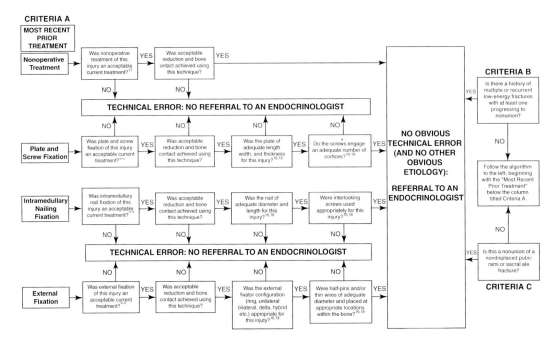

Fig. 2.5 Flowchart for endocrinology referral for patients with nonunion of a fracture. From Brinker, Mark R., et al. "Metabolic and endocrine abnormalities in patients with nonunions." *Journal of Orthopaedic Trauma*, vol. 21, no. 8, 2007, pp. 557–570

[45, 46]. However 68% of patients with nonunions have demonstrated having irregularities in these labs. Some patients (almost 25%) with these abnormal labs may achieve union with just correcting the abnormal labs [44].

Protein deprivation has shown to have an adverse effect on fracture healing [47]. Serum level albumin, total lymphocyte and transferrin should be obtained and if the levels are below normal limits a nutritional consultation is recommended [48]. It is imperative that this is identified and reversed with optimization occurring prior to revision surgery if possible. Reversal of the malnourished state is shown to increase bone mineralization promoting a larger and stronger fracture callus during the healing state [49].

Diabetes has been shown to have detrimental effects in bone healing that lead to decreased callus size, decreased bone formation and decreased mechanical strength [50]. However these effects can be reversed with adequate glycaemic control [51]. Long-term glycaemic control can be monitored with haemoglobin A1c and is best to delay surgery until it approaches 7% [48].

Much like diabetes, hypothyroidism has been shown to cause decreased callus size and bone formation. This is due to the inhibition of endochondral ossification during fracture healing. These effects can be reversed with thyroid supplementation to normalize hormone levels [52].

Hyperthyroidism as well has shown to affect osseous health and healing. Thyrotoxicosis can promote secondary osteoporosis leading to bone that is more prone for hardware failure [53]. Iatrogenic hyperthyroidism, due to oversupplementation, has shown to be present in persistent nonunions [45]. Patients with existing thyroid issues should have a thyroid panel drawn to ensure their medication is being prescribed appropriately. Once again, normalization of these hormones should be achieved prior to revision surgery.

Metabolic abnormalities should be evaluated and addressed as part of the workup for fractures with failed fixation and/or nonunion. If the surgeon neglects this exercise prior to undertaking any revision surgery for the failed fixation/nonunion, they are setting themselves up for continued failure.

Conclusion

For a variety of reasons, fractures fail to heal and become nonunions. If surgical stabilization was used in the initial treatment, failed fixation is not uncommon and almost uniformly needs to be removed and/or revised to obtain bone union. The treating surgeon must remember the cause of nonunion may be multifactorial. First and foremost, septic nonunion must always be ruled out. A thorough preoperative history, physical exam, radiographic studies and laboratory analysis should be undertaken. Additionally, the type of nonunion gives us a clue as to the root cause of nonunion, which can be biological, mechanical, patient related, injury related or even treatment related.

Successful management requires adequate and correct assessment of any/all discernible cause(s) of the nonunion. These include eradicating infection, correcting metabolic abnormalities, adequately stabilizing the bone, introducing biology with bone grafting, cell-based therapies, biological adjuvants and finally restoring a sound vascular environment. Nonunion surgery remains a difficult clinical entity that will challenge your professional acumen and require adherence to sound biological/mechanical principles to adequately restore limb alignment/function and achieve a successful outcome.

References

1. Zura R, Xiong Z, Einhorn T, et al. Epidemiology of fracture nonunion in 18 human bones. JAMA Surg. 2016;151(11):e162775. https://doi.org/10.1001/jamasurg2016.2775. Pub 2016 Nov 16
2. Marsell R, Einhorn TA. The biology of fracture healing. Injury. 2011;42(6):551–5. https://doi.org/10.1016/j.injury.2011.03.031.
3. Gerstenfeld LC, Alkhiary YM, Krall EA, et al. Three-dimensional reconstruction of fracture callus morphogenesis. J Histochem Cytochem. 2006;54(11):1215–28.
4. Pape HC, Giannoudis PV, Grimme K, et al. Effects of intramedullary femoral fracture fixation: what is the impact of experimental studies in regards to the clinical knowledge? Shock. 2002;18(4):291–300.
5. Cho HH, Kyoung KM, Seo MJ, et al. Overexpression of CXCR4 increases migration and proliferation of human adipose tissue stromal cells. Stem Cells Dev. 2006;15(6):853–64.
6. Rahn BA. Bone healing: histologic and physiologic concepts. In: Fackelman GE, editor. Bone in clinical orthopedics. Stuttgart/New York: Thieme; 2002. p. 287–326.
7. Marsell R, Einhorn TA. The role of endogenous bone morphogenetic proteins in normal skeletal repair. Injury. 2009;40(Suppl 3):S4–7. [PubMed: 20082790]
8. Ketenjian AY, Arsenis C. Morphological and biochemical studies during differentiation and calcification of fracture callus cartilage. Clin Orthop Relat Res. 1975;107:266–73. [PubMed: 48443]
9. Shapiro F. Cortical bone repair. The relationship of the lacunar-canalicular system and intercellular gap junctions to the repair process. J Bone Joint Surg Am. 1988;70(7):1067–81.
10. Kaderly RE. Primary bone healing. Semin Vet Med Surg (Small Animal). 1991;6(1):21–5.
11. Einhorn TA. The cell and molecular biology of fracture healing. Clin Orthop Relat Res. 1998;355(Suppl):S7–21.
12. Norris BL, Lang G, Russell TAT, Rothberg DL, Ricci WM, Borrelli J Jr. Absolute versus relative fracture fixation: impact on fracture healing. J Orthop Trauma. 2018;32(Suppl 1):S12–6.
13. Checketts JX, Dai Q, Zhu L, Miao Z, Shepherd S, Norris BL. Readmission rates after hip fracture: are there prefracture warning signs for patients most at risk of readmission? J Am Acad Orthop Surg. 2020;28(24):1017–26.
14. Pivec R, Issa K, Kapadia BH, et al. Incidence and future projections of periprosthetic femoral fracture following primary total hip arthroplasty: an analysis of international registry data. J Long Term Eff Med Implants. 2015;25(4):269–75.
15. Perren SM. Physical and biological aspects of fracture healing with special reference to internal fixation. Clin Orthop Relat Res. 1979;138:175–96.
16. Kfuri M, Fogagnolo F, Pires RE. Biomechanics of plate and screw constructs for fracture fixation. In: Crist BD, Borrelli Jr J, Harvey EJ, editors. Essential biomechanics for orthopedic trauma: a case-based guide. Springer International Publishing; 2020. p. 171–8.
17. Törnkvist H, Hearn TC, Schatzker J. The strength of plate fixation in relation to the number and spacing of bone screws. J Orthop Trauma. 1996;10(3):204–8.
18. Kempf I, Grosse A, Beck G. Closed locked intramedullary nailing. Its application to comminuted fractures of the femur. J Bone Joint Surg Am. 1985;67(5):709–20.
19. Bhandari M, et al. Variability in the definition and perceived causes of delayed unions and nonunions: a cross-sectional, multinational survey of orthopaedic surgeons. J Bone Joint Surg Am. 2012;94(15):1091–6.

20. Bell A, et al. Nonunion of the Femur and Tibia: an update. Orthop Clin North AM. 2016;47(2):365–75.
21. Olszewski D, et al. Fate of patients with a "surprise" positive culture after nonunion surgery. J Orthop Trauma. 2016;30(1):19–23.
22. Amorosa LF, et al. A single-stage treatment protocol for presumptive aspetic diaphyseal non-unions: a review of outcomes. J Orthop Trauma. 2013;27(10):582–6.
23. Arsoy D, et al. Outcomes of presumed aspetic long-bone nonunions with postive intraoperative cultures through a single-stage surgical protocol. J Orthop Trauma. 2018;32(Suppl 1):S35–9.
24. Metsemakers WJ, Morgenstern M, McNally MA, Moriarty TF, McFadyen I, Scarborough M, Athanasou NA, Ochsner PE, Kuehl R, Raschke M, Borens O, Xie Z, Velkes S, Hungerer S, Kates SL, Zalavras C, Giannoudis PV, Richards RG, Verhofstad MHJ. Fracture-related infection: a consensus on definition from an international expert group. Injury. 2018;49:505–10.
25. Wang Z, et al. Usefullness of serum D-dimer for pre-operative diagnosis of infected nonunion after open reduction and internal fixation. Infect Drug Resist. 2019;12:1827–31.
26. Zhao X-Q, et al. Interleukin-6 versus common inflammatory biomarkers for diagnosing fracture-related infection: utility and potential influencing factors. J Immunol Res. 2021;14:616–38.
27. Brinker MR, et al. Utility of common biomarkers for diagnosing infection in nonunion. J Orthop Trauma. 2021;35(3):121–7.
28. van den Kieboom J, et al. Diagnostic accuracy of serum inflammatory markers in late fracture-related infection. Bone Joint J. 2018;100-B(12):1542–50.
29. Sigmund IK, et al. Limited diagnostic value of serum inflammatory biomarkers in the diagnosis of fracture-related infections. Bone Joint J. 2020;102-B(7):904–11.
30. Browner BD, Jupiter JB, Krettek C, Anderson PA, et al., editors. Chapter 25: skeletal trauma: basic science, management, and reconstruction. 5th ed. Saunders/Elsevier; 2009. p. 643–61.
31. Hoffmeier KL, et al. Choosing a proper working length can improve the lifespan of locked plates. A biome-chanical study. Clin Biomech. 2011;26(4):405–9.
32. Ricci WM, et al. Risk factors for failure of locked plate fixation of distal femur fractures: an analysis of 335 cases. J Orthop Trauma. 2014;28(2):83–9.
33. Chen G, et al. Computational investigations of mechanical failures of internal plate fixation. Proc Inst Mech Eng H. 2010;224(1):119–26.
34. Wheatley BM, et al. Effects of NSAIDs on bone healing: a meta-analysis. J Am Acad Orthop Surg. 2019;27(7):330–6.
35. Zawawy HB, et al. Smoking delays chondrogenosis in a mouse model of closed tibia fracture healing. J Orthop Res. 2006;24:2150–8.
36. Little CP, et al. Failure of surgery for the scaphoid non-union is associated with smoking. J Hand Surg (Br). 2006;31:252–5.
37. Hak DJ, et al. Success of exchange reamed intramed-ullary nailing for femoral shaft nonunion or delayed union. J Orthop Trauma. 2005;14:178–82.
38. Castillo RC, et al. Impact of smoking on fracture heal-ing and risk of complications in limb-threating open tibia fracture. J Orthop Trauma. 2005;19(3):151–7.
39. Scolaro JA, et al. Cigarette smoking increases compli-cations following fracture: a systemic review. J Bone Joint Surg Am. 2014;96(8):674–81.
40. Chakkalakal DA. Alcohol-induced bone loss and deficient bone repair. Alcohol Clin Ex Res. 2005;29(12):2077–90.
41. Chakkalakal DA, et al. Inhibition of bone repair in a rat model for chronic and excessive alcohol consump-tion. Alcohol. 2005;36(3):201–2014.
42. Elmali N, et al. Fracture healing and bone mass in rats fed on liquid diet containing ethanol. Alcohol Clin Exp Res. 2002;26(4):509–13.
43. Schemitsch LA, et al. Prognostic factors for reop-eration after plate fixation of the midshaft clavicle. J Orthop Trauma. 2015;29(12):533–7.
44. Brinker MR, et al. Metabolic and endocrine abnor-malities in patients with nonunions. J Orthop Trauma. 2007;21(8):557–70.
45. Holick MF. High prevalence of vitamin D inade-quacy and implications for health. Mayo Clin Proc. 2006;81(3):353–73.
46. Bogunovic L, et al. Hypovitaminosis D in patients schedule to undergo orthopedic surgery: a single-center analysis. J Bone Joint Surg. 2010;92(13):2300–4.
47. Day SM, DeHeer DH. Reversal of the detrimen-tal effects of chronic protein malnutrition on long bone fracture healing. J Orthop Trauma. 2001;15(1):1947–53.
48. Cross MB, et al. Evaluation of malnutrition in orthopaedic surgery. J Am Acad Orthop Surg. 2014;22(3):193–9.
49. Hughes MS, et al. Enhanced fracture and soft tissue healing by means of anabolic dietary supplementa-tion. J Bone Joint Surg Am. 2006;88(11):2386–94.
50. Kayal RA, et al. Diminished bone formation during diabetic fracture healing is related to the premature resorption of cartilage associated with increased osteo-blastic activity. J Bone Miner Res. 2007;22(4):560–8.
51. Kayal RA, et al. Diabetes causes the accelerated loss of cartilage during fracture repair which is reversed by insulin treatment. Bone. 2009;44(2):357–63.
52. Urabe K, et al. Inhibition of endochondral ossification during fracture repair in experimental hypothyroid rats. J Orthop Res. 1999;17(6):920–5.
53. Bassett JHD, Williams GR. Role of thyroid hormones in skeletal development and bone maintenance. Endocr Rev. 2016;27(2):135–87.

General Considerations: Analysis of Failure of Fixation: A Stepwise Approach

3

Volker Alt, Markus Rupp, and Siegmund Lang

Introduction

Failure of fracture fixation constructs can result in breakage of the fracture fixation device, loss of stable bone purchase of screws, displacement of the fragments with loss of fracture reduction and/or even plastic deformity of the implant. There are several reasons for fracture fixation failure with biomechanical, biological and infection causes being among the most relevant ones. Some of them are under the control of the surgeon, e.g., reduction of the fracture, stability of the osteosynthesis etc., whereas others, such as patient compliance, bone, and wound healing disturbances are not (or at least not fully). Herein, our aim is to provide a stepwise approach for the analysis of failed fracture fixation with a focus on malalignment, fracture fixation constructs, and patients' compliance. Theoretical backgrounds will be worked up and several clinical cases will be presented and discussed to help the reader to avoid fracture fixation failures in the future.

The Concept of "Race Between Bone Healing and Construct Failure"

The overall goal of fracture treatment is to achieve fracture healing and bony consolidation in good alignment and to restore pre-fracture activities with high quality of life for the patient. In order to achieve this, surgical treatment of fractures includes adequate reduction of the fracture and the use of stable fracture fixation devices to allow for successful healing. The purpose of the implants for fracture fixation is to maintain the stability of the fracture during the bone healing process in order to promote the bone to return to its normal and stable biomechanical state. Surgical implants undergo and underlie the principle of material fatigue, like all other mechanically loaded materials, and have a finite number of load cycles until failure. This means that implants will only be able to maintain the required stability for bone healing for a certain amount of time, and not forever. In cases of "normal," undisturbed and timely fracture healing, this is not critical as the bone healing process will gradually take over biomechanical stability and result in a consolidated stable bone before material fatigue occurs (Fig. 3.1a).

However, in cases of healing disturbances, bone healing will result in delayed healing or non-union, which means that the stability cannot be restored by the bone itself. This also means that mechanical loading is still on the implant and

V. Alt (✉) · M. Rupp · S. Lang
Department of Trauma Surgery, University Hospital Regensburg, Regensburg, Germany
e-mail: volker.alt@ukr.de; markus.rupp@ukr.de; siegmund.lang@ukr.de

© The Author(s), under exclusive license to Springer Nature Switzerland AG 2024
P. V. Giannoudis, P. Tornetta III (eds.), *Failed Fracture Fixation*,
https://doi.org/10.1007/978-3-031-39692-2_3

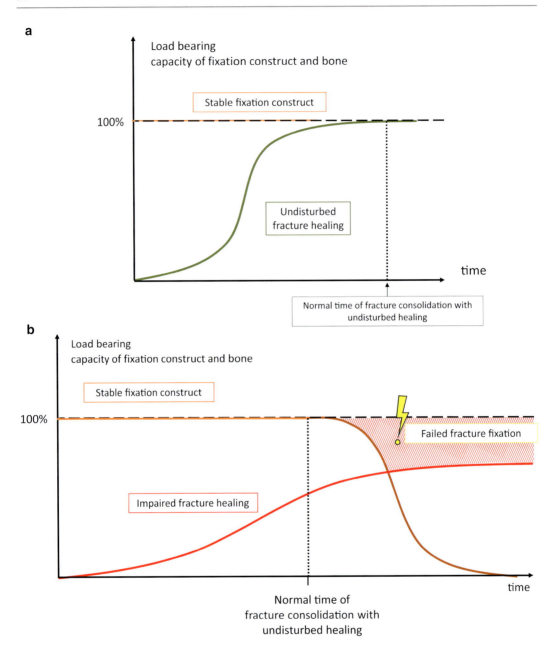

Fig. 3.1 General illustration of the "race between bone healing and construct failure". In case of normal undelayed bone healing, bone healing with stable consolidation will lead to restoration of full-weight bearing capacity of the bone before the fixation construct fails (**a**). In this illustrated case, immediate full weight bearing capacity postoperatively by the fixation construct is assumed. In case of delayed bone healing, the bone will not be able to restore full-weight bearing capacity in normal time and the construct will lose mechanical stability over time, which can result in failure of the fracture fixation construct due to fatigue (**b**). The construct will fail under loading, which is above the decreasing loading capacity of the implant and above the mechanical stability of the unhealed bone

can result in significant material fatigue with breakage of the implant. This phenomenon is well characterized by the term "race between bone healing and construct failure" or in other words "race between biology and mechanics" (Fig. 3.1b).

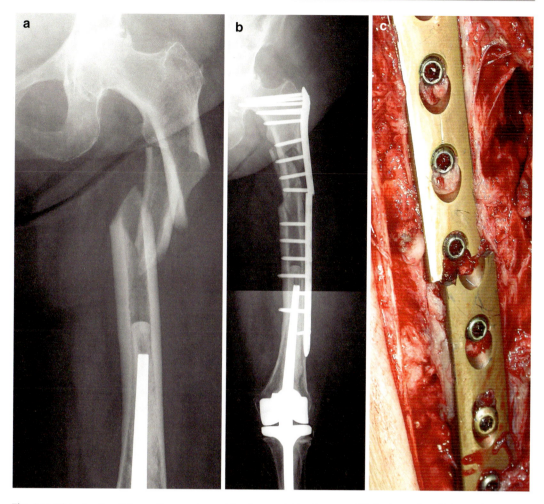

Fig. 3.2 Plate fixation failure after angular stable plate fixation in a proximal periprosthetic femur fracture (**a**) Mulitfragmentary subtrochanteric femur fracture with an indwelling cemented revision knee prosthesis. (**b**) X-ray with fracture fixation faliure with breakage of the angular stable plate most likely due to insufficient reduction and varus malalignment of the fracture 3 months after fixation (**c**) Intraoperative finding with plate breakage in the middle part of the plate

Given the above-mentioned principle of the "race between bone healing and construct failure," it is important to state here that the breakage of the implant is in the very most cases, in which adequate reduction and stable fixation were performed, not due to the general insufficiency or low quality of the implant but due to disturbed bone healing with mechanical overloading and subsequent failure of the implant over time (Fig. 3.2).

The "Diamond Bone Concept" and General Principles of Bone Healing

As fixation constructs have only a finite number of loading cycles until failure, adequate bone healing with restoration of the biomechanical stability is essential before construct failure occurs. Therefore, fracture and bone healing play an important role in understanding of fracture fixation failure.

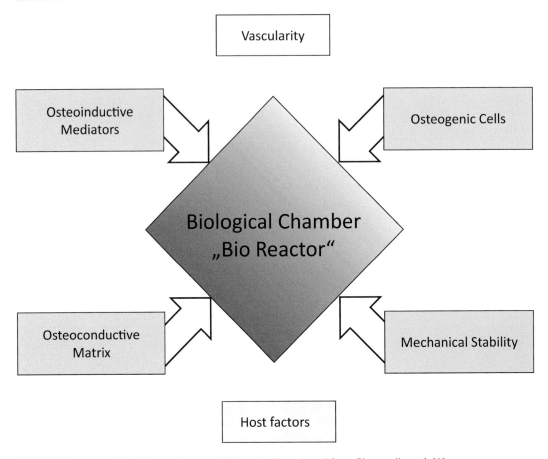

Fig. 3.3 Illustration of the 'diamond concept' of bone healing adapted from Giannoudis et al. [1]

Fracture healing is an orchestrated process that requires the interplay between different cell types, molecules and other important preconditions, such as mechanical stability. These aspects have been framed in the so-called "diamond bone concept" for fracture and bone healing (Fig. 3.3) [1].

This concept covers the three osteoconductive, osteoinductive, and osteogenic key elements for bone healing as well as mechanical stability, vascularity, and also host factors, such as diabetes and smoking. If all pre-conditions are given, the fracture will heal with any healing disturbances and without fracture fixation failure.

The diamond bone concept is not only helpful to explain successful bone healing but also for the analysis of failed fracture healing. Failure of fracture healing is still an important fact in orthopedic trauma as around 8–10% of fractures fail to heal despite modern treatment concepts, e.g., for intramedullary nailing of diaphyseal fractures of the femur and tibia [2, 3]. There are several factors that impair bone healing, which can be divided into patient-dependent, such as diabetes or smoking, and non-patient dependent, such as type of fracture [4]. Mechanical aspects are among the most relevant risks for fracture healing impairment and include fracture fixation by the surgeon as alignment of the fragments and the fracture fixation construct significantly determine the further course of fracture healing.

Types of Bone Healing

The type of bone healing is only a theoretical explanation of the cellular and molecular processes to restore bone stability after a fracture but

3 General Considerations: Analysis of Failure of Fixation: A Stepwise Approach

an important factor to understand both success and failure of fracture fixation as different fixation techniques rely on different healing principles. The understanding of bone healing principles in the context of the underlying osteosynthesis is therefore essential for the analysis of fracture fixation failure.

In general, there are two types of bone healing: direct (primary) and indirect (secondary) healing [5]. Direct healing is uncommonly a natural process of fracture healing as it requires 100% anatomical reduction of the fracture ends without any gap formation and rigid fixation with only minimal strain. In fixation constructs, stability determines strain. Strain is defined as change in the fracture gap divided by the fracture gap ($\Delta L/L$) [6]. A distinction is made between absolute and relative stability. Strain and consequently stability determine the type of fracture healing. Strain less than 2% results in primary bone healing [7] and strain of 2–10% results in secondary bone healing [8]. In general, strain greater than 10% does not permit bone formation due to substantial instability and results in delayed healing and subsequent non-union.

Direct Bone Healing

Direct healing can further be distinguished into contact and gap healing. The aim of both processes is to re-establish an anatomical and biomechanically stable lamellar bone structure. Direct healing can only be achieved after anatomical reduction and rigid fixation with interfragmentary compression, e.g., by compression plating or by interfragmentary screw fixation with or without the additional use of a neutralizing plate. The anatomical and biomechanical prerequisite for contact healing is a gap between bone ends of less than 0.01 mm and interfragmentary strain of less than 2% [7]. If these conditions are met, cutting cones are formed at the ends of the osteons at the fracture site [9]. At a rate of 50–100 µm/day osteoclasts at the tips of the cutting cones generate longitudinal cavities that cross the fracture line by providing pathways for the penetration by blood vessels [10]. This results in the simultaneous generation of a bony union and the restoration of Haversian systems

formed in an axial direction [11, 12]. The restored Haversian systems allow infiltration of osteoblastic precursor cells carried by blood vessels [10, 13]. The bridging osteons later mature by direct remodeling to mechanically stable lamellar bone. Direct fracture healing proceeds without the formation of a periosteal callus.

In contrast to contact healing, bony union and Haversian remodeling do not occur simultaneously in gap healing. Again, anatomical reduction and stable conditions are requirements with gaps less than 800 µm to 1 mm [11]. The fracture site is primarily filled by lamellar bone oriented perpendicular to the longitudinal axis [14]. This primary bone structure is then gradually replaced by longitudinal revascularized osteons carrying osteoprogenitor cells. These differentiate into osteoblasts that produce lamellar bone on each surface of the gap [7]. Due to its perpendicular arrangement to the long axis of the gap, this lamellar bone is mechanically weak. After this initial phase, which lasts 3–8 weeks, the secondary remodeling phase follows resembling the contact healing cascade with cutting cones [7].

Indirect Bone Healing

Indirect fracture healing is the most common form of fracture healing and occurs in non-operative fracture treatment and operative treatment using less-rigid constructs that allow for slight motion at the fracture site and callus formation. Both endochondral and intramembranous ossification occur within the fracture depending on strain and vascularity level at different zones of the fracture site [15]. During endochondral ossification, cartilage is formed, calcified and finally replaced by bone during callus maturation. Intramembranous ossification occurs through direct osteoblast-mediated bone formation by mesenchymal stem cell differentiation [16]. Other than in direct bone healing, anatomical reduction and rigidly stable conditions are not required. Micromotion and (partial) weight bearing enhance indirect bone healing, but too much motion and/or load can result in delayed healing or non-union [17]. In surgically treated fractures, this type of healing is found in intramedullary nailing, external fixation and bridge plate fixation [18, 19].

The reason for the very most cases of failed fracture fixation constructs can be identified with the help of the "diamond bone concept" and the principles of bone healing. Therefore, these will be used for the stepwise approach for the analysis of failed fracture fixation in this book chapter with a focus on malalignment, fracture fixation construct and patient compliance.

Fracture Fixation Failure Due to Malalignment

Good alignment or malalignment of fracture fragments can have several consequences for bone healing, the further functional outcome and the overall quality of life of the patient. First, correct alignment of the major fragments needs to be ensured for uneventful fracture healing as missing bone contact and large fracture gaps end up in impaired and delayed healing with the development of non-union. Second, even if bone healing itself is ensured with good contact with the fracture fragments, malalignment of the fragments with axis and/or rotational deviation can still occur and will result in a consolidated but malaligned bone. Depending on the functional outcome, this malalignment is acceptable or not for the patient, and revision surgery for axis and/or rotational correction should be considered. This chapter will only focus on the first aspect with insufficient reduction with missing bone contact and large fracture gaps as the second one will result in consolidated bone with axis deviation without fracture fixation failure (Fig. 3.4).

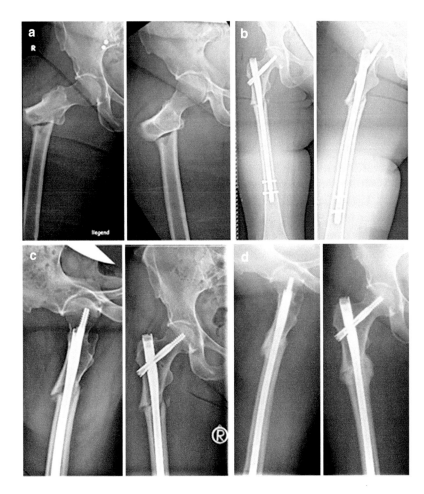

Fig. 3.4 Clinical case example with malalignment after closed reduction of an atypical subtrochanteric femoral fracture in a 66-year-old female (**a**) with a cephalomedullary nail (**b**). Despite considerable recurvatum and additional slight varus malalignment, there is sufficient contact between the fragments (**b**) allowing for successful fracture healing with some callus and bridging callus formation with 3 of 4 cortices after 3 (**c**) and 12 months (**d**) without implant failure, respectively. Patient shows normal gait and good function of the right hip with no need for surgical revision

As mentioned above, fracture healing requires an adequate alignment of the major fracture fragments as large fracture gaps impair bone healing with the risk of delayed healing and non-union [20] with the further risk of fixation failure (Fig. 3.1b).

Adequate alignment must be considered individually for each anatomical region and each type of fracture type fixation depending on the associated underlying type of bone healing, which is determined by the type of fixation. In the case of rigid fixation of a juxta-articular fracture with an anatomical locking plate, anatomical alignment of the major articular fragments by correct reduction is not only a pre-requisite for the avoidance of post-traumatic osteoarthritis but also for successful fracture healing. Furthermore, adequate alignment of fracture fragments with relevant biomechanical function with good interfragmentary contact in correct angulation between the fragments is critical. This is of importance, e.g., for the calcar region of the proximal humerus and of the proximal femur. Inadequate reduction with subsequent fixation of a malreduced fracture will often result in fracture fixation failure as bone healing will be impaired (Fig. 3.5).

For rigid plate fixation, the above-mentioned gaps of less than 0.01 [7] mm for contact healing and gaps less than 800 μm to 1 mm [11] for gap healing should be achieved by open reduction and subsequent fracture fixation with absolute stability. Otherwise, there is an elevated risk for impaired direct bone healing with subsequent fixation construct failure.

The situation is different in metaphyseal or shaft fractures treated by closed reduction and intramedullary nailing or bridge plating technique as indirect bone healing relies on an "untouched" fracture hematoma with subsequent callus formation. Here, no anatomical reduction of the fracture is required as callus formation can

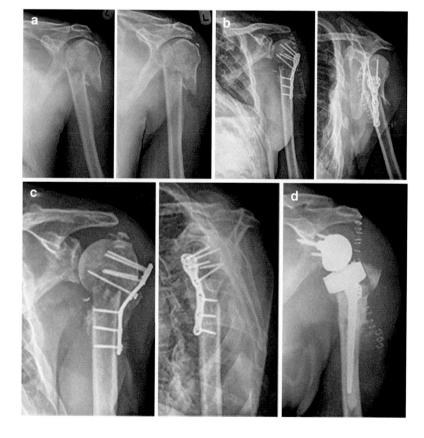

Fig. 3.5 Clinical case example of a 78-year old male with a dislocated subcapital humeral fracture (**a**) and malalignment after open reduction and locking plate fixation with an anatomical proximal humerus plate (**b**). In the postoperative ap view, the calcar region is not anatomically reduced (**b**) and there is also an anterio-posterior malalignment in the axial view (**b**). This results in delayed bone healing and failure of the fixation construct with plastic deformation of the plate and screw breakage (**c**). The case was revised by a reverse total shoulder arthroplasty (**d**)

bridge distances of several millimeters. However, closed reduction and fragment alignment should also be performed in an optimal way to achieve the best anatomical preconditions for healing. In case of critical fracture gaps, delayed bone healing with subsequent fracture fixation can certainly also occur after intramedullary nailing or bridge plating.

Besides direct bone contact, correct angulation between the fracture fragments is of importance in avoid bone healing disturbances. Varus deformity seems to be deleterious for fracture healing, particularly at the proximal humerus [21] and femur [22].

Fracture Fixation Failure Due to Insufficient Fixation Constructs

The race between bone healing and fixation construct failure has been introduced before in this chapter. The failure of the fracture fixation device is mainly due to insufficient biomechanical stability of the construct and is mostly due to two causes: (1) wrong type of implant or (2) incorrect technical application of the implant. In the case of unstable fracture fixation with insufficient construct stiffness due to unsuitable implants, fixation failure is mostly unavoidable (Figs. 3.6 and 3.7).

Plating and nailing are by far the most relevant internal fracture fixation techniques and the respective implants withstand general material and bone healing principles but also individual technical and biomechanical details that contribute to the biomechanical stability of the construct.

In general, construct stiffness must neither be too high nor too low but should be adequate in relation to the fracture pattern. As mentioned above, if absolute stability is targeted with anatomical reduction of the fracture, a rigid fixation should be used, whereas so-called bridge plating relies on flexible fixation with relative stability.

For plating techniques, the underlying principle of plating is of importance both for the preoperative planning and the intraoperative

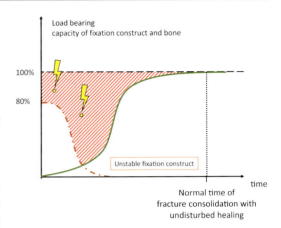

Fig. 3.6 Influence of unstable fracture fixation construct on fixation failure. In insufficient fracture fixation, there is often a reduced load-bearing capacity of the construct right from the beginning (here: only 80% of the desired 100%). This unstable fixation constructs loses further biomechanical stability under mechanical loading and will fail for loading that is above the implant loading capacity and above the mechanical stability of the unhealed bone. This often occurs in early fracture fixation failure

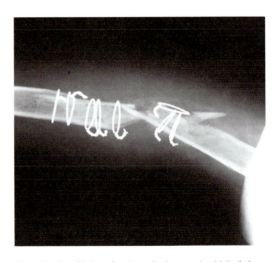

Fig. 3.7 Insufficient fixation of a humeral midshaft fracture in a 14-year-old boy due to wrong implant choice with multiple cerclages and insufficient biomechanical support with subsequent fixation failure

technical accuracy. Absolute stability with rigid fixation should be differentiated versus flexible fixation with relative stability. These two principles determine other important properties, such as the type of plate, plate length, working length of the plate, screw locking options, screw length and screw density are relevant (Table 3.1).

3 General Considerations: Analysis of Failure of Fixation: A Stepwise Approach

Table 3.1 Fixation construct failures

		Plates	Nails
General implant parameters	Type of implant	Neutralization plate	Reamed
		Buttress plate	Unreamed
		Locking plate	
	Length of implant	Plate length	Nail length
Specific implant parameters		Working length	Nail diameter
		Plate-screw density	Type of locking
		Number of screws	Number of locking bolts
		Number of plates: Single vs. double plating	

Plating

Type of Plates

As mentioned above, the type of the used plate mainly depends on the desired plating concept and healing pattern of the fracture. Absolute stability is mainly achieved by compression in anatomically reduced fractures. Compression can be either achieved by lag screws and additional neutralization (or: protection) plating or by compression plating itself. The first principle relies on the protection of the lag screw against torsional and bending forces, e.g., in ankle fractures of the distal fibula. Buttress plating with its resistance against deforming forms in anatomically reduced articular fracture in combination with compression screw fixation, e.g., in tibial plateau fractures, can also be considered as a type of protection plating.

Compression plating uses eccentric screw hole positioning for compression of the fragments over the plate. Typical indications for compression plating with absolute stability are anatomically reduced forearm shaft fractures. Neutralization and compression plating were traditionally performed by generic plates that could also be contoured to fit the fractured bone.

All these plates rely on friction by the screws on the bone surface for biomechanical stabilization of the fractures. Reconstruction plates are easy to contour but are often not strong enough for the fixation of long bones or even the clavicle (Fig. 3.8).

Anatomic reduction often requires an open approach to the fracture site and is mostly associated with a certain degree of soft tissue damage including periosteum stripping that can compromise fracture healing. This drawback led to the development of alternative and modern plating techniques, such as the bridging plating technique.

Bridge plating relies on the concept of flexible fixation with subsequent secondary fracture healing in which the load-bearing plate spans an area of comminution of the fracture. This technique allows for minimally invasive plate osteosynthesis (MIPO) as anatomic reduction of the fracture is not required and the plate can be introduced and fixed by small or even stab incisions. This concept is mainly translated via locked plating with anatomic precontoured plates and angular stability between the screw and the plate. Locked plating is generally considered advantageous in osteoporotic fractures [23, 24] and also difficult metadiaphyseal fractures are good indications for locked plating [25]. A crucial role in bride plating remains the adequate reduction to avoid malalignment and subsequent fracture healing disturbances as limited exposure does not allow for direct open reduction maneuvers at the fracture site. Reduction can only be controlled by intraoperative fluoroscopic imaging as there is no direct visual control of the fracture area. This should always be considered in bridge plating techniques. A further key element in bridge plating is that the construct must not be too stiff as too little micromotion at the fracture impairs callus formation. Construct stiffness in bridge plating is controlled by the plate type itself, plate length and working length of the construct as well as by screw placement strategies.

Plate Length

For all types of plating techniques, the length of the plate is critical as it significantly contributes to the overall stability of the plate fixation con-

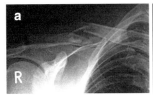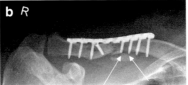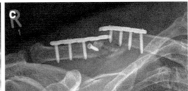

Fig. 3.8 Plate fixation failure due to unstable fixation construct in a multifragmentary clavicular midshaft fracture with a reconstruction plate. (**a**) Mulitfragmentary clavicular midshaft fracture in a 40-year-old male. (**b**) Plate fixation with a reconstruction plate and lag screw fixation on the lateral aspect of the fracture. Medial fixation of the plate shows only unicortical anchorage of the two lateral screws of the 4 medial screws (arrows). (**c**) Plate breakage after 6 months with strong callus formation in the delayed fracture healing zone as a sign of instability

struct. Longer plates can effectively disperse forces with a higher overall construct stability, which is true for both neutralization and bridge plating [26, 27]. Too short plates are often responsible for fracture fixation failure as the resulting strain at the fracture exceeds the tolerable level for fracture healing.

The so-called plate span width defines the ratio between the length of the plate and the fracture length (Fig. 3.9). In general, a plate span width of 3–4 is recommended in comminuted fractures with long fracture lines and >8–10 in simple fractures with short fracture lines [28, 29]. These ratios enable a good pre-operative estimation of the required plate length.

Working Length of the Plate

The working length of the plate is defined by the distance of the first screw proximal (medial) and the first screw distal (lateral) (Fig. 3.9) to the fracture site and is one of the most important surgeon-controlled factors for the flexibility of the construct as it significantly determines stability and micromotion at the fracture site. This is of importance as the construct's stiffness must neither be too low nor too high as both would lead to impaired healing and subsequent fixation failure. In conventional compression plating, screws should be placed in near-near in relation to the fracture site and far-far strategy in relation to the plate ends in in order to maximize the space between the fracture site and the plate ends [26]. Also, for locked plating, the two fracture-neighboring screws should also be as close as possible to the fracture site [24].

Number of Screws and Plate-Screw Density

The number of screws within the plate and their location in the plate are crucial. The general principle is to use three screws on either side of the fracture. This is also true to bridge plating with locking plates in comminuted fractures with the addition that in locations with high torsional forces, e.g., in the humerus or in the forearm, three to four screws on each side of the fracture should be applied.

The plate-screw density is defined as the number of screws relative to the total number of holes in the plate. A plate-screw density of <0.5 is recommended for locked plating to avoid too stiff constructs. In general, plate-screw density at meta-epiphyseal fragments should be >0.5 for sufficient stabilization of shorter fragments, whereas the ratio can be <0.5 in the stable diaphysis [24] (Fig. 3.9).

Number of Plates: Single Vs. Double Plating

In periprosthetic fractures and comminuted extra- or intraarticular fractures, the use of two plates can be beneficial. In these difficult-to-stabilize fractures, double plating was shown to have higher stability under axial and torsional loading compared to unilateral plating [30, 31]. The double-plating concept is currently mainly applied in distal femur fractures in geriatric patients, but large-scale randomized clinical trials are still missing [32].

Fig. 3.9 Important characteristics of plate fixation: plate length, working length, and plate screw density. (Adopted from: Stoffel et al., 2003)

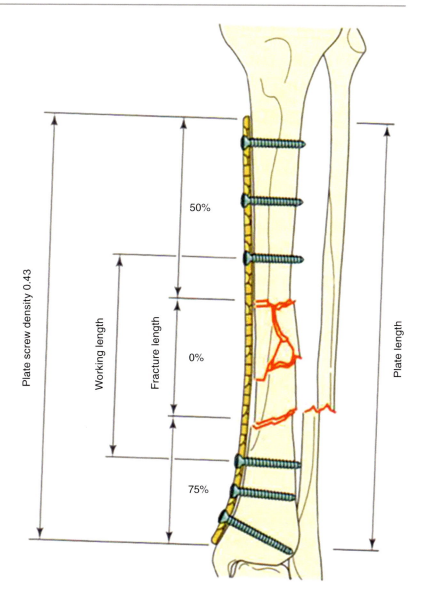

Nailing

Intramedullary nailing has been widely accepted for the standard of care treatment of diaphyseal fracture of the femur, tibia and even the humerus. Furthermore, proximal femur and proximal humerus fractures are often treated with intramedullary implants with additional screw fixation of the articular fragment. Pre-conditions for successful fracture healing in intramedullary are adequate reduction and good placement of the nail, which mainly depends on the correct entry point of the nail. Like in plate fixation, other important factors in intramedullary nailing, such as type of nail, nail length, nail diameter, type of locking, and number of locking bolts/screws, are key elements for the fixation construct stability (Table 3.1).

Type of Nail: Reamed Vs. Unreamed Nails

Nails can be introduced into the intramedullary canal either using the reamed or unreamed technique. In the first, a guide wire is placed into the intramedullary canal after the reduction of the fracture. This guide wire is then used for cannulated reamers to ream the intramedullary to facilitate the introduction of the nail itself. The nail is also cannulated and inserted via the guide wire. Attention should be paid to the reaming procedure itself, as reaming can enhance the pressure and the temperature in the intramedullary canal, which can be associated with fat thromboembolism or heat necrosis [33, 34]. If done extensively, the reaming procedure can lead to bone loss, particularly in the isthmus of the bone, with a negative impact on the stability of the nail osteosynthesis. Therefore, reaming should generally be done with caution, and the concept of "gentle reaming" has now been widely accepted [35, 36]. The unreamed technique relies on the direct introduction of a solid nail into the intramedullary canal. Reaming usually allows the use of larger nails in diameter due to the pre-treatment of the canal, which can be beneficial for the stability of the construct [37].

Nail Length

For diaphyseal long bone fractures, the nail should span the most part of the entire length of the bone from the typical entry point to the far fragment. For epi-metaphyseal fractures, the nail length is often pre-determined by the typical commercially available implants, e.g., for the proximal humerus or proximal femur. A clear analysis of the fracture type is essential for the correct choice of the nail length as short nails are often associated with fracture fixation failure, e.g., in subtrochanteric fracture [38]. These fractures are often misinterpreted as pertrochanteric fractures and short cephalo-medullary nails are

used, which are too short and often cause catastrophic fracture fixation failure.

Nail Diameter

The diameter of the nail significantly contributes to the overall stiffness of the nailing construct. Enlargement of the diameter from 9 to 11 mm in tibial nailing was shown to increase the stiffness in a cadaveric study between 20–50% and up to 80% in static and dynamic compression, respectively [39]. The authors concluded that the nailing with the largest possible diameter after minimal reaming should be done.

If a nail with a too narrow diameter is used, the construct will often fail due to insufficient stiffness (Fig. 3.10).

Type of Locking and Number of Locking Bolts/Screws

Nails can either be statically or dynamically locked depending on the fracture and primary stability of the fracture. Dynamic locking is believed to promote micromotion at the fractures site with a positive effect on the fracture healing process. Transverse or short oblique fractures are deemed axially stable, for which dynamic locking can be applied [40, 41]. Long oblique fractures or fractures with comminution zones should be statically locked due to its higher primary stability compared to dynamic locking [39].

The number of locking screws is also of relevance as fixation of small fragments, e.g., in distal tibial nailing with higher primary stability can be improved [42].

Recently, the concept of locked locking has been introduced in intramedullary nailing allowing for angular stable fixation of the locking bolts [43].

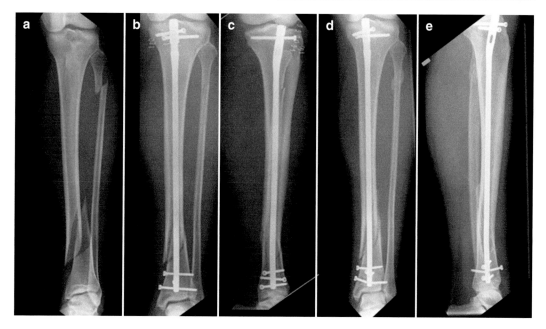

Fig. 3.10 Fracture fixation failure of an unreamed tibia nail. (**a**) Tibia-fibula fracture with spiroid fracture of the distal tibial shaft. Post-operative X-ray (**b**: ap, **c**: lateral view) after good reduction of the fracture and implantation of an unreamed tibia nail of 8 mm diameter and distal locking with 3 locking bolts. Implant failure with breakage of all 3 distal locking bolts after 5 months most likely due to inadequate implant choice with a too narrow diameter of the nail with subsequent insufficient fixation construct stiffness (**d**: ap, **e**: lateral view)

Fracture Fixation Failure Due to Incompliance of the Patient

The compliance with post-operative protocols is essential for successful consolidation of the fracture in order to ensure adequate protection of the fracture site and the fracture fixation construct for unimpaired fracture healing. The goal in fracture fixation is to achieve post-operative full weight bearing as tolerated for the patient. This reduces both the risk for (early) fracture fixation failure and enhances fracture healing due to biomechanical stimulation of the fracture gap. Furthermore, today, full weight bearing as tolerated can often be achieved by modern fracture fixation techniques, such as intramedullary nailing and also for some types of locking plates for certain fracture types.

However, there is still a significant amount of fracture fixation constructs that do not allow for full weight bearing after surgery. This mainly concerns standard plate fixation of the lower extremity fractures, such as distal femoral, tibia and ankle fractures. In these cases, the construct stiffness is not sufficient to tolerate high loadings and the osteosynthesis needs to be "protected" by partial weight bearing for a certain amount of time. This mainly refers to the first six post-operative weeks and relies on the assumption that starting bone healing will gradually contribute to the overall stability and that load is transferred not only via the implant but also via the restabilized bone that will reduce the stress on the implant. This period of partial weight bearing is essential and requires the patient to comply with those restrictions as forces that exceed the stability of the construct will result in fracture fixation failure (Fig. 3.11).

In certain patient groups, compliance with post-operative protocols after fracture surgery is challenging. Recent findings suggest that elderly patients seem to be unable to maintain weight-bearing restrictions [44–46]. Kammerlander et al. demonstrated with the help of insole force

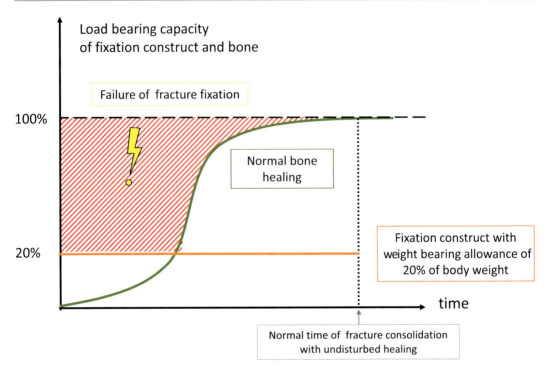

Fig. 3.11 Influence of patient compliance on fixation failure. If patients do not comply with post-operative recommendations for partial weight bearing (e.g. partial weight bearing of 20% of body weight), the fixation construct will fail as neither the construct nor the unhealed bone will be able to bear this overloading. Overloading can either be caused by single high impact or repetitive lower impact energy due to patient incompliance

sensor measuring that patients aged 75 years or older are unable to comply with weight-bearing restrictions as recommended [47]. The same is true for patients with dementia or other mental problems. Furthermore, patients with polyneuropathia of the lower extremity with the absence of biofeedback from the loading of the limb are at risk. Even young and healthy individuals are often not able to properly follow weight-bearing instructions after surgery for fractures of the lower extremity [48] (Fig. 3.12).

Non-compliance with weight-bearing restrictions can result in catastrophic fixation failures, including soft-tissue problems, subsequent infections and amputations (Figs. 3.8 and 3.9). This underscores the importance of the primary stability of the fracture fixation construct and surgeons should provide the patient with a stable fracture fixation construct whenever possible. If patient's comorbidities make non-compliance likely, additional protection aspects with avoidance of any weight bearing of the limb by the use of a wheelchair or additional plaster or cast immobilization should be considered.

3 General Considerations: Analysis of Failure of Fixation: A Stepwise Approach   51

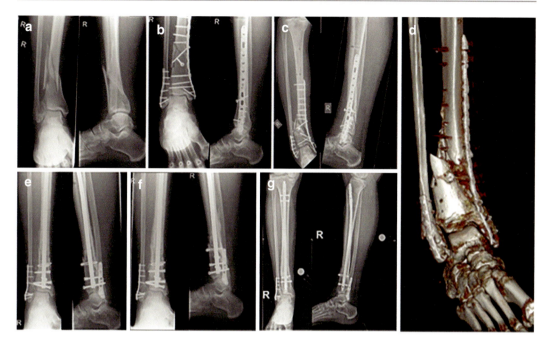

Fig. 3.12 Fracture fixation failure of a distal tibia-fibula fracture after plate fixation due to patient's incompliance. A 54-year-old male sustained a distal tibia-fibula fracture (**a**) that was adequately fixed with locked plate fixation of the distal tibia and conventional plate fixation of the distal fibula (**b**). Partial weight bearing of 20 kg for 6 weeks was advised. Patient returned 2 weeks after fixation with catastrophic fracture fixation failure with severe dislocation (**c, d**). Reason for failure was patient's incompliance due to an underlying Korsakow's syndrome. The patient was revised with an antegrade nail for the tibia and re-plating of the distal fibula (**e**). The leg was additionally immobilized with a cast for 6 weeks. The fracture then showed uneventful fracture healing at 6 months (**f**) with full consolidation at 12 months (**g**)

Stepwise Approach for Analysis of Fixation Failure

In the case of fracture fixation failure, the analysis of the "why and how" did the fixation fail is of high relevance. The before mentioned factors alignment of the fracture, fracture fixation and patient's compliance belong to the most critical parameters of such an analysis. For a stepwise approach, the questions below help to systemically address these parameters:

1. Was the fracture well reduced with a good alignment of the fragments?
2. Was the implant choice correct?
3. Was the fixation done technically correct?
4. Was the patient's compliance sufficient?

Each question has multiple dimensions as several parameters contribute to the answers and have been presented in the last paragraphs and are summarized in Table 3.2. The correct questions will deliver the correct answers and will help to guide the surgeon through the clinical history and X-rays of the patient.

Table 3.2 Areas and questions for stepwise approach of fracture fixation failure

Area	Question	Implication for healing
Alignment	Was the fracture reduced well?	Does alignment of the fragments allow for successful fracture healing?
Fixation construct	Was the implant choice correct?	Does the type of implant provide sufficient stability for successful fracture healing?
	Was the fixation done technically correct?	Is the underlying principle of fracture healing for the chosen implant respected?
		Does the technical implementation with the chosen implant provide sufficient stability for successful fracture healing?
Patient's compliance	Was patient's compliance sufficient?	Does the patient's behavior allow for successful healing?

Summary: Lessons Learned

Fracture fixation failure is in most cases a devastating complication for the patient as it often requires revision surgery, prolongation of the treatment and results in significant reduction in patient's quality of live. There are several facts that can lead to fracture fixation failure and malalignment, unsuitable implant selection or incorrect technical application and patient's incompliance are amongst the most relevant ones. Other factors, such as infection or other biological or host-related problems are beyond the scope of this chapter. A thorough analysis will in most cases identify the underlying cause or even a combination of causes for failure. The chapter tried to provide surgeons with an armamentarium for the crucial assessment of fracture fixation failure. This is of utmost importance for both revision surgery of the underlying case and to avoid further failures in comparable cases in primary fixation in the future.

References

1. Giannoudis PV, Einhorn TA, Marsh D. Fracture healing: the diamond concept. Injury. 2007;38:S3–6. https://doi.org/10.1016/S0020-1383(08)70003-2.
2. Rupp M, Biehl C, Budak M, Thormann U, Heiss C, Alt V. Diaphyseal long bone nonunions - types, aetiology, economics, and treatment recommendations. Int Orthop. 2018;42:247–58. https://doi.org/10.1007/s00264-017-3734-5.
3. Hak DJ, Fitzpatrick D, Bishop JA, Marsh JL, Tilp S, Schnettler R, et al. Delayed union and nonunions: epidemiology, clinical issues, and financial aspects. Injury. 2014;45(Suppl 2):S3–7. https://doi.org/10.1016/j.injury.2014.04.002.
4. Andrzejowski P, Giannoudis PV. The 'diamond concept' for long bone non-union management. J Orthop Traumatol. 2019;20:21. https://doi.org/10.1186/s10195-019-0528-0.
5. Marsell R, Einhorn TA. The biology of fracture healing. Injury. 2011;42:551–5. https://doi.org/10.1016/j.injury.2011.03.031.
6. Rice C, Christensen T, Bottlang M, Fitzpatrick D, Kubiak E. Treating tibia fractures with far cortical locking implants. Am J Orthop (Belle Mead NJ). 2016;45:E143–7.
7. Shapiro F, Cortical bone repair. The relationship of the lacunar-canalicular system and intercellular gap junctions to the repair process. J Bone Joint Surg Am. 1988;70:1067–81.
8. Perren SM. Fracture healing: fracture healing understood as the result of a fascinating cascade of physical and biological interactions. Part I. An attempt to integrate observations from 30 years AO research. Acta Chir Orthop Traumatol Cechoslov. 2014;81:355–64.
9. Slatter DH. Textbook of small animal surgery. Elsevier Health Sciences; 2003.
10. Einhorn TA. The cell and molecular biology of fracture healing. Clin Orthop Relat Res. 1998;355S:S7–21. https://doi.org/10.1097/00003086-199810001-00003.
11. Kaderly RE. Primary bone healing. Semin Vet Med Surg Small Anim. 1991;6:21–5.
12. Rahn BA. Bone in clinical orthopaedics. Philadelphia, PA: WB Saunders; 1982.
13. Greenbaum MA, Kanat IO. Current concepts in bone healing. Review of the literature. J Am Podiatr Med Assoc. 1993;83:123–9. https://doi.org/10.7547/87507315-83-3-123.
14. Schenk RK, Hunziker EB. Bone formation and repair. IL: The American Academy of Orthopaedic Surgeons Rosemont; 1994.
15. Gerstenfeld LC, Alkhiary YM, Krall EA, Nicholls FH, Stapleton SN, Fitch JL, et al. Three-dimensional reconstruction of fracture callus morphogenesis. J Histochem Cytochem. 2006;54:1215–28. https://doi.org/10.1369/jhc.6A6959.2006.

16. Doblaré M, García JM, Gómez MJ. Modelling bone tissue fracture and healing: a review. Eng Fract Mech. 2004;71:1809–40. https://doi.org/10.1016/j.engfracmech.2003.08.003.
17. Green E, Lubahn JD, Evans J. Risk factors, treatment, and outcomes associated with nonunion of the midshaft humerus fracture. J Surg Orthop Adv. 2005;14:64–72.
18. Pape H-C, Giannoudis PV, Grimme K, van Griensven M, Krettek C. Effects of intramedullary femoral fracture fixation: what is the impact of experimental studies in regards to the clinical knowledge? Shock. 2002;18:291–300. https://doi.org/10.1097/00024382-200210000-00001.
19. Perren SM. Evolution of the internal fixation of long bone fractures. J Bone Joint Surg Br. 2002;84-B:1093–110. https://doi.org/10.1302/0301-620X.84B8.0841093.
20. Claes L. Improvement of clinical fracture healing - what can be learned from mechano-biological research? J Biomech. 2021;115:110148. https://doi.org/10.1016/j.jbiomech.2020.110148.
21. Solberg BD, Moon CN, Franco DP, Paiement GD. Locked plating of 3- and 4-part proximal humerus fractures in older patients: the effect of initial fracture pattern on outcome. J Orthop Trauma. 2009;23:113–9. https://doi.org/10.1097/BOT.0b013e31819344bf.
22. Sanders R, Swiontkowski M, Rosen H, Helfet D. Double-plating of comminuted, unstable fractures of the distal part of the femur. J Bone Joint Surg Am. 1991;73:341–6.
23. Gardner MJ, Griffith MH, Demetrakopoulos D, Brophy RH, Grose A, Helfet DL, et al. Hybrid locked plating of osteoporotic fractures of the humerus. J Bone Joint Surg Am. 2006;88:1962–7. https://doi.org/10.2106/JBJS.E.00893.
24. Stoffel K, Dieter U, Stachowiak G, Gächter A, Kuster MS. Biomechanical testing of the LCP—how can stability in locked internal fixators be controlled? Injury. 2003;34(Suppl 2):B11–9. https://doi.org/10.1016/j.injury.2003.09.021.
25. Kregor PJ, Stannard JA, Zlowodzki M, Cole PA. Treatment of distal femur fractures using the less invasive stabilization system: surgical experience and early clinical results in 103 fractures. J Orthop Trauma. 2004;18:509–20. https://doi.org/10.1097/00005131-200409000-00006.
26. Sanders R, Haidukewych GJ, Milne T, Dennis J, Latta LL. Minimal versus maximal plate fixation techniques of the ulna: the biomechanical effect of number of screws and plate length. J Orthop Trauma. 2002;16:166–71. https://doi.org/10.1097/00005131-200203000-00005.
27. Rozbruch SR, Müller U, Gautier E, Ganz R. The evolution of femoral shaft plating technique. Clin Orthop Relat Res. 1998;354:195–208. https://doi.org/10.1097/00003086-199809000-00024.
28. Gautier E, Sommer C. Guidelines for the clinical application of the LCP. Injury. 2003;34(Suppl 2):B63–76. https://doi.org/10.1016/j.injury.2003.09.026.
29. Smith WR, Ziran BH, Anglen JO, Stahel PF. Locking plates: tips and tricks. J Bone Joint Surg Am. 2007;89:2298–307. https://doi.org/10.2106/00004623-200710000-00028.
30. Park K-H, Oh C-W, Park I-H, Kim J-W, Lee J-H, Kim H-J. Additional fixation of medial plate over the unstable lateral locked plating of distal femur fractures: a biomechanical study. Injury. 2019;50:1593–8. https://doi.org/10.1016/j.injury.2019.06.032.
31. Fontenot PB, Diaz M, Stoops K, Barrick B, Santoni B, Mir H. Supplementation of lateral locked plating for distal femur fractures: a biomechanical study. J Orthop Trauma. 2019;33:642–8. https://doi.org/10.1097/BOT.0000000000001591.
32. Sheridan GA, Sepehri A, Stoffel K, Masri BA. Treatment of B1 distal periprosthetic femur fractures. Orthop Clin North Am. 2021;52:335–46. https://doi.org/10.1016/j.ocl.2021.05.001.
33. Giannoudis PV, Snowden S, Matthews SJ, Smye SW, Smith RM. Temperature rise during reamed tibial nailing. Clin Orthop Relat Res. 2002;395:255–61. https://doi.org/10.1097/00003086-200202000-00031.
34. Wenda K, Runkel M, Degreif J, Ritter G. Pathogenesis and clinical relevance of bone marrow embolism in medullary nailing—demonstrated by intraoperative echocardiography. Injury. 1993;24(Suppl 3):S73–81. https://doi.org/10.1016/0020-1383(93)90011-t.
35. Rommens PM, Küchle R, Hofmann A, Hessmann MH. Intramedullary nailing of metaphyseal fractures of the lower extremity. Acta Chir Orthop Traumatol Cech. 2017;84(5):330–40.
36. Rudloff MI, Smith WR. Intramedullary nailing of the femur: current concepts concerning reaming. J Orthop Trauma. 2009;23:S12–7. https://doi.org/10.1097/BOT.0b013e31819f258a.
37. Chapman MW. The effect of reamed and nonreamed intramedullary nailing on fracture healing. Clin Orthop Relat Res. 1998;355S:S230–8. https://doi.org/10.1097/00003086-199810001-00023.
38. Viberg B, Eriksen L, Højsager KD, Højsager FD, Lauritsen J, Palm H, et al. Should pertrochanteric and subtrochanteric fractures be treated with a short or long intramedullary nail?: A multicenter cohort study. J Bone Joint Surg Am. 2021;103:2291–8. https://doi.org/10.2106/JBJS.20.01904.
39. Penzkofer R, Maier M, Nolte A, von Oldenburg G, Püschel K, Bühren V, et al. Influence of intramedullary nail diameter and locking mode on the stability of tibial shaft fracture fixation. Arch Orthop Trauma Surg. 2009;129:525–31. https://doi.org/10.1007/s00402-008-0700-0.
40. Krettek C, Schulte-Eistrup S, Schandelmaier P, Rudolf J, Tscherne H. Osteosynthesis of femur shaft fractures with the unreamed AO-femur nail. Surgical

technique and initial clinical results standard lock fixation, vol. 97. Der Unfallchirurg; 1994. p. 549–67.

41. Krettek C, Schandelmaier P, Tscherne H. Nonreamed interlocking nailing of closed tibial fractures with severe soft tissue injury. Clin Orthop Relat Res. 1995;315:34–47.

42. Gong F, Wang K, Dang X, Wang L. Study of the impact of the number of distal locking bolts on the biomechanical feature of locking intramedullary nails. Zhongguo Xiu Fu Chong Jian Wai Ke Za Zhi. 2005;19:58–60.

43. Höntzsch D, Blauth M, Attal R. Angle-stable fixation of intramedullary nails using the angular stable locking system® (ASLS). Oper Orthop Traumatol. 2011;23:387–96. https://doi.org/10.1007/s00064-011-0048-4.

44. Braun BJ, Veith NT, Rollmann M, Orth M, Fritz T, Herath SC, et al. Weight-bearing recommendations after operative fracture treatment-fact or fiction? Gait results with and feasibility of a dynamic, continuous pedobarography insole. Int Orthop. 2017;41:1507–12. https://doi.org/10.1007/s00264-017-3481-7.

45. Vasarhelyi A, Baumert T, Fritsch C, Hopfenmüller W, Gradl G, Mittlmeier T. Partial weight bearing after surgery for fractures of the lower extremity – is it achievable? Gait Posture. 2006;23:99–105. https://doi.org/10.1016/j.gaitpost.2004.12.005.

46. Chiodo CP, Macaulay AA, Palms DA, Smith JT, Bluman EM. Patient compliance with postoperative lower-extremity non-weight-bearing restrictions. JBJS. 2016;98:1563–7. https://doi.org/10.2106/JBJS.15.01054.

47. Kammerlander C, Pfeufer D, Lisitano LA, Mehaffey S, Böcker W, Neuerburg C. Inability of older adult patients with hip fracture to maintain postoperative weight-bearing restrictions. J Bone Joint Surg Am. 2018;100:936–41. https://doi.org/10.2106/JBJS.17.01222.

48. Eickhoff AM, Cintean R, Fiedler C, Gebhard F, Schütze K, Richter PH. Analysis of partial weight bearing after surgical treatment in patients with injuries of the lower extremity. Arch Orthop Trauma Surg. 2022;142:77–81. https://doi.org/10.1007/s00402-020-03588-z.

Acromioclavicular Joint Dislocation Failed Fixation

4

Paul Cowling

History of Previous Primary Failed Treatment

This is the case of a 46-year-old fit and well male who sustained multiple injuries from a climbing accident out of area. He was taken by air ambulance to the local trauma centre and his injuries included a left femoral fracture, which received an immediate intramedullary nail, multiple left-sided rib fractures with bilateral pneumothoraces, a minor head injury, a thoracic spine injury requiring fixation 5 days after the accident, as well as this left shoulder acromioclavicular (ACJ) Grade V injury. Following resuscitation, he had his femur and thoracic spine stabilised within the first 48 hours. The ACJ injury had been ade-quately visualised on plain radiographs at the time of initial injury (Fig. 4.1), and quite reasonably had been left until 14 days following the accident until surgical intervention. At that point, an open ACJ ligament reconstruction had been performed using a suture button type fixation passed around the coracoid (Fig. 4.2). Subsequently, 17 days after the accident he was repatriated to our centre for further management. Following a short hospital stay, he was discharged home 23 days following the accident.

However, over the course of the next 10 weeks, whilst he was attempting to mobilise with the aid of crutches for her femoral fracture, it was noticed that his left shoulder gradually became deformed over the superior aspect (Fig. 4.3).

P. Cowling (✉)
Department of Trauma and Orthopaedic Surgery, Leeds Teaching Hospitals NHS Trust, Leeds, UK
e-mail: paulcowling@nhs.net

© The Author(s), under exclusive license to Springer Nature Switzerland AG 2024
P. V. Giannoudis, P. Tornetta III (eds.), *Failed Fracture Fixation*,
https://doi.org/10.1007/978-3-031-39692-2_4

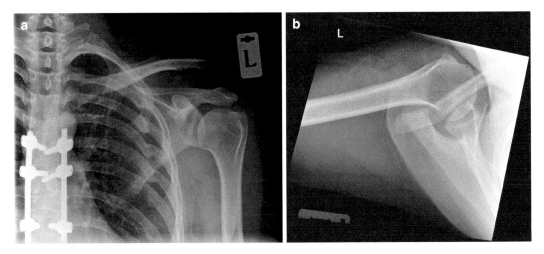

Fig. 4.1 (**a**) Anteroposterior (AP) and (**b**) axial radiographs of initial left acromioclavicular injury

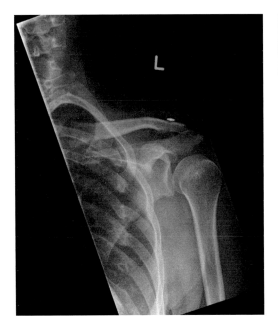

Fig. 4.2 Initial AP shoulder post-operative image demonstrating acceptable reduction and fixation of the ACJ

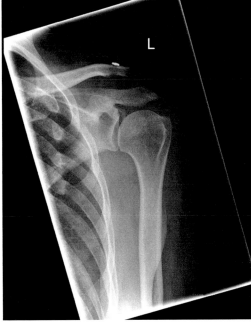

Fig. 4.3 Plain AP left shoulder radiograph performed at 8 weeks following initial fixation, demonstrating loss of reduction of the ACJ

Evaluation of the Aetiology of Failure of Fixation

This case demonstrates failure of reconstruction over a time period of the initial 2–3 months. Consideration of the reason for failure is vitally important with these injuries, to determine the means of correction.

In this specific case, it was presumed that a suture fixation technique was performed around the coracoid, with a cortical button placed on the superior clavicle. The original position certainly seemed acceptable, and the patient described no issues in the initial phase of her rehabilitation. However, a gradual loss of position was noted by the patient, with recognition of a deformity over the ACJ with a high-riding clavicle (Fig. 4.3). Symptoms of crepitus on movement were also noted.

It was, therefore, felt that the failure in this case had been mechanical in nature, due to the patient requiring loading on the shoulder to help mobilise with crutches following his femoral fixation from the initial accident. He was still using crutches and/or a stick several weeks following the intramedullary fixation of the femur as there had been a delayed union of the femur, and it was felt this prolonged period of upper limb weight-bearing had contributed to the failure of fixation as there was no adequate time to allow ligament healing.

Clinical Examination

The clinical examination of the ACJ following surgery involves full exposure of both shoulders to compare either side. Generally, the examination progressed through the common 'look' 'feel' 'move' stepwise process.

The focus of any clinical examination following stabilisation of an ACJ dislocation would be on the mode of failure suspected. In the case of infection, scrutiny of the scar for any erythema, subcutaneous collection or wound breakdown is important. In this case, the scar was well healed with no signs of erythema or infection, but the deformity that had appeared was concerning the patient.

It is then necessary to observe the ACJ itself: in this case, no acute change of position was noted, but a gradual alteration leading to an obvious prominence of the distal clavicle.

Palpation over the distal clavicle, acromion and coracoid (if possible) can determine any areas of pain, abnormal anatomy or the palpation of metalwork or other surgical implant used in the initial fixation. Tenderness over the distal clavicle or acromion may point towards inflammation, osteolysis or damage caused by fixation failure, e.g. pull-out of sutures or graft. This patient did have pain over the distal 1/3 of the clavicle, and generalised tenderness throughout the region of the ACJ as well as where the CC ligaments would be situated. As the ACJ now sits in an obviously dislocated position (Fig. 4.4), it is important to note whether the distal clavicle can be reduced: this may point towards structures damaged, such as the deltopectoral fascia. In this case, pressure over the distal clavicle, as well as

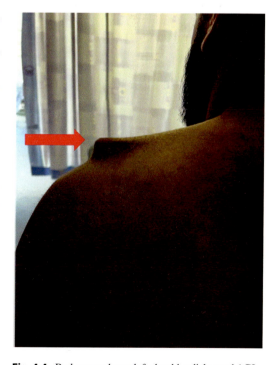

Fig. 4.4 Red arrow shows left shoulder dislocated ACJ

elevation of the arm/scapula revealed pain, demonstrated the ability to fully reduce the distal clavicle, as well as pain.

Recording of the range of movement of the arm, particularly the posture of the ACJ during movement, as well as any pain or other symptoms during motion is important. In this case, the patient demonstrated a reduction in range in abduction and flexion, which was met with intermittent crepitus over the superior aspect of the shoulder. Cross body adduction highlighted the deformity. It was difficult to assess the amount of movement in an anteroposterior direction, but it seemed more mobile than one would expect.

Finally, careful examination and documentation of the neurovascular status of the upper limb is a requirement: in the patient's case, he was fully intact.

Diagnostic-Biochemical and Radiological Investigations

In order to ascertain the nature of the failure, plain film images are required to investigate for the most frequent mechanisms of fixation failure, particularly mechanical failure and loss of reduction of the ACJ. In this case, it had become obvious that a loss of reduction had occurred on plain radiographs by 10 weeks following fixation (Fig. 4.3).

Traditionally, to image the ACJ, a standard antero-posterior clavicle view as well as a 30-degree caudal view is important. This will allow assessment of the acromioclavicular and coracoclavicular distance to determine if reduction has been lost following the previous surgery. Generally, if there is >8 mm acromioclavicular distance, and >13 mm coracoclavicular distance, there is a loss of ACJ alignment. An axillary view would allow assessment of any displacement of the clavicle posteriorly in keeping with a Rockwood IV injury. However, a Zanca view allows focussed evaluation of the ACJ and distal clavicle. This is an antero-posterior view focusing upon the distal clavicle and ACJ performed with a 10-degree cephalic tilt.

Initially, the patient elected not to proceed with further surgical intervention to the failed ACJ fixation, citing the fact that she was still struggling to mobilise on her healing left femoral fracture, so felt he would like to be more confident with this, and past the point of requiring walking aids before any form of operative intervention on his shoulder.

The patient then returned 4 weeks later, at 14 weeks following the initial fixation. At this point, he was walking freely and the femur had healed. Further radiographs were performed, unfortunately demonstrating worsening migration of the ACJ, as well as lysis around the cortical button and suture tunnel through the distal clavicle (Fig. 4.5).

With this lysis now visible, further tests were felt necessary to investigate infection as a cause for failure. Blood tests investigating infection included a white cell count (8.9 × 10^9/L), C-reactive protein (76 mg/L). A computed tomography (CT) of the ACJ depicted the lysis and loss of reduction in more detail and was able to more accurately demonstrate the position of the initial fixation and suture passage through the distal clavicle (Fig. 4.6).

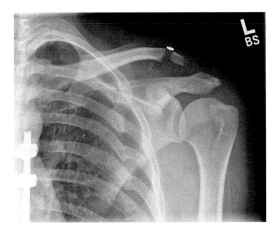

Fig. 4.5 Plain radiograph performed at 12 weeks following initial fixation, demonstrating worsening of the displacement along with significant lysis in the distal clavicle around the cortical button

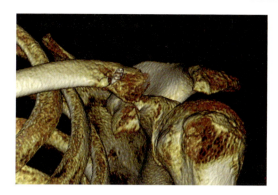

Fig. 4.6 Three-dimensional reconstruction CT images of the ACJ, demonstrating bone lysis around the cortical button and displacement of the ACJ

Preoperative Planning

From the results of the patient's investigations, it was felt that infection could have contributed to the failure of the ACJ fixation. In our institution, in such cases of infected fixation, a multidisciplinary approach is taken. Therefore, in a meeting with surgeons, microbiologists and radiologists, a surgical plan was put into place. A discussion occurred with the patient about the outcomes of the investigations, and he agreed that now was time for surgical intervention to be considered. It was felt that further delay may lead to fracture of the distal clavicle through the area of lysis, and therefore making operative intervention much more challenging.

It was decided to embark upon a two-stage process of surgical intervention. In the first stage, debridement of the ACJ would occur, removal of all surgical implants including cortical button and suture material, x5 deep tissue samples for microbiology, and curettage of the lysis of the distal clavicle. Then depending upon the microbiological sampling, a course of antibiotics would be provided to the patient for a period of 6–8 weeks, before proceeding with the second stage of fixation.

It was felt necessary to await the outcome following first-stage debridement to decide the definitive fixation technique, as it may be that due to necessary extensive debridement, several options may be required.

Revision Surgery

First-Stage Revision Surgery

The patient was positioned in a beach-chair position, with draping to allow access to the anterior and posterior areas of the ACJ. An arm support is used to be able to position the arm where required, and aid the reduction of the ACJ. The initial longitudinal incision just inferior to the distal clavicle was used to access the ACJ, with the skin edges excised. Though the author's preferred approach to the distal clavicle and ACJ is a 'sabre' type transverse incision, it was felt at only 3 months since the initial procedure that performing as new incision could compromise wound healing.

A 'deltoid turndown approach' is utilised: this is at the medial raphe between deltoid and pectoralis major, with a triangular detachment performed. This not only allows for spacious approach to the coracoid, but also for strong closure following fixation, which has been demonstrated to add further stability to the repair.

The ACJ was found dislocated, and the distal clavicle mobile. The cortical button itself was easily removed, but the attached suture passing through the clavicle and around the coracoid was more difficult to retrieve. This required dissection down to the superior aspect of the coracoid in the infra-clavicular tissue around the CC ligaments. It was found that the suture had failed within the tunnel or around the suture button, as no suture material was found within or around the button, and was all infraclavicular and still around the coracoid. Eventually all material was removed.

The lytic area of the distal clavicle was then debrided using a 3.5 mm drill and a curette. Furthermore, the distal end of the clavicle (approximately the last 5 mm) was excised using an oscillating saw in order to aid eventual reduction and fixation. Five deep tissue samples, including bone from the distal clavicle, bone from the lytic region and tissue from the infraclavicular area were sent for microbiological culture and sensitivity testing. Further debridement of the surrounding tissues, including the superior and inferior surface of the clavicle was then undertaken, along with rigorous lavage of the surgical site. Closure of the wound with monofilament sutures was performed.

A broad-spectrum antibiotic in the form of teicoplanin was commenced following surgery. Unfortunately, after prolonged cultures, a *Cutibacterium* isolate was seen in three of the five deep tissue specimens, sensitive to clindamycin. The antibiotic regime was subsequently changed to clindamycin 450 mg 6 hourly for 6 weeks. This type of organism is most commonly found as an infective agent in upper limb surgery, and often doesn't mount a huge systemic or even local response, such as in this patient's case: the wound was dry and pristine prior to revision surgery with no obvious systemic features of infection.

Inflammatory markers were monitored throughout the patient's treatment following the first stage, along with monitoring for symptoms of diarrhoea, a side effect of this regimen, which might necessitate alternative antibiotic treatment. Imaging was also performed, noting the lytic region remodelling following debridement and antibiotic treatment (Fig. 4.7).

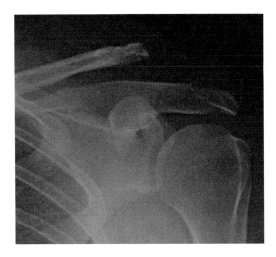

Fig. 4.7 Plain radiograph demonstrating the appearance of the ACJ following the first-stage procedure of debridement and removal of surgical implant

Second-Stage Revision Surgery

This was performed when the patient was 2 weeks following the conclusion of the 6 weeks of antibiotic management. Inflammatory markers had revealed a normal white cell count ($6.8 \times 10^9/L$)) and CRP of 15 mg/L. The scar had healed well with no erythema.

The same surgical set up and approach was performed. Because it was felt that the distal clavicle lytic region around the previous suture fixation had remodelled sufficiently, a combined fixation approach was considered, using a hook plate augmented with a synthetic graft (Ligament Augmentation and Reconstruction System (LARS™) ligament, Corin, Cirencester, UK). This graft is made from polyethylene terephthalate, chosen for its good biocompatibility and biomechanical characteristics [1].

This technique was chosen as there was still concern that though the lysis had improved, there was still weakness in the distal clavicle: 'spreading the load' through this region with the fixation was deemed necessary. Furthermore, a combination of fixation would allow a 'belt and braces' to the fixation, hopefully providing rigidity in the stabilisation.

Further tissue specimens were taken for microbiology to guide any post-operative antibiotic therapy: however, the surgical site appeared pristine, and eventually proved negative for any further bacterial growth. The first part of this approach was to reduce the distal clavicle back down into the ACJ. This was performed more easily with the debridement of the distal end of the clavicle. Elevation of the arm, with downward pressure on the clavicle allowed reduction and temporary fixation using a transfixing 1.6 mm Kirschner-wire from the acromion into the distal clavicle. The LARS™ ligament was then passed around the coracoid using a side specific suture passer placed from medial to lateral close to the coracoid to prevent neurovascular injury. The drill holes for the interference screw fixation are ordinarily at the isometric points where the conoid and trapezoid ligaments would usually be found: in this case, care was taken to provide satisfactory distance between the new drill holes and the previously used drill hole from the initial failed fixation. Luckily, as depicted on the pre-operative CT scan, the placement of the new drill holes was not too far from the intended position.

With tension on the synthetic ligament, the interference screws were tightened, ensuring good hold and stable reduction of the ACJ. The free ends of the synthetic ligament were then tied anteroinferior to the distal clavicle so as to not irritate the skin overlying the distal clavicle. The temporary reduction K-wires could now be removed as the synthetic ligament was holding the reduction.

This construct was able to hold the ACJ in a reduced position, and the stability could be assessed on the operating table. However, due to the concern of previously noted lysis through the distal clavicle, a hook plate was used to augment the repair. The difficulty with using a hook plate in addition to the synthetic ligament was positioning of the plate over the interference screws and ligament ends. As can be noted in Fig. 4.8, the plate is not flush with the distal clavicle but held well enough with three screws into the clavicle, avoiding the synthetic ligament. The hook, having been anteroinferior to the acromion, provided additional support in the anteroposterior stability of the reconstructed ACJ.

The deltotrapezial fascia was closed meticulously to gain further stability around the ACJ, with wound closure performed with an absorbable suture.

Due to concern regarding the possible erosion of the acromion reported with use of a hook plate, initially the patient was restricted in post-operative activities with the physiotherapy team: full active internal and external rotation was allowed with the elbow by the side, but abduction and forward flexion was restricted to a maximum of 90 °.

The hook plate remained in situ for 3 months, before removal was performed. The ACJ has remained stable, and the patient returned to full range of motion and function in the shoulder by 6 months following the second-stage procedure.

Summary: Lessons Learned

Historically, certain methods of ACJ reconstruction have been linked to specific means of failure. However, as this case has hopefully demonstrated, infection should also never be excluded, and investigations may be required to ensure the correct diagnosis.

Early fixation methods of ACJ dislocation included the use of percutaneous insertion of a screw through the clavicle into the coracoid, with the aim of reducing the space between the coracoid and the clavicle via compression: this became eponymously known as 'Bosworth Screw' fixation [2]. Despite being widely accepted as the method of fixation at the time, it proved technically challenging, with studies demonstrating failure by the screw missing the coracoid, as well as late screw failure, and subluxation after screw removal [3]. It was proven that as there is movement between the coracoid and clavicle of approximately 5 °, fatigue and ultimately failure of screw fixation would eventually be inevitable with this method of treatment [4]. This necessitated a second procedure for screw removal, so essentially, patients undergoing this technique of fixation were consenting for two operations.

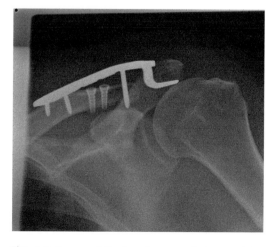

Fig. 4.8 Images following the second-stage revision using a combination of hook plate fixation, LARS™ ligament and autologous hamstring graft

This was the same finding with hook plate fixation: This plate is fixed with several screws to the distal clavicle, with the 'hook' component of the plate then placed resting on the under surface of the acromion in the subacromial space, thus reducing a dislocated ACJ. However, there is high incidence of acromial erosion, necessitating a second operation for removal [5]. However, this method does provide good results with ACJ reconstruction. As we found in this case, a hook plate is also an excellent option for revision of failed fixation.

In 1972, Weaver and Dunn described a procedure involving excision of the distal clavicle, and transferring the coraco-acromial (CA) ligament, often with a small amount of acromial bone still attached to the proximal end, fixing the bone into the cut end of the distal clavicle [6]. A subsequent modification was added by Copeland to stabilise the clavicle on the acromion with an additional augmentation, often a suture, around the coracoid and over the clavicle [7]. However, it has been found that when this augmentation was performed with GORE-TEX loop or Dacron graft, an inflammatory reaction could occur, providing symptoms of persistent anterolateral shoulder pain and osteolysis of the distal clavicle [8, 9]. Other methods of failure of the Weaver-Dunn technique include failure of the CA ligament transfer to heal, leading to recurrent instability, and tunnel widening of the passage through the distal clavicle of the drill holes for suture fixation [10].

Additional more historical fixation methods involved reduction in the displaced ACJ, and fixation with two Kirschner wires passed from the acromion into the distal clavicle. This practice has largely fallen out of favour due to numerous reports of wires migrating to the lungs, spinal canal, subclavian artery and aorta [11]. It also appears within the literature that most neurovascular injuries took place due to migration of Kirschner wires or pins in early methods of ACJ stabilisation [11].

Since the Weaver-Dunn technique came to prominence, other so-called 'anatomical' reconstructions have since been described. The aim of these procedures is to reconstruct the CC ligaments. Initial versions of this procedure used autologous graft, such as semitendinosus tendon, gracilis or toe extensor graft [12]. There are a number of specific techniques described, ranging from passing the graft around the coracoid and over the clavicle; fixing the graft into the base of the coracoid with a biotenodesis screw, then doubling it over and passing it through drill holes in the distal clavicle and using interference screws to tension and hold the graft; or passage of a doubled over graft into the coracoid via drill hole, and then through the distal clavicle and the acromion in an attempt to recreate the anatomy of the CC ligaments [13]. This is the design of the LARS™ ligament we used for the revision surgery, but it can be utilised just as well as the sole fixation in the primary repair.

Though the outcomes of these procedures are generally very good, failure of these anatomic reconstructions has been described in several ways: Lee et al. described midsubstance tears of the graft and fractures at the coracoid base [12]; Miller et al. described fracture of the distal clavicle, fracture through a more medial clavicle bone tunnel [14].

A number of recent techniques described now involve suture fixation involving either screw fixation or a cortical button, with the aim of recreating the CC ligaments. This use of synthetic material to pass either around or through the coracoid and then around or through the clavicle to reduce and stabilise an ACJ dislocation has gained popularity as the synthetic ligament reconstruction has been shown to have good tensile strength, promotes tissue ingrowth and avoids sacrifice of the native coracoacromial ligament for reconstruction [15]. Such reconstructions have produced excellent outcomes, with few complications [16, 17], but in the few failures noted in the literature, the most commonly reported is suture breakage or the suture button migrating through the coracoid [13]. In the case of our patient, the primary failure was with suture breakage at the clavicle side rather than the coracoid, coupled with infection.

Arthroscopic ACJ stabilisations or arthroscopically assisted stabilisations have also increased in recent years. The arthroscopic portion of the procedure is described as allowing for accurate placement of the drill hole through the coracoid base for button placement. It has also been stated that performing a diagnostic arthroscopy of the glenohumeral joint at the time of ACJ stabilisation may allow for other procedures to be performed: it has been shown that high-grade ACJ dislocations can be associated with traumatic concomitant glenohumeral joint pathology in up to 15% of cases [18]. Various specific techniques have been described, but with such a new and evolving surgical technique, description of outcomes and failures in the literature are limited. That said, some of the published studies noted early failure caused by cutting of the suture loop through the cortex of the clavicle, with eccentric drilling through the anterior cortex thought to be one of the important causes. Partial loss of reduction was seen with clavicular osteolysis associated with the clavicular button [19]. A review of complications following arthroscopic fixation of ACJ separations found residual shoulder/ACJ pain or hardware irritation occurred at a rate of 26.7%. The rate of coracoid/clavicle fracture was 5.3% and occurred most commonly with techniques utilising bony tunnels. Loss of AC joint reduction occurred in 26.8% of patients [20].

In conclusion, many types of ACJ dislocation do not require surgical intervention at the time of initial injury. However, when surgery is indicated, failure of fixation is rare. In some cases, despite this failure, re-operation may not be mandatory. In cases where surgical intervention in the presence of fixation failure is required, the technique required will depend upon the mode of failure. The most common salvage procedure is the use of either a synthetic graft or an autologous tendon graft to recreate the CC ligaments, to which a hook plate may be used as an augment if there is concern about bone stock or the hold of any graft.

References

1. Trieb K, Blahovec H, Brand G, et al. In vivo and in vitro cellular ingrowth into a new generation of artificial ligaments. Eur Surg Res. 2004;24:148–51.

2. Bosworth BM. Complete acromioclavicular dislocation. N Engl J Med. 1949;241:221–5.
3. Tsou P. Percutaneous cannulated screw coracoclavicular fixation for acute acromioclavicular dislocations. Clin Orthop. 1989;243:112–21.
4. Rockwood CA Jr. Injuries to the acromioclavicular joint. In: Rockwood Jr CA, Greem DP, editors. Fractures in adults. 2nd ed. Philadelphia PA: JB Lippicott; 1984. p. 860–910.
5. Sim E, Schwarz N, Hocker K, et al. Repair of complete acromioclavicular separations using the acromioclavicular-hook plate. Clin Orthop. 1995;314:134–42.
6. Weaver JK, Dunn HK. Treatment of acromioclavicular injuries, especially complete acromioclavicular separations. JBJS. 1972;54-A:1187.
7. Copeland S. Operative shoulder surgery. New York: Churchill Livingstone; 1995.
8. Jones HP, Lemos MJ, Schepsis AA. Salvage of failed acromioclavicular joint reconstruction using autogenous semitendinosus tendon from the knee. Am J Sports Med. 2001;29:234–7.
9. Jones HP, Lemus MJ, Schepsis AA. Salvage of failed acromioclavicular joint reconstruction using autogenous semitendinosus tendon from the knee. Surgical technique and case report. Am J Sports Med. 2001;29(2):234–7.
10. Tauber M, Eppel M, Resch H. Acromioclavicular reconstruction using autogenous semitendinosus tendon graft: results of revision surgery in chronic cases. J Shoulder Elb Surg. 2007;16:429–33.
11. Lemos MJ, Tolo ET. Complications of the treatment of the acromioclavicular and sternoclavicular joint injuries, including instability. Clin Sports Med. 2003;22:371–85.
12. Lee SJ, Nicholas SJ, Akizuki KH, et al. Reconstruction of the coracoclavicular ligaments with tendon grafts. Am J Sports Med. 2003;31:648–54.
13. Geaney LE, Miller MD, Ticker JB, et al. Management of the failed AC joint reconstruction: causation and treatment. Sports Med Arthrosc Rev. 2010;18:167–72.
14. Turman KA, Miller CD, Miller MD. Clavicular fracture following anatomic coracoclavicular ligament reconstruction with tendon graft: a report of 3 cases. J Bone Joint Surg Am. 2010;96(2):1526–32.
15. Jeon I-H, et al. Chronic acromioclavicular separation: the medium term results of coracoclavicular ligament reconstruction using braided polyester prosthetic ligament. Injury. 2007;38(11):1247–53.
16. Wright J, et al. Stabilisation for the disrupted acromioclavicular joint using a braided polyester prosthetic ligament. J Orthop Surg (Hong Kong). 2015;23(2):223–8.
17. Younis F, et al. Operative versus non-operative treatment of grade III acromioclavicular joint dislocations and the use of SurgiLig: a retrospective review. Ortop Traumatol Rehabil. 2017;19(6):523–30.
18. Pauly S, et al. Prevalence of concomitant intraarticular lesions in patients treated operatively for high-

grade acromioclavicular joint separations. Knee Surg Sports Traumatol Arthrosc. 2009;17(5):513–5.

19. Zhang L-F, et al. Arthroscopic fixation of acute acromioclavicular joint disruption with TightRopeTM: outcome and complications after minimum 2 (2e5) years follow-up. J Orthop Surg. 2017;25(2):230949901668449.

20. Woodmass JM, Esposito JG, Ono Y, et al. Complications following arthroscopic fixation of acromioclavicular separations: a systematic review of the literature. Open Access J Sports Med. 2015;10(6):97–107.

Failed Fixation of Clavicle Fracture

5

Brian J. Page and William M. Ricci

Anatomical Site

Clavicle fractures are very common injuries with a high incidence. They represent 2.6–4% of all fractures [1–5]. Historically, in the 1960s, many clavicle fractures were treated non-operatively with reported non-union rates hovering around 1% [6–8]. At that time, the non-union rate was considered higher in clavicle fractures treated with surgery than in clavicle fractures treated non-operatively [6, 7]. Currently, the reported non-union rate after conservatively treated clavicle fractures is considerably higher than early reports and many surgeons report improved functional outcomes after surgical treatment [2, 9–12]. However, it remains that most non-displaced clavicle fractures, regardless of location, are typically managed non-operatively [2, 6, 7, 13–15].

The clavicle is unique in many facets compared to other long bones. It is the only long bone to ossify via intramembranous ossification. It is the first bone in the body to ossify gestationally,

in the fifth week of fetal life, and the last bone to complete ossification. However, like other long bones, its primary ossification is located centrally and there are two secondary ossification centers—one at each end of the clavicle. The medial ossification center is responsible for approximately 80% of the longitudinal growth and the lateral ossification center is responsible for approximately 20% [16].

The clavicle has several functional purposes. First, it serves as a base for muscular attachments. It also struts the glenohumeral joint in the parasagittal plane stabilizing the shoulder joint and the range of grasp in the three-dimensional space for the hand. It provides for arm-trunk power above the shoulder level. It protects the brachial plexus and vascular structures of the neck and extremities. Lastly, it provides a cosmetic function providing a gentle curve to the base of the neck [16].

Clavicle fractures have historically been classified by location according to three segments of equal length—lateral, midshaft, and medial thirds. This has classically been without any three-dimensional criteria or reference to anatomic structures [17]. However, newer data suggest the segments are unequal in length with the middle clavicle comprising the greatest length of the segments (Fig. 5.1) [17]. The clavicle is better represented by two inverse curves creating an "s" shape that enables the clavicle to absorb stress [18]. The first curve (medial) is more than half of

B. J. Page (✉)
Department of Orthopedic Surgery, Maimonides Medical Center, Brooklyn, NY, USA

W. M. Ricci
Orthopaedic Trauma Service, Hospital for Special Surgery and New York-Presbyterian Hospital, Orthopaedic Surgery, Weill Cornell Medical College, New York, NY, USA
e-mail: ricciw@hss.edu

© The Author(s), under exclusive license to Springer Nature Switzerland AG 2024
P. V. Giannoudis, P. Tornetta III (eds.), *Failed Fracture Fixation*,
https://doi.org/10.1007/978-3-031-39692-2_5

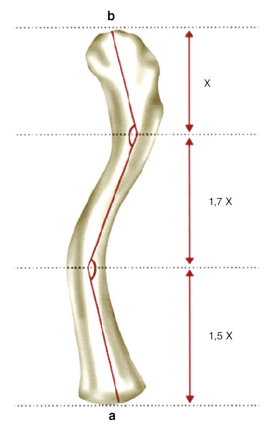

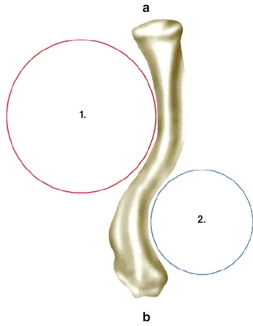

Fig. 5.1 Clavicle segments (lateral, midshaft, and medial) are unequal in length. The middle clavicle is the largest segment

Fig. 5.2 The clavicle is represented by two inverse curves creating an "s" shape. The first curve (medial) is more than half of the length of the clavicle and is convex anteromedially; the second curve (lateral) has a radius that is half the size of the first curve and is convex posterolaterally

the length of the clavicle and is convex anteromedially; the second curve (lateral) has a radius that is half the size of the first curve and is convex posterolaterally (Fig. 5.2) [18].

Clavicle fractures most commonly involve the midshaft region, approximately 69% of the time [1, 8]. Lateral clavicle fractures and medial clavicle fractures have a considerably lower incidence accounting for 28 and 3% of clavicle fractures, respectively [1]. Risk factors for non-union of clavicle fractures include fracture shortening of 1.5–2 cm, female sex, smoking, fracture comminution, fracture displacement, older age patients, severe initial trauma, soft tissues interposition, open fractures, polytrauma, inadequate initial immobilization, and unstable lateral fractures [8, 16, 19]. However, in general, non-union rates vary based on fracture location, fracture energy, and fracture morphology. An example of this is seen in medial clavicle fractures, which are typically high-energy injuries with a relatively high risk for non-union compared to lower energy injuries. The non-union rates of medial clavicle fractures also vary if they are non-displaced or displaced. Non-displaced medial clavicle fractures have a non-union rate of 7% and displaced medial clavicle fractures have a non-union rate of 14–20% [1, 10, 20–22].

Avoiding failure of fixation of clavicle fractures is particularly challenging due to the deforming forces on the fracture fragments that implants are required to withstand until fracture union. The weight of the arm and the pull of the pectoralis major muscle produce an inferior and medial force to the lateral clavicle, respectively. The sternocleidomastoid muscle creates a superior force vector medially on the clavicle (Fig. 5.3) [16]. Fixation methods chosen must be able to withstand these forces until fracture union.

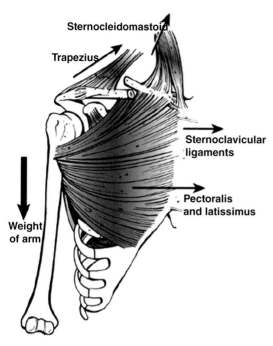

Fig. 5.3 Deforming forces on clavicle fractures

Elevation of the arm imparts forces on the clavicle that fracture fixation methods must also be able to withstand until fracture union. During elevation of the arm, the clavicle angles upward by approximately 30 degrees, posteriorly by approximately 35 degrees, and rotates about its longitudinal axis as much as 50 degrees [23]. These motions subject the clavicle to bending moments in the coronal and sagittal planes that stress the implants until fracture union.

Other challenges in avoiding fixation failure are due to the compositional characteristics of the bone that are innate to the clavicle. The anatomic middle third of the clavicle is largely cortical bone, with sparce cancellous bone, and few soft tissue attachments [24]. Cortical bone heals slower than cancellous bone prolonging the duration the implants must withstand the deforming forces until fracture union compared with metaphyseal fractures [25].

In practice, operative indications for clavicle fractures vary between providers. However, the literature reports indications for operative treatment that include (1) >2 cm displacement; (2) open fracture; (3) extensive soft tissue damage; (4) neurovascular compromise; (5) high-energy mechanisms with high-energy injury patterns (floating shoulder, shoulder impaction, polytrauma); (6) symptomatic malunions and non-unions; (7) improve cosmesis [4, 17]. This list of operative indications is highly specific; however, it can be generalized to clavicle fractures that are at modest risk for non-union, to restore anatomy, to maximize function and to improve cosmesis relative to non-operative management.

Non-operatively managed clavicle fractures have traditionally been treated in the figure-of-eight brace, but newer literature suggests elbow-to-body sling had similar results with improved tolerance and ease of use [26, 27]. Non-operatively managed clavicle fractures almost universally heal with some degree of malunion; however, symptomatic malunion is uncommon [8, 28].

Operatively managed fractures have been treated primarily via plate osteosynthesis and occasionally with intramedullary fixation. Plate osteosynthesis and intramedullary fixation both encompass a large variety of implants. Plate osteosynthesis has been considered the gold standard fixation option for midshaft clavicle fractures [17]. In modern practice, there are a large variety of plate types used for midshaft clavicular fracture fixation including reconstruction plates, dynamic compression plates (DCPs), mini-fragment plates and pre-contoured plates. Each of these types may or may not have locking capability.

Reconstruction plates were historically the primary plating option. They would be contoured intra-operatively by the surgeon to fit the highly curved bony anatomy. These plates are much less commonly used today in favor of modern pre-contoured plating options. Complications have developed secondary to the strength of the plate, which has a high incidence of failed fixation. These plates are too thin and malleable (notched edges) resulting in a less rigid plate that can be unable to withstand the deforming forces on the fracture (Fig. 5.4). Failure rates with single-plating reconstruction plates have been reported to be as high as 53%. Dynamic compression

Fig. 5.4 Progression of plate failure from bending those ultimate leads to breakage of the plate

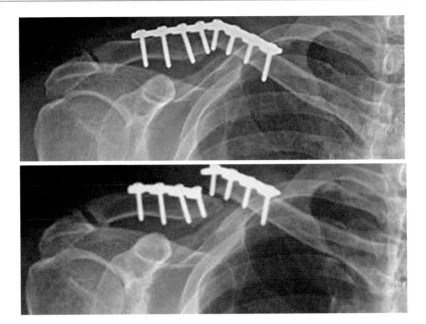

plates (DCPs) and other similar plates have offered increased plate strength but multiplane contouring of the plate to the clavicle is extremely difficult. Many surgeons, therefore, began to dual-plate clavicle fractures to increase multiplanar strength and in-turn reduce the failure risk [29–32]. Modern dual-plating techniques have a much lower failure rate than reconstruction plates alone with reports of failure rates in the range of 2–3% [29].

Newer anatomic plates have offered significantly easier plate application and significantly less contouring. However, there is still a wide variation in mismatch, and they often still require contouring for proper application to the clavicle. Compared with reconstruction plates, these plates are typically more robust and can withstand greater deforming forces [17]. Like reconstruction plates, anatomic plates have the option to be locked or nonlocked. Plates with locked screws have been shown to have lower failure rates in clavicle fractures [33]. Studies have also shown that bicortical locked screws have lower failure rates than unicortical locked screws in clavicle fractures [34].

There are many different intramedullary fixation options. These are much less commonly used than they were in the past due to a relatively high failure rate compared to plate fixation devices. Like other mechanical devices, intramedullary devices vary in their strength due to design differences. Solid fixation devices have been shown to be stronger than cannulated fixation devices. Studies have shown that fixation of midshaft clavicle fractures with cannulated screws may lead to early failure because the device may have inadequate mechanical strength [35]. Additionally, in comparison to plate osteosynthesis, intramedullary devices have been shown to be inferior when rotational stiffness is required [29].

Etiology of Failure of Fixation

Failure of fracture fixation is typically secondary to one of two causes, excluding infectious etiology, fracture non-union and/or inappropriate implant selection (Fig. 5.5). An infectious etiology must always be considered and ruled out, but this is outside the scope of this text.

Clavicle non-union is a common cause of failed fixation in clavicle fractures. Risk factors for non-union include intrinsic and extrinsic factors. Intrinsic factors include age, smoking and female gender [19]. Extrinsic factors include dis-

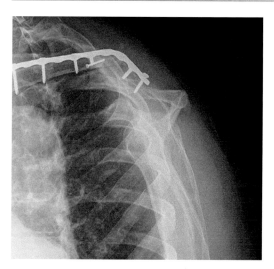

Fig. 5.5 Example of implant failure. The plate is bent and the screws are beginning to pull out

placement, shortening, soft tissue interposition, open fractures, polytrauma and inadequate initial immobilization [16, 19]. Clinicians use a variety of criteria to define a non-union. Typically, a non-union is defined as a fracture that is not healed by 6–9 months and a delayed union is defined as a fracture that is not healed between 3–6 months [16]. However, in practice, many clinicians treat unhealed fractures as non-unions at earlier timeframes. Non-union inevitably leads to failure of fixation because the implant(s) fatigue due to the mechanical load via stress transfer. This stress transfer to the plate and screws will ultimately end in breakage and/or loosening of the implant(s).

Blood supply to the clavicle may also be a factor in development of non-union. In the anterior part of the middle segment of the clavicle the blood supply is purely periosteal, from the thoracoacromial artery via the pectoralis major and deltoid muscles. Therefore, care to preserve midshaft periosteum during dissection may mitigate non-union risk for fractures in this area [36]. The posterior clavicle vascularization is received from the suprascapular artery via periosteal branches and a nutrient branch lending to greater healing potential and lower non-union rates [36].

Another common cause for implant failure is selection of the incorrect implant for the fracture being treated. Plates that are too thin and malleable may lead to early breakage, bending and/or the backing out of screws. A plate that may be appropriate in a younger patient with anatomical cortical reduction may not be appropriate for a geriatric patient with a comminuted fracture pattern. Understanding the fracture personality and quality of bone of the patient is essential.

Clinical Examination

Failed hardware in clavicle fracture fixation rarely presents asymptomatically in patients. Patient's often experience disability due to pain at the fracture/non-union site, altered shoulder mechanics and/or compressive lesions on the brachial plexus or vascular structures (Fig. 5.6) [16]. Symptoms most often result from prominent loose screws, broken or bent plates and/or deformity of the shoulder. Symptoms present as tenderness to palpation, gross motion, crepitus, pain, and/or paresthesias [8].

When evaluating patients with pain after clavicle fracture surgery, it is important to take a careful history and perform a thorough physical exam. Asking questions regarding the onset of pain, change in function, change in shoulder contour, recent trauma, and recent illnesses can aid in making a diagnosis. A thorough physical exam can aid the clinician in making the correct diagnosis by examining the patient for shoulder asymmetry, prominent screws/plates, gross motion at the fracture/non-union site, and any evidence of infection.

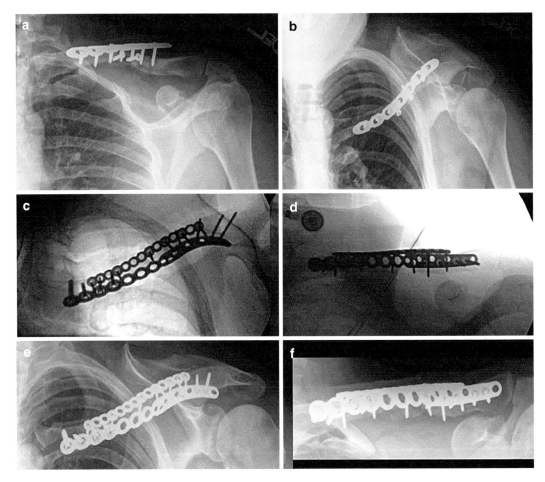

Fig. 5.6 This is a 37-year-old male patient who presents with pain and clicking 1 year status post-open reduction internal fixation of a clavicle fracture. (**a**, **b**) clinical film; (**c**, **d**) intra-operative films; (**e**, **f**) 5 months follow-up

Diagnostic

When a patient presents with pain and a history of a previously treated clavicle fracture, failed fixation should be ruled out. All patients being worked up for failed fixation require plane radiographs of the clavicle. There are multiple images that can be obtained, but most commonly a plane anteroposterior X-ray is obtained. Additional images that may be helpful are clavicle inlet and outlet films (aka serendipitous views), which are performed by obtaining images with craniocaudal tilt and caudocranial tilt, respectfully. Shortening is difficult to accurately assess on unilateral plain X-rays. Therefore, a bilateral clavicle X-ray and/or CT is more useful to evaluate shortening. Additionally, inferior displacement is commonly underestimated on supine films; therefore, obtaining films in the upright position may be beneficial [37].

Plain X-ray images typically can confirm the diagnosis and aid in understanding fragment locations and failed implant locations. However, sometimes the implant failure is subtle (i.e., screw loosening) and degree of healing difficult to evaluate using plain X-rays alone. This may be secondary to the location of the prior implants obstructing the visualization of fracture union or it may be secondary to the severity of fracture comminution. Therefore, in cases where failed fixation is not obvious, but the clinical concern remains elevated, a CT scan may add valuable information. It may also be helpful given the curved shape and small diameter of the bone, but sometimes it may be obscured by metal artifact. Other advanced imaging modalities such as MRIs are not typically useful.

All patients that are being worked up for failed fixation require a general lab workup to rule out infection as the etiology. This varies slightly by institution, but in general a complete blood count (CBC), erythrocyte sedimentation rate (ESR), and C-reactive protein (CRP) are sufficient. Additionally, most surgeons will obtain deep cultures at time of revision surgery. Other biochemical tests are not generally warranted.

removal sets should be available. Scrutiny of preoperative studies will aid in assuring all screws are removed prior to attempting to remove plates. Intra-operative fluoroscopy is used to localize buried or otherwise not visible implants and used to confirm removal. If possible, if is helpful to know the metallurgy of the implants used to better prepare for implant removal. Titanium locking screws more commonly strip with removal or are found to be cold-welded to the plate than stainless steel locked screws. Carbide drill bits can also be useful to remove screws that are cold-welded into the plate.

Formulation of Preoperative Planning

After a diagnosis of a clavicle aseptic non-union with failed fixation is made, a careful and detailed surgical plan should be formulated. Typically, this is initiated with clinical X-rays that were previously obtained and supplemented with bilateral CT scans of the clavicles. Three-dimensional reconstruction images may be formatted, which can be very helpful in understanding fracture morphology. These images allow direct measurements of both clavicles to determine the degree of shortening and the location of displaced fractured implants. Pre-operative plans can be created using tracing paper or more modern operative planning software if the surgeon desires.

At the time of revision surgery, it is helpful to know which implants where previously used to assure removal instruments are available. If the existing implants cannot be identified, universal

New Implant Selection

In general, revision clavicle surgery for failed fixation requires an increase in implant rigidity compared to the previous surgery. This may be done with either 1 or 2 implants in various sizes and plate categories. If a single plate is to be used, this will typically be a 3.5 mm plate on either the superior or anteroinferior surface of the clavicle. If two plates are used, a 3.5 mm plate may be supplemented with an additional 2.7 or 2.4 mm plate placed orthogonal to the first plate. Occasionally, in a small statured person, dual 2.7 mm plates or a 2.7 mm plate and a 2.4 mm plate may be sufficient. Orthogonal plating may be useful in maintaining reduction and it increases torsional strength; good outcomes with dual-plating have been reported [38–40]. It may be helpful to have precontoured plates available to help recreate the "S"-shape of the normal clavicle using the plate contour as a template (Figs. 5.7 and 5.8).

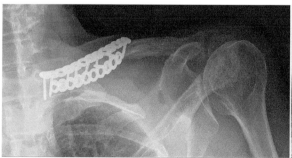
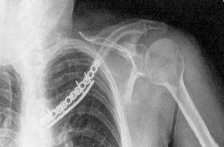

Fig. 5.7 An example of a plating construct for a medial clavicle non-union

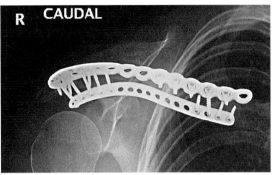 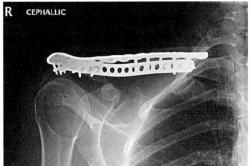

Fig. 5.8 An example of a plating construct for a lateral clavicle non-union

Need for Bone Grafting

Bone grafting in revision clavicle fracture surgery is not absolutely necessary [41]. If two healthy surfaces of bone are available for compression, length is satisfactory and the patient is a good host, then it may not be required. Multiple studies have reported excellent clinical results in treating clavicle non-unions without bone graft [42–45]. However, intercalary tricortical autograft is commonly needed when bone defects are present. This may be used to help obtain union and restore anatomic length [16]. Cancellous autograft can also be supplemented at the margins of the fragments. Autogenous iliac crest bone graft is still considered to be the gold standard because of its osteogenic, osteoconductive, and osteoinductive properties, but other anatomic donor sites and allograft options may be used if needed [24]. Disadvantages to autograft include limited volume of bone available, increased operative time, increased blood loss, and donor site morbidity [46–49]. Other graft options include vascularized fibular autograft, non-vascularized fibular autografts, allografts, and bone graft substitutes but these have limited roles in the treatment of clavicle non-union [50, 51].

Revision Surgery

A stepwise approach is used in addressing failed fracture fixation:

1. The revision surgery is typically performed through the previous surgical approach, which is typically through a previous transverse incision. Care must be taken to preserve native tissue for an adequate closure at the end of the case.
2. Anatomical landmarks are used to assist to accurately access and adjust length and rotation before prior implants are removed. Once length is either established or landmarks are marked based on your pre-operative plan, the previous implants can then be removed.
3. Five tissue samples are obtained and sent to microbiology to rule out indolent infection.
4. Debridement of non-union is performed in multiple rounds. This is typically initiated with a curette and pituitary rongeur. Once the edges are free of soft tissue a burr is used to freshen the bone edges until bleeding bone edges are visualized.
5. The canal is opened in both directions either with a curette if the canal is maintained or a drill bit if bone has grown over the fracture edges.
6. A provisional reduction is the obtained with reduction clamps and/or provisional plates. K-wire fixation in hard diaphyseal cortical clavicle bone has limited utility and can cause heat necrosis.
7. With a provisional reduction obtained, the final implant selection may be determined. Initial small/thin reduction plates are applied to whichever surface (anterior/inferior or

superior) is most amenable given the location of the reduction clamps. A more robust plate is then applied to the opposite surface from the reduction plate. When deciding on the relative location of thin and thick plates in a dual-plate construct, consideration should also be given to the fracture obliquity so that dynamic compression is through the thicker plate.

8. If bone graft is needed, it should be harvested after a provisional reduction is obtained. Timing of the bone graft harvest is such that it can be used and implanted soon after harvest so that it does not lose biologic activity by being at room temperature for a prolonged period.

9. The previously selected plates are then applied to the clavicle. If structural graft is used, it is compressed to the native bone with the plates and screws or a tensioning device. Additionally, at least one screws is placed through the graft to avoid migration. Cancellous graft can then be placed around the non-union margins.

10. A standard multi-layered closure is then performed.

11. Post-Operative Protocol:
    (a) Immediately post-operative
        (i) Coffee-cup weightbearing
        (ii) Active range of motion of the shoulder, elbow, forearm, and hand
        (iii) Overhead motion avoided for the first 4 weeks
    (b) First follow-up appointment: ~2 weeks post-op
        (i) Wound check and suture removal
        (ii) No images are typically obtained at this visit
    (c) Second follow-up appointment: ~6 weeks post-op
        (i) X-rays are obtained
        (ii) Overhead motion is initiated following clinical and radiographic evaluation typically at this point
    (d) Further follow-up: Until union and clinical improvement

Summary: Lessons Learned

Clavicle fractures are common injuries with a relatively high incidence of non-union compared to other fractures. An appropriate understanding of clavicle fracture deforming forces (i.e., weight of the arm, pull of the pectoralis major muscle, and pull of the sternocleidomastoid muscle), degrees of motion about the clavicle (i.e., bending moments in the sagittal and coronal planes), and compositional characteristics of the bone (i.e., high quantity of cortical bone) may aid in mitigating the risk of non-union after the index surgery. Additionally, an understanding of the fracture morphology and the patient treated should guide early treatment in acute fractures. Historical plate designs were typically thin and malleable, whereas modern plating designs tend to be stronger and are often pre-contoured lending to more fatigue resistance and ease of plate application. Dual-plating options offer increased rigidity and fatigue resistance, which may further mitigate failure of fixation.

Failure of fracture fixation of clavicle fractures is typically secondary to one of two causes, fracture non-union, and/or inappropriate implant selection, excluding infectious etiology. Failed hardware in clavicle fracture fixation rarely presents asymptomatically in patients. Symptoms most often result from prominent loose screws, broken or bent plates, and/or deformity of the shoulder. Symptoms present as tenderness to palpation, gross motion, crepitus, pain, and/or paresthesias [8].

If failed fracture fixation is identified, appropriate workup should be started immediately. This should always include an infectious workup to rule out an infectious etiology. Radiographs and bilateral CT scans of the clavicle may aid in the diagnosis of failed fixation and may be used in surgical planning for revision surgery.

A thorough pre-operative plan and an inventory of the necessary equipment enable a successful revision surgery. Revision surgery can be performed with various options of plate types, plate locations, plate quantities, bone graft (structural or non-structural), and augmentation with suture and tendon allografts as needed depending on the fracture morphology, location and biological needs. A stepwise surgical approach is best to optimize the possibility of a successful revision clavicle surgery.

References

1. Robinson CM. Fractures of the clavicle in the adult. Epidemiology and classification. J Bone Joint Surg Br. 1998;80(3):476–84.
2. Canadian Orthopaedic Trauma Society. Nonoperative treatment compared with plate fixation of displaced midshaft clavicular fractures. A multicenter, randomized clinical trial. J Bone Joint Surg Am. 2007;89(1):1–10.
3. Smeeing DPJ, van der Ven DJC, Hietbrink F, et al. Surgical versus nonsurgical treatment for midshaft clavicle fractures in patients aged 16 years and older: a systematic review, meta-analysis, and comparison of randomized controlled trials and observational studies. Am J Sports Med. 2017;45(8):1937–45.
4. Frima H, van Heijl M, Michelitsch C, et al. Clavicle fractures in adults; current concepts. Eur J Trauma Emerg Surg. 2020;46(3):519–29.
5. Johnson EW, Collins HR. Nonunion of the clavicle. Arch Surg. 1963;87:963–6.
6. Neer CS 2nd. Nonunion of the clavicle. J Am Med Assoc. 1960;172:1006–11.
7. Rowe CR. An atlas of anatomy and treatment of midclavicular fractures. Clin Orthop Relat Res. 1968;58:29–42.
8. Martetschläger F, Gaskill TR, Millett PJ. Management of clavicle nonunion and malunion. J Shoulder Elb Surg. 2013;22(6):862–8.
9. McKee RC, Whelan DB, Schemitsch EH, McKee MD. Operative versus nonoperative care of displaced midshaft clavicular fractures: a meta-analysis of randomized clinical trials. J Bone Joint Surg Am. 2012;94(8):675–84.
10. Robinson CM, Goudie EB, Murray IR, et al. Open reduction and plate fixation versus nonoperative treatment for displaced midshaft clavicular fractures: a multicenter, randomized, controlled trial. J Bone Joint Surg Am. 2013;95(17):1576–84.
11. Woltz S, Krijnen P, Schipper IB. Plate fixation versus nonoperative treatment for displaced midshaft clavicular fractures: a meta-analysis of randomized controlled trials. J Bone Joint Surg Am. 2017;99(12):1051–7.
12. Woltz S, Stegeman SA, Krijnen P, et al. Plate fixation compared with nonoperative treatment for displaced midshaft clavicular fractures: a multicenter randomized controlled trial. J Bone Joint Surg Am. 2017;99(2):106–12.

13. Van der Meijden OA, Gaskill TR, Millett PJ. Treatment of clavicle fractures: current concepts review. J Shoulder Elb Surg. 2012;21(3):423–9.
14. Lazarides S, Zafiropoulos G. Conservative treatment of fractures at the middle third of the clavicle: the relevance of shortening and clinical outcome. J Shoulder Elb Surg. 2006;15(2):191–4.
15. Rasmussen JV, Jensen SL, Petersen JB, Falstie-Jensen T, Lausten G, Olsen BS. A retrospective study of the association between shortening of the clavicle after fracture and the clinical outcome in 136 patients. Injury. 2011;42(4):414–7.
16. Jones GL, McCluskey GM, Curd DT. Nonunion of the fractured clavicle: evaluation, etiology, and treatment. J South Orthop Assoc. 2000;9(1):43–54.
17. Ropars M, Thomazeau H, Huten D. Clavicle fractures. Orthop Traumatol Surg Res. 2017;103(1S):S53–9.
18. Bachoura A, Deane AS, Wise JN, Kamineni S. Clavicle morphometry revisited: a 3-dimensional study with relevance to operative fixation. J Shoulder Elb Surg. 2013;22(1):e15–21.
19. Liu W, Xiao J, Ji F, Xie Y, Hao Y. Intrinsic and extrinsic risk factors for nonunion after nonoperative treatment of midshaft clavicle fractures. Orthop Traumatol Surg Res. 2015;101(2):197–200.
20. Salipas A, Kimmel LA, Edwards ER, Rakhra S, Moaveni AK. Natural history of medial clavicle fractures. Injury. 2016;47(10):2235–9.
21. Throckmorton T, Kuhn JE. Fractures of the medial end of the clavicle. J Shoulder Elb Surg. 2007;16(1):49–54.
22. Robinson CM, Court-Brown CM, McQueen MM, Wakefield AE. Estimating the risk of nonunion following nonoperative treatment of a clavicular fracture. J Bone Joint Surg Am. 2004;86(7):1359–65.
23. Simpson NS, Jupiter JB. Clavicular nonunion and malunion: evaluation and surgical management. J Am Acad Orthop Surg. 1996;4(1):1–8.
24. Boehme D, Curtis RJ, DeHaan JT, Kay SP, Young DC, Rockwood CA. Non-union of fractures of the midshaft of the clavicle. Treatment with a modified Hagie intramedullary pin and autogenous bone-grafting. J Bone Joint Surg Am. 1991;73(8):1219–26.
25. Han D, Han N, Xue F, Zhang P. A novel specialized staging system for cancellous fracture healing, distinct from traditional healing pattern of diaphysis corticalfracture? Int J Clin Exp Med. 2015;8(1):1301–4.
26. Ersen A, Atalar AC, Birisik F, Saglam Y, Demirhan M. Comparison of simple arm sling and figure of eight clavicular bandage for midshaft clavicular fractures: a randomised controlled study. Bone Joint J. 2015;97-B(11):1562–5.
27. Andersen K, Jensen PO, Lauritzen J. Treatment of clavicular fractures. Figure-of-eight bandage versus a simple sling. Acta Orthop Scand. 1987;58(1):71–4.
28. Smekal V, Attal R, Dallapozza C, Krappinger D. Elastic stable intramedullary nailing after corrective osteotomy of symptomatic malunited midshaft clavicular fractures. Oper Orthop Traumatol. 2011;23(5):375–84.

29. Chiu YC, Huang KC, Shih CM, Lee KT, Chen KH, Hsu CE. Comparison of implant failure rates of different plates for midshaft clavicular fractures based on fracture classifications. J Orthop Surg Res. 2019;14(1):220.

30. Woltz S, Duijff JW, Hoogendoorn JM, et al. Reconstruction plates for midshaft clavicular fractures: a retrospective cohort study. Orthop Traumatol Surg Res. 2016;102(1):25–9.

31. Shin SJ, Do NH, Jang KY. Risk factors for postoperative complications of displaced clavicular midshaft fractures. J Trauma Acute Care Surg. 2012;72(4):1046–50.

32. Mirzatolooei F. Comparison between operative and nonoperative treatment methods in the management of comminuted fractures of the clavicle. Acta Orthop Traumatol Turc. 2011;45(1):34–40.

33. Renfree T, Conrad B, Wright T. Biomechanical comparison of contemporary clavicle fixation devices. J Hand Surg Am. 2010;35(4):639–44.

34. Little KJ, Riches PE, Fazzi UG. Biomechanical analysis of locked and non-locked plate fixation of the clavicle. Injury. 2012;43(6):921–5.

35. Wang SH, Lin HJ, Shen HC, Pan RY, Yang JJ. Biomechanical comparison between solid and cannulated intramedullary devices for midshaft clavicle fixation. BMC Musculoskelet Disord. 2019;20(1):178.

36. Havet E, Duparc F, Tobenas-Dujardin A-C, Muller J-M, Delas B, Fréger P. Vascular anatomical basis of clavicular non-union. Surg Radiol Anat. 2008;30(1):23–8.

37. Backus JD, Merriman DJ, McAndrew CM, Gardner MJ, Ricci WM. Upright versus supine radiographs of clavicle fractures: does positioning matter? J Orthop Trauma. 2014;28(11):636–41.

38. Sadiq S, Waseem M, Peravalli B, Doyle J, Dunningham T, Muddu BN. Single or double plating for nonunion of the clavicle. Acta Orthop Belg. 2001;67(4):354–60.

39. Stufkens SA, Kloen P. Treatment of midshaft clavicular delayed and non-unions with anteroinferior locking compression plating. Arch Orthop Trauma Surg. 2010;130(2):159–64.

40. Michel PA, Katthagen JC, Heilmann LF, Dyrna F, Schliemann B, Raschke MJ. Biomechanics of upper extremity double plating. Z Orthop Unfall. 2020;158(2):238–44.

41. Baker JF, Mullett H. Clavicle non-union: autologous bone graft is not a necessary augment to internal fixation. Acta Orthop Belg. 2010;76:725–9.

42. Khan SA, Shamshery P, Gupta V, Trikha V, Varshney MK, Kumar A. Locking compression plate in long standing clavicular nonunions with poor bone stock. J Trauma. 2008;64(2):439–41.

43. O'Connor D, Kutty S, McCabe JP. Long-term functional outcome assessment of plate fixation and autogenous bone grafting for clavicular non-union. Injury. 2004;35(6):575–9.

44. Olsen BS, Vaesel MT, Søjbjerg JO. Treatment of midshaft clavicular nonunion with plate fixation and autologous bone grafting. J Shoulder Elb Surg. 1995;4(5):337–44.

45. Zhang J, Yin P, Han B, Zhao J, Yin B. The treatment of the atrophic clavicular nonunion by double-plate fixation with autogenous cancellous bone graft: a prospective study. J Orthop Surg Res. 2021;16(1):22.

46. Jones AL, Bucholz RW, Bosse MJ, et al. Recombinant human BMP-2 and allograft compared with autogenous bone graft for reconstruction of diaphyseal tibial fractures with cortical defects. A randomized, controlled trial. J Bone Joint Surg Am. 2006;88(7):1431–41.

47. Arrington ED, Smith WJ, Chambers HG, Bucknell AL, Davino NA. Complications of iliac crest bone graft harvesting. Clin Orthop Relat Res. 1996;329:300–9.

48. Robertson PA, Wray AC. Natural history of posterior iliac crest bone graft donation for spinal surgery: a prospective analysis of morbidity. Spine (Phila Pa 1976). 2001;26(13):1473–6.

49. Sasso RC, LeHuec JC, Shaffrey C, Spine Interbody Research Group. Iliac crest bone graft donor site pain after anterior lumbar interbody fusion: a prospective patient satisfaction outcome assessment. J Spinal Disord Tech. 2005;18(Suppl):S77–81.

50. Lenoir H, Williams T, Kerfant N, Robert M, Le Nen D. Free vascularized fibular graft as a salvage procedure for large clavicular defect: a two cases report. Orthop Traumatol Surg Res. 2013;99(7):859–63.

51. Riggenbach MD, Jones GL, Bishop JY. Open reduction and internal fixation of clavicular nonunions with allograft bone substitute. Int J Shoulder Surg. 2011;5(3):61–7.

Failed Fixation of Proximal Humerus Fracture

6

David Limb

Aetiology of Failed Fixation

A consideration of the aetiology of failed fixation in the proximal humerus invites contemplation on the indications for fixation in the first place. The gut instinct of many on looking at a radiograph showing a displaced fracture is to recommend surgical management, usually by reduction and internal fixation of some sort. The reduction methods can be closed or open. The fixation may involve sutures, absorbable implants, pins, plates, screws or intramedullary devices alone or in combination. What is undoubted is that in most cases the radiological alignment of the fracture can be improved. The postoperative radiograph looks as though the shoulder should function better for the patient and therefore measurements of outcome reported by the patient (rather than measured from a radiograph by the surgeon) should be better. Increasingly, randomised controlled trials suggest that in many, or even most, cases we do not actually make a difference [1–3] and in some we make the patient worse. In this chapter, we will be considering how to salvage the latter situation—the challenge, therefore, is to research which patients with which fractures are actually likely to benefit from surgery. Currently, it seems,

a large proportion do not, and that is not the best use of resources. Even some of those patients with an X-ray image that shows perfect reduction report an outcome no better than some patients with a significant malunion.

What then are the main aetiological factors leading to failed fixation? We can consider patient-related, fracture-related and surgery-related causes, though there is overlap and often more than one cause [4, 5].

Patient-related factors are those which affect bone healing, those which affect the strength of fixation and those that reduce resistance to infection. Internal fixation provides temporary stability at least to resist deforming forces until sufficient healing has occurred to resist physiological forces. Sometimes there is no intention to resist significant physiological loading for several weeks (e.g. percutaneous wires), whilst in other cases the intention is to allow loading as quickly as possible (some locking plates and intramedullary nails).

Patient factors that affect bone healing include diabetes and smoking.

Patient factors that affect the strength of the fixation are those that cause diminished bone quality, notably osteoporosis.

Patient factors that affect resistance to infection include any form of immune deficiency, but the most prevalent in the western world are diabetes and smoking.

D. Limb (✉)
Trauma and Orthopaedic Surgery, Leeds Teaching Hospitals Trust, Chapel Allerton Hospital, Leeds, UK
e-mail: david.limb@nhs.net

© The Author(s), under exclusive license to Springer Nature Switzerland AG 2024
P. V. Giannoudis, P. Tornetta III (eds.), *Failed Fracture Fixation*,
https://doi.org/10.1007/978-3-031-39692-2_6

Note that there is limited scope for modifying the majority of these factors once the fracture has occurred—stopping smoking will be helpful as time elapses, but smokers who abstain from the point of fracture still have worse overall outcomes.

Fracture-related causes are those that affect the initial strength of fixation and those that have an effect on healing times. Prominent in both respects are factors related to the energy of injury. Initial stability of the construct is significantly greater if the fracture can be anatomically reduced to allow load transmission from one fragment to another rather than relying on the plate. This is much more difficult in multifragmentary fractures and impossible if there is bone loss. Higher energy injuries also take longer to heal, prolonging the time for which reliance is placed on the fixation, therefore increasing the likelihood of fixation failure. Indirectly related to energy of injury is the fracture pattern—if fracture lines lead to impaired blood supply or devascularisation of major fracture fragments (e.g. anatomical neck fractures), then not only does fracture healing prolong but the risk of avascular necrosis is substantially increased. In some proximal humerus fracture patterns, such as dislocations associated with anatomic neck fractures, or more commonly 3- and 4-part fracture dislocations, the risk is so high that currently arthroplasty is often favoured as the primary treatment.

Surgery-related factors are related to deficiencies in decision making (fixation of fractures that cannot be reduced adequately or have such a high risk of complications such as avascular necrosis (AVN) or infection that failure was predictable) or technique. Anatomic reduction is not essential for all fractures—if any part of the fracture line is visible on the postoperative X-ray, even as a thin line, the reduction is not, by definition, anatomical. However, it is desirable and it is also important to avoid fixation with significant malreduction. This can cause immediate problems with rehabilitation, increase the risk of failure of fixation and, even if the fracture heals, increase the risk of screw cut-out, avascular

necrosis and poor outcomes in terms of function and pain.

Whatever the cause of failure of fixation the result is the same—an unhappy patient with a stiff, painful shoulder who looks to you to improve the situation for them. In this chapter, we will look at a case of internal fixation that developed avascular necrosis and went on the treatment by arthroplasty.

Clinical Examination

Inspection is important as it may show prominent metalwork, will reveal any scars related to the original trauma, indicate the surgical approach to fracture fixation and the state of wound healing, with clues as to whether infection has been an issue in the past even if there are no active signs. Deltoid wasting can be due to disuse of a painful shoulder or denervation due to axillary nerve injury.

The majority of proximal humerus fractures will have been approached via a deltopectoral route, but a more lateral scar could indicate an anterosuperior approach or a deltoid splitting approach, and the relationship of the axillary nerve to the scar and the fixation device should be worked out (ideally by obtaining the operation note of the original surgery). The issues going through the surgeons mind are 'can I reuse a previous scar without compromising my planned surgery, and if not can I make a new approach that doesn't compromise the skin' and 'is the skin quality good enough to allow healing after another operation.' If unsure about the latter, then involving a colleague from plastic surgery may be appropriate, and this should also be taken into account in deciding whether surgery is in the best interests of the patient after all. If there are signs of ongoing infection, then this requires a multidisciplinary team approach.

In the case, we are considering there was fortunately a well-healed deltopectoral scar and by using the same scar we could approach the proximal humerus with minimal risk to the axillary nerve.

Palpation of any unexpected prominence can reveal whether this is the fixation device, commonly appearing anterosuperiorly in failed proximal humerus fixations, or bone that is either a result of malunion or is a normal landmark, such as the coracoid or acromion, thrown into relief by deformity. Palpation will also reveal any tenderness (of metalwork, normal landmarks or the shoulder or acromioclavicular joints).

In our case, the deltoid was thin and there was a slightly tender anterosuperior prominence that was the remains of the humeral head and attached fixation device brought to the front by internal rotation contracture of the shoulder.

Moving the joint will reveal the range of motion and identify if any parts of the range are painful. Almost all patients with failed fixation will have some, usually substantial, deficits in motion and at least end-range pain. This is usually why they are asking you to do something about it!

Our patient had about 50 degrees of combined elevation, an internal rotation contracture of 30 degrees and could internally rotate to reach the buttock. Only the end of the range of motion was painful, increasing significantly if attempted passive movement beyond the active range was tested.

Investigations

In most cases of failed fixation of the proximal humerus, a plain anteroposterior (AP) and axial radiograph will provide most, if not all, of the information needed for successful management. However, it is important to ensure that the whole management pathway is clear and if not, to consider whether further imaging, blood or pathology tests are required.

A plain X-ray can give a sufficient picture to plan many interventions. If there are loose screws or screws penetrating the humeral head, then a plan can be instituted to remove these, even if it may need an image intensifier to identify the appropriate screw in theatre. In our case, a four-part fracture was initially managed by open reduction and internal fixation using a locking plate (Fig. 6.1a and b) but AVN has caused collapse of the humeral head around the fixation

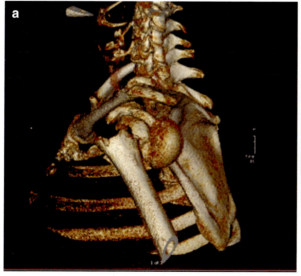
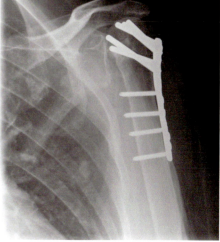

Fig. 6.1 (**a** and **b**) The patient's original injury—a displaced proximal humeral fracture with dislocation. The patient was considered rather young for a primary arthroplasty, therefore, initial management was open reduction and internal fixation with a locking plate

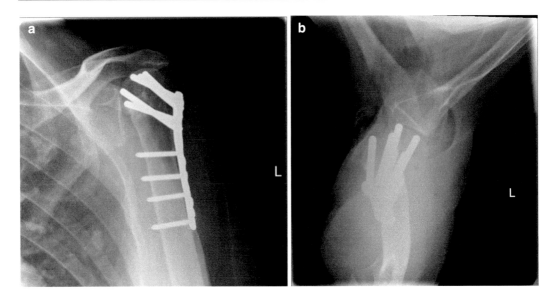

Fig. 6.2 (**a** and **b**) The patient continued to complain of pain and AVN led to penetration of the humeral head though there was no damage to the glenoid

pegs, leading to penetration of the head, but there is no significant damage to the glenoid (Fig. 6.2a and b). The subacromial space is narrow and this usually means that the cuff is torn, though after trauma this can occur if the tuberosities are reduced and fixed non-anatomically with a gap between subscapularis and supraspinatus. A plain X-ray may in itself give sufficient information to allow a revision fixation and grafting of an ununited surgical neck component with increasing deformity. However, if the state of union of other fragments is unsure or the extent of bone loss, then a computed tomography (CT) may be considered. Some cases of AVN may be planned for revision to an anatomic arthroplasty. Nonetheless, if the state of the bone stock, particularly in the glenoid, is unclear, then CT may again be needed and many would consider it essential before proceeding to total anatomic, or increasingly commonly reverse, shoulder arthroplasty. CT is less often needed for elucidating the biology of nonunion, unlike nonunion in long bones. Vascularity issues in the proximal humerus almost always manifest as AVN and humeral head collapse.

Magnetic resonance (MR) imaging is less useful than may be thought. Many proximal humeral fractures appear to have avascular necrosis on imaging taken soon after fixation, only to go on to heal uneventfully with no clinical or radiological evidence of AVN. It is useful, however, if infection is suspected. MR does give an indication as to the integrity of the rotator cuff and can, therefore, be important if revision fixation or osteotomy is considered, and especially if anatomic arthroplasty is being contemplated. Ultrasound can, in many cases, provide this information quickly and more cheaply, but not if there is deformity of the tuberosities or rotation of the humeral head, which can make ultrasound very difficult to perform and interpret. As technology develops it is possible MR and Ultrasound may have increased indications in the future [6].

Infection within the differential diagnosis is also the main reason why a range of other investigations may be considered ranging from simple blood tests such as the full blood count, through established inflammatory markers to a range of new indicators in various states of clinical assessment. Biopsy may be indicated to obtain tissue samples and although aspiration may be helpful, open biopsy of multiple specimens using clean instrument sets for each is far more accurate and if arthroplasty is being contemplated will help plan antibiotic management in one- or two-stage arthroplasty implantation.

Preoperative Planning

Preoperative planning is intimately linked to investigations—investigations will determine if there is sufficient articular surface, rotator cuff and bone stock to manage a nonunion by revision internal fixation with or without bone grafting. If arthroplasty is being considered CT is particularly useful, though can be degraded by metalwork in situ. Removal of metalwork as the first stage in dealing with failed fixation, particularly if arthroplasty is being considered, is well worth considering. In any event the radiographs, but preferably the operation note from the primary procedure, will indicate the type of implant that has to be removed and plans can be made to ensure the correct size(s) and type(s) of screwdriver(s) and any kit for removing, for example, intramedullary nails, is available.

CT can help predict problems such as occlusion or deformity of the medullary canal that could interfere with stem insertion, head/shaft deformity that can affect the seating of the metaphyseal component of an arthroplasty, heterotopic bone and displaced, separated tuberosity fragments that could interfere with range of movement, glenoid deficiencies and scapular deformities that might interfere with glenoid component insertion and alignment. The scan also allows templating and, if necessary, the creation of patient-specific guides or prosthetic components.

Implant Selection

After determining the operative strategy, which could involve revision fixation with or without grafting, but in our case replacement arthroplasty, implant selection can take place. Shoulder arthroplasty is available in both anatomic and reverse variants. Anatomic replacement can be in hemiarthroplasty form or total arthroplasty, and the humeral component can be resurfacing, stemless or stemmed. However, all of these rely on a functional rotator cuff. Reverse arthroplasty is a form of total arthroplasty and although the humeral stem length can vary, stemmed components are the norm. Reverse arthroplasty does not require a functional rotator cuff, and when it first began to be used for trauma it was indicated for the elderly who were assumed to have a deficient rotator cuff [7]. However, it can still be carried out in the presence of a rotator cuff and in trauma cases there is some evidence that preserving the tuberosities and their attached cuff tendons improves the functional outcome [8].

Irrespective of whether or not the rotator cuff is intact (as shown in our case on an ultrasound scan) and functioning well (difficult to tell in our case because of stiffness but there was some fatty atrophy of the supraspinatus muscle belly on ultrasound scanning, suggesting a degree of chronic dysfunction), the patient themselves has to be considered in the decision-making algorithm. It has been observed that shoulder replacement in general, when carried out in patients under 60, is significantly likely to need revision in the patient's lifetime. Over the age of 80 the prosthesis is very likely to outlast the patient. Anatomic shoulder replacements are associated with better functional scores, but the main reason for revision of anatomic shoulder replacements in the UK National Joint Registry is rotator cuff failure (see—https://reports.njrcentre.org.uk/). In elderly patients, therefore, the cuff is likely to be of poorer quality and a reverse prosthesis is likely to last the patient's lifetime, so a reverse prosthesis is most often selected [9]. In a young, higher demand patient, the cuff is likely to be of better quality and revision is more likely to be required in the future, irrespective of the prosthesis used; therefore, an anatomic replacement is more likely to be appropriate.

In our case, the patient was 75 years old and independent, but with no high demands such as sporting pastimes, and there was evidence of rotator cuff deficiency; therefore, a reverse total shoulder replacement was selected.

Surgery

The patient was involved throughout in debates about the risks and rewards and the impact of imaging findings. They were happy to proceed with revision of the failed internal fixation to a reverse total shoulder arthroplasty. Preoperative examination and blood tests, along with a consideration of the clinical course since the original surgery and the current imaging, meant that there was no suspicion of infection. A one-stage procedure was, therefore, chosen, removing the locking plate and screws and inserting a reverse total shoulder replacement under the same anaesthetic.

Anaesthesia consisted of an interscalene block and general anaesthesia. The interscalene block effectively deals with pain control both during and after surgery; therefore, the general anaesthetic can be very light, allowing rapid patient recovery after surgery. Prophylactic antibiotics are administered before surgery starts according to local policy. The patient was placed in the Beach chair position with the arm draped free.

The surgical approach mirrors that used in the original surgery—the previous scar is reopened and deepened to the deltopectoral interval (Fig. 6.3). The cephalic vein may or may not have been preserved in the primary surgery, and sometimes landmarks and planes can be difficult to identify. If there is any difficulty, it is useful to simply extend the skin wound by 1 or 2 cm and utilise a region not previously disturbed, and therefore with preserved fat and tissue planes, to direct one to the humeral shaft in the subdeltoid plane and the coracoid process with its attached conjoint tendon.

Having identified these landmarks, the subdeltoid region can be opened, following round the humeral shaft and releasing scar tissue from this in an upwards and lateral direction until one is all the way around the shaft and tuberosities, exposing the plate. The dissection can then be continued above the plate to enter the subacromial space and sharp dissection may be needed to release subacromial scar. Rotating the free arm reveals planes of movement, which are the planes that have to be released to properly expose the proximal humerus. In the same plane, dissecting medially will take one beneath the conjoint tendon on the superficial surface of subscapularis and care has to be taken beneath the conjoint tendon not to threaten the musculocutaneous nerve.

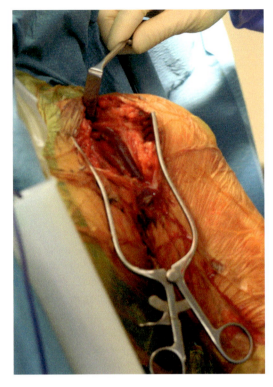

Fig. 6.3 The original deltopectoral approach was reused to allow access to the proximal humerus for removal of the metalwork, then the glenohumeral joint for arthroplasty

Once the proximal humerus has been adequately exposed, a process which often improves the range of movement in any event, the defunct metalwork can be removed. After removing all screws/pegs from the plate, a check should be made for strong suture material such as fibre wire which may have been used to fix the rotator cuff and tuberosities to the plate through specifically designed holes in the plate. Any such sutures have to be at least cut, if not removed, to allow the plate to be lifted out.

After removal of the metalwork, attention can be paid to the arthroplasty. Depending on the state of the rotator cuff, whether it is intact and mobile, a decision can be made as to whether an osteotomy of the lesser tuberosity is to be carried out in order to preserve and repair the subscapularis afterwards, or whether the cuff is to be sacrificed. In our case, the cuff was completely deficient above the prosthesis and the remaining cuff anterior and posterior was scarred and stiff, so a decision was taken to excise it. Of course, this improves access to the glenohumeral joint which can then be dislocated and, using appropriate jigs, the flattened and necrotic humeral head can be removed at the correct level and angle to accommodate the planned humeral stem. Using the broaches and jigs appropriate for the device to be used, the humeral canal can be prepared and usually a trial stem can be left within the canal, with a flat plate attached to it that sits on the cut surface and protects it whist the glenoid is prepared.

Access to the glenoid is achieved in the same way as it is in primary arthroplasty—even in primary osteoarthrosis the capsule is often scarred and thick, and obtaining a good release around the glenoid is essential to allow the humeral shaft to be retracted backwards and inferiorly to allow access to the glenoid.

If the glenoid has been damaged by projecting screws, for example, managing the glenoid can become complex with a need for patient-specific guides or augments to the glenoid component. However, in most cases this is not necessary and after trauma, such as in the case we are managing, there may even be residual cartilage on the glenoid that needs reaming to the subchondral bone surface.

Preparation and insertion of the glenoid should be carried out using the specific instruments for the prosthesis to be inserted. The glenosphere should be placed low on the glenoid and not in the central position used for the glenoid component of an anatomic shoulder. Slight inferior overhang of the glenosphere is one measure that reduces the risk of impingement and scapular notching, with the possibility of early loosening. After inserting the glenosphere, a polyethylene liner of appropriate size to fit the glenosphere and produce adequate tension in deltoid can be fixed to the stem. The joint is then reduced and, if it was planned, the subscapularis and other components of the rotator cuff can be repaired around the prosthesis (not needed in our case). After a thorough washout and check for stability through range of movement, the shoulder can be reduced.

The deltopectoral interval should close as retractors are removed and only the fat and skin layers need closing.

Postoperative Management

The intention of arthroplasty is to allow early functional movement and although the patient will need a sling until their interscalene block has worn off, they should be allowed to use their arm for activities of daily living as soon as that has occurred. Drains are not usually needed nor are postoperative antibiotics. An X-ray is taken after surgery to confirm satisfactory postoperative appearances (Fig. 6.4a and b). The patient can usually be discharged from hospital within 24 h of surgery, but loaded use of the arm is restricted at first, being gradually resumed over 3 months after surgery.

There is a difference in the complication rates after anatomic and reverse total shoulder replacement—a reverse prosthesis carries a higher risk of infection and dislocation than an anatomic prosthesis. The risk of revision is higher in the first 3 years after implantation, but beyond 9 years anatomic shoulder replacements overtake reverse shoulders in terms of revision rate. Postoperative review should account for this, with exercises and their progression supervised by a physiotherapist and the patient warned to report back quickly if there is any redness, discharge, pain or loss of movement. However, if a postoperative X-ray taken before discharge is satisfactory, no further imaging is usually necessary in the first year or two after surgery if the patient progresses satisfactorily with their rehabilitation. Outpatient review can, therefore, be arranged according to local protocols—our patient was contacted for telephone review 6 weeks after surgery and attended physiotherapy once a month for a review of rehabilitation exercises. She was seen after 1 year and X-rays at this stage were compared to postoperative films and deemed suitable for the patient to be followed up in a virtual clinic thereafter, with X-rays after 2 more years and patient reported outcome measures

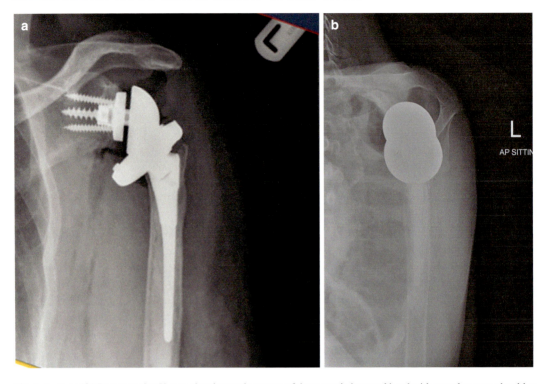

Fig. 6.4 (**a** and **b**) Postoperative X-rays showing replacement of the necrotic humeral head with a total reverse shoulder arthroplasty

compared to the previous year to flag up any deterioration that might trigger a face-to-face review.

Summary: Lessons Learned

This patient underwent open reduction and internal fixation of a displaced proximal humerus fracture in which there was no contact between the shaft and head fragments; therefore, this is not the sort of fracture that was considered in the ProfHer trial [1] (which suggested no difference between operatively and nonoperatively treated proximal humerus fractures in the majority of cases). Unfortunately, AVN ensued and of course if this could have been predicted, then arthroplasty would have been considered as the primary operation. However, it is better to restore the natural joint than to replace it and this was attempted but failed due to collapse of the humeral head, penetration of pegs into the glenohumeral joint and failure of the rotator cuff. In the future, we might develop algorithms to identify those patients in whom this is an inevitability and those who are more likely to retain their natural joint, but for now cases such as ours will continue to arise.

Once failure had manifest itself the decision-making process was one of recognising that arthroplasty was the only real operative option, and balancing then the relative risks and rewards of the various variants of anatomic and reverse shoulder replacement. Unlike many cases in which revision of a fracture fixation is contemplated, the revision of fixation to an arthroplasty, particularly in the shoulder, is a decision-making process that intimately involves the patient right down to the variant of implant to be used. Securing union after previous failed fixation of a fracture can be followed by removal or retention of the implant and no significant consequences for the patient. Revision to an arthroplasty, however, leaves the patient with an articulation subject to wear for the rest of their lives and may, even if completely successful, require further revision surgery in the future.

References

1. Handol H, Brearley S, Rangan A, et al. The ProFHER (PROximal fracture of the humerus: evaluation by randomisation) trial - a pragmatic multicentre randomised controlled trial evaluating the clinical effectiveness and cost-effectiveness of surgical compared with non-surgical treatment for proximal fracture of the humerus in adults. JAMA. 2015;313(10):1037–47.
2. Handol H, Keding A, Corbacho B, et al. Five-year follow-up results of the PROFHER trial comparing operative and non-operative treatment of adults with a displaced fracture of the proximal humerus. Bone Joint J. 2017;99-B(3):383–92.
3. Beks RB, Ochen Y, Frima H, et al. Operative versus nonoperative treatment of proximal humeral fractures: a systematic review, meta-analysis, and comparison of observational studies and randomized controlled trials. J Shoulder Elb Surg. 2018;27(8):1526–34.
4. Krappinger D, Bizzotto N, Riedman S, et al. Predicting failure after surgical fixation of proximal humerus fractures. Injury. 2011;42(11):1283–8.
5. Goudie EB, Robinson MC. Prediction of nonunion after nonoperative treatment of a proximal humeral fracture. J Bone Joint Surg. 2021;103(8):668–80.
6. Nicholson JA, Yapp AZ, Keating JF, et al. Monitoring of fracture healing. Update on current and future imaging modalities to predict union. Injury. 2021;52(S2):S29–34.
7. Bufquin T, Hersan A, Hubert L, et al. Reverse shoulder arthroplasty for the treatment of three- and four-part fractures of the proximal humerus in the elderly - a prospective review of 43 cases with a short-term follow-up. J Bone Joint Surg. 2007;89B(4):516–20.
8. Al Yaseen M, Smart Y, Seyed-Safi P, et al. Effect of implant size, version and rotator cuff tendon preservation on the outcome of reverse shoulder arthroplasty. Cureus. 2022;14(6):e25741.
9. Hussey MM, Hussey SE, Mighell MA. Reverse shoulder arthroplasty as a salvage procedure after failed internal fixation of fractures of the proximal humerus. Bone Joint J. 2015;97B:967–72.

Failed Fixation of the Humeral Neck Fracture

7

Carol A. Lin and Milton T. M. Little

Anatomical Location

The humeral neck is the zone of metaphyseal bone at the junction between the cranial portion of the humeral shaft and the caudal portion of the tuberosities and humeral head. It is notable for being a transitional zone between two clusters of tendon attachments that impart significant displacing forces. Proximally, the humeral head tuberosities are the attachment points for the muscles of the rotator cuff, while distally, the deltoid, pectoralis major, teres major, and latissimus dorsi impart proximal translation, extension, adduction, and internal rotation forces, respectively [1]. While the humeral head often remains rotationally neutral within the glenohumeral joint because of balanced internal and external rotation forces, the unopposed tension of the supraspinatus in displaced fractures may pull the fracture into varus alignment, and the forces at the proximal shaft frequently result in anterior translation, apex anterior as well as varus angulation, and fracture shortening (Fig. 7.1).

C. A. Lin (✉) · M. T. M. Little
Department of Orthopaedic Surgery, Cedars-Sinai
Medical Center, Los Angeles, CA, USA
e-mail: Carol.Lin@cshs.org; Milton.Little@cshs.org

© The Author(s), under exclusive license to Springer Nature Switzerland AG 2024
P. V. Giannoudis, P. Tornetta III (eds.), *Failed Fracture Fixation*,
https://doi.org/10.1007/978-3-031-39692-2_7

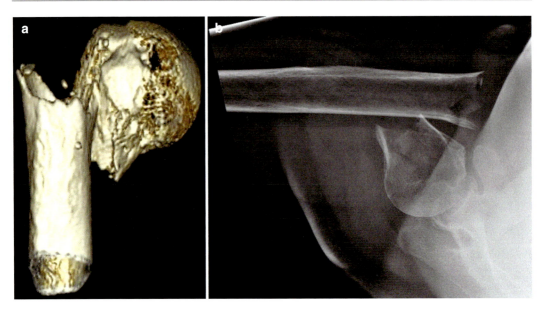

Fig. 7.1 Displaced fracture of the humeral neck. (**a**) 3D reconstruction of CT scan of the shoulder shows proximal migration of the shaft and (**b**) axillary lateral shows apex anterior angulation and translation. (Courtesy of C Moon)

Etiology of Failure of Fixation

Due to the strong unbalanced tendinous forces involved in displaced fractures of the surgical neck, osteosynthesis of fractures requires a thorough understanding of the pathoanatomy of the injury to resist these forces following fixation. The most common mechanisms of failure of fixation include varus collapse, screw penetration of the humeral head, tuberosity displacement, and avascular necrosis [2]. An anatomic restoration of the medial column is critical to preventing loss of reduction and failure of fixation [3]. Multiple biomechanical and clinical studies have shown that the use of an intramedullary nail [4], intramedullary structural support of the medial surgical neck with allograft fibula or bone cement [5–9], and/or appropriate placement of locking screws into the inferior humeral head [10–12] significantly enhances the stability of the fracture fixation construct (Fig. 7.2). The most common causes for fixation failure include fracture patterns at high risk for avascular necrosis (AVN) [2], fractures with inadequate bone for fixation in the humeral head [13], varus malreduction [5], advanced age, and poor bone quality [2, 5] (Fig. 7.3).

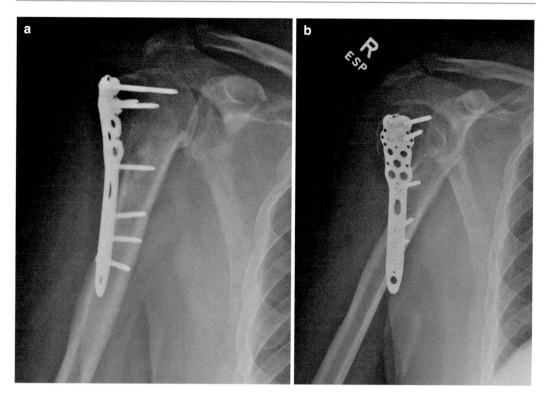

Fig. 7.2 Failure of fixation 3 months postoperatively. Note the (**a**) lack of medial column screw placement or intramedullary support, medial translation, and (**b**) extension deformity. (Courtesy of M Stone)

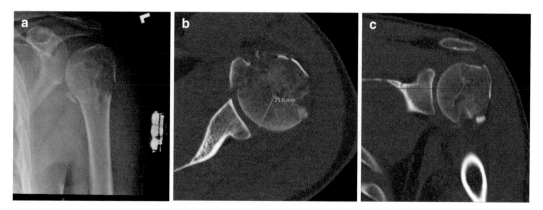

Fig. 7.3 Displaced fracture in a 62-year-old type 1 diabetic. Note the (**a**) varus displacement and absence of medial metaphyseal bone attached to the humeral head, (**b**) borderline amount of bone available in the humeral head for fixation, and (**c**) involvement of the lesser and greater tuberosities making this a complex four-part fracture. Arthroplasty should be considered in this patient given the high risk of fixation failure and AVN

Clinical Examination

A detailed history and physical exam should be performed on any patient presenting with failure of fixation of the humeral neck. Medical conditions such as diabetes, inflammatory arthropathies, osteoporosis, renal disease, cardiac disease, and immunosuppressive conditions should be assessed to assist with surgical decision-making and general perioperative risk. Similarly, a detailed social history including tobacco and recreational drug use and housing status should be obtained. The patient should be asked about any evidence of infection such as wound healing complications or treatment with oral or intravenous (IV) antibiotics. Prior surgical details and operative reports should be obtained whenever possible to identify implants and surgical approach. The patient's active medication list should be confirmed with careful attention paid to opioids, anti-inflammatory, and adjunct pain medication use. A clear understanding of the patient's functional goals can be very helpful in guiding the decision-making process.

The affected shoulder should be careful evaluated for functional deficits in both strength and range of motion compared to the intact side. Any neurological deficits in the extremity should be carefully documented. Surgical scars should be noted and evaluated for any evidence of active infection. Additionally, one should assess the patient's shoulder function prior to their previous surgical procedure in terms of rotator cuff function, impingement, or functional limitations.

Diagnostic Evaluation

The patient should be evaluated for both acute and chronic infection on presentation. In addition to the history and physical, evidence of infection can be ascertained via a complete blood count and inflammatory serologic markers though these values alone may not be sensitive in cases of chronic indolent infection [14, 15]. In high-risk cases or if considering arthroplasty, a shoulder aspiration or even image-guided percutaneous bone biopsy may be considered.

Endocrine abnormalities should also be considered in fixation failures, particularly those concerning vitamin D and calcium. Brinker et al. recommended a detailed laboratory panel based on a high rate of endocrinopathies found in their 2007 nonunion cohort [16].

Advanced imaging can be very helpful in preoperative planning or to aid with surgical decision-making. Metal artifact reduction sequences for both computed tomography (CT) and magnetic resonance imaging (MRI) can provide a significant amount of information regarding remaining intact bone for fixation or rotator cuff integrity for arthroplasty (Fig. 7.4). If there is a concern for neurological injury, an electromyographic (EMG) study may be obtained to confirm or complement the physical exam and may determine whether the patient is a candidate for reverse total shoulder arthroplasty.

7 Failed Fixation of the Humeral Neck Fracture

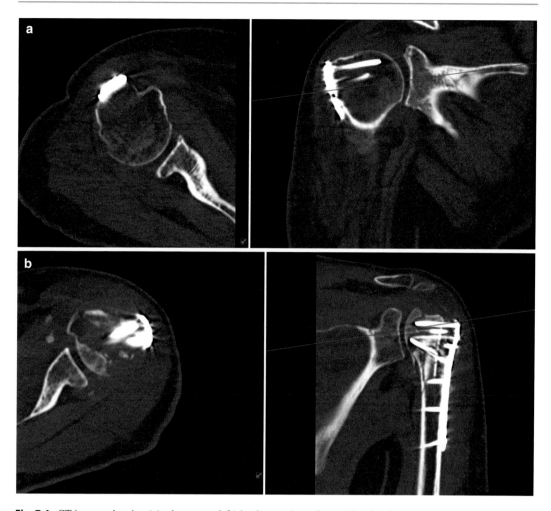

Fig. 7.4 CT images showing (**a**) adequate and (**b**) inadequate bone for revision fixation

Preoperative Planning

Once the patient's diagnostic evaluation is complete, and it has been determined that surgical management of the failed humeral neck is in line with the patient's functional goals, the surgeon may proceed with preoperative planning.

Whenever possible, the patient's prior operative reports and imaging should be used to identify any hardware that is currently implanted so that the proper screwdrivers can be obtained. However, these records are not often available, and as such universal screw removal sets, broken screw removal sets, straight and curved osteotomes, and straight and angled curettes are very useful to remove unidentified or overgrown hardware. Occasionally, if the hardware cannot be identified, no available screwdrivers will fit, or if the locked screws are cold-welded into the plate, high-speed metal-cutting disks or burrs may be necessary to cut through old implants. The use of sterile lubricant during burring can be helpful at limiting metal debris contamination of the soft tissues. In cases of incarcerated intramedullary rods, long, thin, flexible osteotomes, such as those used to remove cemented hip stems, and removal sets specifically designed for intramedullary rods may be necessary.

The presence of old incisions or wounds around the shoulder and implant choice may influence what surgical approach is used. Additionally, the robust vascularity of the shoulder often allows for multiple incisions, though in general it is best to avoid creating long, narrow skin bridges [17]. The deltopectoral approach to the shoulder is an extensile intermuscular and internervous approach that is the most used approach for the shoulder and useful for a wide variety of open procedures [18]. However, the deltopectoral approach has limited access to the posterior structures, is not often in line with access for intramedullary nailing or placement of a lateral plate, and often requires violation of the subscapularis for intra-articular fragments without lesser tuberosity involvement. For this reason, the deltoid splitting approach has been described as an alternative approach. It has been shown to be successful for fixation fractures with diaphyseal extension as well as intra-articular involvement, though it may place the axillary nerve at greater risk [19–22].

In situations where the patient has an active infection or there is a very strong concern for one, then it is best to proceed in a staged fashion with removal of all implants first with high-quality intraoperative cultures or frozen section prior to inserting new implants. In grossly infected failures of fixation, a temporizing antibiotic spacer or beads may be necessary to obtain adequate infection control combined with antibiotic-coated plates or nails for boney stabilization.

Implant Selection

If the patient has a healed malunion but function is acceptable and the main concern is articular penetration of screws, then a simple screw and plate removal is adequate. For cases where function and alignment are unacceptable, a thorough consideration of the reason for failure (Fig. 7.5) and status of remaining bone is critical. Based on the presumed mode of failure, the surgeon may elect to revise the fixation with a nail or plate where there is adequate bone for fixation or convert to arthroplasty in cases of poor bone or AVN (Fig. 7.4). If there is robust bone in the majority of the humeral head despite prior fixation, revision to either plate with appropriately placed medial calcar screws with or without augmentation or use of an intramedullary nail is reasonable (Fig. 7.6a and b). Current studies suggest that at least 25-mm humeral head thickness is necessary for adequate fixation [13]. In contrast, where there is little bone in the head for revision fixation or if the quality of the bone is suspect, arthroplasty may be the most appropriate choice

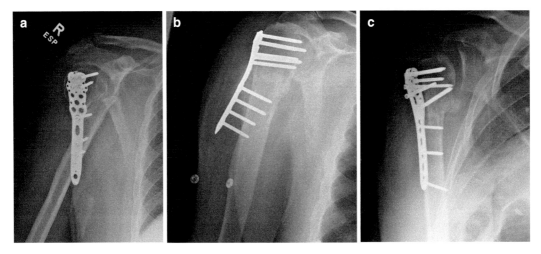

Fig. 7.5 Modes of failure: (**a**) loss of reduction from lack of medial column support; (**b**) loss of reduction from pullout of locked screws in osteoporotic diaphysis; and (**c**) loss of fixation from AVN of the head

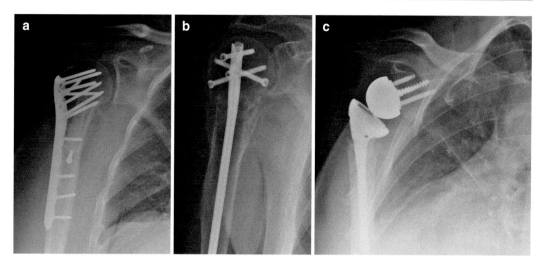

Fig. 7.6 (**a**) Revision fixation with plate and intramedullary strut allograft augmentation; (**b**) revision fixation with intramedullary nail; and (**c**) revision to reverse total shoulder arthroplasty

(Fig. 7.6c). In all situations, it is important to preoperatively template to anticipate implant size and type, as well as placement and location of screws in the humeral head for appropriate purchase. Additionally, it is critical to discuss the patient's goals of treatment and desired level of function with secondary surgical intervention.

Bone Grafting

Because of the robust vascularity of the shoulder, atrophic nonunions are rare, and most explanations for fixation failure can be traced back to improper implant selection, inadequate reduction, or inadequate fixation construct [5]. Autograft, allograft, and tricalcium phosphate have all been described in the management of bone voids for proximal humerus nonunions with equivalent healing rates, though the use of autograft may result in shorter healing times [23, 24].

Structural allografts or injectable tricalcium phosphate for bone augmentation has been shown to increase the rigidity of a construct and decrease the rate of screw cut-out [6, 10, 25]. In particular, the use of fibular shaft allograft to create an intramedullary support of the medial calcar has been shown to significantly increase stiffness and failure load even in the presence of medial bone loss [10].

Surgery

The patient in Fig. 7.2 presented 3 months after initial open reduction internal fixation with a locking plate through a deltoid split approach. There were no signs or indications of an infection. A CT scan showed adequate bone in the humeral head for revision fixation (Fig. 7.4a).

The patient was placed in the beach chair position and a deltopectoral approach was used. The prior plate was removed without incident. Following plate removal, the patient was found to have an intercalary spiral oblique segment of the proximal humeral shaft, which had not healed. This was anatomically reduced and lagged. The biceps tendon was noted to be frayed and so was released from its groove and origin for later tenodesis.

A fibula shaft allograft was then contoured and trimmed to fit into the medullary canal. A hand reamer was inserted into the head retrograde to create a space for the allograft in the humeral head in line with the humeral shaft. The fibula allograft was carefully tamped into place while being stabilized and manipulated with a threaded Steinmann pin (Fig. 7.7a). Initially the allograft was difficult to insert into the humeral shaft and caused distraction at the nonunion site (Fig. 7.7b) and so was trimmed further for ease of

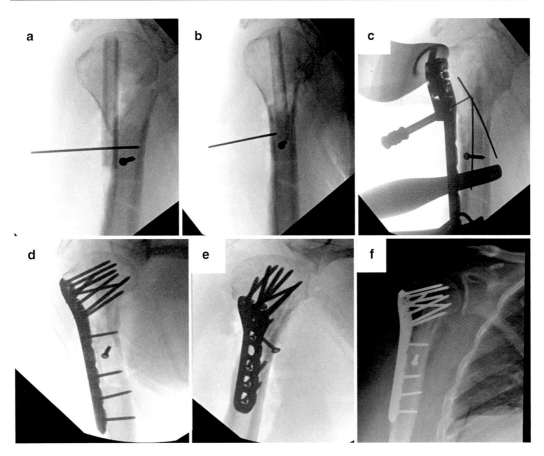

Fig. 7.7 Intraoperative fluoroscopy of revision plate fixation with intramedullary strut graft. (**a**) Insertion of the contoured fibula shaft allograft into the humeral head using a threaded Steinmann pin as a joystick. (**b**) Insertion of the base of the fibular shaft allograft into the humeral shaft with the allograft pinned in place and resting on the previously inserted lag screw. (**c**) Application of a proximal humeral locking plate using the medial support screws as a reference for height. Final fluoroscopic views show anatomic restoration of neck angle (**d**) and sagittal alignment (**e**) with union at 1 year (**f**)

insertion. Note that insertion of the intramedullary allograft alone significantly improved sagittal and coronal alignment. The allograft was placed medially in the shaft and medial head to provide additional medial column support. The allograft was then pinned in place while the locking plate was positioned for optimal inferomedial support screw placement (Fig. 7.7c). Shaft screws were placed to compress the plate to bone followed by placement of locking screws in the head through the fibular allograft and inferomedial support screw placement reestablishing after the anatomic valgus neck shaft angle (Fig. 7.7d) and sagittal alignment (Fig. 7.7e).

Postoperatively, the patient was allowed immediate full passive range of motion and allowed to begin weight bearing at 6 weeks. The patient had 90% recovery of his range of motion compared to the other side with complete union at 1 year (Fig. 7.7f).

Summary: Lessons Learned

Failed fixation of the humeral neck is a challenging diagnosis that is frequently the result of inadequate fixation due to poor bone quality or a suboptimal fixation strategy. A detailed failure analysis is necessary for surgical decision-making and subsequent implant choice. In revision fixation, restoration of the anatomic neck shaft angle and correction of sagittal malalignment are critical for a good outcome. Once the alignment is restored, appropriate medial calcar support either through the use of an intramedullary implant, structural allograft, or locking screw placement is necessary to maintain the reduction and facilitate early mobilization for an optimal recovery.

References

1. Duparc F. Malunion of the proximal humerus. Orthop Traumatol Surg Res. 2013;99:S1–S11.
2. Solberg BD, Moon CN, Franco DP, Paiement GD. Locked plating of 3- and 4-part proximal Humerus fractures in older patients: the effect of initial fracture pattern on outcome. J Orthop Trauma. 2009;23:113–9.
3. Gardner MJ, et al. The importance of medial support in locked plating of proximal humerus fractures. J Orthop Trauma. 2007;21:185–91.
4. Yoon RS, et al. A comprehensive update on current fixation options for two-part proximal humerus fractures. Injury. 2014;45:510–4.
5. Krappinger D, et al. Predicting failure after surgical fixation of proximal humerus fractures. Injury. 2011;42:1283–8.
6. Schliemann B, et al. How to enhance the stability of locking plate fixation of proximal humerus fractures? An overview of current biomechanical and clinical data. Injury. 2015;46:1207–14.
7. Berkes MB, Little MTM, Lorich DG. Open reduction internal fixation of proximal humerus fractures. Curr Rev Musculoskelet Med. 2013;6:47–56.
8. Matassi F, et al. Locking plate and fibular allograft augmentation in unstable fractures of proximal humerus. Injury. 2012;43:1939–42.
9. Little MTM, et al. The impact of preoperative coronal plane deformity on proximal humerus fixation with endosteal augmentation. J Orthop Trauma. 2014;28:338–47.
10. Katthagen JC, et al. Biomechanical effects of calcar screws and bone block augmentation on medial support in locked plating of proximal humeral fractures. Clin Biomech. 2014;29:735–41.
11. Padegimas EM, et al. Defining optimal calcar screw positioning in proximal humerus fracture fixation. J Shoulder Elb Surg. 2017;26:1931–7.

12. Mehta S, Chin M, Sanville J, Namdari S, Hast MW. Calcar screw position in proximal humerus fracture fixation: don't miss high! Injury. 2018;49:624–9.
13. Stern L, Gorczyca MT, Gorczyca JT. Preoperative measurement of the thickness of the center of the humeral head predicts screw cutout after locked plating of proximal humeral fractures. J Shoulder Elb Surg. 2021;30(1):80–8. https://doi.org/10.1016/j.jse.2020.03.047. Epub 2020 Jun 9. PMID: 33317705.
14. Govaert GAM, et al. Diagnosing fracture-related infection: current concepts and recommendations. J Orthop Trauma. 2020;34:8–17.
15. Brinker MR, Macek J, Laughlin M, Dunn WR. Utility of common biomarkers for diagnosing infection in nonunion. J Orthop Trauma. 2021;35:121–7.
16. Brinker MR, O'Connor DP, Monla YT, Earthman TP. Metabolic and endocrine abnormalities in patients with nonunions. J Orthop Trauma. 2007;21:14.
17. Memarzadeh K, Sheikh R, Blohmé J, Torbrand C, Malmsjö M. Perfusion and oxygenation of random advancement skin flaps depend more on the length and thickness of the flap than on the width to length ratio. Eplasty. 2016;16:e12.
18. Chalmers PN, Van Thiel GS, Trenhaile SW. Surgical exposures of the shoulder. J Am Acad Orthop Surg. 2016;24:250–8.
19. Gardner MJ. Deltoid-splitting approach. J Orthop Trauma. 2022;36:158.
20. Gardner MJ, Boraiah S, Helfet DL, Lorich DG. The anterolateral acromial approach for fractures of the proximal humerus. J Orthop Trauma. 2008;22:132–7.
21. Westphal T, Woischnik S, Adolf D, Feistner H, Piatek S. Axillary nerve lesions after open reduction and internal fixation of proximal humeral fractures through an extended lateral deltoid-split approach: electrophysiological findings. J Shoulder Elb Surg. 2017;26:464–71.
22. Berkes MB, et al. Intramedullary allograft fibula as a reduction and fixation tool for treatment of complex proximal humerus fractures with diaphyseal extension. J Orthop Trauma. 2014;28:e56–64.
23. Zastrow RK, Patterson DC, Cagle PJ. Operative management of proximal humerus nonunions in adults: a systematic review. J Orthop Trauma. 2020;34:492–502.
24. Yamane S, Suenaga N, Oizumi N, Minami A. Interlocking intramedullary nailing for nonunion of the proximal humerus with the straight nail system. J Shoulder Elb Surg. 2008;17:755–9.
25. Egol KA, et al. Fracture site augmentation with calcium phosphate cement reduces screw penetration after open reduction–internal fixation of proximal humeral fractures. J Shoulder Elb Surg. 2012;21:741–8.

Humeral Shaft Fracture: Failed Intramedullary Nail Fixation

8

Ashley Lamb, Ian Hasegawa, and Joshua L. Gary

History of Previous Primary Failed Treatment

Humeral shaft fractures are relatively common injuries treated by orthopedic surgeons and account for 1.3–3% of all fractures [1]. Although many of these injuries can be successfully treated with nonoperative management, absolute and relative indications for operative treatment exist. These indications may include anatomic location of fracture, unacceptable alignment with closed treatment, patient's ability to comply with nonoperative management, open fractures, associated vascular injury, brachial plexopathy, polytrauma, ipsilateral forearm fractures, and/or patient preference for surgical treatment.

Humeral intramedullary (IM) nailing provides fixation without violating the periosteal blood supply adjacent to the fracture fragments when closed reduction techniques are used. Open approaches for reduction may still be done prior to instrumentation with a nail. Proper patient selection, fracture characteristics, and meticulous surgical technique are essential to the success of this procedure. Although intramedullary devices were first described by Kuntscher in the 1940s [2, 3], humeral intramedullary nailing was disseminated by Seidel with the addition of distal locking fins that aimed to improve rotational control [3]. Nonlocked devices such as K-wires, flexible nails, and Enders nails have largely been abandoned secondary to inability of rotational control predisposing the fracture to increased strain [1]. Humeral intramedullary nailing became increasingly popular in the 1990s as surgical techniques evolved and there was a trend toward minimally invasive surgery. Distal locking screws were introduced in the early 2000s, which significantly improved rotational control of the construct and improved reliability of fixation. Although humeral IM nail rotational control was improved with the addition of locking screws, axial and rotational stability remains decreased compared to plates [4]. Humeral IM nail usage among surgeons has been down trending in the recent decade with a significant decline in use [5]. Gottschalk et al. hypothesized that the decline in humeral IM nail use was multifactorial including implant cost, device specifics, and recent literature describing increased shoulder pain and nonunions compared to open reduction and internal fixation (ORIF) [5].

A. Lamb
Keck School of Medicine USC,
Los Angeles, CA, USA

I. Hasegawa
John A. Burns School of Medicine, University of Hawai'i, Honolulu, HI, USA
e-mail: iangh@hawaii.edu

J. L. Gary (✉)
Department of Orthopaedic Surgery, Keck School of Medicine of the University of Southern California, Los Angeles, CA, USA

© The Author(s), under exclusive license to Springer Nature Switzerland AG 2024
P. V. Giannoudis, P. Tornetta III (eds.), *Failed Fracture Fixation*,
https://doi.org/10.1007/978-3-031-39692-2_8

Evaluation of the Etiology of Failure of Fixation

Failed fixation with humeral IM nails can be attributed to mechanical properties, biologic factors, or be multifactorial. The humerus is subject to more rotatory forces and less axial loading; thus, this is the force that can most jeopardize fixation. Biomechanically, intramedullary nail fixation provides a load sharing device. Interlocking screws through the nail provide a counter to the rotational forces seen at the humerus. Clinical results utilizing locked humeral IM nails have not been as successful as similar constructs utilized in the lower extremities [6]. The literature regarding fixation failure after intramedullary nailing of humeral shaft fractures is scant and based primarily on retrospective case series. Nonetheless, these studies highlight two key causes of failure: insufficient construct stability and fracture distraction. Fracture distraction has been a common reported cause of humeral shaft nonunion after intramedullary nailing. The etiology can be iatrogenic or secondary to insufficient axial stability. Iatrogenic fracture distraction can occur during antegrade nail insertion due to the rapid narrowing of the medullary canal from proximal to distal [7–9]. Canal diameters of less than 8 mm have been noted in several studies [9, 10], and smaller diameter nails would provide decreased stability. In a retrospective series of 111 humeral shaft fractures treated with first- and second-generation nails, fracture distraction was noted in 14 cases (12.6%), five of which went on to delayed union or nonunion [10]. All five of these fractures were locked in distraction greater than 4 mm. On the other hand, late fracture distraction may occur from the lack of axial compression because the humerus is a nonweight-bearing bone [11]. The humerus is subject to gravitational downward forces, increasing distraction strain at the fracture site, which may contribute to nonunion formation [6, 12]. This is in contrast to the axially loaded force seen in the lower extremities with the use of intramedullary devices [6, 12]. Tsourvakas [13] reported two humeral shaft nonunions after intramedullary nailing secondary to late fracture distraction. Both fractures were initially locked with a gap less than 3 mm. However, at follow-up, both gaps were noted to be greater than 6 mm [13].

Proximal and distal third diaphyseal fractures are at particular risk for intramedullary fixation failure due to insufficient construct stability. Failure rates have ranged between 0 and 50% [4]. Fractures of the proximal third diaphysis, or intermuscular zone [14, 15], are subject to high deforming forces from the pectoralis major, deltoid, and latissimus dorsi insertions. This leads to a typical valgus medialized proximal segment and shortened distal segment. Varus deformity can also occur when the main fracture line is distal to the deltoid insertion. Similar to proximal femur fracture fixation, longer implants with fixed-angular stability are needed to withstand these rotational forces over time. In many instances, however, humeral nail length is limited by the restraints of the distal humerus medullary canal [9]. Additionally, early generation nails consisted of limited proximal and distal interlocking options (e.g., single, uniplanar, and dynamic locking). Nail length and angular stability have also been a concern for distal third diaphyseal fractures. Metsemakers et al. reported two failures after intramedullary nailing [16]. In one case, the short working length of the nail in the distal segment led to toggling of the distal humerus with subsequent widening of the canal, loosening of the screw, and finally a peri-implant fracture. In the second case, late fracture distraction occurred after the distal interlocking screw loosened.

Clinical Examination

In patients with humeral shaft nonunion, subjective complaints of pain at the fracture site and difficulty with repetitive movements are the main reported factors [17]. Clinical evaluation should begin with inspection and evaluation of the skin. Inspection of incisions for location of prior surgical approach is important as they may be used or extended for surgical revision. Erythema, warmth, or discoloration should be noted and give warning that underlying indolent infection may be present. Drainage or sinus tracts should be documented and almost certainly imply underlying infection [18]. Tenderness or discomfort about the fracture site should be documented. A thorough neurovascular exam including gross motor strength grading from 0 to 5, sensation throughout the upper extremity, and distal perfusion should also be noted. Active and passive range of motion at the shoulder to include flexion, extension, abduction, internal rotation, and external rotation should also be evaluated. The passive arc of motion may hinder retrieval of the nail if unable to position the arm in the appropriate collinear trajectory of the original insertion point. Antegrade humeral IM nails utilize a start point that may jeopardize the integrity of the rotator cuff; therefore, evaluation and special testing of the rotator cuff musculature is recommended. Shoulder impingement from antegrade humeral nailing is a known complication and should be evaluated in these patients. In addition, preoperative function of the peripheral motor and sensory nerves should be assessed. Radial nerve palsies are present in 10–20% of patients at initial presentation with humeral shaft fractures [3]. Radial nerve palsies manifest with wrist drop, difficulty extending the fingers, and sensory loss about the dorsal and radial hand. After fixation with humeral IM nails, postoperative palsies are relatively rare, but have been documented at rates <3% [3]. The axillary nerve is at risk with the placement of proximal interlocking screws and the radial nerve is at risk with the placement of transverse distal interlocking screws. Gross motion about the fracture site or around the implant is important to recognize as this could portend delayed union or nonunion.

Diagnostic-Biochemical and Radiological Investigations

Standard orthogonal AP and lateral views of the humerus should be obtained. Radiographs should be assessed for bone quality, implant position, nail and interlocking screw integrity, and evidence of hardware loosening. Alignment and rotation of the humerus should be evaluated, not-ing any deformity that may be present contributing to the failure of the current construct and to address at the time of revision. Interfragmentary diastasis, if present, should be noted. Nonunion characteristics should be documented and provide the treating surgeon insight into the method of failure. The type of nonunion, hypertrophic versus oligotrophic versus atrophic, should first be defined. Hypertrophic nonunions demonstrate hypertrophic and sclerotic fracture margins with abundant callus formation. Hypertrophic nonunions are often present in the setting of malalignment or mechanical instability and indicate a perfused and preserved biologic environment that permits fracture healing. Atrophic nonunions demonstrate osteopenic characteristics at the fracture margins with absent callus formation. Atrophic nonunions have compromised vascular supply and/or a disrupted biologic environment that prevents normal fracture healing. Radiographs should also be assessed for evidence of osteonecrosis of the humeral head, pathologic fracture, and extent of bone loss [17]. CT may be a useful modality to evaluate bony healing when fracture characteristics and consolidation are difficult to assess on radiographs. In a retrospective series of failed humeral intramedullary nailing, Allende found that 34% of failures demonstrated atrophic nonunions and 66% demonstrated oligotrophic nonunions [4]. In the setting of atrophic nonunions, the local fracture environment may have poor vascularity and will have a higher chance for superimposed infection [18]. Prior infection should be evaluated with a standardized protocol including complete blood count (CBC), C-reactive protein (CRP), and erythrocyte sedimentation rate (ESR) as elevated ESR and CRP have been found to be independent risk factors in the setting of nonunion [19]. When using CBC, ESR, and CRP, Stucken et al. [19] reported that based on the number of abnormal lab values (0, 1, 2, and 3), the predicted probability of infection was 20, 19, 56, and 100%, respectively. Infection should be addressed and eradicated prior to definitive revision for successful treatment and ultimate union. Fracture healing is a complex symphony of metabolic pathways, that, if disrupted, can lead to impaired healing and potential nonunion [20]. Metabolic status should be evaluated with a basic metabolic panel (BMP) to assess any underlying medical conditions that may be contributing to the nonunion [17, 20]. Protein deficiency, vitamin D deficiency, calcium abnormalities, and thyroid/parathyroid disorders are known modifiable risk factors that should be addressed for optimal bone healing [20]. Bone stock and working length of revision construct should be considered. A "windshield wiper effect" at humerus nonunion site in the setting of intramedullary nailing can compromise bone stock and lead to osteolysis [6] presenting the treating surgeon with limitations for fixation in the face of revision.

Preoperative Planning

Removal of hardware can be a challenge. Formulation of a preoperative plan with the appropriate equipment available is crucial for success. Preoperative radiographs should be analyzed for the integrity of the intramedullary nail and note any signs of failure or hardware breakage. With identification of the implant, system-specific removal devices can be obtained to aid the surgeon with interlocking screw removal and nail extraction. If implant-specific devices are not available, a universal extraction device such as the SHUKLA Nail (S9NAIL) Universal IM Nail Extraction System (formerly known as the Winquist) can be used. The SHUKLA Nail Extraction System device has a multitude of extraction attachments including a conical extractor that can be threaded into the nail and a solid nail removal device in which trephines cut into the outer aspect of the nail allowing for removal. There are several different size hook options that can be utilized to retrieve the nail or broken pieces of the nail by engaging the interlocking holes within the nail. If the intramedullary nail is broken, there are many described techniques for the retrieval [21]. Abdelgawad et al. [21] described eight different methods for extraction of broken nails. Of the methods described, the most common and easily reproducible is a technique of interference fit with a ball-tipped guidewire that is passed past the tip of the nail and a second smooth guidewire passed past the tip, creating a friction fit [21, 22]. As the ball-tipped wire is removed, the nail is retrieved. A universal large fragment screwdriver can be utilized to remove interlocking screws that may be present. In the setting of broken screws, a variety of techniques have been described for removal [22]. The Synthes Screw Removal Set has a variety of extraction attachments including a reverse thread conical screw attachment that can cut into a screw head for removal, and a trephine that can cut around the screw if necessary. Hak et al. [22] describe the usefulness and effectiveness of screw extractors, trephines, and extraction bolts for removing stripped or broken screws. Broken screws may also be advanced out by impaction with a Steinmann pin [22].

New Implant Selection

Patient and fracture failure characteristics should determine implant selection for revision. For failed humeral IM nails, options include hardware removal with plate osteosynthesis, exchange nailing, and plate augmentation to the current construct. Each revision construct has a unique set of properties and advantages and the decision should be tailored to the individual situation.

Plating

Hardware removal and plate osteosynthesis afford the surgeon opportunity to correct malalignment, evaluate the nonunion site, apply bone graft, and compress or bridge across the fracture site. Compression plate osteosynthesis for the treatment of humeral shaft nonunions, with the goal of primary bone healing, has achieved excellent results reported in literature [17]. McKee et al. [6] reported a series of patients who underwent humeral IM nail with nonunion. In this series, nine of nine patients who were treated with IM nail removal and compression plating with bone grafting progressed to union [6]. This option allows for correction of angular or rotational deformities that contribute to the failure of the primary construct and provides improved rotational stability. If necessary, shortening osteotomy with compression plate osteosynthesis may be performed. Limb length discrepancy in the arm is well tolerated up to 3 cm [23].

Exchange Nailing

Exchange nailing is an option when the diameter of the primary humeral IM nail is mismatched with the isthmus of the humerus, lacking stability of the construct. However, based on current literature, exchange nailing of the humerus has been well established to not produce good results [6, 12, 24–26]. A few studies have reported small cohorts of patients who have undergone exchange nailing [12]. Robinson [24] demonstrated two of five patients who ultimately achieved union following exchange nailing. McKee et al. [6] reported four of ten patients who underwent exchange nailing, three of ten who had open bone grafting, of whom only two of four patients ultimately achieved union. This is compared to nine of nine (100%) union rate in the same series of patients who underwent plate fixation after failed humeral IM nail, which demonstrates the superiority of plate fixation. The authors hypothesized that failure of exchange nailing could be a result of the osteolysis and loss of bone from failure of the locking screws [6, 12]. Flinkkila [25] reported three of 13 patients who achieved union after exchange nail. Lin [26] described 22 of 23 patients who achieved union after the exchange nail. It should be noted that all in this series had bone autograft applied at the nonunion site and 83% had interfragmentary wiring at the nonunion site. Unsuccessful humerus exchange nailing is hypothesized to be multifactorial and likely due to the bone loss at the nonunion site, cortical thinning due to windshield wiper effect, and absence of cyclical loading in humerus [6, 27].

Based on this evidence, exchange nailing has a limited role in revision surgery for failed humeral IM nailing.

Plate Augmentation (Plating without Nail Removal)

Plate augmentation to a humeral IM nail construct is a viable option in the setting of rotational instability. The intramedullary nail maintains load sharing and bending strength and the addition of a plate augments rotational stability of the humerus. In a series of 37 patients with humeral nonunion in the setting of IM nailing, Gessmann et al. [28] described a successful 97% union rate at 6 months with plate augmentation. In this series, no deep infections or wound complications were reported. Patients demonstrated pain-free shoulder and elbow range of motion at 14 months postoperatively [28].

Need for Bone Grafting

Autogenous bone grafting has been successful in treating humerus nonunions [6, 17, 27, 29]. Autogenous bone graft may be harvested from the iliac crest (or other anatomic sites for harvest such as the proximal tibia) or from the intramedullary canal of long bones with the Synthes Reamer-Irrigator-Aspirator (RIA) system. The RIA system collects both a solid and a liquid graft from canal reamings that are filtered from waste products. Both the solid and liquid graft are rich in mesenchymal stem cells [30]. The RIA system has the advantage of acquiring larger volumes of bone graft and stem cells with less donor site morbidity compared to iliac crest bone graft [17, 30]. In patients with a large cortical defect with the need for biologic augmentation, free vascularized fibula graft provides mechanical and physiologic support [17]. Allograft may be considered in patients who will not tolerate donor site morbidity or in the setting of augmenting autograft.

Revision Surgery

Patient Presentation

A 17-year-old male patient presented to the emergency department with right arm pain after sustaining a ballistic injury from a shotgun. He was reaching into the back seat of his truck when his shotgun had an accidental discharge. He reported numbness about the radial nerve distribution and inability to extend his fingers.

Examination demonstrated a 6-cm ballistic entrance wound about the anteromedial arm and two large exit wounds on the posterolateral aspect of the arm with exposed muscle and bone (Fig. 8.1). He was noted to have a dense radial nerve palsy upon sensory and motor examination but was otherwise intact in all other distributions. There was no evidence of vascular injury with a 2+ radial pulse and hand that was warm and well perfused. Radiographs demonstrated a highly comminuted midshaft diaphyseal humerus fracture.

Initial Management

The patient was taken to the operating room on the day of presentation for debridement and irrigation with stabilization of the fracture with external fixator placement. The wounds were systematically debrided of nonviable tissue and deemed appropriate for primary closure. Multiple large, devitalized bony fragments were removed. The radial nerve segmental defect was identified and the proximal and distal ends were tagged with Prolene sutures. He was continued postoperatively on intravenous cefazolin for 48 h for open fracture management.

The patient returned to the operating room (OR) on hospital day 4 for repeat debridement, external fixator removal, and antegrade humeral IM nail placement (Fig. 8.2). The posterolateral traumatic wound was reopened and was exploited for the placement of an antibiotic cement spacer in the large segmental defect for the purpose of the Masquelet technique. There was no evidence of infection or necrotic tissue noted. The radial

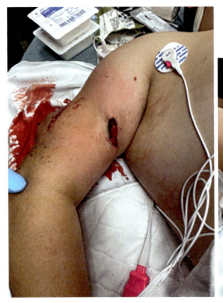
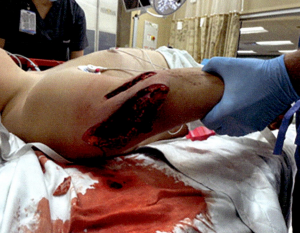

Fig. 8.1 Entry and exit ballistic wounds about the right humerus. (Image courtesy of Dr. Joshua L. Gary)

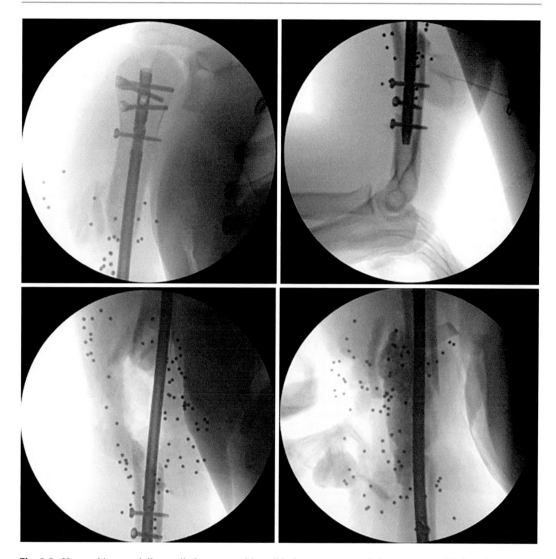

Fig. 8.2 Humeral intramedullary nail placement with antibiotic cement spacer in large segmental defect. (Image courtesy of Dr. Joshua L. Gary)

nerve deficit was explored with a hand specialist, who did not believe that nerve grafting would provide chance for meaningful functional recovery and planned delayed tendon transfers for improved function.

Due to large void/dead space, a Jackson-Pratt (JP) flat drain was placed within the wound to prevent fluid collection and was maintained for 8 weeks postoperatively (Fig. 8.3). He tolerated the procedure well and was encouraged to range his shoulder and elbow. His weightbearing was limited to activities of daily living (ADLs) and less than 5 lb.

The patient returned to the operating room 12 weeks postoperatively for the second stage of the Masquelet technique (Fig. 8.4). Synthes RIA was passed in a retrograde fashion within the patient's right femur for harvest of corticocancellous autogenous bone graft. A large volume of graft was obtained. Posterolateral wound about the humerus was again opened. Membrane surrounding the cement spacer was encountered and incised. Cement spacer was removed and bone graft was placed within the membrane that had formed around the large defect. No evidence of infection was encountered

Fixation Failure

The patient returned for follow-up 8 months postoperatively with increasing pain about the fracture site. Imaging demonstrated evidence of oligotrophic nonunion demonstrating minimal fracture consolidation and evidence of hardware failure with a distal interlocking screw backing out (Fig. 8.5). Infectious workup with CBC, BMP, ESR, and CRP was all within normal limits and there were no clinical signs of infection.

Revision Surgery

After discussion and shared decision-making with the patient, he returned to the operating room 10 months postoperatively for revision fixation and nonunion repair. The patient was placed on a radiolucent operating table with the right arm able to be extended off the edge of the bed and the nail was removed without complication. Of note, the most distal interlocking screw had broken and only the head of the screw was removed. The proximal aspect of the nail was cleared of soft tissue and bony debris, and an extraction bolt was threaded into the nail. The nail was back-slapped out of the humerus without complication. Vascularized free fibula graft was harvested from the ipsilateral lower leg and preserved on the back table. The anterolateral approach with proximal deltopectoral extension was made along the length of the arm gaining access to the nonunion site and providing adequate exposure of the proximal and distal aspect of the bone. Free fibula graft was introduced into the medullary canal of the humerus through the nonunion site and the vascular pedicle was anastomosed. Free fibula graft was utilized to provide both structural and biologic support of the nonunion. A bridging construct with dual plating of the humerus was performed utilizing 3.5-mm plates applied to the lateral and anteromedial surfaces of the humerus spanning the nonunion segment with appropriate working length. A long

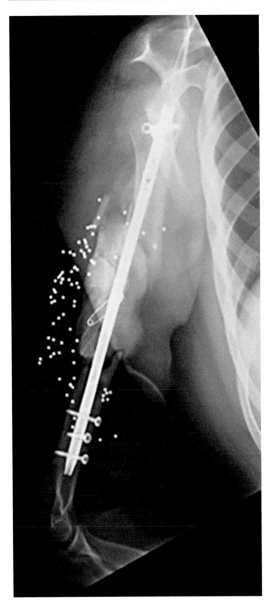

Fig. 8.3 8 weeks postoperatively with intact construct, maintained alignment, and JP drain in place. (Image courtesy of Dr. Joshua L. Gary)

during this procedure. He tolerated the procedure well and returned to ADLs 2 weeks postoperatively. His initial postoperative course was uneventful and the patient returned to activity without limitation (other than those associated with his radial nerve deficit) for several months.

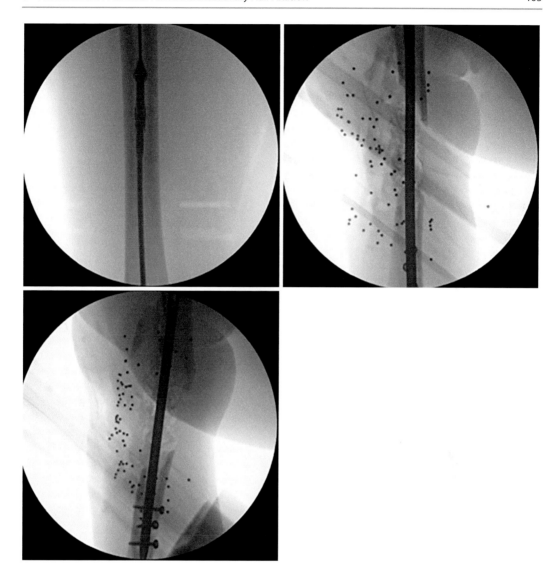

Fig. 8.4 RIA passage within femoral canal and second stage of the Masquelet technique with spacer removal and application of autogenous bone graft. (Image courtesy of Dr. Joshua L. Gary)

proximal humerus plate was chosen for lateral fixation to allow for proximal screw cluster fixation into the humeral head (Fig. 8.6). There was no evidence of infection at the time of revision surgery. Surgical wounds were closed primarily without undue tension. Soft dressing and a fracture brace were applied and the patient was encouraged to maintain gentle elbow and shoulder range of motion throughout the recovery process. The patient progressed to right upper extremity weightbearing as tolerated at 6 weeks postoperatively after revision surgery.

At 1 year postoperatively from revision surgery, the patient was doing well. His surgical incisions were healed and he reported no pain or signs of infection. Radiographs demonstrated bony union without evidence of hardware failure. He had full and painless range of motion about the shoulder and elbow. He was able to perform ADLs without pain about the humerus. He returned to baseball pitching (with his contralateral throwing arm) and subjectively reported a good outcome.

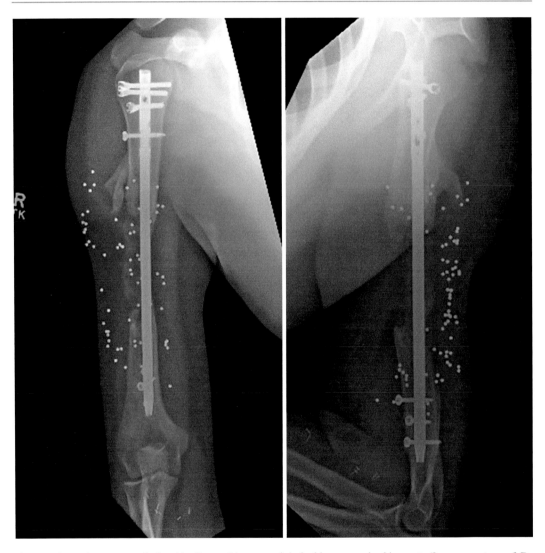

Fig. 8.5 8 months postoperatively with oligotrophic nonunion demonstrating minimal fracture consolidation and evidence of hardware failure with the proximal most distal interlocking screw backing out. (Image courtesy of Dr. Joshua L. Gary)

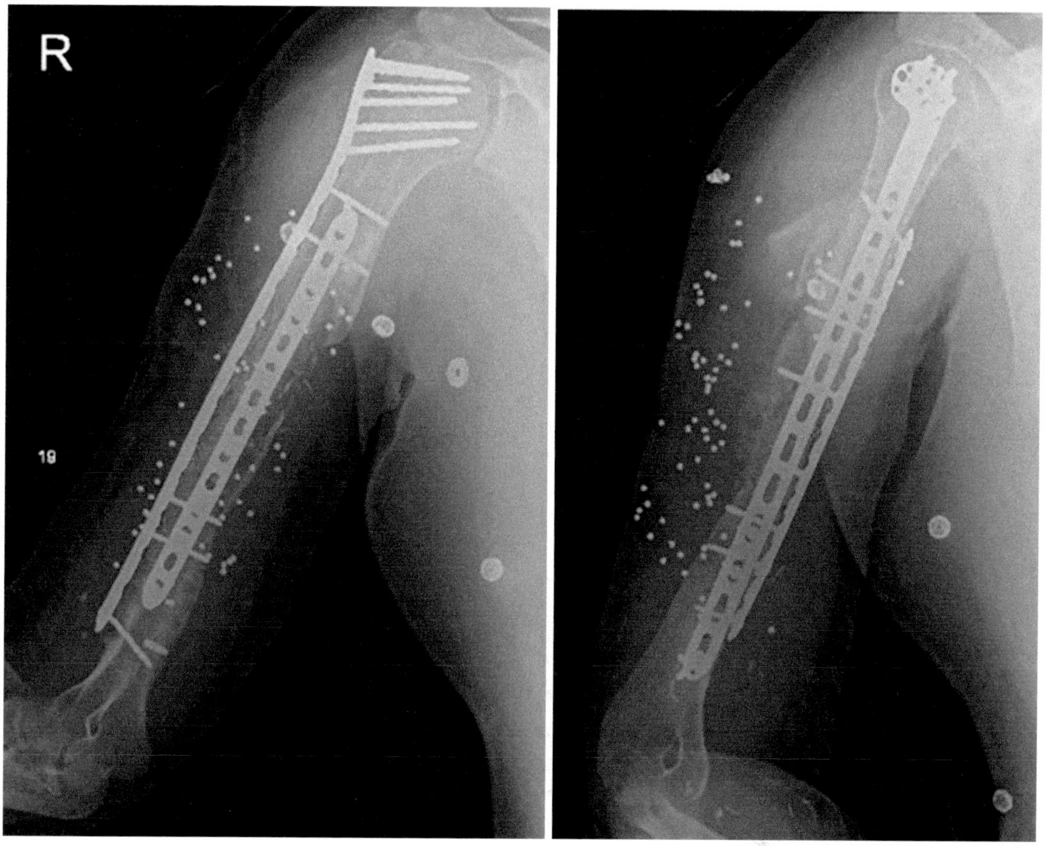

Fig. 8.6 Revision construct of the right humerus with free fibula graft and dual plating. (Image courtesy of Drs. Joshua L. Gary, Kyle Woerner, and Andrew M. Choo)

Summary: Lessons Learned

This case demonstrates a complex injury with a challenging clinical course to address. The patient had a large zone of soft tissue injury with a sizable segmental bone defect. Initial fixation with an intramedullary device was chosen to limit surface implants in a large, ballistic wound that would be prone to infection and potential wound complications. Meticulous systematic debridement and primary soft tissue closure at the initial procedure were critical for maintaining a clean environment for healing. Our patient was fortunate to have no evidence of infection throughout his clinical course. His initial fixation was successful for 8 months postoperatively until he presented with hardware failure and nonunion. A decision was made to proceed with open repair and plating to allow for enhanced biomechanical stability and direct access to the nonunion site for grafting. Free fibula graft was chosen to provide structural and biologic support at the nonunion site. Since revision, the patient has had a successful postoperative course and has returned to ADLs and recreational activities without pain.

References

1. Updegrove GF, Mourad W, Abboud JA. Humeral shaft fractures. J Shoulder Elb Surg. 2018;27(4):e87–97.
2. Kuentscher G. Intramedullary splinting. Med Bull U S Army Force Europe Theater Off Theater Chief Surg. 1947;3(2):5–8.
3. Pidhorz L. Acute and chronic humeral shaft fractures in adults. Orthop Traumatol Surg Res. 2015;101(1 Suppl):S41–9.

4. Allende C, Paz A, Altube G, Boccolini H, Malvarez A, Allende B. Revision with plates of humeral nonunions secondary to failed intramedullary nailing. Int Orthop. 2014;38(4):899–903.

5. Gottschalk MB, Carpenter W, Hiza E, Reisman W, Roberson J. Humeral shaft fracture fixation: incidence rates and complications as reported by American Board of Orthopaedic Surgery Part II candidates. J Bone Joint Surg Am. 2016;98(17):e71.

6. McKee MD, Miranda MA, Riemer BL, Blasier RB, Redmond BJ, Sims SH, Waddell JP, Jupiter JB. Management of humeral nonunion after the failure of locking intramedullary nails. J Orthop Trauma. 1996;10(7):492–9.

7. Rommens PM, Kuechle R, Bord T, Lewens T, Engelmann R, Blum J. Humeral nailing revisited. Injury. 2008;39(12):1319–28.

8. Cole PA, Wijdicks CA. The operative treatment of diaphyseal humeral shaft fractures. Hand Clin. 2007;23(4):437–48. vi

9. Drew AJ, Tashjian RZ, Henninger HB, Bachus KN. Sex and laterality differences in medullary humerus morphology. Anat Rec (Hoboken). 2019;302(10):1709–17.

10. Baltov A, Mihail R, Dian E. Complications after interlocking intramedullary nailing of humeral shaft fractures. Injury. 2014;45(Suppl 1):S9–S15.

11. Lammens J, Bauduin G, Driesen R, Moens P, Stuyck J, De Smet L, Fabry G. Treatment of nonunion of the humerus using the Ilizarov external fixator. Clin Orthop Relat Res. 1998;353:223–30.

12. Brinker MR, O'Connor DP. Exchange nailing of ununited fractures. J Bone Joint Surg Am. 2007;89(1):177–88.

13. Tsourvakas S, Alexandropoulos C, Papachristos I, Tsakoumis G, Ameridis N. Treatment of humeral shaft fractures with antegrade intramedullary locking nail. Musculoskelet Surg. 2011;95(3):193–8.

14. McKee MD. Fractures of the shaft of the humerus. In: Bucholz RW, Heckman JD, Court-Brown C, editors. Rockwood and Green's: fractures in adults, vol. 6. Philadelpha, PA: Lippincott Williams & Wilkins; 2006. p. 1117–59.

15. Stedtfeld HW, Biber R. Proximal third humeral shaft fractures: a fracture entity not fully characterized by conventional AO classification. Injury. 2014;45(Suppl 1):S54–9.

16. Metsemakers WJ, Wijnen V, Sermon A, Vanderschot P, Nijs S. Intramedullary nailing of humeral shaft fractures: failure analysis of a single centre series. Arch Orthop Trauma Surg. 2015;135(10):1391–9.

17. Cadet ER, Yin B, Schulz B, Ahmad CS, Rosenwasser MP. Proximal humerus and humeral shaft nonunions. J Am Acad Orthop Surg. 2013;21(9):538–47.

18. Bassiony AA, Almoatasem AM, Abdelhady AM, Assal MK, Fayad TA. Infected non-union of the humerus after failure of surgical treatment: management using the orthofix external fixator. Ann Acad Med Singap. 2009;38(12):1090–4.

19. Stucken C, Olszewski DC, Creevy WR, Murakami AM, Tornetta P. Preoperative diagnosis of infection in patients with nonunions. J Bone Joint Surg Am. 2013;95(15):1409–12.

20. Brinker MR, O'Connor DP. The biological basis for nonunions. JBJS Rev. 2016;4(6):e3.

21. Abdelgawad AA, Kanlic E. Removal of a broken cannulated intramedullary nail: review of the literature and a case report of a new technique. Case Rep Orthop. 2013;2013:461703.

22. Hak DJ, McElvany M. Removal of broken hardware. J Am Acad Orthop Surg. 2008;16(2):113–20.

23. Rutgers M, Ring D. Treatment of diaphyseal fractures of the humerus using a functional brace. J Orthop Trauma. 2006;20(9):597–601.

24. Robinson CM, Bell KM, Court-Brown CM, McQueen MM. Locked nailing of humeral shaft fractures. Experience in Edinburgh over a two-year period. J Bone Joint Surg Br. 1992;74(4):558–62.

25. Flinkkilä T, Ristiniemi J, Hämäläinen M. Nonunion after intramedullary nailing of humeral shaft fractures. J Trauma. 2001;50(3):540–4.

26. Lin J, Chiang H, Chang DS. Locked nailing with interfragmentary wiring for humeral nonunions. J Trauma. 2002;52(4):733–8.

27. Singh J, Kalia A, Khatri K, Dahuja A. Resistant nonunion of humerus after intramedullary nailing treated with locking compression plate with bone grafting with nail in situ and shoulder spica: a case report. J Orthop Case Rep. 2017;7(5):80–3.

28. Gessmann J, Königshausen M, Coulibaly MO, Schildhauer TA, Seybold D. Anterior augmentation plating of aseptic humeral shaft nonunions after intramedullary nailing. Arch Orthop Trauma Surg. 2016;136(5):631–8.

29. Ziveri G, Biase CF. A case report of humeral nail breakage after 11 years secondary to shaft nonunion: treatment with autogenous iliac crest bone graft and compression plate. J Orthop Case Rep. 2019;10(1):89–92.

30. Cox G, McGonagle D, Boxall SA, Buckley CT, Jones E, Giannoudis PV. The use of the reamer-irrigator-aspirator to harvest mesenchymal stem cells. J Bone Joint Surg Br. 2011;93(4):517–24.

Failure of Plate Fixation of Humeral Shaft Fractures

9

Emmanuele Santolini and Peter V. Giannoudis

History of Previous Primary Failed Treatment

A 25-year-old normally fit and well female student fell off a 5-feet ladder landing onto her left upper limb, while she was abroad.

She sustained a closed, neurovascularly intact, isolated left distal third humeral diaphyseal fracture, with a medial butterfly fragment visible at the plain radiographs (Fig. 9.1a). Initially the left humerus of the patient was immobilized with an above elbow backslab and then admitted to hospital for further management (Fig. 9.1b).

After 2 days, the fracture was surgically treated. The patient was positioned in lateral decubitus position and the distal humeral shaft was approached via a posterior triceps-splitting approach. It was stabilized with a seven-hole nonlocking dynamic compression plate (DCP) plate using both 3.5-mm screws and cerclage wires.

Postoperative instructions included early passive and active motion of the shoulder and elbow to prevent elbow stiffness, avoiding load bearing or exercise against resistance for 6 weeks.

After the surgery, the patient was repatriated and referred to our department for further management.

At the 3-month follow-up, the patient presented with persistent pain around the distal humerus together with some clicking sensation at the mobilization of the elbow. X-rays showed loosening of the metal work and no significant evidence of bony formation especially through the main oblique fracture line (Fig. 9.2a, b). Consequently, according to the clinical and radiographical picture, the patient was booked and planned for revision of the fixation.

E. Santolini
Academic Department of Trauma and Orthopaedics,
School of Medicine, University of Leeds, Leeds, UK

P. V. Giannoudis (✉)
Academic Department of Trauma and Orthopaedics,
School of Medicine, University of Leeds, Leeds, UK

NIHR Leeds Biomedical Research Center, Chapel
Allerton Hospital, Leeds, UK

© The Author(s), under exclusive license to Springer Nature Switzerland AG 2024
P. V. Giannoudis, P. Tornetta III (eds.), *Failed Fracture Fixation*,
https://doi.org/10.1007/978-3-031-39692-2_9

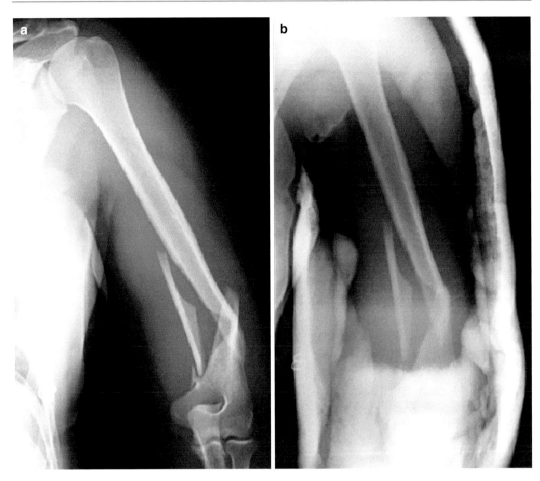

Fig. 9.1 (**a**) Anteroposterior (AP) plain radiograph of the left humerus showing a distal third shaft fracture with a medial butterfly fragment. (**b**) AP radiograph of the fracture after application of a temporary plaster above elbow backslab

9 Failure of Plate Fixation of Humeral Shaft Fractures

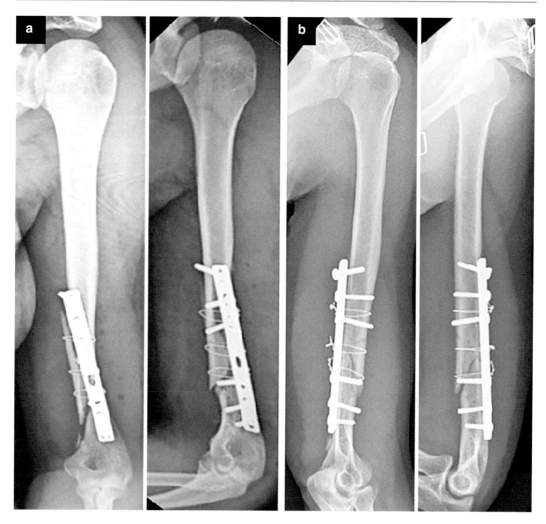

Fig. 9.2 (**a** and **b**) AP and lateral views of humeral shaft fracture fixation performed with a 3.5-mm standard plate held with screws and cerclage wires at the 3-month follow-up showing loosening of the metal work and no evidence of fracture healing across the fracture line

Evaluation of the Aetiology of Failure of Fixation

Plate fixation for the treatment of humeral shaft fracture has been shown to be effectively able to provide healing in more than 98% of the fractures [1]. However, some cases fail to achieve bony union due to several causes such as poor fixation biomechanics, violation of fracture biology, occurrence of further trauma and the onset of infection. In the presented case, the cause of failure can be attributed to the poor biomechanics of the fixation related to the plate selected and the method of stabilization as it can be observed from the immediate postoperative radiographs taken. The goal of plate fixation in case of simple and wedge humeral shaft fractures, especially with regard to fractures affecting the distal third of the shaft, is indeed the achievement of absolute stability of the fracture [2]. This is best achieved by the anatomic reduction of the fracture fragments and the application of interfragmentary compression obtained with lag screws. The lag screws are then protected by the use of a

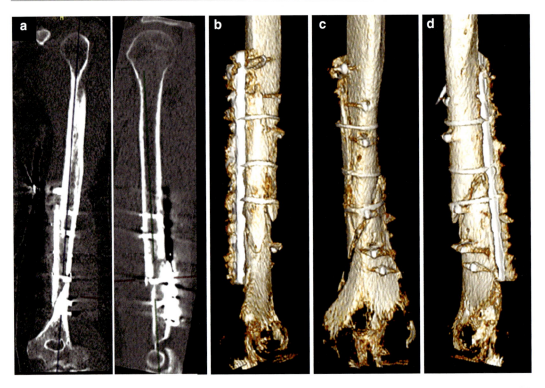

Fig. 9.3 CT of the left humerus at the 3-month follow-up showing the absence of significant bony formation across both the main oblique and the accessory butterfly fracture lines in the coronal and sagittal reformatting (**a**) and in the medial (**b**), volar (**c**) and lateral (**d**) views of the three-dimensional (3D) volume rendering reconstructions. The 3D images also show that the most proximal screw is unicortical not piercing the far cortex (**b, c**) and how the attempted interfragmentary screw is through the main oblique fracture line failing to compress it and further displacing it (**c, d**)

neutralization plate, which should provide enough stability to counteract the displacing forces—especially bending and torsional—applied to this segment of the humerus. For this reason, a 4.5-mm or a thick 3.5-mm plate of at least eight-hole length is usually utilized. The plate must then be fixed with a number of screws able to provide at least six to eight cortices fixation per each main fracture fragment [3, 4]. In the presented case, the fracture is not anatomically reduced and rather than lag screws, cerclage wires were used to control both the butterfly and the main oblique fracture lines. Cerclage wires are not able to provide adequate interfragmentary compression and are not able to resist torsional forces. In addition, an attempt of positioning a lag screw has been done with one of the distal screws inserted through the plate. It fails to provide interfragmentary compression as the screw is not perpendicular to the fracture line, and further displaces the fracture (Fig. 9.2). Therefore, the first mechanical problem leading to failure/loosening of fixation and impaired healing is the lack of absolute stability. Further, another mechanical issue identified is represented by the neutralization plate itself. It is indeed a normal width 3.5-mm seven-hole plate, but fixed to bone only with five cortices proximally (two bicortical and one unicortical screws) and four cortices distally (two bicortical screws) (Fig. 9.3). The plate is therefore not strong and long enough to adequately neutralize the displacing forces acting onto the fracture, leading to implant failure following the mobilization of the upper limb. In

Clinical Examination

At the 3-month follow-up, the patient presented with increasing dull pain around the distal humerus, especially during mobilization of the upper limb. In addition, she complained of sensation of instability and clicking of the bone main segments during active and passive range of motion of the elbow. Surgical scar was unremarkably healed without any redness, discharge or other signs of infection.

Diagnostic-Biochemical and Radiological Investigations

Three months after surgery, blood tests were obtained to rule out the possible presence of infection. White cell count and C-reactive protein levels were found to be within the normal ranges.

Further, a left upper limb computed tomography (CT) scan was performed to better investigate the characteristics of the fracture and of the fixation, to confirm the absence of significant bony formation across the fracture site and to appropriately plan the revision surgery (Fig. 9.3).

Preoperative Planning

The revision surgery consisted of the following steps:

1. Removal of metalwork—plate and screws and cerclage wires.
2. Anatomical reduction of the fracture and new internal fixation with lag screws and neutralization plate.

Implants/equipment required:

- Bacterial cultures as a routine practice to rule out infection.
- Reduction clamps.
- 3.5- and 2.5-mm drill bits for the positioning of 3.5-mm lag screws
- A posterolateral 3.5-mm thick distal humeral plate.

We were expecting that the removal of metalwork would have allowed us to properly visualize the fracture fragments in order to be able to anatomically reduce and fix them with lag screws and a neutralization plate (Plan A). Nevertheless, in the scenario of an excessive comminution not suitable for anatomical reduction and absolute stability, we were ready to perform bridging plate technique in order to allow the fracture to heal by secondary bone healing according to the relative stability principles (Plan B).

We did not plan to provide any bone graft enhancement or biological stimulation, as we believed that the cause of failure was purely mechanical.

Revision Surgery

Revision surgery was performed under general anaesthesia and peripheral block with the patient in a right lateral decubitus with the left arm supported by a dedicated arm support and under the guidance of image intensifier. A posterior triceps-splitting surgical approach was performed over the previous incision. Soft tissues were dissected by layers and tissue samples sent for routine cultures. Radial nerve was identified and protected in the proximal part of the extended wound throughout the procedure. Metalwork was removed and the fracture was found to be grossly mobile at distal portion of the prior butterfly fragment, as seen on CT. Thorough washout and debridement of the soft tissues and of the nonunion site was performed: the humeral canal was reopened with a 3.5-mm drill and fracture ends

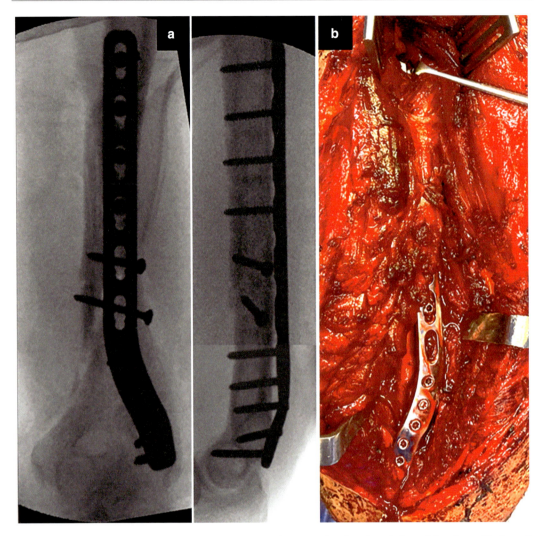

Fig. 9.4 Fluoroscopic and intraoperative images of the revision surgery. (**a**) AP and lateral views of the distal humeral shaft showing the fixation with two independent lag screws and the dedicated locking neutralization plate. (**b**) Intraoperative image of the dorsal aspect of the humerus showing the relation of the plate with the soft tissues and the presence of the radial nerve crossing the surgical field within the triceps fibres on the top of the image

freshened. Fracture was then reduced with dedicated clamps and fixed with two 3.5-mm independent lag screws and a posterolateral 3.5-mm thick distal humeral locking plate, held proximally with four bicortical nonlocking screws and distally with three bicortical and two unicortical locking screws under image intensifier guidance (Fig. 9.4).

At the 3-month follow-up following the revision surgery, the patient presented pain-free to the outpatient clinic, with a symmetric arm and elbow compared to the contralateral side. A full range of motion was apparent. X-rays taken on the same day confirmed the healing of the fracture with no concerns with regard to the implants (Fig. 9.5).

9 Failure of Plate Fixation of Humeral Shaft Fractures

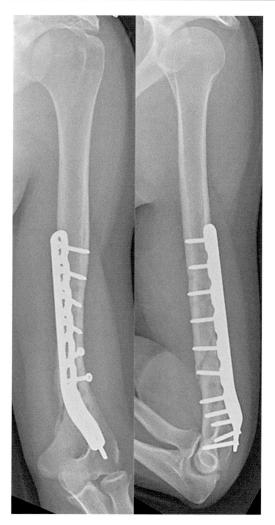

Fig. 9.5 AP and lateral views of the revision plate fixation at the 3-month follow-up showing the radiological assessment of fracture healing

Summary: Lessons Learned

Humeral shaft fractures are subjected to great displacing forces and this is especially true if we refer to fractures of the distal third. When surgery is selected as the indicated treatment strategy, a mechanical stable fixation according to the principles of osteosynthesis should be performed, in order to allow the fracture to maintain adequate stability until fracture union occurs. Intramedullary nailing constructs have been used with mixed results particularly for distal one-third humeral shaft fractures (retrograde nailing). In the case presented, in any event the fracture was too distal and there was a butterfly segment prohibiting such an option to be considered.

Plate fixation was the choice of treatment but failure to correctly apply the principles of fracture fixation led to an inadequate mechanical stability, which caused failure of the fixation.

References

1. Gottschalk MB, Carpenter W, Hiza E, Reisman W, Roberson J. Humeral shaft fracture fixation: incidence rates and complications as reported by American Board of Orthopaedic Surgery Part II Candidates. J Bone Joint Surg Am. 2016;98:e71.
2. van de Wall BJM, Theus C, Link BC, van Veelen N, van de Leeuwen RJH, Ganzert C, et al. Absolute or relative stability in plate fixation for simple humeral shaft fractures. Injury. 2019;50:1986–91.
3. Nowak LL, Dehghan N, McKee MD, Schemitsch EH. Plate fixation for management of humerus fractures. Injury. 2018;49(Suppl 1):S33–S8.
4. Spiguel AR, Steffner RJ. Humeral shaft fractures. Curr Rev Musculoskelet Med. 2012;5:177–83.
5. Singh AK, Narsaria N, Seth RR, Garg S. Plate osteosynthesis of fractures of the shaft of the humerus: comparison of limited contact dynamic compression plates and locking compression plates. J Orthop Traumatol. 2014;15:117–22.

Distal Humerus Failed Plate Fracture Fixation

10

Chang-Wug Oh and Peter V. Giannoudis

History of Previous Primary Failed Treatment

A 61-year-old female patient was admitted to the local hospital after falling two steps landing onto her left elbow. Her medical history was unremarkable. She was a nonsmoker and had not taken any medication for bone protection. On admission, trauma primary and secondary surveys revealed an isolated left distal humerus fracture with comminution over the medial and lateral columns and intra-articular extension (Fig. 10.1).

The fracture was closed and there was no distal neurovascular deficit. An above-elbow splint was applied in the emergency department for temporarily stabilisation and pain relief. She was admitted to the orthopaedic ward for definitive reconstruction. A computed tomography (CT) scan of the left elbow was not obtained. The following day she was taken to the operating room and through a medial and a lateral approach she had the fracture stabilised with a lateral and medial plate. Two days later, postoperative radiographs revealed a compromised fixation (lateral column: unreduced fracture stabilised with a short plate having one screw in each bone fragment; the medial plate last screw was not in bone), Fig. 10.2.

The drain was removed 2 days after surgery and the patient was discharged home the third day. She was seen at 2 weeks in the outpatient clinic. New radiographs taken showed the fixation to have become loose and the medial distal plate screw to have been backed out (Fig. 10.3).

The surgical team decided to proceed with revision of the fixation, and 2 weeks later after the wound had settled down using the same approaches the plates were removed. However, difficulties were encountered with the reconstruction and it was decided to stabilise the fracture with two medial and two lateral K-wires (Fig. 10.4).

Subsequently, the fixation became loose and one of the medial wires backed out through the skin and it was removed.

At 10 weeks following surgery, she was referred to our institution with failed fixation and healthy looking medial and lateral wounds (Fig. 10.5).

C.-W. Oh
Department of Trauma & Orthopaedic Surgery,
School of Medicine, Kyungpook National University
Hospital, Daegu, South Korea
e-mail: cwoh@knu.ac.kr

P. V. Giannoudis (✉)
Academic Department of Trauma and Orthopaedics,
School of Medicine, University of Leeds, Leeds, UK

NIHR Leeds Biomedical Research Center, Chapel
Allerton Hospital, Leeds, UK

© The Author(s), under exclusive license to Springer Nature Switzerland AG 2024
P. V. Giannoudis, P. Tornetta III (eds.), *Failed Fracture Fixation*,
https://doi.org/10.1007/978-3-031-39692-2_10

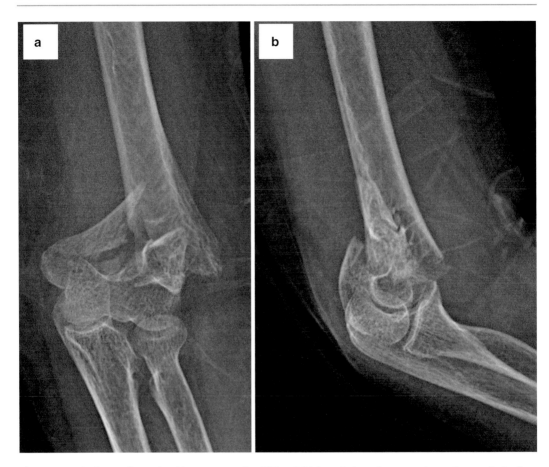

Fig. 10.1 Left elbow radiographs: (**a**) anteroposterior (AP) and (**b**) lateral views demonstrating an intra-articular fracture with comminution with posterior medial displacement

10 Distal Humerus Failed Plate Fracture Fixation

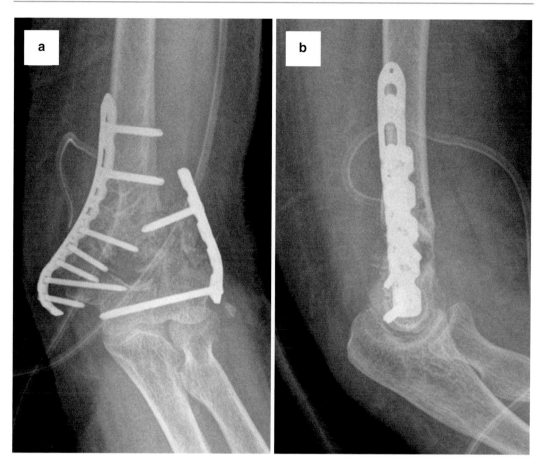

Fig. 10.2 Left elbow radiographs: (**a**) AP and (**b**) lateral views demonstrating a compromised fixation with a drain in situ

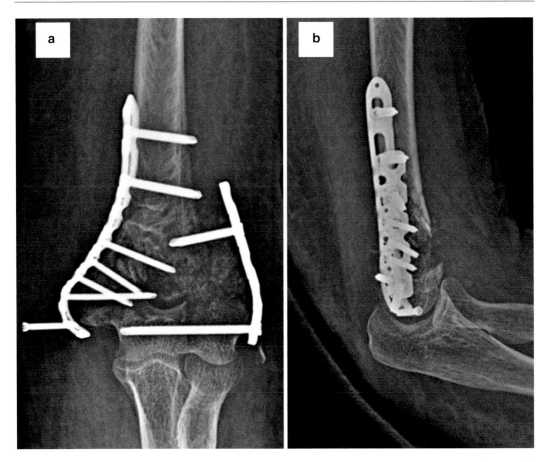

Fig. 10.3 Left elbow radiographs: (**a**) AP and (**b**) lateral views demonstrating loosening of the fixation with the medial distal screw backing out

10 Distal Humerus Failed Plate Fracture Fixation

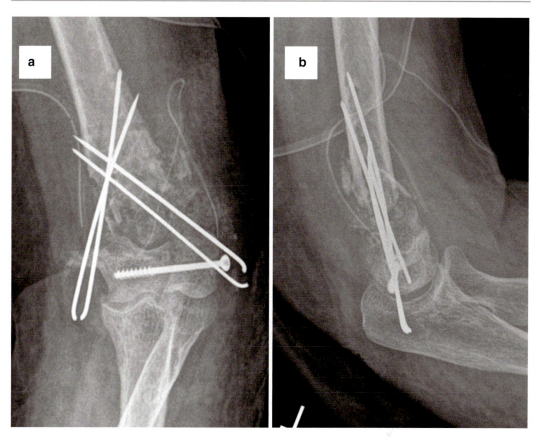

Fig. 10.4 Left elbow radiographs: (**a**) AP and (**b**) lateral views demonstrating revision of fixation with two medial and two lateral K-wires

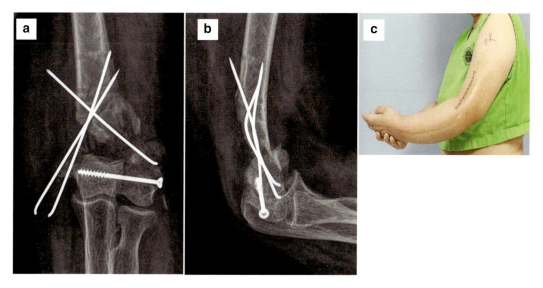

Fig. 10.5 Left elbow radiographs at 10 weeks: (**a**) AP and (**b**) lateral views demonstrating failure of the K-wire fixation. (**c**) Clinical photo of the left elbow showing the healthy lateral incision

Evaluation of the Aetiology of Failure of Fixation

The initial left elbow postoperative radiographs (Fig. 10.2) demonstrate that the fracture was not reduced anatomically and there was a residual valgus deformity. In addition, both columns of the elbow were stabilised with poor fixation as there were only two screws on the lateral column (one on each fragment) and two screws to each proximal and distal fragment on the medial column. Following the revision of the fixation made, the stability of the fixation was further weakened as two K-wires were inserted on each of the medial and lateral columns of the elbow (Fig. 10.3). Both attempts of stabilisation were associated with suboptimal fixation leading to the subsequent failure. The surgical team failed to obey to the principles of intra-articular fracture fixation being restoration of the mechanical axis, anatomical reduction of the articular surface, stable fixation of the articular segment, stable connection of the articular segment to the metaphysis of the affected bone (humerus in this case) and early mobilisation for preservation of cartilage and restoration of the arc of joint movement.

Clinical Examination

At the 10-week follow-up, the wounds were healthy (Fig. 10.5). There was no evidence of infection. There was no redness or erythema. No distal neurovascular deficit was present. Left elbow movements were limited due to pain and the presence of instability. The medial wires were palpable through the skin but not visible.

Diagnostic-Biochemical and Radiological Investigations

In this case it was important to exclude the presence of low-grade infection. Haematological and biochemical investigations were requested, which revealed a normal white blood count, erythrocyte sedimentation rate (ESR) and C-reactive protein (CRP). From the clinical examination, biochemical and haematological investigations were caried out and there was no evidence of infection.

The plain radiographs taken (Fig. 10.5) were complemented with a left elbow computed tomography scan to allow a more detailed evaluation of the local environment (Fig. 10.6).

10 Distal Humerus Failed Plate Fracture Fixation

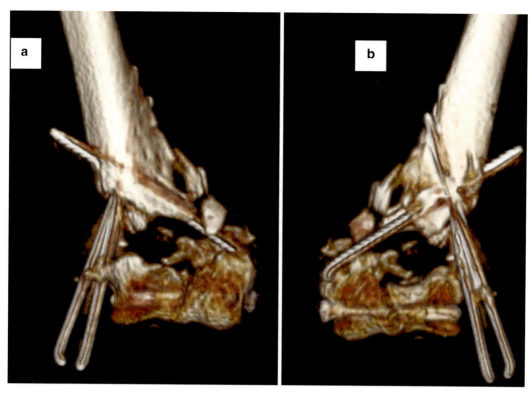

Fig. 10.6 Left elbow three-dimensional (3D) reconstruction: (**a**) anterior and (**b**) posterior views showing the distal humerus nonunion and K-wire failed fixation

Preoperative Planning

Following the analysis of failure of the fixation, the preoperative plan implemented included:

1. Utilisation of a posterior approach to the distal humerus through an olecranon osteotomy for removal of K-wires and removal of the subchondral screw.
2. Visualisation and protection of the ulnar nerve throughout the procedure.
3. Cleaning the previous fracture planes for reduction of the intra-articular component of the fracture and insertion of lag screws.
4. Sending tissue samples to microbiology to exclude low-grade infection.
5. Anatomical reattachment of the articular segment to the metaphysis with K-wires prior to definitive fixation.
6. Osteosynthesis of the lateral column with application a posterior lateral plate.
7. Osteosynthesis of the medial column with a medial plate.
8. Reduction of the osteotomised olecranon fragment and stabilisation with tension band wiring and a one-third semitubular plate to prevent backing out of the K-wiring.

The Depuy-Synthes anatomical distal humerus combi-hole plates were selected for fracture fixation. They have the options of either locking or nonlocking screw insertion.

In case that following reduction and fixation of the left elbow fragments bone voids were present, autologous iliac crest bone graft would be harvested from the left iliac crest supporting the process of osteogenesis and bone repair. For this reason, small osteotomes were also requested in case that bone grafting would be necessary.

Revision Surgery

Under general anaesthesia, the patient was placed in the lateral decubitus position on a standard table with the left elbow hanging overusing a supporting device attached to the table in a flexed position. The patient was administered one dose of intravenous prophylactic antibiotics (flucloxacillin and gentamycin). We prefer to use a tourniquet. Following prepping and draping of both the left iliac crest and the left elbow, a posterior incision over the distal humerus was made down to the triceps, which curves around the tip of the olecranon, thus minimising the exertion of skin pressure at the incision after wound closure. Then the ulnar nerve was identified by dissection on the medial side and was isolated with a sling.

A chevron olecranon osteotomy is performed with its apex being made at the bare area of the olecranon fossa. Then the triceps fascia is incised and mobilised both medially and laterally while protecting the ulnar and radial nerves. The tip of the olecranon was then held and isolated with a wet swab, proximally allowing good visualisation of the distal humerus articular surface (Fig. 10.7).

The previous lag screw was removed. The articular fragments were mobilised, and the articular surface was cleaned and reduced with pointed reduction forceps. Tissue samples were sent to microbiology.

Two 3.5-mm lag screws were inserted for fixation of the intercondylar fracture. Subsequently, using two K-wires the articular block was reduced and was connected to the metaphysis (Fig. 10.8).

Initially a posterolateral six-hole anatomical combi plate was applied for fixation of the lateral column. The medial column was stabilised with an eight-hole medial combi anatomical plate. During the reconstruction process, a defect area was apparent on the medial distal metaphyseal region (Fig. 10.9).

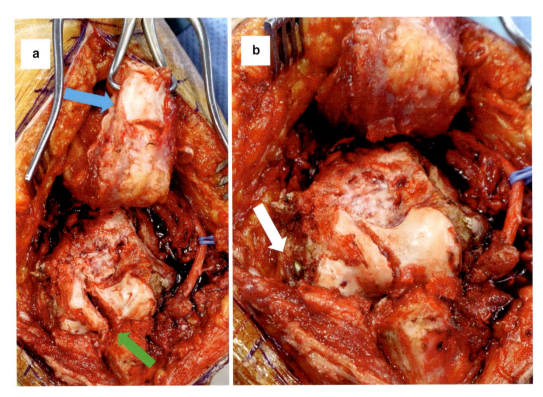

Fig. 10.7 Intraoperative picture showing: (**a**) ulnar nerve being retracted with a blue vascular sling; blue arrow: osteotomised olecranon fragment held with reduction forceps and being retracted proximally; green arrow: intra-articular extension of the fracture; and (**b**) white arrow: the screw previously used for fixation of the intra-articular component prior to its removal

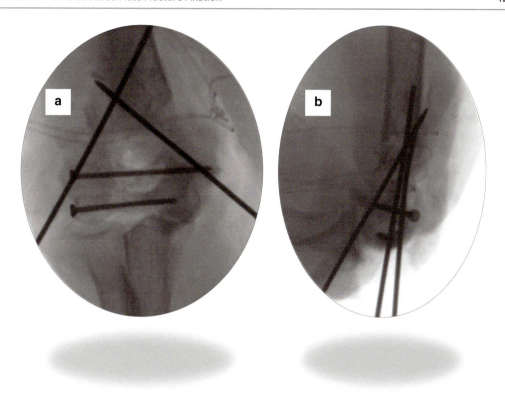

Fig. 10.8 Intraoperative image of the left elbow: (**a**) AP and (**b**) lateral views showing reduction of the distal humerus with K-wire insertion over the medial and lateral columns

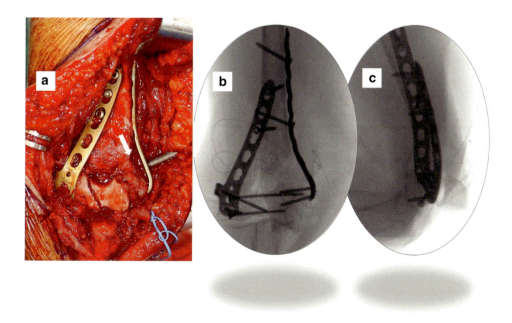

Fig. 10.9 (**a**) Intraoperative picture showing stabilisation of the fracture with a posterolateral and medial column plate. The white arrow shows the bone defect area on the medial metaphyseal area. (**b**) AP and (**c**) lateral fluoroscopic images of the left distal humerus showing fixation of the fracture with the plates

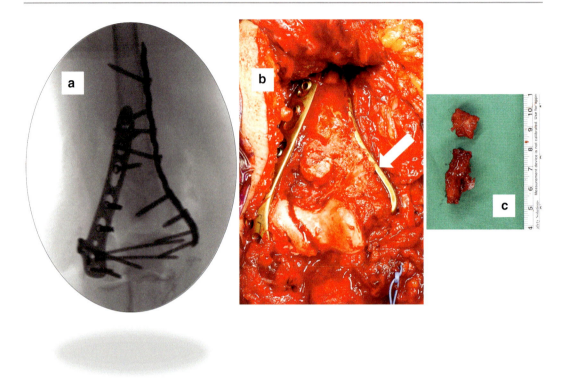

Fig. 10.10 (**a**) AP fluoroscopic image of left distal humerus showing fixation of the fracture with the plates and the reconstruction of the medial column bone defect area with iliac crest bone graft. (**b**) Intraoperative picture showing the presence of the bone graft in the previous medial bone defect area (white arrow). (**c**) Intraoperative image of the autologous iliac crest bone graft harvested from the left pelvic iliac crest

Iliac crest bone graft was harvested from the left iliac crest and was inserted in the area of the bone defect (Fig. 10.10).

Reduction of the fracture and implant positioning and appropriate screw length were checked with the image intensifier prior to fixation of the olecranon osteotomy. The olecranon osteotomy was then reduced with a pointed reduction forceps and was stabilised with tension band wiring. A six-hole one-third semitubular plate was applied with its proximal end siting at the top of K-wires to minimise the risk of wires backing out (Fig. 10.11).

The ulnar nerve was not anteriorly transposed but was left in its natural place. After a drain was inserted, the wound was closed in layers, 1/0; 2/0 PDS and 3/0 S/C stich for the skin. The pelvic iliac wound was closed with 1/0; 2/0 PDS and 3/0 nylon for the skin. A wound dressing was applied. The tourniquet was released (tourniquet time: 1 h 50 min) and a dressing was applied to the wound. The arm was rested in a collar and cuff.

The patient has a good postoperative course without the development of any complications. Neurovascularly, she remained intact. The drain was removed at the second postoperative day. The following day she had postoperative radiographs and a CT scan and was discharged home (Fig. 10.12).

She was seen in the outpatient clinic at 12 days for wound check and removal of stiches. The microbiology samples were all negative for any

10 Distal Humerus Failed Plate Fracture Fixation

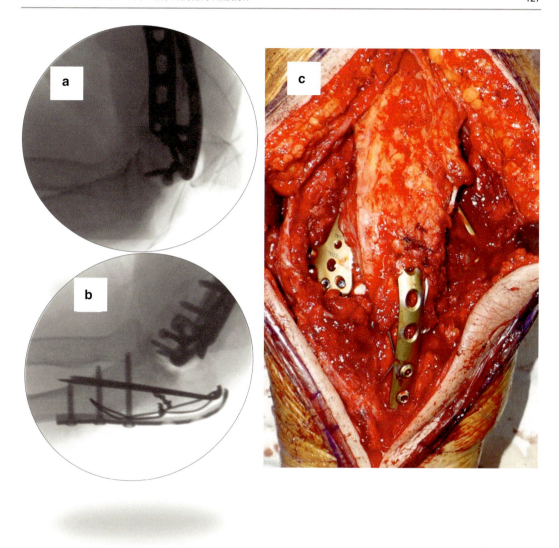

Fig. 10.11 (**a**) and (**b**) Fluoroscopic images of the left elbow showing fixation of the olecranon osteotomy with tension band wiring and the one-third semitubular plate.
(**c**) Intraoperative image showing the one-third semitubular plate placed over the olecranon osteotomy.

pathogens. She then started gentle mobilisation of the elbow joint. She was sent to physiotherapy at 4 weeks. She was seen at regular intervals in the outpatient clinic. The fracture united at 12 weeks following surgery. At the final follow-up, 10 months after surgery, she had an excellent range of elbow motion (she lacked only 15° of full elbow extension; flexion and supination/pronation were full and pain-free) and radiographs showed union without radiological features of ectopic bone formation or implant loosening (Fig. 10.13).

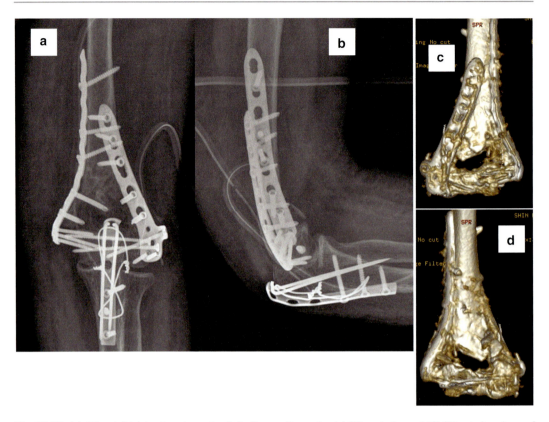

Fig. 10.12 (**a**) AP and (**b**) lateral postoperative left elbow radiographs. (**c**) 3D posterior and (**d**) 3D anterior views of the distal humerus showing the final result of reconstruction with safe placement of the metalwork

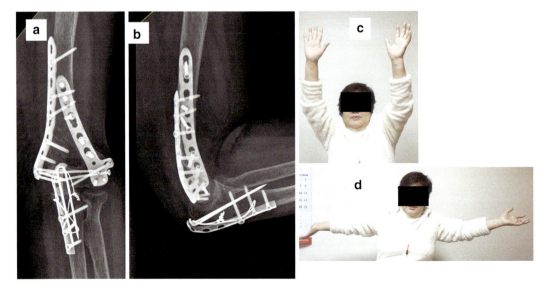

Fig. 10.13 (**a**) AP and (**b**) lateral left elbow radiographs 10 months after surgery showing osseous healing with no metalwork failure. (**c**) and (**d**) Images showing left elbow and shoulder function

Summary: Lesson Learned

Management of distal humerus fractures, particularly intra-articular with comminution, continues to be challenging injuries to reconstruct.

The goal of fracture treatment is the same like any other intra-articular fracture focusing on restoring rotation and the mechanical axis, anatomical joint reduction and fixation and early range of motion to minimise the development of joint stiffness and functional impairment. Acquisition of computed tomography is of paramount importance for accurate evaluation of the fracture lines and position of the metalwork.

When there exists comminution of the articular surfaces, angular, stable plate fixation (bridging plates) should be considered particularly in elderly patients with compromised bone stock. Plate configuration in 90° or 180° positioning as long as they are placed according to the principles of fracture fixation of periarticular fractures can be both successful. In comminuted fractures, or when revision surgery is required, an olecranon osteotomy approach can provide good exposure of the articular surface, facilitating anatomic reduction and easy placement of subchondral lag screws.

Overall, in this case the principles of fixation of intra-articular fractures were not followed leading to mal-reduction and inappropriate selection of implants for fixation inhibiting stable fixation and early range of motion. The subsequent revision performed addressed all the issues that were overlooked (fracture reduction, stable fixation) and loss of bone continuity by the implantation of autologous bone grafting. The revision of fixation strategy that was applied in this case should be considered when surgeons are dealing with analogous situations of failure of fixation of distal humerus fractures.

Further Reading

Lauder A, Richard MJ. Management of distal humerus fractures. Eur J Orthop Surg Traumatol. 2020;30(5):745–62. https://doi.org/10.1007/s00590-020-02626-1. Epub 2020 Jan 21.

Moursy M, Wegmann K, Wichlas F, Tauber M. Distal humerus fracture in patients over 70 years of age: results of open reduction and internal fixation. Arch Orthop Trauma Surg. 2022;142(1):157–64. https://doi.org/10.1007/s00402-020-03664-4.

O'Driscoll SW. The triceps-reflecting anconeus pedicle (TRAP) approach for distal humeral fractures and nonunions. Orthop Clin North Am. 2000;31(1):91–101.

O'Driscoll SW, Sanchez-Sotelo J, Torchia ME. Management of the smashed distal humerus. Orthop Clin North Am. 2002;33(1):19–33, vii 2. Shin SJ, Sohn HS, Do NH. A clinical comparison of two different double plating methods for intraarticular distal humerus fractures. J Shoulder Elb Surg. 2010;19(1):2–9.

Schneider MM, Nowak TE, Bastian L, et al. Tension band wiring in olecranon fractures: the myth of technical simplicity and osteosynthetical perfection. Int Orthop. 2014;38(4):847–55.

Yetter TR, Weatherby PJ, Somerson JS. Complications of articular distal humeral fracture fixation: a systematic review and meta-analysis. J Shoulder Elbow Surg. 2021;30(8):1957–67. https://doi.org/10.1016/j.jse.2021.02.017.

Failed Fixation of Olecranon Fractures

11

Hüseyin Bilgehan Çevik and Peter V. Giannoudis

History of Previous Primary Failed Treatment

A 72-year-old male presented to the local hospital with an elbow injury after a slip and fall onto his outstretched right arm. He presented to the local hospital and complained of right elbow pain with a restricted passive range of motion and no active elbow extension. On physical examination, the skin was intact with a palpable gap over the olecranon, and he was neurovascularly intact distally. Radiographs of the right elbow demonstrated a displaced olecranon fracture (Fig. 11.1). An above-elbow splint cast was applied for comfort initially.

Later the same day, he was taken to the operating room for fixation. Using a posterior skin incision, the fracture ends were debrided, and the fracture was reduced with small, pointed reduction forceps. The fracture was then stabilised with tension band wiring using two parallel intramedullary 1.6 mm Kirschner wires (K-wires) and a 1.0-mm tension-band wire loop (Fig. 11.2). The following day, post-operative radiographs revealed distraction at the fracture site (loss of reduction), which was unacceptable. Following discussion with the patient, revision open reduction internal fixation (ORIF) was decided and carried out 3 days later. Using the old incision, the metal hardware was removed, and after debridement of the fracture edges, tension band wiring was performed again. The patient was discharged home, having had an uneventful post-operative course. He was seen in the outpatient clinic 10 days later when the wound was found to be clean, but radiographs taken demonstrated that the olecranon fracture was not reduced, and the tension band wiring fixation had failed again (Fig. 11.3).

The patient was then referred to our clinic for further management.

H. B. Çevik
Department of Orthopaedics and Traumatology,
Ankara Etlik City Hospital, University of Health
Sciences, Ankara, Turkey

P. V. Giannoudis (✉)
Academic Department of Trauma and Orthopaedics,
School of Medicine, University of Leeds, Leeds, UK

NIHR Leeds Biomedical Research Center, Chapel
Allerton Hospital, Leeds, UK

© The Author(s), under exclusive license to Springer Nature Switzerland AG 2024
P. V. Giannoudis, P. Tornetta III (eds.), *Failed Fracture Fixation*,
https://doi.org/10.1007/978-3-031-39692-2_11

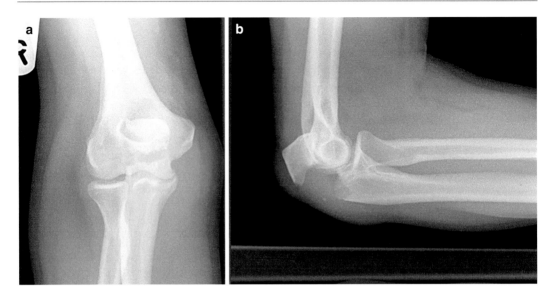

Fig. 11.1 (**a**) AP and (**b**) Lateral radiograph demonstrating a fracture of the right olecranon

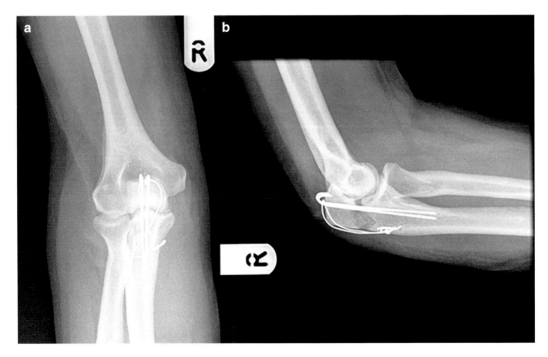

Fig. 11.2 (**a**) AP and (**b**) Lateral postoperative radiographs demonstrating an unreduced right olecranon fracture and failed tension band wiring

11 Failed Fixation of Olecranon Fractures

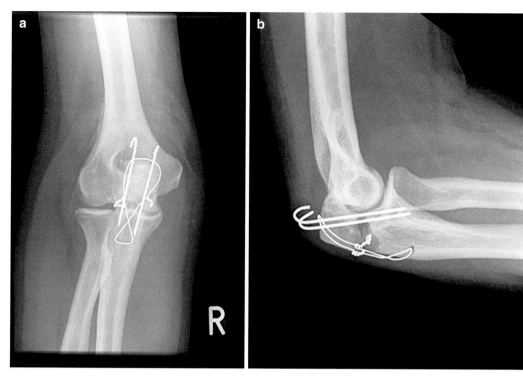

Fig. 11.3 (**a**) AP and (**b**) Lateral postoperative radiographs demonstrating displaced right olecranon fracture with failed tension band construction

Evaluation of the Aetiology of Failure of Fixation

Tension band wiring is accepted as the standard treatment for isolated, displaced two-part transverse olecranon fractures, being performed quickly, being economical, and having biomechanical and clinical results comparable to the plate-screw configuration [1]. However, there are technical pitfalls associated with tension band wiring. In the first surgery, intramedullary placement of K-wires instead of anterior transcortical fixation was performed, which may have caused the tension band wiring structure to be unstable [2]. However, intramedullary placement of k-wires may be acceptable if the fracture is properly reduced and the figure of the eight loops has been adequately tensioned [3]. During the second surgery, the subsequent failure can be attributed to either inadequate reduction or insufficient wire tensioning and/or both.

Clinical Examination

On examination, this patient was hesitant to move the elbow due to pain after the first two surgeries. The surgical incision was healthy with no signs of infection. The elbow joint, which was painful with active movement, allowed the gravity-assisted extension but not flexion. In addition, a crepitation sound was noticeable in passive flexion. The distal neurovascular examination was normal.

Diagnostic-Biochemical and Radiological Investigations

As the patient was systemically well and the wound was healthy, it was decided not to carry out any haematological investigations to screen for infection markers. Moreover, since the cause of failure was evident in the radiographs, obtaining further imaging was unnecessary.

Preoperative Planning

As the patient had already made two attempts to stabilise the fracture with tension band wiring, it was felt that another method of fixation would be more appropriate. It was decided, therefore, to proceed with plate fixation. Such a technique would provide adequate fracture stability to facilitate an early range of motion.

Revision Surgery

Ten days later, revision surgery was carried out. The patient was placed in the supine position with a high arm tourniquet. Prophylactic (one dose of flucloxacillin 1 g and gentamycin 500 mg) intravenous antibiotics prior to inflation of the tourniquet were prescribed.

The previous incision in the midline of the elbow was utilised and extended distally by 3 cm to facilitate plate fixation. The failed metal hardware (2 k-wires and a tension wire) at the fracture site was removed, and the fracture was irrigated and debrided. Then the olecranon fracture was reduced with two small pointed reduction forceps. After the articular reduction was confirmed under fluoroscopy, fixation was performed with a 3.5-mm plate (ALPS plating system, Zimmer Biomet®) of appropriate length and six cortical screws (Fig. 11.4). On examination, the elbow was stable, and therefore wound was closed in layers (2/0 Vicryl; 3/0 monocryl). Postoperatively, the patient was instructed to wear a sling for 2 weeks for wound healing and resolution of soft tissue swelling. At the postoperative second-week follow-up visit, active range of motion of the elbow was allowed as tolerated (Fig. 11.5).

Afterwards, active maximum flexion and extension were allowed. Radiographic fracture healing was observed in the sixth postoperative week. His radiographs in the sixth month demonstrated good bony union and congruent humeroulnar joint, yet no complication regarding his second revision fixation (Fig. 11.6). At this point, the patient had a painless full functional capacity.

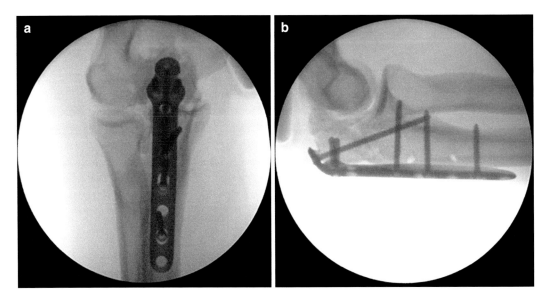

Fig. 11.4 (**a**) Intraoperative AP and (**b**) Lateral fluoroscopy images demonstrating revision fixation with plate fixation

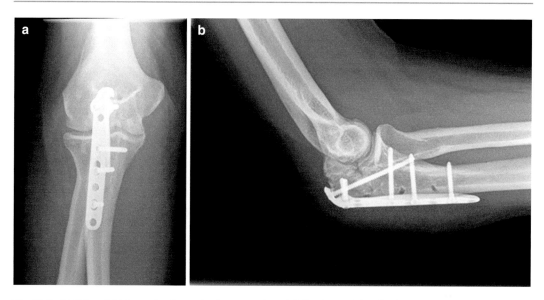

Fig. 11.5 (**a**) AP and (**b**) Lateral radiograph taken second week following revision fixation demonstrating maintenance of the reduced position with no peri-implant complication

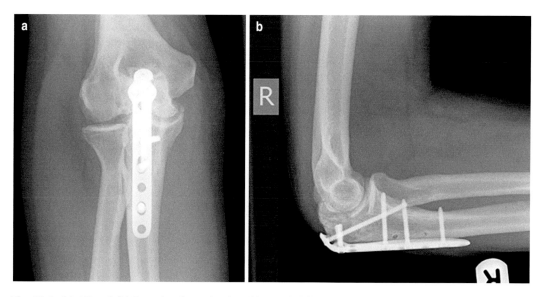

Fig. 11.6 (**a**) AP and (**b**) Lateral radiograph taken 6th month following revision fixation demonstrating congruent elbow joint

Summary: Lessons Learned

This case summarises the clinical course of an elderly patient who presented with two early failures of tension band wiring fixation of the olecranon, a common standard treatment for transverse olecranon fractures. The tension band wiring fixation converts tensile forces on the dorsal side of the olecranon into compression forces at the joint line during flexion. This simple and economical method is usually successful if applied optimally, which was not the case.

In order to avoid such failures, the following recommendations can be made:

- Anatomical reduction is essential with maintenance of reduction until completion of reconstruction.
- Transcortical rather than intramedullary positioning of the K-wires is recommended to avoid revision surgery in tension band wiring fixation.
- Transcortical K-wires should be positioned as close to the joint as possible to provide adequate compression forcing at the joint line.
- The figure of eight loops must be tight enough to convert tensile forces into compression forces.

We choose to use the plating technique for revision surgery. Plating olecranon fixation creates a more stable fixation than tension band fixation, requiring fewer revision surgeries and hardware removal after fracture healing.

Plating of olecranon fractures has been associated with good results in the literature, but complications have also been reported including symptomatic prominent hardware, infection, wound dehiscence and joint stiffness.

Recommendations for successful plating of olecranon fractures including:

- Anatomical reduction and fixation of the olecranon fracture should be achieved with absolute stability of the articular surface, preserving the blood supply to soft tissues and bone.
- Early and safe mobilisation and rehabilitation of the elbow joint should be priority.

In conclusion, care should be taken to follow the basic principles of tension band wiring. In this case, final revision surgery with plate fixation was successfully performed after two consecutive tension band wiring failures.

References

1. Hume MC, Wiss DA, Olecranon fractures. A clinical and radiographic comparison of tension band wiring and plate fixation. Clin Orthop Relat Res. 1992;285:229–35.
2. Schneider MM, Nowak TE, Bastian L, et al. Tension band wiring in olecranon fractures: the myth of technical simplicity and osteosynthetical perfection. Int Orthop. 2014;38(4):847–55.
3. Duckworth AD, Carter TH, Chen MJ, Gardner MJ, Watts AC. Olecranon fractures: current treatment concepts. Bone Joint J. 2023;105-b(2):112–23.

Failed Fixation of Capitellum Fractures

12

Paul L. Rodham, Vasileios Giannoudis, and Peter V. Giannoudis

History of Previous Primary Failed Treatment

A fit and well 18-year-old male presented to the local hospital following a fall from his pushbike. He complained of right elbow pain with restricted range of movement with radiographs demonstrating a displaced fracture of the right capitellum (Fig. 12.1). A CT scan of the right elbow was performed to better detail the anatomy of the injury and confirmed a displaced, minimally comminuted right capitellum fracture, which had flexed through 90° and was no longer contained by the radial head (Fig. 12.2).

Following a discussion with the patient, an open reduction and internal fixation were performed at 10 days following injury. Fixation was performed via a Kaplan approach and the fracture fragment was reduced and fixed with two 2.4 mm headless compression screws (Fig. 12.3). Postoperatively he was advised to avoid loading of this arm for 6 weeks but was encouraged to per-

form a range of motion exercises from the first post-operative day, which were guided by the outpatient physiotherapy service.

He was seen in the clinic at a month following the operation at which time he had minimal pain and had near full elbow flexion and extension, and full pronosupination. Radiographs taken at this point demonstrated maintenance of the position of the capitellum, with no change to the position of the headless compression screws (Fig. 12.4). He was therefore discharged to the physiotherapy with the advice to continue avoiding weight-bearing activities for a further 2 weeks.

Unfortunately, a day following his outpatient clinic appointment, he vaulted a wall using his right arm for support and hyper-extended his elbow. He presented to the A&E department at this time complaining of increased pain in his right elbow, swelling and reduced range of movement. Repeated radiographs demonstrated pull out of the headless compression screws with vertical translation of the capitellum (Fig. 12.5).

P. L. Rodham · V. Giannoudis
Academic Department of Trauma and Orthopaedics, School of Medicine, University of Leeds, Leeds, UK
e-mail: p.rodham@nhs.net; vasileios.giannoudis@nhs.net

P. V. Giannoudis (✉)
Academic Department of Trauma and Orthopaedics, School of Medicine, University of Leeds, Leeds, UK

NIHR Leeds Biomedical Research Center, Chapel Allerton Hospital, Leeds, UK

© The Author(s), under exclusive license to Springer Nature Switzerland AG 2024
P. V. Giannoudis, P. Tornetta III (eds.), *Failed Fracture Fixation*,
https://doi.org/10.1007/978-3-031-39692-2_12

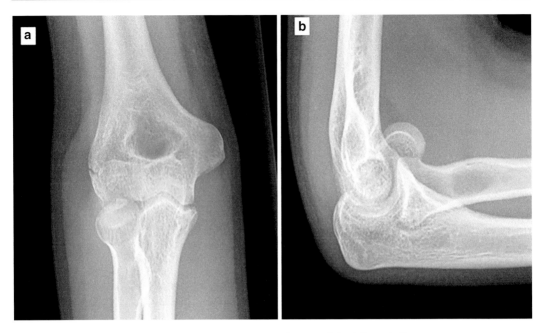

Fig. 12.1 (**a**) AP and (**b**) Lateral radiograph demonstrating a fracture of the right capitellum

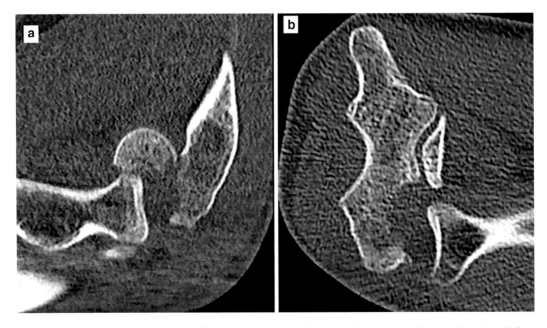

Fig. 12.2 (**a**) Sagittal and (**b**) coronal CT reformatted images demonstrating a minimally comminuted capitellum fracture that was rotated through 90° to sit anterior to the radial head

12 Failed Fixation of Capitellum Fractures

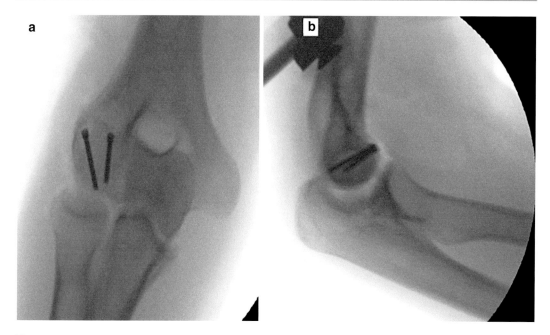

Fig. 12.3 (**a**) AP and (**b**) Lateral intraoperative images demonstrating reduction and fixation of the capitellum with two 2.4 mm headless compression screws

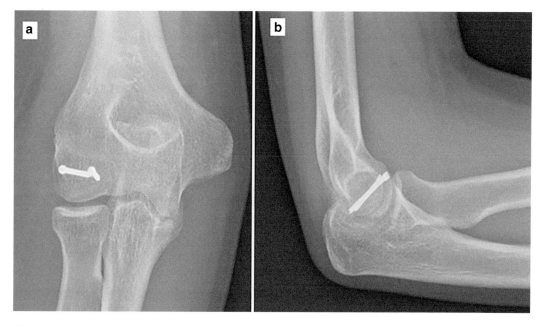

Fig. 12.4 (**a**) AP and (**b**) Lateral radiograph taken from clinic follow-up one month following surgery demonstrating maintenance of the position of the capitellum and no change to the position of the headless compression screws

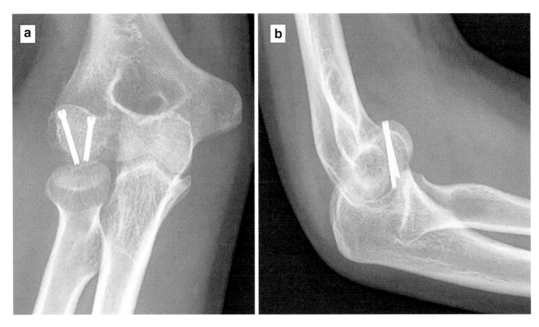

Fig. 12.5 (**a**) AP and (**b**) Lateral radiograph taken the day following final clinic appointment demonstrating pull out of the headless compression screws and vertical translation of the capitellum

Evaluation of the Aetiology of Failure of Fixation

The capitellum is particularly sensitive to shear due to its shape, which translates its centre of rotation anteriorly away from the majority of the humeral bone stock. As an intra-articular fracture, these injuries should be treated with anatomic reduction and compression; however, the fixation must also withstand the higher shear stresses experienced by the capitellum. This is of particular importance when loading the elbow whilst in extension. In this case, the original compression screws were placed oblique to the fracture plane, orientated inferiorly; as opposed to being applied perpendicular to the fracture plane. This made the fixation less resistant to shear forces which when combined with an early return to weight bearing in extension led to the early failure of this fixation.

Clinical Examination

On assessment, this patient was hesitant to move the elbow at all due to pain. His surgical scars were well healed and there was minimal swelling. He had good movements of both the shoulder above and the hand and wrist below. His distal neurovascular examination was normal.

Diagnostic-Biochemical and Radiological Investigations

Given the clear history of a repeated injury with no clinical evidence of injury, blood investigations were not required in this case. Consideration was given to the acquisition of a CT scan prior to embarking on revision surgery; however, it was felt that this would contribute little additional information to what would not otherwise be directly visible at the time of surgery.

Preoperative Planning

A discussion was undertaken with the patient as to the potential options moving forward. Non-operative treatment whilst possible would lead to an unsatisfactory outcome. Revision surgery would include the opening of the fracture site, removal of the 2.4 mm headless compression screws, reduction of the fracture and fixation with 3.5 mm screws perpendicular to the plane of the fracture. Revision fixation would mandate direct access to the fracture site and therefore percutaneous closed reduction with screw insertion from the posterior aspect would not be possible, nor would an arthroscopic approach. The patient was counselled that should there be excessive comminution or poor bone quality then excision of the fragments would be performed.

Revision Surgery

The patient was positioned supine on the table with an arm board. A high-arm tourniquet was applied and inflated for the duration of the revision procedure. Prophylactic antibiotics were given prior to the inflation of the tourniquet.

The previous incision was re-opened and extended distally by 1 cm to facilitate access. A plane posterior to the previous Kaplan approach was opened and developed to allow access to the fracture whilst also protecting the insertion of the lateral collateral ligament. The fracture site was found to have a small amount of callus within which was debrided to free up the capitellar fragment.

The original 2.4 mm screws were removed following which the capitellum was reduced and held with two K-wires perpendicular to the plane of the fracture (Figs. 12.6 and 12.7). The articular reduction was confirmed under direct vision and with the image intensified following which two 3.5 headless compression screws with a continuously varying pitch achieved maximal compression (Figs. 12.8 and 12.9).

Under examination, the elbow was stable and therefore closed in layers. Post-operatively the patient was instructed to wear a sling for 2 weeks but was able to flex from 90 to maximal

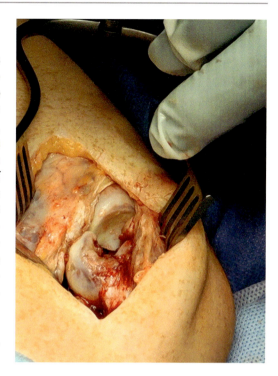

Fig. 12.6 The capitellum fragment was approached through the original incision, and mobilised to facilitate reduction

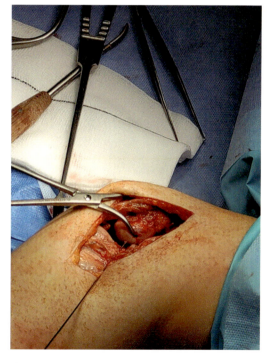

Fig. 12.7 Once mobilised the capitellum fragment was reduced and held with a pointed reduction clamp, at which point two K-wires were passed orthogonal to the plane of the fracture

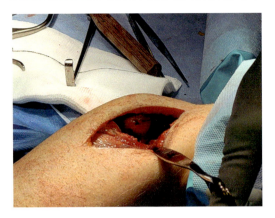

Fig. 12.8 Once an acceptable reduction was attained on image intensifier, two headless compression screws were passed achieving good compression

flexion with no restrictions on pronosupination. At 2 weeks, he began to work on passive extension achieving a flexion-extension arc from 45° to 120° by the 4-week mark. By eight weeks, he achieved a flexion-extension arc of 30–130° and had full pronosupination. His radiographs at 12 weeks demonstrated a small amount of heterotopic ossification adjacent to the radial head; however, no complication regarding his revision fixation (Fig. 12.10). At this point, weight-bearing activities were resumed through this limb, guided by the physiotherapists.

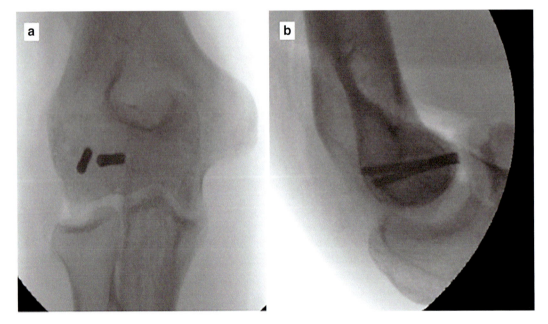

Fig. 12.9 (**a**) Intraoperative AP and (**b**) Lateral image intensifier images demonstrating revision fixation with 3.5 mm headless compression screws with continuously variable pitch

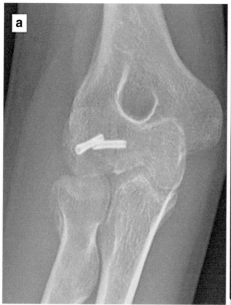 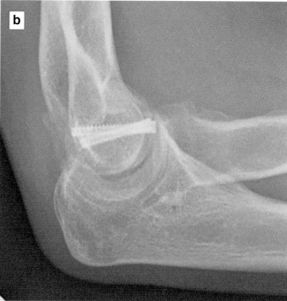

Fig. 12.10 (a) AP and (b) Lateral radiograph taken 12 weeks following revision fixation demonstrating maintenance of the reduced position with no peri-implant complication. A small amount of heterotopic bone is visible adjacent to the radial neck

Summary: Lessons Learned

This case summarises a young patient who presented with an early failure of headless compression screw fixation of the capitellum, which was utilised to treat a shear-type injury. It is important to consider the need to compress these injuries not only to achieve primary bone healing due to the intra-articular element of this fracture, but also to resist the shear forces to which the capitellum is subjected. Care should also be taken to clearly instruct the patients as to the postoperative weight-bearing protocol and the rationale for this in order to reduce the risk of overuse early in rehabilitation. This case was successfully revised utilising larger screws orientated perpendicular to the fracture plane with a continuously variable pitch allowing maximal compression and maximal resistance to shear.

Further Reading

Bayam L, Arshad M, Kumar P, Wykes P, Warner J, Hodgson S. A review of outcomes following surgical fixation of adult capitellum fractures: a six-year case series. Acta Orthop Belg. 2020;86(3):8–16.

Bellato E, Giai Via R, Bachman D, Zorzolo I, Marmotti A, Castoldi F. Coronal shear fractures of the distal humerus. J Funct Morphol Kinesiol. 2022;7(1):7. https://doi.org/10.3390/jfmk7010007.

Elkowitz SJ, Kubiak EN, Polatsch D, Cooper J, Kummer FJ, Koval KJ. Comparison of two headless screw designs for fixation of capitellum fractures. Bull Hosp Jt Dis. 2003;61(3-4):123–6.

Ruchelsman DE, Tejwani NC, Kwon YW, Egol KA. Open reduction and internal fixation of capitellar fractures with headless screws. Surgical technique. J Bone Joint Surg Am. 2009;91(Suppl 2 Pt 1):38–49. https://doi.org/10.2106/JBJS.H.01195.

Failed Fixation of Radial Head Fractures

13

Charalampos G. Zalavras and John M. Itamura

Introduction

Open reduction internal fixation (ORIF) of displaced radial head fractures typically results in fracture healing and a good clinical outcome when anatomic reduction and stable fixation are achieved and early postoperative motion is initiated [1]. However, fixation failure after radial head ORIF has not been well described in the literature.

This chapter will summarize what we currently know about the rate and risk factors for failed fixation of radial head fractures and then present an algorithm for the assessment and management of this challenging complication.

Fixation Failure Incidence and Risk Factors

Comminuted fractures of the radial head are subject to early fixation failure, especially in the setting of elbow or forearm instability [2–4].

C. G. Zalavras (✉) · J. M. Itamura
Department of Orthopaedics, Keck School of Medicine, University of Southern California, LAC+USC Medical Center, Los Angeles, CA, USA

The Kerlan Jobe Institute at White Memorial Medical Center, Cedars Sinai Medical Center, Los Angeles, CA, USA
e-mail: zalavras@usc.edu

Ring et al. reported that none of 15 patients with an isolated, non-comminuted type-2 radial head fracture had an unsatisfactory result compared to 4 of 15 patients with a comminuted Mason type-2 fracture (these four patients had fractures associated with a fracture-dislocation of the forearm or elbow) and 13 of 14 patients with a Mason Type-3 comminuted fracture with more than three articular fragments [3].

Reinhardt et al. identified 7520 patients in a database review and found that ORIF of radial head/neck fractures had fewer complications and reoperations in simple fractures without an associated elbow dislocation. Interestingly, the rate of reoperation in fractures with an associated elbow dislocation was 45%, which underscores the complex task of achieving stable fixation that can withstand the increased mechanical requirements when other elbow stabilizing structures are injured [5].

Furthermore, osteoporosis compromises the stability of the fixation construct and patient nutritional deficiencies and comorbidities may delay or arrest the healing process and eventually lead to fixation failure.

Assessment

Detailed clinical, imaging, and laboratory assessment of the patient is necessary to determine the reasons for fixation failure and help devise a

---

© The Author(s), under exclusive license to Springer Nature Switzerland AG 2024
P. V. Giannoudis, P. Tornetta III (eds.), *Failed Fracture Fixation*,
https://doi.org/10.1007/978-3-031-39692-2_13

management plan, based on factors pertaining to the radial head, the elbow and forearm, the upper extremity in general, and the patient.

This chapter focuses on aseptic causes of fixation failure, so we will not present details on the diagnosis of infectious complications, but infection should always be considered in the presence of failed fixation, even in the absence of any clinical suspicion [6].

Clinical Assessment

Elbow pain and limited motion of the elbow and forearm are usual symptoms reported by patients with failed fixation of the radial head. The patient should be asked whether an elbow dislocation took place at the time of the initial injury.

Inspection of the elbow will reveal the location of previous incision(s) that has to be taken into account when planning revision surgery. Any erythema and/or drainage should be noted.

Palpation may elicit tenderness over the radial head. Tenderness over the wrist and/or interosseous membrane of the forearm suggests an Essex-Lopresti injury that is often missed in patients with radial head fractures.

Elbow flexion and extension, as well as forearm pronation and supination, are documented paying attention to the presence of crepitus, clicking, or a hard stop suggesting intra-articular protrusion of implants. Complete lack of forearm rotation may indicate transfixion of the radial head/neck to the proximal ulna by screws that are too long.

Posterolateral rotatory instability indicates posterior subluxation of the radial head and alerts the examiner to the presence of elbow instability due to associated injuries of other stabilizing structures.

The neurovascular status of the upper extremity should be carefully assessed and documented. It is important to determine the current impact of the injury/surgery on the patient's function. The degree of pain and loss of motion after failed fixation of the radial head may vary from patient to patient but also the functional status and demands of each patient vary considerably. For example, a similar condition on the dominant extremity of a young manual laborer may have a vastly different impact compared to an elderly, retired, low-demand individual.

Imaging

Careful evaluation of good-quality plain radiographs of the elbow will clarify several important factors about the injury and previous surgery.

- Radial head: Is there a nonunion or malunion of the radial head? Is there comminution?
- Implants: Are the existing implants broken or loose? Or are they intact with loss of fixation and displacement of the radial head fragment(s)? Are there screws penetrating into the proximal radio-ulnar joint (PRUJ), the radiocapitellar joint, or the proximal ulna? Is a plate positioned outside of the safe zone or too proximally? What exactly are the implants used, so as to have the appropriate extraction tools available?
- Elbow: Are the radiocapitellar and ulnohumeral joints reduced? Is there evidence of a coronoid fracture?
- Bone quality: Does the bone quality appear compromised?

Wrist radiographs of the injured side should be obtained when an Essex-Lopresti injury is suspected to assess shortening/proximal migration of the radius. Radiographs of the contralateral wrist may be useful for comparison purposes.

Computed tomography scan of the injured elbow may provide further detail on the factors listed above and especially on intra-articular penetration of screws.

Laboratory Studies

Inflammatory markers may be helpful when infection is suspected.

Screening for metabolic abnormalities, e.g., vitamin D deficiency, calcium imbalances, and endocrine abnormalities, e.g., thyroid disorders, should be done in nonunions or when revision of fixation is planned [7].

Metal allergy screening, for example by lymphocyte transformation testing, may be helpful in select patients with pain and implant loosening after other causes (infection, elbow or forearm instability) have been ruled out.

Elbow Arthroscopy

In cases where the fixation implants are still intact but a block to motion exists and imaging studies are indeterminate regarding intra-articular screw penetration or the exact cause for the block to motion, elbow arthroscopy can be helpful.

Preoperative Planning

A preoperative plan tailored to the specific characteristics of the injury and the patient is developed based on the aforementioned detailed assessment. This chapter focuses on aseptic failure of fixation, so we will not discuss our approach when infection is present or suspected.

No Instability & No Block to Motion

This clinical scenario may result from a malunion due to loss of fixation into the radial head fragment. Slight displacement of the radial head into a new position with bone contact with the neck may provide stability, prevent further displacement, and lead to union in this position. In the absence of elbow/forearm instability or block to motion, intervention is not required.

Block to Motion Without Instability

Block to motion may result from displacement of the radial head/neck fracture, implant malpositioning, or both.

Surgery is usually required unless the degree of motion loss is small without a functional impact on the patient.

The surgical plan starts with addressing the current implant (screw revision or implant removal) followed by intraoperative reassess-

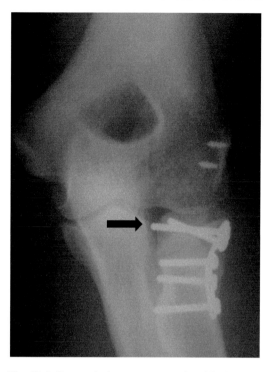

Fig. 13.1 Intra-articular screw penetration (black arrow) into the proximal radio-ulnar joint

ment of elbow and forearm motion. Then we may stop there or proceed with revised fixation or resection of the radial head.

- Screw revision: This is indicated if the block to motion is due to intra-articular penetration of screws (Fig. 13.1), or even transfixion of the radial head/neck to the proximal ulna, due to screws that are too long. The offending screws are revised and if motion is restored we can stop there. If motion is still blocked by a malpositioned implant or a displaced/mal-united radial head, we proceed with one of the following options.
- Implant removal only: This is indicated if the block to motion is due to plate malpositioning and the fracture has healed in an acceptable position.
- Revised fixation: This is an option when the fixation has failed, and the radial head/neck fracture has displaced. Revised fixation is also an option in nonunions or malunions in an unacceptable position (in malunions revised fixation will be done after an intra-articular

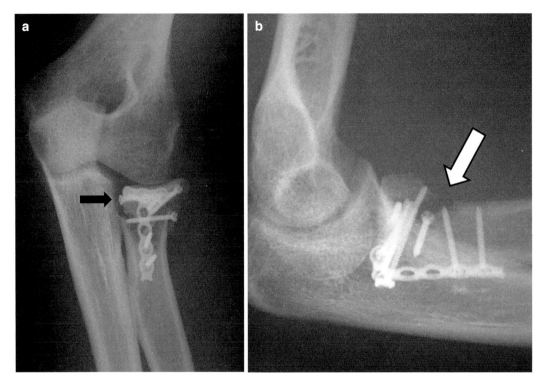

Fig. 13.2 Nonunion of a radial head and neck fracture following ORIF. The fixation has failed to take the fracture to healing and breakage of the plate will follow without further intervention. Note the presence of implant impingement at the lesser sigmoid notch (**a**, black arrow) and the presence of a bone defect at the level of the neck (**b**, white arrow). When fixing these fractures, it is important to place implants in the safe zone and to fill any defects with bone graft. In this case, the implants were removed, and the radial head excised because both the elbow and the forearm were stable

osteotomy). Revised fixation is challenging due to the limited remaining bone stock of the radial head once the existing implants are removed. This option is best reserved for younger patients with a simple fracture and a radial head fragment of adequate size and bone stock to allow for stable fixation. Bone grafting is required to fill any defects created after fragment disimpaction.

- Radial head resection: If the above conditions are not met and stable revised fixation is unlikely in the setting of failed fixation and nonunion (Fig. 13.2a, b) or malunion, radial head resection is indicated. It should be emphasized that radial head resection should not be done in the setting of an unstable elbow or forearm.

Elbow or Forearm Instability

Failed fixation of the radial head in the setting of elbow or forearm instability requires prosthetic replacement.

When elbow instability is present, as in fracture-dislocations of the elbow, other stabilizing structures, such as the lateral collateral ligament and the coronoid process, are injured. In this setting, the reconstructed radial head (either stably fixed or replaced) becomes critically important.

Fracture-dislocations of the elbow are usually associated with comminuted radial head fractures, which would preclude stable fixation. However, after failed fixation, it would be extremely challenging or impossible to achieve stable fixation with revision osteosynthesis even in simple fracture patterns [4]. Much of the previously available bone stock has been already lost due to the insertion of the previous implants and the displacement of the fracture after the previously unstable fixation.

Moreover, the surgeon should prepare a plan to address any associated injuries, for example by repair or reconstruction of the lateral collateral ligament or fixation of a large coronoid fragment. Also, the surgeon should be ready to address any residual instability, for example by a hinge external fixator.

The aforementioned preoperative planning is essential, but the surgeon needs to be aware that in some cases the best course of action may only become apparent during surgery. For example, subtle elbow or forearm instability may not be evident before and may be demonstrated during surgery with the assistance of fluoroscopy. Furthermore, a fracture that appeared to be simple may prove to be more complex, or an initial attempt to revise the fixation may not result in adequate stability. Therefore, the surgeon should always be prepared to proceed with the replacement of the radial head in these cases.

The plan and the potential for intra-operative plan modifications should be discussed with the patient and informed consent should include all potential procedures. Furthermore, all surgical trays and implants that may potentially be used should be available. These include implant extraction tools, fixation implants (headless compression screws, anatomic radial head plates, other mini plates, and screws), and radial head replacement implants.

Revision Surgery

The surgical approach is usually performed through the existing skin incision and the deeper interval depends on the specifics of each case. If the elbow is stable, an extensor split anterior to the fibers of the lateral collateral ligament is utilized. If elbow instability is present, a Kocher or Wrightington approach that allows improved access to the radial head and the lateral collateral ligament is required.

Based on the algorithm outlined in the preoperative planning section, the existing implants are removed, the elbow and forearm are carefully assessed under direct visualization and fluoroscopy, and the next step is determined.

Technical Tips for Revision ORIF

The radial head fragment is reduced with a dental pick and the fracture site is carefully inspected for any voids secondary to bone loss at the previous surgery or cancellous bone impaction at the level of the neck (Fig. 13.2b). Small voids can be filled with cancellous autograft from the adjacent proximal ulna or cancellous allograft chips but the presence of bone loss may dictate a change of the plan to prosthetic replacement instead of revised fixation.

The radial head fragment is provisionally held in place with a clamp and Kirschner wires. If headless cannulated screws will be used, the guide wires for the screws can be used for provisional fixation.

Plate fixation requires careful placement of the plate in the safe zone to avoid impingement and precise screw length [4] (Figs. 13.1 and 13.2a). The forearm should be maximally pronated and supinated to ensure that the plate is appropriately placed. Following fixation, the elbow and forearm should be ranged to ensure that no screw penetration into a joint space has occurred, especially into the PRUJ.

Technical Tips for Prosthetic Replacement

Avoidance of excessive diameter and height of the radial head prosthesis is essential. It is helpful to reconstruct the radial head at the back table and use it as a template. The diameter of the prosthesis should correspond to the inner and not the outer diameter of the native radial head. The radial head trial should articulate well with the lesser sigmoid notch without the superior aspect of the implant protruding more proximally.

Fluoroscopic evaluation of the radial head prosthesis is also useful to assess both the diameter of the implant, especially when the native radial head is comminuted or fragments are missing, and its height. The superior aspect of the implant should be in line with the lesser sigmoid notch and 2 mm distal to the coronoid.

In cases of Essex-Lopresti injuries, the surgeon should verify that the ulnar variance at the wrist has been restored to that of the contralateral side and modify the height of the implant appropriately.

Soft Tissue Considerations

Radial head fractures are very rarely associated with soft tissue compromise or loss and the wound is primarily closed uneventfully. Consultation with a plastic or hand surgeon is needed in the event of local soft tissue injury.

Postoperative Protocol

- Excision: Motion is initiated immediately to avoid any stiffness.
- Revised fixation: Motion is initiated in a week, but weight bearing is avoided for 6 weeks. After that progressive use of the extremity for activities of daily living is started with resumption of full weight bearing in 12 weeks.
- Replacement: Motion is initiated in 1–2 weeks with the use of a hinge elbow brace while

avoiding any varus stress on the elbow. Overhead range of motion of the elbow with the patient supine is helpful as gravity helps maintain the elbow reduced. Weight bearing is avoided for 6 weeks with progressive use of the extremity for activities of daily living after that. Resumption of full weight bearing in 12 weeks.

References

1. King GJ, Evans DC, Kellam JF. Open reduction and internal fixation of radial head fractures. J Orthop Trauma. 1991;5(1):21–8.
2. Ring D. Radial head fracture: open reduction-internal fixation or prosthetic replacement. J Shoulder Elb Surg. 2011;20(2 Suppl):S107–12.
3. Ring D, Jaime Quintero J, Jupiter JB. Open reduction and internal fixation of fractures of the radial head. J Bone Joint Surg Am. 2002;84(10):1811–5.
4. King GJW. Fractures of the radial head. In: Wolfe SW, Pederson WC, Kozin SH, editors. Green's operative hand surgery. Elsevier; 2022.
5. Reinhardt D, Toby EB, Brubacher J. Reoperation rates and costs of radial head arthroplasty versus open reduction and internal fixation of radial head and neck fractures: a retrospective database study. Hand (N Y). 2021;16(1):115–22.
6. Olszewski D, Streubel PN, Stucken C, Ricci WM, Hoffmann MF, Jones CB, Sietsema DL, Tornetta P 3rd. Fate of patients with a "surprise" positive culture after nonunion surgery. J Orthop Trauma. 2016;30(1):e19–23.
7. Brinker MR, O'Connor DP, Monla YT, Earthman TP. Metabolic and endocrine abnormalities in patients with nonunions. J Orthop Trauma. 2007;21(8):557–70.

Forearm Fracture Failed Fixation

14

John A. Scolaro

History of Previous Primary Failed Treatment

Patient is a 23-year-old right-hand dominant male, construction laborer, who initially sustained a closed injury to his right forearm following a motorcycle trauma 1 month prior to presentation. The patient was initially treated at an outside facility where plain radiographs showed a diaphyseal radius and ulna fracture (Figs. 14.1 and 14.2). The patient was taken to the operating room the day following presentation for surgical fixation of his forearm fracture.

Surgical operative report described a volar approach to the radial shaft and a dorsal approach to the ulna. The procedure was performed under a tourniquet. The radius was exposed along its entire length and an 8-hole 3.5-mm reconstruction plate was placed on the radial shaft in bridge mode across the fracture after length, alignment, and rotation had been established. Six cortices of nonlocking fixation were obtained on either side of the fracture. The ulna was similarly exposed along its entire length and an 8-hole 3.5-mm reconstruction plate was placed on the ulnar shaft in bridge mode across the fracture after length, alignment, and rotation had been established.

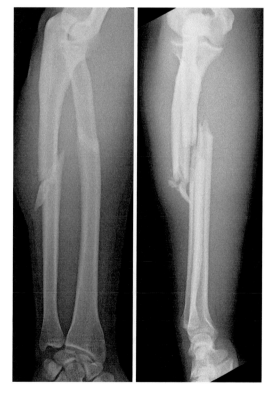

Figs. 14.1 and 14.2 Anteroposterior (AP) and lateral (Lat) radiographs from initial injury showing fractures of the radial and ulnar diaphysis

Six cortices of nonlocking fixation were obtained on either side of the fracture (Figs. 14.3 and 14.4).

The patient was placed in a sugar tong splint following primary closure of both surgical

J. A. Scolaro (✉)
Department of Orthopaedic Surgery, University of California, Irvine, Orange, CA, USA
e-mail: jscolaro@hs.uci.edu

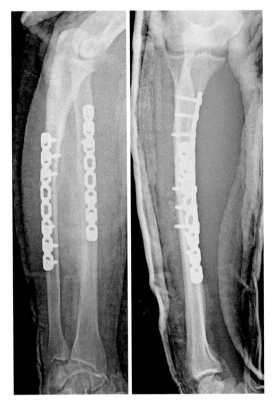

Figs. 14.3 and 14.4 Immediate postoperative AP and lateral radiographs showing reconstruction style plate fixation of radial and ulnar diaphysis

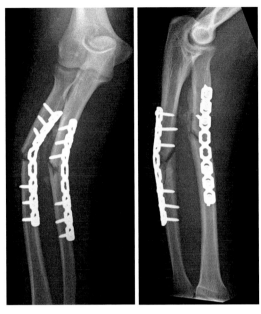

Figs. 14.5 and 14.6 AP and lateral radiographs 1 month following surgery showing acute loss of forearm alignment with bending of both plates

approaches and was made non-weight bearing on the right upper extremity. The patient presented to the outpatient orthopedic clinic 1 month following surgery with pain and deformity in the right upper extremity. He stated that his splint had come off at some point following discharge and he had been using the extremity for select activities of daily living.

Evaluation of the Etiology of Failure of Fixation

Plain radiographs were taken of the patient's right forearm during his outpatient clinic visit 1 month following surgical fixation showed acute loss of alignment of the radius and ulna (Figs. 14.5 and 14.6). On the anteroposterior view, both the radius and ulna had approximately 30° of varus malalignment with apex-radial deformity. On the lateral view, there was loss of radial bow with slight apex ulnar malalignment. The ulna was also malaligned on this view with 15° of apex ulnar deformity.

Close evaluation of the radiographs did not show loss of screw fixation along the radius or ulna. The small fragment nonlocking screws remained well fixed without toggling or loosening. In both the radius and ulna, loss of alignment was the result of plate bending. This occurred at the fracture site in both bones where there was no fixation. The implant originally chosen for fracture fixation is a flexible implant that does not provide appropriate stability, especially when applied in bridge mode. No stability was accomplished through interfragmentary lag screws or plate-generated compression, resulting in a construct that was not rigid enough to allow for physiologic motion or weight bearing of any kind [1–5].

Clinical Examination

Clinical examination of the patient's right forearm showed notable gross deformity and varus angulation, in keeping with the radiographic deformity identified on radiographs. Evaluation of the soft tissues revealed healed volar and dorsal surgical incisions. There were no erythema, fluctuance, drainage, or areas of wound breakdown. The patient had warm and well-perfused fingertips with palpable 2+ radial and ulnar pulses and brisk capillary refill in all fingertips. The patient had intact and 5/5 strength in the muscular innervations of the anterior interosseous nerve, posterior interosseous nerve, and deep branch of the ulnar nerve. There was fully intact sensation in the ulnar and median nerve distribution; the radial nerve distribution was intact except for a small area of altered sensation along the posterior aspect of the dorsal thumb in the distribution of the radial sensory nerve.

The patient had tenderness to palpation along the midportion of the radius and ulna. There was no tenderness about the elbow or the wrist. He was able to actively flex his elbow to 90° and extend to 10°. He had active pronation to 10° and active supination to 15°. Passive motion was painful past the above-noted limits.

Diagnostic-Biochemical and Radiological Investigations

Initial injury and postoperative radiographs from the outside institution were not initially available and were requested prior to surgical revision surgery. Noting that there had been failure of the plate to provide appropriate stability, without loss of screw fixation, it was determined that plate deformation occurred through primarily a bending moment. There was less likely to be a significant rotational component to the deformity if the length, alignment, and rotation were deemed to be appropriate at the index surgical procedure. There was some ectopic bone formation about the interosseous membrane in the 1-month post-operative radiographs, but this was not bridging. There was no notable osseous heal-ing or consolidation at the radial or ulnar fracture site. Understanding the primary deformity, lack of healing, and presence of early callus and ectopic bone, a computed tomography scan was not deemed to be indicated. Similarly, there was no role for magnetic resonance imaging. Plain radiographs of the contralateral, unaffected forearm were obtained for templating purposes.

Laboratory investigation included a complete blood count, C-reactive protein, and erythrocyte sedimentation rate to assess for inflammation and/or infection. In addition, a complete metabolic workup was performed. This included a thyroid cascade to evaluate for thyroid dysfunction and pre-albumin/albumin to evaluate for any nutritional deficiency.

Preoperative Planning

Preoperative plan involved supine patient positioning and the use of a radiolucent hand table. A nonsterile tourniquet would be used. Initial exposure and removal of both implants to allow for realignment were planned. The operative report from the outside facility noted the manufacturer and type of implants used but a broken screw removal set would be available if needed. The volar surgical approach would be made first to remove the implants from the radial shaft. Then the direct dorsal approach to the ulna would be made to remove the implants from the ulnar shaft. The ulna shaft would be mobilized using an elevator or similar instrumentation to allow for revision reduction and fixation of the radial shaft [6–8].

Previous forearm fixation failure was due to the selection of inappropriately flexible implants. There was no indication of bone loss and preoperative radiographs indicated that direct cortical reads may be available to set anatomic length, alignment, and rotation. Thus, the goal was for anatomic reduction of the radius first with multiple clamps and the use of minifragment 2.0 mm or 2.4 mm screws placed using the lag technique. Then, a 3.5-mm limited compression dynamic compression plate (LC-DCP) that exceeded the length of the previously placed reconstruction style plate was to be used as a neutralization plate or compression plate if the fracture pattern allowed. This would eliminate the possibility of any stress riser at a previous screw hole and provide instrumented bone for fixation proximal and distal to the previous plate location. Six cortices of nonlocking fixation on either side of the fracture were planned but the option to use locking screws if there was poor fixation or overlap of old and new screw paths.

After the radius was addressed, the ulna would be addressed using the same principles outlined for the radius. If a good cortical read was available and amenable for a lag screw, a minifragment screw or screws would be used. An LC-DCP plate that exceeded the previous plate length would then be used in neutralization or compression mode if an amenable transverse or oblique fracture was present. Similarly, the plan was for six cortices of fixation on either side of the fracture with nonlocking screws; locking screws would be used if necessary.

Intraoperative radiographs would be utilized as needed to assess length alignment and rotation of the forearm. The proximal and distal radioulnar joint would also be assessed to ensure revision forearm fixation did not result in subluxation or dislocation at either end of the forearm. Hemostasis would be achieved after deflation of the tourniquet, the drain would be placed as needed and primary closure would be performed with deep absorbable and superficial non-absorbable suture. The patient would be placed in a soft dressing after surgery. No weight bearing would be allowed but immediate range of motion would be started.

New Implant Selection

Implants previously placed in this case were 3.5 mm small fragment reconstruction-style plates. These are flexible implants uncommonly used in isolation to provide rigid fixation in diaphyseal radius and ulna fractures. In addition, with no inherent stability at the fracture site with lag screws or interfragmentary compression, these implants were placed in bridge mode, resulting in a construct with inappropriately low stiffness.

The new implants chosen were 3.5 mm small fragment LC-DCP) plates, which are stiffer implants and can appropriately be used in bridge or neutralization mode for diaphyseal forearm fractures. In addition, as noted in the preoperative plan, the chosen length would exceed the length of the initial implants to avoid the creation of a stress riser at a previous screw hole.

Need for Bone Grafting

In this case, the goal was anatomic reduction and interfragmentary compression of the fracture as the injury was closed and there was no reported bone loss. Therefore, there was no plan to use autogenous or allograft bone. In addition, based on close evaluation of the patient's preoperative radiographs, there was some indication that an interosseous synostosis was already forming and there was no desire for excessive graft material to be used unless necessary.

Revision Surgery

The patient was taken to the operating room and positioned supine with a nonsterile tourniquet on the upper arm. A hand table was used. Following preparation and draping of the right upper extremity and surgical time-out, the arm was exsanguinated using a compressive wrap, and the tourniquet was elevated. The volar approach was performed first using the previous surgical incision. The brachioradialis, radial artery, and superficial radial nerve were all identified and retracted radially. The pronator teres and flexor carpi radialis were retracted ulnarly. The pronator teres and supinator were identified about the plate and the previous plate was removed without difficulty. Next, the subcutaneous ulnar exposure was made using the previous skin incision. The extensor carpi ulnaris and the flexor carpi ulnaris were retracted to expose the plate and the implants were removed without difficulty. At this point, the ulnar fracture was mobilized using an elevator and attention was directed back to the radius.

The volar approach was utilized again for the evaluation of the fracture. A direct cortical read was available at the fracture site and a 2.4-mm

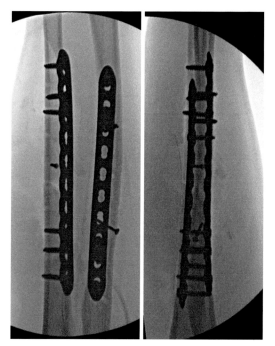

Figs. 14.7 and 14.8 AP and lateral intraoperative fluoroscopic images showing restoration of forearm alignment, with independent lag screw fixation and rigid LC-DCP plate fixation

screw was placed using the lag technique. Next, the radial bow was evaluated, and a 10-hole LC-DCP) was placed and balanced on the radial diaphysis. It was positioned such that it extended beyond the previous screw holes from the original hardware. The plate was precontoured and compression was generated through the eccentric placement of a nonlocking screw. Two bicortical nonlocking screws were placed on either side of the fracture and one locking screw was placed proximally and distally as the bone had been previously drilled adjacent to these screw positions. The ulnar approach was used to visualize and reduce the fracture. A 2.0-mm minifragment screw was placed using the lag technique across a small cortical fragment to then create a compressible surface. Similar to the radial shaft, the plate was slightly precontoured and compression was generated through an eccentrically placed nonlocking screw. Two bicortical nonlocking screws were placed on either side of the fracture and one locking screw was placed proximally and distally (Figs. 14.7 and 14.8).

The tourniquet was let down at 120 min, hemostasis was achieved, and a small Hemovac drain was placed deep into the volar closure. The forearm fascia was not closed, and the skin was closed with subcutaneous absorbable suture and superficial nonabsorbable suture. The patient was placed in a soft noncompressible dressing before being awakened. Postoperatively he was made non-weight bearing, received a single dose of perioperative antibiotics, and was allowed immediate elbow flexion and extension, forearm rotation, and full wrist and hand range of motion as tolerated. The drain was removed 24 h following surgery and the patient was discharged from the hospital.

Summary: Lessons Learned

In this case, a simple closed diaphyseal radius and ulna fracture were fixed with implants that were not sufficiently rigid to allow for an immediate range of motion. It is unclear whether patient noncompliance with initial non-weight-bearing restrictions was a factor in the early failure. Some evidence does exist regarding immediate weight bearing on plated both bone forearm fractures using rigid fixation with small fragment plates and eight cortices of fixation on either side of the fracture [9]. Knowing the initial fracture was closed and there was no bone loss, the goal was anatomic reduction and rigid fixation. This was accomplished by interfragmentary compression and the use of plates that were both longer and more rigid. This allowed for immediate range of motion and full weight bearing was allowed at 6 weeks with evidence of healing (Figs. 14.9 and 14.10). The patient did develop an incomplete radiographic radioulnar synostosis but this was not symptomatic for him and did not require any further surgical intervention by the last follow-up at 8 months (Figs. 14.11 and 14.12) [10].

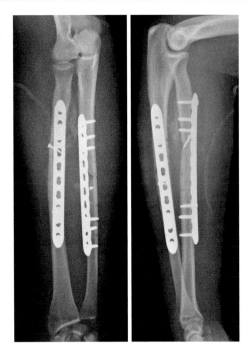

Figs. 14.9 and 14.10 Immediate postoperative AP and lateral radiographs from revision surgery

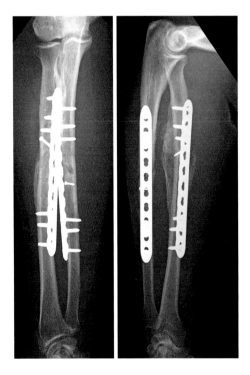

Figs. 14.11 and 14.12 AP and lateral radiographs at 8 months showing maintenance of alignment and complete osseous healing of the radial and ulnar diaphysis

References

1. Anderson LD, Sisk D, Tooms RE, Park WI 3rd. Compression-plate fixation in acute diaphyseal fractures of the radius and ulna. J Bone Joint Surg Am. 1975;57(3):287–97.
2. Chapman MW, Gordon JE, Zissimos AG. Compression-plate fixation of acute fractures of the diaphyses of the radius and ulna. J Bone Joint Surg Am. 1989;71(2):159–69.
3. Schulte LM, Meals CG, Neviaser RJ. Management of adult diaphyseal both-bone forearm fractures. J Am Acad Orthop Surg. 2014;22(7):437–46.
4. Droll KP, Perna P, Potter J, Harniman E, Schemitsch EH, McKee MD. Outcomes following plate fixation of fractures of both bones of the forearm in adults. J Bone Joint Surg Am. 2007;89(12):2619–24.
5. Leung F, Chow SP. Locking compression plate in the treatment of forearm fractures: a prospective study. J Orthop Surg (Hong Kong). 2006;14(3):291–4.
6. Schemitsch EH, Richards RR. The effect of malunion on functional outcome after plate fixation of fractures of both bones of the forearm in adults. J Bone Joint Surg Am. 1992;74(7):1068–78.
7. Chia DS, Lim YJ, Chew WY. Corrective osteotomy in forearm fracture malunion improves functional outcome in adults. J Hand Surg Eur Vol. 2011;36(2):102–6.
8. Jayakumar P, Jupiter JB. Reconstruction of malunited diaphyseal fractures of the forearm. Hand (N Y). 2014;9(3):265–73.
9. Marchand LS, Horton S, Mullike A, Goel R, Krum N, Ochenjele G, O'Hara N, O'Toole RV, Eglseder WA, Pensy R. Immediate weight bearing of plated both-bone forearm fractures using eight cortices proximal and distal to the fracture in the polytrauma patient is safe. J Am Acad Orthop Surg. 2021;29(15):666–72.
10. Bergeron SG, Desy NM, Bernstein M, Harvey EJ. Management of posttraumatic radioulnar synostosis. J Am Acad Orthop Surg. 2012;20(7):450–8.

Distal Radius K-Wiring Failed Fracture Fixation

15

Michael G. Kontakis and Peter V. Giannoudis

History of Previous Primary Failed Treatment

A physically active 68-year-old male patient fell on his left hand and sustained a dorsally displaced distal radius and ulna fracture (Fig. 15.1a). Figure 15.1b shows the result after the second unsuccessful reduction attempt at the emergency department. There is a dorsal angulation of 40°, positive ulnar variance and flattening of the radial inclination at the frontal projection. The decision was made to treat the fracture surgically, thus the patient was discharged from the hospital and planned for manipulation and pinning under anaesthesia.

Three days later, the patient was readmitted. Using a fracture table, in the supine position and using an arm extension, he underwent manipulation and pinning (K-wire fixation) as per Kapandji under general anaesthesia. Firstly, a satisfactory length was achieved with manual axial traction and contra-traction with the forearm in full pronation. A 1.6-mm K-wire was introduced from the lateral side and restored the radial inclination as seen on the frontal projection. A dorsal 1.6-mm K-wire further stabilized the fracture by levering the fracture back in neutral alignment in the sagittal plane; the alignment was secured by advancing the wires to the proximal cortex, (Fig. 15.2). A dorsal splint was applied.

The patient returned to the clinic 10 days later for radiologic and clinical control. The dorsal pin was removed because the skin around the insertion site was inflamed, the dorsal splint was changed to a lightweight circumferential cast and new X-rays were taken (Fig. 15.3). There was a shortening of the radius and the sagittal alignment and coronal alignment were lost. Oral antibiotics were prescribed to the patient, and he was planned for admission and revision of the fixation within a week.

M. G. Kontakis
Academic Department of Trauma and Orthopaedics,
School of Medicine, University of Leeds, Leeds, UK

Department of Surgical Sciences, Orthopaedics,
Uppsala University, Uppsala, Sweden

P. V. Giannoudis (✉)
Academic Department of Trauma and Orthopaedics,
School of Medicine, University of Leeds, Leeds, UK

NIHR Leeds Biomedical Research Center, Chapel
Allerton Hospital, Leeds, UK

© The Author(s), under exclusive license to Springer Nature Switzerland AG 2024
P. V. Giannoudis, P. Tornetta III (eds.), *Failed Fracture Fixation*,
https://doi.org/10.1007/978-3-031-39692-2_15

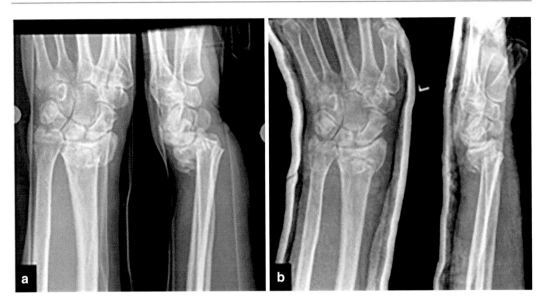

Fig. 15.1 (a) AP and lateral wrist showing a distal radius and ulna fracture, the radius has a dorsal displacement of almost 90°. (b) Post-reduction AP and lateral X-rays of the wrist following the second closed reduction attempt

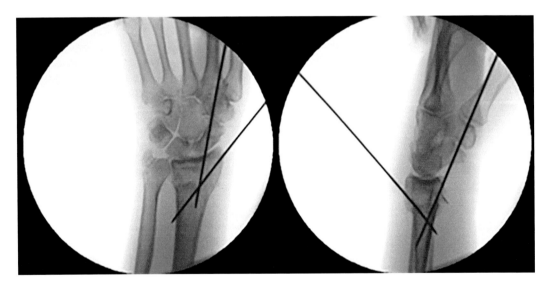

Fig. 15.2 Intraoperative AP and lateral X-rays after percutaneous pinning of the fracture. Satisfying alignment has been achieved

15 Distal Radius K-Wiring Failed Fracture Fixation

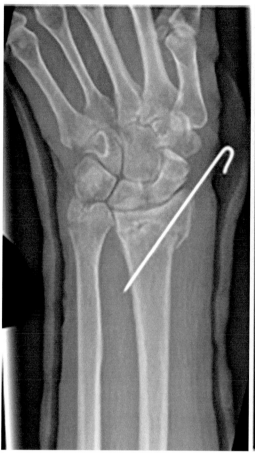 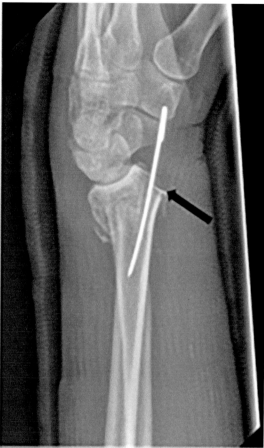

Fig. 15.3 AP and lateral left wrist radiographs showing loss of reduction 10 days postop. The dorsal pin was removed due to soft tissue infection. The pin at the radial styloid is intact but it cannot provide resistance to the dorsal displacement of the distal fragment (arrow)

Evaluation of the Aetiology of Failure of Fixation

Although closed manipulation followed by K-wires bears a relatively low risk for loss of reduction at 6 weeks and a low risk for further surgery up to 12 months [1], it might not provide sufficient stability in osteoporotic or unstable fractures. Marked dorsal displacement after closed reduction, the existence of comminution, a concomitant ulnar fracture and elderly patients are all features that characterize unstable distal radius fractures. Infection and non-compliance, or re-injury postop might also lead to loss of fixation. The patient was 68 years old (probably osteoporotic), the sagittal alignment could not be restored with closed manipulation alone, and there was comminution at the dorsal cortex (Fig. 15.1). The case was further complicated by a soft tissue infection that warranted the removal of the dorsal pin, the radial pin arguably did not provide enough stability on its own for the distal fragment, as shown in the lateral projections (Figs. 15.2 and 15.3).

Traditionally, the K-wires are introduced through the fracture gap dorsally and radially and then are angled and advanced in order to restore the sagittal and the coronal alignment as buttresses [2]. Another option is to use two K-wires passing through the tip of the radial styloid, pointing proximally and medially, anchored at the volar and dorsal cortex [3, 4]. Care should be taken not to injure the superficial branch of the radial nerve and the long abductor and the extensors of the thumb. In the present case, the radial pin was placed too volarly at the level of the distal fragment (Figs. 15.2 and 15.3), which provided little if any resistance at all to the dorsally displacing forces at the absence of the dorsal pin.

Clinical Examination

There was redness and swelling around the entry site of the dorsal pin without any purulent discharge. The patient was not febrile and denied any chills, he complained however of a dull pain at the dorsum of the wrist. The hand had normal capillary refill time, normal sensation to the touch, no numbness, or paraesthesia in the fingers; the motor branches of the radial, medial and ulnar nerve were tested with satisfactory power.

Diagnostic-Biochemical and Radiological Investigations

Blood tests were obtained, the CRP and WBC were within normal limits. Less than two weeks had passed since the fracture was manipulated and pinned, thus a reduction in theatre would still be feasible.

Preoperative Planning

1. Removal of the radial pin and fracture fixation with a volar plate. In the event of deep infection, use an external fixator instead.
2. The impacted dorsal cortex will result in a bone defect when reduced; the defect should be filled with bone substitute for stability.

Implants/Equipment Required

- Bacterial cultures in case of deep infection.
- Image intensifier is necessary for intraoperative imaging.
- Distal radius volar locking plating system (DVR-ZimmerBiomet).
- Bone substitute for the bone void dorsally anticipated (hydroset bone cement, Stryker).

The initial plan would be to address the coronal and sagittal malalignment with a volar plate (plan A) and fill the bone void with a bone cement. If there is a deep infection, then an external fixator should be used instead of a plate (plan B). The bone defect can be filled in that case with antibiotic-carrying bone analogues (e.g., Cerament-G® or Stimulan®).

Revision Surgery

Under general anaesthesia, the volar aspect of the distal radius was exposed through an incision over the FCR tendon, as per Henry approach (Fig. 15.4a, b).

There was no evidence of deep infection. The fracture was reduced with two K-wires in a Kapandji fashion (Fig. 15.5).

A distal locking volar T-plate was placed volarly, parallel to the longitudinal axis of the radius (Fig. 15.6).

In the lateral projection, the bone defect on the dorsal cortex is evident (Fig. 15.7a). A stab incision is made dorsally over healthy skin, the extensor tendons are bluntly undermined and the cavity is defined well with a periosteal elevator. Afterwards, using a syringe, the hydroset was injected in the bone void area (Fig. 15.7a, b). This is necessary to provide stability and support for the distal fragment so as not to lose the sagittal alignment. A dorsal cast was applied, and the patient returned to the outpatient clinic 2 weeks afterwards for new X-rays and wound control (Fig. 15.7c).

15 Distal Radius K-Wiring Failed Fracture Fixation

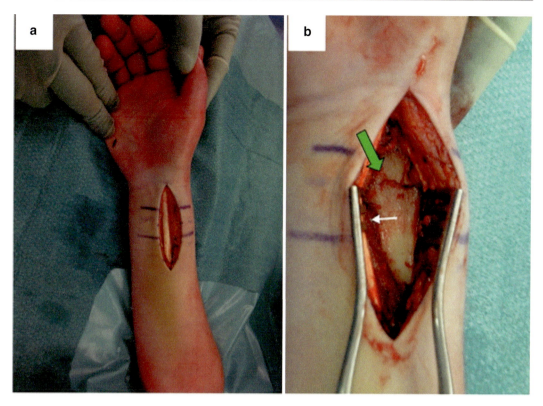

Fig. 15.4 (**a**) Intraoperative picture showing the volar approach and the Flexor carpi radialis (FCR) tendon. (**b**) Exposure of the fracture having being realigned (white arrow FCR; green arrow fracture line)

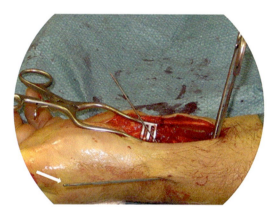

Fig. 15.5 Intra-operative picture showing the fracture to have been reduced with K-wires (white arrow showing the radial styloid wire maintaining fracture reduction)

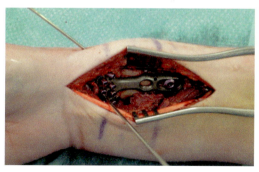

Fig. 15.6 Intra-operative picture showing stabilization of the fracture with the volar locking plate

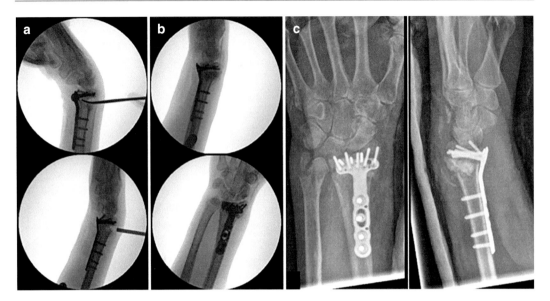

Fig. 15.7 (**a**) Intraoperative X-rays of the fixated fracture; a periosteal elevator helps the dissection down to the defect area and then a syringe is passed. (**b**) The cavity is filled with hydroset bone cement. The sagittal and the coronal alignment are restored. (**c**) AP and lateral X-rays of the wrist two weeks postop, the alignment is maintained

Summary: Lessons Learned

Surgical fixation of distal radius fractures in geriatric patients has not been shown to provide superior long-term functional results in comparison to non-operative treatment [5]. However, that might not be the case for older patients who are active and have high functional demands; in these cases, one could advocate surgical fixation if closed reduction is not satisfactory. In our case, fixation with a distal locking volar plate should have been the first treatment, given the underlying osteoporosis and the unstable characteristics of the fracture.

References

1. Costa ML, Achten J, Ooms A, Png ME, Cook JA, Lamb SE, Hedley H, Dias J. Surgical fixation with K-wires versus casting in adults with fracture of distal radius: DRAFFT2 multicentre randomised clinical trial. BMJ. 2022;376:e068041.
2. Haentjens P, Casteleyn PP. The Kapandji pinning technique for the treatment of fractures of the distal radius. Oper Orthop Traumatol. 1996;8(1):20–30.
3. Tang P, Ding A, Uzumcugil A. Radial column and volar plating (RCVP) for distal radius fractures with a radial styloid component or severe comminution. Tech Hand Up Extrem Surg. 2010;14(3):143–9.
4. Sanders L, Johnson N, Dias JJ. Kirschner wire fixation in dorsally displaced distal radius fractures: a biomechanical evaluation. J Wrist Surg. 2022;11(01):021–7.
5. Hassellund SS, Williksen JH, Laane MM, Pripp A, Rosales CP, Karlsen Ø, Madsen JE, Frihagen F. Cast immobilization is non-inferior to volar locking plates in relation to QuickDASH after one year in patients aged 65 years and older: a randomized controlled trial of displaced distal radius fractures. Bone Joint J. 2021;103-B(2):247–55.

Distal Radius Plate Failed Fixation

16

Mitch Rohrback, Erik Slette, Austin Hill, and David Ring

History of Previous Primary Failed Treatment

The distal radius is a common site of fracture due to the combination of diminished bone quality from the effects of osteoporosis and age-associated decreased agility sufficient for more frequent falls while maintaining the ability to extend the arm to help break the fall. The vast majority of fractures heal, so the goal of treatment is alignment for function, comfort, and aesthetics.

Operative treatment has moved from pin and external fixation to internal volar locking plate fixation over the last few decades [1, 2]. Pins often provide inadequate fixation, particularly in osteoporotic bone [3]. The problem with external fixation is often inability to obtain and maintain reduction and alignment, and supplementation with pins, bone graft, and bone substitute was attempted [4–7]. These fixation tactics merit attention given the recent, high-level, data showing no difference in patient-reported outcomes between pin and volar plate fixation [8]. Since the

loss of fixation is straightforward for pinning constructs, in this chapter, we focus on the loss of fixation with a volar locking plate construct.

Volar locking plate fixation usually provides adequate stability and merits attention to limited implant prominence [9] and no errant screws either irritating tendons or in the joint [10]. Loss of fixation is most common with small articular fragments in shearing or compression-type fractures [11], loss of fixation of the volar lunate facet in particular. Loss of fixation with bending (extra-articular fractures) is often related to technical inadequacies in the fixation [12].

Case Introduction

Patient 1: A 55-year-old woman fell from a standing height and fractured her right distal radius (Fig. 16.1a, b). The fracture was a volar shearing fracture with articular fragmentation and a small volar lunate facet fragmentation. Fixation was achieved through an FCR exposure using a volar plate and screws.

Patient 2: A 28-year-old man fell from a height and fractured his right distal radius (Fig. 16.2a, b). The fracture was a complete articular fracture with sagittal and coronal fracture lines and metaphyseal comminution (AO C3.2). Initial

---

M. Rohrback · E. Slette · A. Hill · D. Ring (✉)
Department of Surgery and Perioperative Care, Dell Medical School, Austin, TX, USA
e-mail: David.Ring@austin.utexas.edu

© The Author(s), under exclusive license to Springer Nature Switzerland AG 2024
P. V. Giannoudis, P. Tornetta III (eds.), *Failed Fracture Fixation*,
https://doi.org/10.1007/978-3-031-39692-2_16

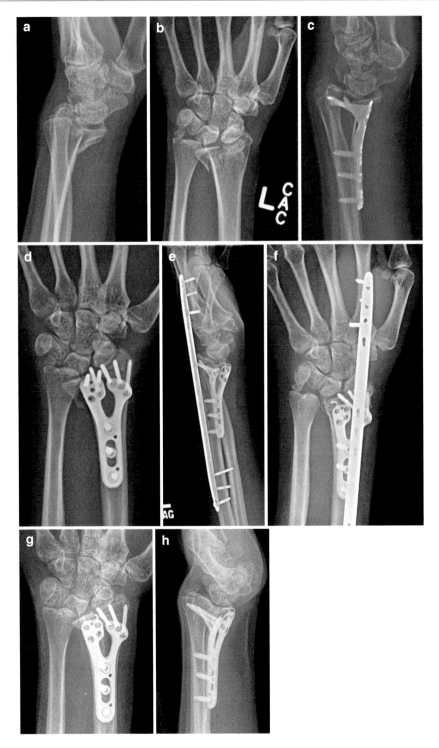

Fig. 16.1 Case 1: (**a**, **b**) Pre-operative radiographs. (**c**, **d**) Fixation failure post-operative radiographs, index surgery. (**e**, **f**) Case 1, revision surgery. (**g**, **h**) Post-bridge plate removal

16 Distal Radius Plate Failed Fixation

fixation with a volar plate through an FCR exposure achieved a good reduction (Fig. 16.2c, d).

Patient 3: A 42-year-old woman presented after a motorcycle versus truck accident with multiple upper and lower extremity fractures including a right closed intra-articular distal radius fracture with meta-diaphyseal extension and distal radioulnar joint dislocation (Fig. 16.3a, b). The fracture was approached using a standard volar FCR approach. Significant meta-diaphyseal comminution was noted. The radius fracture and the dorsally dislocated ulna were reduced with traction and manipulation. Radial length was restored with axial traction and the distal radius was pinned in place. A plate designed for the volar surface of the distal radius and extending into the diaphysis proximally was used to secure the fracture, bridging the meta-diaphyseal comminution (Fig. 16.3c, d). The DRUJ was aligned under image intensification and did not dislocate with forearm rotation. The wrist was splinted post-operatively.

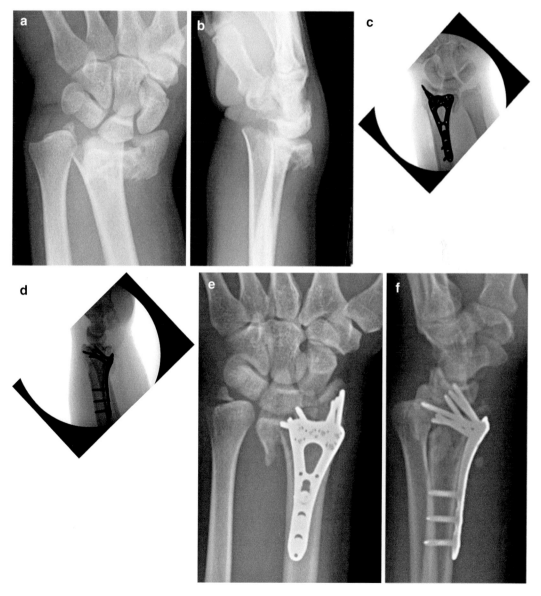

Fig. 16.2 Case 2: (**a**, **b**) Pre-operative radiographs. (**c**, **d**) Intraoperative fluoroscopy images, index surgery. (**e**, **f**) Follow-up radiographs with failed fixation, one week post-index surgery. (**g**, **h**) Case 2, revision surgery. (**i**, **j**) Post bridge plate, hardware removal

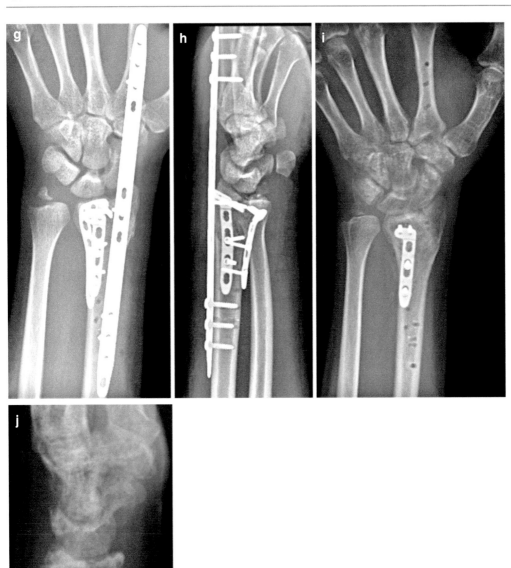

Fig. 16.2 (continued)

16 Distal Radius Plate Failed Fixation

Fig. 16.3 Case 3: (**a**, **b**) Pre-operative radiographs. (**c**, **d**) Intraoperative fluoroscopy images. (**e**, **f**) Failed fixation, five weeks post-index surgery. (**g**, **h**) Case 3, revision surgery. (**i**, **j**) Post-op follow-up radiographs

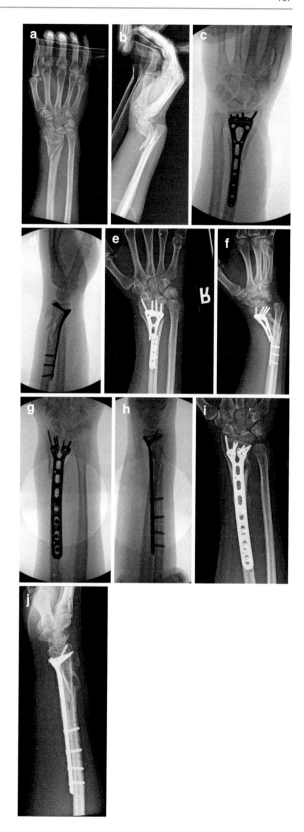

Evaluation of the Etiology of Failure of Fixation

Bending Fractures

Loss of volar locking plate fixation of bending type, extra-articular fractures of the distal radius are usually related to fragmentation of the metaphyseal cortex, osteoporosis, and inadequate fixation. Key technical elements of volar locking plate fixation include having the locking screws relatively close to the subchondral bone without being in the joint. The screws should extend sufficiently dorsal without penetrating the dorsal cortex. Fractures can collapse and bend dorsally over short screws that are only about half the anteroposterior width of the bone. Proximal fixation is less problematic, but occasionally loosens, so it is wise to always use three screws proximally, particularly with poor-quality bone, with the third screw in the diaphysis where there is better-quality bone.

Shearing Fractures

Volar shearing fractures may feature a small volar articular marginal fragment that is often fragmented. The volar lunate facet fragment in particular can be problematic in both shearing and compression fractures [12–14]. It is the site of origin of the long and short radiolunate ligaments–some of the most important stabilizers of the radiocarpal articulation. It is a small and thin protrusion from the volar articular margin that can be difficult to secure with internal fixation [15]. Central articular impaction and fracture and rotation of the dorsal articular fragment (complete articular volar shearing pattern fractures) can contribute to the forces encouraging subluxation of the carpus volarly along with the volar lunate facet fragment [16–19].

Compression Fractures

Loss of alignment and fixation of compression fractures combines the elements of bending and shearing fractures. The fracture can collapse at the metaphyseal level for the reasons mentioned and also due to greater difficulty obtaining secure fixation due to the fragmentation of the distal, articular fragments. The volar lunate, and less commonly the dorsal lunate fragment, can also escape fixation and become misaligned.

Patient 1: On the first post-operative radiographs, 2 weeks after surgery, it was noted that the volar lunate facet fragment had dislocated around the edge of the volar plate (Fig. 16.1c, d).

Patient 2: A repeat radiograph at the first post-operative visit 1 week after injury identified loss of fixation of the volar lunate facet fragment (Fig. 16.2e, f). The carpus had dislocated with that fragment. What seemed like adequate fixation was inadequate likely due to the combined articular and metaphyseal fragmentation. With AO C3.2 and 3.3 fractures, the bone is not sharing the forces trying to displace the fracture and the plate and screws must do all the work. Even two good screws in that fragment could not, on their own, resist the forces driving the volar lunate facet fragment proximally and volarly.

Patient 3: Patient returned for outpatient follow-up roughly 5 weeks after her index operation. She reported increased pain and new deformity to the right wrist after a heavy object fell on her right forearm. Radiographs demonstrate a broken plate just distal to the zone of metaphyseal comminution (Fig. 16.3e, f). The location of failure through the oblong hole in the proximal aspect of the plate likely represents a construct that was unable to withstand the bending forces across the hardware. The patient may have progressed weight bearing in the right arm early out of necessity given her bilateral lower extremity injuries.

Clinical Examination

Loss of fixation is not typically apparent on physical examination. This is in part due to swelling and bruising. If the radius shortens, the distal ulna may be prominent giving the sense of radial deviation of the wrist. If the carpal subluxates volarly, that may be visible on exam depending on the swelling.

Deformity might increase pressure on the median nerve, and these are often high-energy injuries at risk of acute carpal tunnel syndrome, so examine the nerve carefully.

Diagnostic-Biochemical, and Radiological Investigations

Radiographs are the standard method of surveillance for distal radius fractures after fixation. They are relatively low cost and provide sufficient information in most cases undergoing routine healing. Implant position and fracture malalignment can be monitored using radiographs. Advanced imaging is not typically needed or recommended for routine surveillance.

For potential problems not clear on radiographs, advanced imaging such as computed tomography (CT) scan with or without 3D reconstructions can be useful. Non-contrast CT scans can be useful to assess fracture healing when investigating a nonunion or delayed bone healing situation. CT scans in conjunction with 3D reconstructions are valuable in assessing fracture fragment position and alignment, particularly for articular fractures.

Distal radius fractures rarely lack the biological capacity to heal, have a high rate of healing without operative intervention, and may have trouble healing when metaphyseal and diaphyseal fragmentation leads to a bone gap when the fracture is realigned [20]. However, if there is clinical concern for atrophic nonunion as a contributor to implant failure, a metabolic work-up can be considered, including vitamin D, CMP, and TSH. Patient factors that may impede fracture healing (diabetes control, tobacco use, etc.) should be optimized.

Preoperative Planning

Appropriate orthogonal radiographs of the distal radius should be obtained. In instances where restoration of (patient-specific) ulnar variance may be challenging to interpret, contralateral wrist radiographs may be obtained. Non-contrast CT scans can be valuable when assessing a delayed union or nonunion. In the operating room, either a mini c-arm or standard c-arm is utilized to guide fracture reduction, plate positioning, and screw placement.

Revision surgery for loose or broken implants around a fracture often benefits from techniques and equipment beyond that available in the standard distal radius system. Identifying the manufacturer of the prior implants via operative reports or imaging and request for the manufacturer's specific screwdriver is very helpful. In addition, a general screw removal set and broken screw removal set with multiple drive recesses and extraction instruments for intact and damaged screws should be available.

Implant removal and revision fracture fixation often benefit from a more extensile approach and exposure than the initial surgery, and the patient should anticipate a more extensive incision. Second, depending on the timing of the revision surgery in relation to the primary surgery and the degree of deformity after loosening or breakage of fixation, the patient should be prepared for potential limitations and harms from the second surgery. Similar to second surgeries to remove implants, the potential for neurovascular, tendon, and muscle injury is incrementally higher depending on the region [21]. While there is concern regarding peripheral nerve catheter application for the management of distal radius fractures in the acute setting secondary to masking of post-traumatic acute carpal tunnel syndrome or forearm compartment syndrome, peripheral nerve blocks may be relatively safe in the revision setting as they may reduce post-operative discomfort and narcotic utilization.

Implant Selection

Loosening or breakage of fixation often indicates that the initial construct was inadequate (technical shortcomings) or there was inadequate biology (remaining dead bone or infection) not addressed at the time of the index operation.

Altered Plate/Screw Construct

Loss of fixation due to hardware failure, either broken plate or screw pull-out, indicates that the initial construct may have been at a biomechanical disadvantage. Alteration of the volar plate and screw construct can come in many forms. There is some variability in volar plate implants between vendors in terms of plate stiffness as well as proximal and distal fixation options. Fixation failure such as plate breakage or proximal screw pull-out is often due to insufficient working length of the construct, delayed union, or both. Distal fixation failure is typically related to fracture pattern, poor bone quality, or lack of supplemental fixation.

Fragment-Specific Fixation

The concept of fragment-specific plating techniques (each fragment receives its own, specific fixation) gained favor for the fixation of specific articular fragments with fragmentation in both the coronal and sagittal planes (AO Type C3 fractures). Nowadays, most fractures can be adequately secured with a volar locking plate, occasionally augmented by a dorsal plate. The fragment-specific concept may be used in the unusual circumstances when a radial styloid fragment is difficult to control with a volar plate alone when a dorsal ulna fragment is markedly displaced, and for small volar lunate facet fragments [22]. Fixation of the volar lunate facet has been investigated extensively due to its importance in resisting volar carpal subluxation. Multiple fixation strategies to address the volar lunate facet fragment have been described in the literature including wire-loop fixation, spring wire fixation, volar hook plate, and pre-contoured plates designed to capture the distal articular fragments [14, 23–26].

Dorsal Distraction Plate

A dorsal distraction plate can provide much greater distraction/ligamentotaxis and neutraliza-

tion than an external fixator due to the mechanical advantages of being directly adjacent to the bone. It also provides some dorsal buttressing of articular fragments [27]. It is typically used for fractures with combined articular and metaphyseal (AO C3.2) or metaphyseal and diaphyseal fragmentation (AO C3.3). For most Type C fractures, a separate volar exposure and fixation are needed for adequate control of the volar lunate facet fragment. Most extra-articular fractures with extensive fragments (e.g., AO A3.3) can be secured with a long plate with a good articular head with numerous locking screws. The distraction plate can also be used with shearing fractures to maintain the carpus in position either indirectly by holding the hand and carpus in place or directly with a screw through the distraction plate into the capitate.

Augments (Grafting)

The evidence does not provide consensus on the indications for the use of bone graft and substitutes for distal radius fractures. In the past, bone graft and graft substitutes were commonly used to fill bone voids in the metaphysis to support the reduction and speed healing within the time that an external fixator could be maintained [28, 29]. Some studies indicate that augmentation with graft or substitute has improved radiographic alignment but links to function and overall outcomes are limited [30].

Bone graft and bone graft substitutes can support articular fragments, impacted central articular fragments in particular. Once replaced into position, there is a metaphyseal defect behind the fragment. These fragments are often too small to be well controlled by subchondral support screws. A large amount of bone graft substitute can impede healing at the metaphyseal level, but a small amount is acceptable.

Revision Surgery

Patient 1: Revision construct (Fig. 16.1e, f). After bridge plate removal (Fig. 16.1g, h).

An attempt was made to hold the carpus up with a distraction plate and hold the volar lunate facet fragment with a hook extension to the plate. But without a screw directly in the capitate, the distraction plate did not hold the carpus up as well as hoped. And the hook plate kept the lunate facet fragment from escaping, but the lunate was now articulating with the impacted area of the articular surface relatively volar. Our interpretation is that there is some volarward rotation of the dorsal articular surface and some central/volar articular impaction, and the carpus has "slid" down this "ramp" into the articular impaction and away from the more preserved dorsal articular surface, without completely dislocating. Even with a screw in the capitate, it is probably necessary to push the impacted central articular fragments into a more anatomic position that can reduce the forces encouraging the carpus to subluxate volarly. After pushing them in place, through the metaphyseal fracture line, and against the carpus, the fragments could be stabilized by a combination of subchondral support from locking screws and perhaps bone graft of bone graft substitute.

Patient 2: Revision construct (Fig. 16.2g, h). After bridge plate removal (Fig. 16.2i, j).

The addition of a dorsal distraction plate, holding the carpus and hand in place and reducing the force on the distal radius allows a volar plate to adequately maintain the alignment of the volar lunate facet. AO Type C3.2 and 3.3 fractures should be treated with a distraction plate along with other fixation as needed to get the fragments aligned and stabilized as well as possible. Loss of fixation as in this case can be salvaged by adding the distraction plate.

Patient 3: Revision construct (Fig. 16.3g, h). Post-op follow-up radiograph (Fig. 16.3i, j). The previous 2.4-mm plate and screws were removed and the meta-diaphyseal fracture component was reduced. An extended volar plate with a 3.5-mm diaphyseal thickness was implanted which still permitted a variety of screw options distally but greater resistance to bending failure. Fractures with longer segments of comminution in the meta-diaphysis, particularly in patients with concomitant lower extremity injuries, may require a thicker plate to withstand weight-bearing earlier than standard protocols allow.

Summary: Lessons Learned

Patient 1: A 55-year-old woman experienced loss of fixation of the volar lunate facet after volar plate fixation of a volar shearing fracture. In addition to the potential for escape of small volar lunate facet fragments in volar shearing fractures, surgeons can anticipate and identify central articular impaction, and rotation of the dorsal lunate fragment, both of which can contribute to subluxation and lead to malarticulation of the lunate with the radius. It may be helpful to rotate and elevate these fragments and support them with a distraction plate including a screw in the capitate.

Patient 2: A 28-year-old man who fell from a height experienced loss of fixation of the volar lunate facet after volar plate fixation of a fracture with both articular and metaphyseal fragmentation (AO C3.2). Fractures with complex articular and metaphyseal/diaphyseal fragmentation are at risk for loss of fixation. Surgeons can have a low threshold for using a distraction plate and this should limit fixation failure.

Patient 3: A 42-year-old woman presented after a motorcycle collision with a right intra-articular distal radius fracture, significant meta-diaphyseal extension, and distal radioulnar joint dislocation. The patient also sustained bilateral lower extremity injuries precluding weight bearing for 6 weeks. After a possible repeat traumatic event, the patient presented at 5 weeks with the plate broken in the meta-diaphysis and loss of alignment. It may be that she was bearing weight through the fracture and plate. The fracture was revised to a thicker plate and went on to heal.

References

1. Schneppendahl J, Windolf J, Kaufmann RA. Distal radius fractures: current concepts. J Hand Surg Am. 2012;37(8):1718–25.
2. Mattila VM, Huttunen TT, Sillanpää P, Niemi S, Pihlajamäki H, Kannus P. Significant change in the

surgical treatment of distal radius fractures: a nation-wide study between 1998 and 2008 in Finland. J Trauma. 2011;71(4):939–42; discussion 942–3.

3. Ring D, Jupiter JB. Treatment of osteoporotic distal radius fractures. Osteoporos Int. 2005;16(Suppl 2):S80–4.

4. Trumble TE, Wagner W, Hanel DP, Vedder NB, Gilbert M. Intrafocal (Kapandji) pinning of distal radius fractures with and without external fixation. J Hand Surg Am. 1998;23(3):381–94.

5. Seitz WH Jr, Froimson AI, Leb R, Shapiro JD. Augmented external fixation of unstable distal radius fractures. J Hand Surg Am. 1991;16(6):1010–6.

6. Wolfe SW, Pike L, Slade JF 3rd, Katz LD. Augmentation of distal radius fracture fixation with coralline hydroxyapatite bone graft substitute. J Hand Surg Am. 1999;24(4):816–27.

7. Tyllianakis ME, Panagopoulos A, Giannikas D, Megas P, Lambiris E. Graft-supplemented, augmented external fixation in the treatment of intra-articular distal radial fractures. Orthopedics. 2006;29(2):139–44.

8. Chung KC, Kim HM, Malay S, Shauver MJ, WRIST Group. Comparison of 24-month outcomes after treatment for distal radius fracture: the WRIST randomized clinical trial. JAMA Netw Open. 2021;4(6):e2112710.

9. Soong M, Earp BE, Bishop G, Leung A, Blazar P. Volar locking plate implant prominence and flexor tendon rupture. J Bone Joint Surg Am. 2011;93(4):328–35.

10. Soong M, Got C, Katarincic J, Akelman E. Fluoroscopic evaluation of intra-articular screw placement during locked volar plating of the distal radius: a cadaveric study. J Hand Surg Am. 2008;33(10):1720–3.

11. Beck JD, Harness NG, Spencer HT. Volar plate fixation failure for volar shearing distal radius fractures with small lunate facet fragments. J Hand Surg Am. 2014;39(4):670–8.

12. Arora R, Lutz M, Hennerbichler A, Krappinger D, Espen D, Gabl M. Complications following internal fixation of unstable distal radius fracture with a palmar locking-plate. J Orthop Trauma. 2007;21(5):316–22.

13. Harness NG, Jupiter JB, Orbay JL, Raskin KB, Fernandez DL. Loss of fixation of the volar lunate facet fragment in fractures of the distal part of the radius. J Bone Joint Surg Am. 2004;86(9):1900–8.

14. Chin KR, Jupiter JB. Wire-loop fixation of volar displaced osteochondral fractures of the distal radius. J Hand Surg Am. 1999;24(3):525–33.

15. Andermahr J, Lozano-Calderon S, Trafton T, Crisco JJ, Ring D. The volar extension of the lunate facet of the distal radius: a quantitative anatomic study. J Hand Surg Am. 2006;31(6):892–5.

16. Souer JS, Wiggers J, Ring D. Quantitative 3-dimensional computed tomography measurement of volar shearing fractures of the distal radius. J Hand Surg Am. 2011;36(4):599–603.

17. Souer JS, Ring D, Jupiter JB, Matschke S, Audige L, Marent-Huber M, AOCID Prospective ORIF Distal Radius Study Group. Comparison of AO Type-B and Type-C volar shearing fractures of the distal part of the radius. J Bone Joint Surg Am. 2009;91(11):2605–11.

18. Bolmers A, Luiten WE, Doornberg JN, Brouwer KM, Goslings JC, Ring D, Kloen P. A comparison of the long-term outcome of partial articular (AO Type B) and complete articular (AO Type C) distal radius fractures. J Hand Surg Am. 2013;38(4):753–9.

19. Harness N, Ring D, Jupiter JB. Volar Barton's fractures with concomitant dorsal fracture in older patients. J Hand Surg Am. 2004;29(3):439–45.

20. Fernandez DL, Ring D, Jupiter JB. Surgical management of delayed union and nonunion of distal radius fractures. J Hand Surg Am. 2001;26(2):201–9.

21. Sanderson PL, Ryan W, Turner PG. Complications of metalwork removal. Injury. 1992;23(1):29–30.

22. Geissler WB, Clark SM. Fragment-specific fixation for fractures of the distal radius. J Wrist Surg. 2016;5(1):22–30.

23. Minato K, Yasuda M, Shibata S. A loop-wiring technique for volarly displaced distal radius fractures with small thin volar marginal fragments. J Hand Surg Am. 2020;45(3):261.e1–7.

24. Gavaskar AS, Parthasarathy S, Balamurugan J, Raj RV, Anurag R, Gopinath D. Volar hook plate stabilization of volar marginal fragments in intra-articular distal radius fractures. Injury. 2021;52(1):85–9.

25. Fogel N, Shapiro LM, Roe A, Denduluri S, Richard MJ, Kamal RN. Outcomes of supplementary spring wire fixation with volar plating for volar lunate facet fragments in distal radius fractures. Hand (N Y). 2020;15:1558944720976404.

26. Hayakawa K, Okamoto H, Kojima T, Fukuoka M, Murakami H. Volar RIM plate rarely causes flexor tendon complications in a short period despite its plate prominence over the watershed line: a descriptive study. J Hand Surg Asian Pac Vol. 2021;26(2):194–206.

27. Perlus R, Doyon J, Henry P. The use of dorsal distraction plating for severely comminuted distal radius fractures: a review and comparison to volar plate fixation. Injury. 2019;50(Suppl 1):S50–5.

28. Ozer K, Chung KC. The use of bone grafts and substitutes in the treatment of distal radius fractures. Hand Clin. 2012;28(2):217–23.

29. Tosti R, Ilyas AM. The role of bone grafting in distal radius fractures. J Hand Surg Am. 2010;35(12):2082–4.

30. Handoll HH, Watts AC. Bone grafts and bone substitutes for treating distal radial fractures in adults. Cochrane Database Syst Rev. 2008;2:CD006836.

Perilunate Dislocation Failed Fixation

17

Chrishan Mariathas

History of Previous Primary Failed Treatment

A 24-year-old male car driver involved in a high-speed road traffic collision (RTC), sustained an injury to their non-dominant left wrist and contra-lateral acetabulum.

Primary radiographs of the left wrist injury are shown in Figs. 17.1 and 17.2, clearly demonstrating instability about the lunate with gross scapholunate (SL) interval widening and loss of congruency of the radiocarpal articulation. The lines described by Gilula [1] are clearly disrupted. Note the significant radial dislocation of the scaphoid, which is not typical of the recognised perilunate injury pattern. Fractures to the triquetrum and ulnar styloid are also evident.

At presentation, the patient underwent a manipulation of the injury in the emergency department, resulting in the radiographs shown in Figs. 17.3 and 17.4, and satisfactory initial reduction of the wrist.

Seven days post-injury, once their acetabulum and been surgically managed, the patient underwent surgical stabilisation of his wrist under a regional block and fluoroscopic control. Figures 17.5 and 17.6 shows the final intra-operative imaging before they were placed in a forearm backslab. One week later, routine radiographs (Figs. 17.7 and 17.8) revealed gross disruption of the midcarpal joint, necessitating revision surgery 4 days subsequently.

C. Mariathas (✉)
Leeds Teaching Hospitals NHS Trust, Leeds, UK
e-mail: cmariathas@nhs.net

© The Author(s), under exclusive license to Springer Nature Switzerland AG 2024
P. V. Giannoudis, P. Tornetta III (eds.), *Failed Fracture Fixation*,
https://doi.org/10.1007/978-3-031-39692-2_17

Figs. 17.1 and 17.2 AP and lateral of left wrist demonstrating instability about the lunate with gross scapholunate (SL) interval widening; there is loss of congruency of the radiocarpal articulation and there is significant radial dislocation of the scaphoid. Fractures to the triquetrum and ulnar styloid are also evident

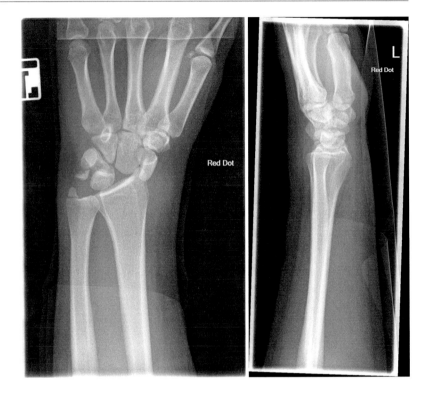

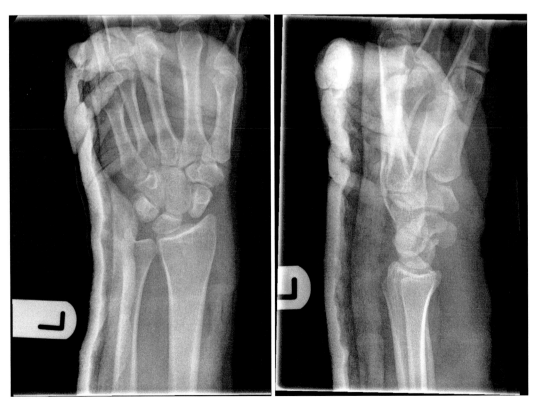

Figs. 17.3 and 17.4 AP and lateral left wrist radiographs post manipulation showing satisfactory initial reduction of the wrist

17 Perilunate Dislocation Failed Fixation

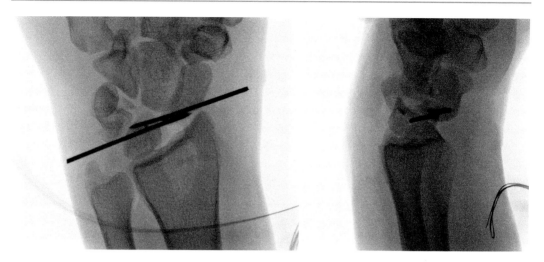

Figs. 17.5 and 17.6 AP and lateral of the left wrist show the final intra-operative imaging before they were placed in a forearm backslab

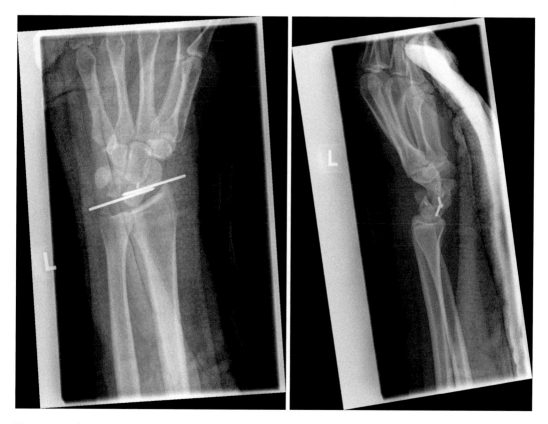

Figs. 17.7 and 17.8 AP and lateral of left wrist of follow-up radiographs a week later revealed gross disruption of the midcarpal joint

Evaluation of the Aetiology of Failure of Fixation

The primary carpal reduction and stabilisation were performed through a dorsal approach to the wrist (between the third and fourth extensor compartments), utilising the radially based ligament sparing arthrotomy popularised by Berger [2]. At the time of the approach, trauma to the dorsal radiocarpal (DRC) ligament was documented. The operative surgeon identified a complex SL ligament tear partly avulsed from the lunate and partly avulsed from the scaphoid. Attempt was made to ensure that the SL diastasis was reduced along with dorsal intercarpal segment instability (DISI) using two 1.6 mm Kirschner wires before surgical repair of the SL ligament with two 2 mm anchors fitted with 4-0 braided, non-absorbable suture.

Figures 17.5 and 17.6 demonstrate just two wires, one inserted from the radial side through the scaphoid, and a second inserted from the ulnar side bypassing the fragmented triquetrum. While these two wires may have been able to stabilise the lunate, they were unable to confer any stability to the midcarpal joint. While the SL diastasis has been decreased, there is still incongruency of the scaphoid with respect to the radius, as well as the capitate. The lateral view shows that the midcarpal (luno-capitate) articulation does not appear to be congruent, with a volar displaced scaphoid.

The presentation radiographs (Figs. 17.1 and 17.2) show a very radially displaced scaphoid, which is not a common component of a perilunate injury. Trying to apply the basic concepts of perilunate instability here appears to have underestimated the injury severity and the likely contribution of extrinsic ligament injury in this case. Another contributor to this could have been the comminuted triquetrum and the disrupted DRC ligament encountered during surgical exposure. This high degree of instability requires a greater level of stabilisation and focus on adequate reduction of the radiocarpal and midcarpal articulations.

Clinical Examination

Following the primary stabilisation procedure, the wrist was swollen to some extent, but all wounds were clean and healthy. Movements of the digits were restricted by swelling; however, the neurological state of the hand was normal. While the patient had been instructed to be kept non-weight bearing through his incomplete cast, it would appear that he had been exposing it to load while trying to transfer from their bed after their acetabular surgery.

Diagnostic-Biochemical and Radiological Investigations

Following the radiographs taken one week post operatively, a CT was performed to help characterise the incongruent luno-capitate joint and the volar displaced scaphoid. It was deemed that, as the injury had been almost three weeks previously, the SL ligament was still amenable to primary repair in the setting of revision surgery.

Preoperative Planning

The revision surgery was planned with the help of the MDT meeting of consultant wrist surgeons and MSK radiologists. As implants had only been inserted 1 week prior, it was felt that there should be no difficulty in K-wire extraction. It was likely that anchors would not be amenable to removal from the carpal bones.

At the time of the MDT, it had been considered that the initial 1.6-mm K-wires may have been a bit too thick and may have contributed to the displaced scaphoid at the time of their insertion, by pushing the scaphoid volarwards. The decision to use more flexible 1.2-mm K-wires during the revision was made, to minimise adversely steering the clearly very unstable scaphoid at the time of wire insertion. An emphasis was placed on needing to stabilise the midcarpal joint with the revision wire configuration, as this was clearly unstable. At least three wires were deemed to be necessary, and again the comminuted triquetrum was thought to be unsuitable to rely upon for the construct.

Bone graft was not applicable to this case due to the predominantly ligamentous nature of this injury.

Revision Surgery

Revision stabilisation was performed under the regional block with fluoroscopic control. The previous dorsal approach was used to the wrist, along with the Berger capsulotomy. Both k-wires were removed and a dorsal wire was used to 'joy stick' the scaphoid into an anatomic position. Three 1.2-mm k-wires were then used to stabilise both the scapholunate interval and the midcarpal joint into more anatomically appropriate positions. Two wires were again used through the proximal carpal row to tray and ensure rotational stability at the SL interval. Figures 17.9 and 17.10 show the final intra-operative fluoroscopy with a reduced scaphoid and reduced midcarpal joint. At this stage, it was noted that one of the sutures holding the avulsed SL ligament had torn out of the soft tissue, therefore an additional anchor was placed into the lunate to re-tension the avulsed SL ligament.

The wires were cut and buried beneath the skin once the dorsal wound was closed, and the patient was placed in an incomplete cast. Again, the patient was advised to not weight bear through the operated wrist. A plan was made for them to be seen 1 week post-revision surgery with fresh radiographs before being put into a full forearm synthetic cast and given permission to forearm weight bear when needed. Their radiographs at this stage are shown in Figs. 17.11 and 17.12.

Eight weeks post-revision surgery, the patient had removed their wires under regional block before commencing aggressive physiotherapy to maximise their wrist range of movement and grip strength. This period of time was to allow for ligamentous healing, both of the scapholunate ligament, but also the evidently injured extrinsic wrist ligaments, to confer stability once the wires were removed.

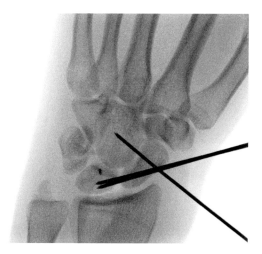 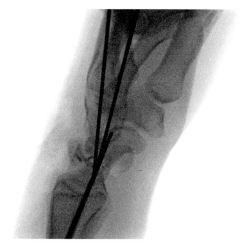

Figs. 17.9 and 17.10 AP and lateral radiographs of the left wrist showing the final intra-operative fluoroscopy with a reduced scaphoid and reduced midcarpal joint. At this stage it was noted that one of the sutures holding the avulsed SL ligament had torn out of the soft tissue, therefore an additional anchor was placed into the lunate to re-tension the avulsed SL ligament

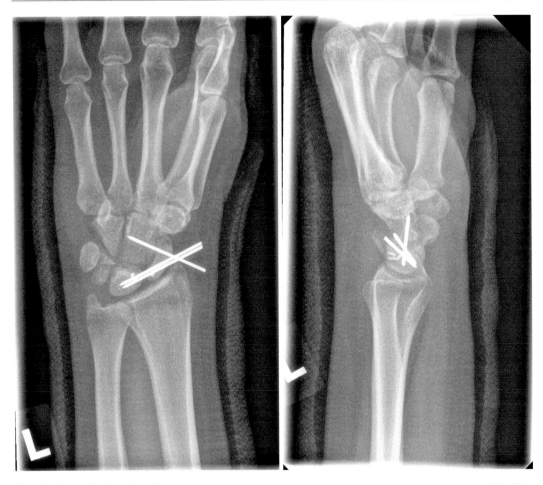

Figs. 17.11 and 17.12 AP and lateral radiographs of the left wrist 1 week after revision surgery showing that the wires were cut and buried beneath the skin and satisfactory reduction of the mid carpal joint and the radio carpal articulation

Summary: Lessons Learned

A key point to appreciate from this case is identifying, from the presentation radiographs (Figs. 17.1 and 17.2), that this injury is not a typical perilunate injury [3]. The surgeon must be weary due to the mechanism and the degree of scaphoid displacement that reduction is likely to be more difficult than a 'run-of-the-mill' injury around the lunate. There must also be an appreciation that there must be adequate stabilisation across the midcarpal joint, and midcarpal reduction must be scrupulously checked on intra-operative imaging.

The operative surgeon must take care not to displace unstable carpal bones when inserting k-wires to help stabilise, but also value the contribution of 'joy-stick' wires to help control unstable small bones within the wrist prior to definitive stabilisation.

This case highlights the importance of checking for displacement post-stabilisation, in this instance 1 week postoperatively. Robust clinical follow-up enabled revision to be undertaken in a timely manner while the wrist was still salvageable and amenable to ligamentous healing. The role of the MDT enabled a clear plan for revision fixation and its timely execution.

References

1. Linn MR, Mann FA, Gilula LA. Imaging the symptomatic wrist. Orthop Clin North Am. 1990;21(3):515–43.
2. Berger RA. The ligaments of the wrist. A current overview of anatomy with considerations of their potential functions. Hand Clin. 1997;13(1):63–82.
3. Mayfield JK, Johnson RP, Kilcoyne RK. Carpal dislocations: pathomechanics and progressive perilunar instability. J Hand Surg. 1980;5(3):226–41. https://doi.org/10.1016/s0363-5023(80)80007-4.

Pelvic Fracture Failed Fixation

18

Nathan Olszewski and Reza Firoozabadi

History of Previous Primary Failed Treatment

A 59-year-old morbidly obese male, with 23-year pack year history of smoking, was involved in a motorcycle collision 6 weeks prior and underwent operative management of his pelvic ring at a Level 1 hospital in North America. He has been non-weightbearing bilateral lower extremities and original imaging was not able to be transferred. He states that his pain has improved over the past 4 weeks, and he rarely takes narcotics. His pain in the back of his pelvis is worse than the pain in the front. Furthermore, he is interested in starting to weightbearing so he can get back to work.

Radiographic evaluation at 6 weeks utilizing 3 views of the pelvis was performed (Fig. 18.1). Radiographs supported a pubic symphysis disruption that was reduced and plated. One of the six small fragment screws was partially backed out. A partially threaded large caliber cannulated screw used in the posterior aspect of the pelvic ring across a left sided Zone 2/3 junction sacral fracture. The screw was showing evidence of strain with slight bend in the middle and haloing around the screw.

Clinical plan at this point was to keep the patient non-weightbearing bilateral lower extremities and obtain imaging in 2 weeks to determine if signs of hardware failure had progressed. The patient missed appointment and presented at 12 weeks postop with significant increase in pain.

Radiographs at 12 weeks demonstrated multiple failed points of fixation at the anterior aspect of the pelvic ring (Fig. 18.2). The sacroiliac (SI) joint was also slightly wider and in retrospective evaluation of his 6-week films, the joint appeared slightly wide then. Significant haloing was also noted around the posteriorly based screw.

N. Olszewski · R. Firoozabadi (✉)
Harborview Medical Center/University of Washington, Seattle, WA, USA
e-mail: Rezaf2@uw.edu

© The Author(s), under exclusive license to Springer Nature Switzerland AG 2024
P. V. Giannoudis, P. Tornetta III (eds.), *Failed Fracture Fixation*,
https://doi.org/10.1007/978-3-031-39692-2_18

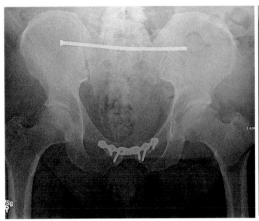 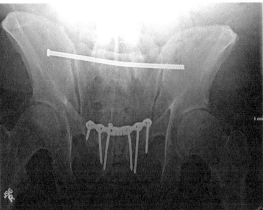

Fig. 18.1 6 week post-op AP and outlet X-rays

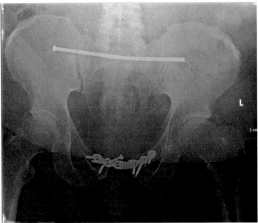 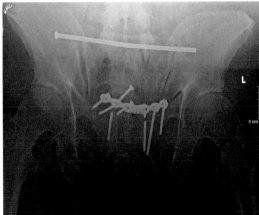

Fig. 18.2 12 week post-op AP and outlet X-rays

Evaluation of the Etiology of Failure of Fixation

This is a challenging case considered the injury pattern and the patient's body mass index (BMI). The etiology leading to hardware failure and nonunion was likely the result of insufficient reduction and fixation posteriorly. This resulted in catastrophic failure of the anterior hardware resulting in a pelvic malunion.

Clinical Examination

On examination he is a super obese appearing male of stated age in a wheelchair (BMI 60). He could transfer from wheelchair to clinic bed with significant increase in pain over the anterior aspect of his pelvis. His anterior-based incision is hidden underneath a pannus, it is well healed. The percutaneous screw insertion site wounds have healed. No other pertinent findings on exam.

Diagnostic-Biochemical, and Radiological Investigations

A computed tomography (CT) scan was ordered and demonstrated a partially threaded screw that was crossing a widened SI joint and a gapped left sided sacral fracture (Fig. 18.3). Furthermore, the symphysis was disrupted.

Infection workup was also performed, and erythrocyte sedimentation rate (ESR), C-reactive protein (CRP), and white blood cell (WBC) were within normal limits. Vitamin D was found to be low at 13.1. Calcium levels were normal. The patient was treated with 2000 U daily for 6 weeks to replete his vitamin D levels.

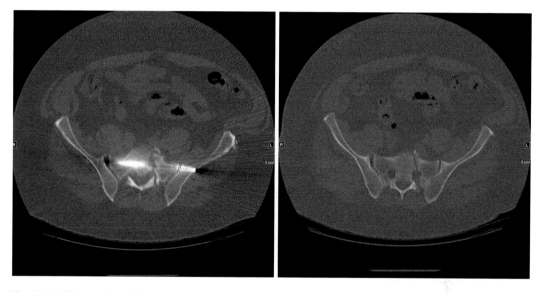

Fig. 18.3 CT posterior pelvic ring with sacral fracture gap and wide right sacroiliac joint

Preoperative Planning

Clinical challenge is failed fracture fixation of the pubic symphysis and posterior pelvic ring in a morbidly obese male at 3 months. This patient has three distinct injuries which have no evidence of healing; a pubic symphysis diastasis, a right sided sacroiliac joint disruption, and a potentially atrophic gapped sacral fracture. The treatment options of the individual components of the injury will be discussed, followed by a summary of the surgical plan.

Anterior Ring Injury

There are several options to be considered regarding the anterior pelvis. Treatment options include non-operative management, external fixation, internal fixation with pedicle screws and bar, and revision internal fixation with plates and screws. Each one offers a different mechanical construct in addition to coming with its own risk benefit profile for this individual patient.

First, given the patient's body habitus and weight, the anterior pelvis could be managed non-operatively to avoid complications associated with surgical intervention. However, non-operative management is likely to result in poor reduction, a greater likelihood of gait disturbance, and overall worse outcomes [1–5]. This patient is at increased risk for developing pelvic pain, symptomatic leg length inequality, and rotational deformity of the lower extremity [1, 2]. Not intervening now could potentially result in an even more difficult surgery as the deformity could worsen and additional scar tissue could form. For these reasons we felt that some form of anterior fixation was needed.

The least invasive surgical intervention anteriorly would be external fixation. Pins can be placed into the iliac crest or into the supracetabular corridor. Risks associated with external fixation include developing a pin site infection, with the potential for development of osteomyelitis, and lateral femoral cutaneous nerve palsy [6–8]. Operative risks are even higher in morbidly obese patients with a BMI of 40 or greater [9].

Additionally, if external fixation was chosen the patient's pannus would likely be rubbing against the external fixation device, limiting the patient's ability to sit up. Hupel et al. showed that anterior external fixation in isolation was unable to provide sufficient stabilization of the pelvic ring in obese patients compared to non-obese patients [10]. Not only is there no literature to support the use of an anterior external fixation device in the setting of revision symphyseal fixation, but it would be unlikely to close the symphysis without opening and removing the scar tissue surgically given the amount of scar tissue that has formed as the patient is 3 months post-op. Given the myriad of complications and the literature demonstrating anterior frames cannot hold the anterior pelvis reduced in obese patients, external fixation was felt to not be a reasonable option for the anterior pelvis.

A minimally invasive form of anterior fixation would be use of pedicle screws with a bar, also known as an in-fix. This would allow for a more stable construct compared to an external fixation device and would also avoid the pin site complications [8, 11]. The patient would also be able to sit upright to a greater extent than a patient in an external fixator. They would not have the external bar rubbing against the pannus or compressing the thighs [12]. However, fixation with pedicle screws and bar would predispose the patient to additional complications such as risk for femoral nerve palsy, deep infection, and heterotopic ossification [6, 11]. Newer techniques have been developed to stiffen the overall construct by adding an additional pedicle screw into the pubic body [8]. Though with this additional pedicle screw it still is not the stiffest construct for the anterior pelvis [7]. Another downside for using an internal fixator is the eventual need for removal of the pedicle screws and bar [6, 8, 11–13].

The most invasive intervention would be an open reduction and internal fixation of the pubic symphysis, which has several advantages. Anterior plating allows for a more anatomic reduction of the symphysis and provides a stiffer construct than the use of pedicle screws and bar [6, 7]. Plating of the anterior symphysis comes with the highest risk of complication, especially in revision cases. Performing an open reduction and internal fixation of the pelvic ring exposes the patient to increased bleeding and risk of deep infection [6]. The dissection of the symphysis is even more difficult in revision cases where scar tissue from previous surgeries can be adherent to the bladder leading to disruption of the bladder wall during dissection, or inadvertently cutting the bladder, or other critical structures such as the corona mortis during the approach. Not only is a revision case more difficult, but the obesity of the patient will add additional challenges to this case. There will be a large amount of soft tissue to dissect, the pannus will make placement of reduction clamps more difficult and will make getting the appropriate trajectory for the symphysis plate screws more difficult. These complications could all be avoided with either an external fixator or internal fixator; however, it is unlikely that the symphysis would be reducible. Opening the symphysis would afford us different reduction techniques such as placing a point-to-point clamp or using a Jungbluth clamp. It was felt that performing an open reduction and internal fixation of the anterior pelvis would provide the best opportunity to obtain an anatomic reduction and provide the most stable construct possible. Also reducing and plating the anterior pelvis would help reduce and stabilize the posterior pelvis. Additionally, opening the anterior pelvis provides the opportunity to add a second plate to increase the stiffness, but this requires additional soft tissue dissection, may prolong the surgery, and increases the bleeding time [14, 15].

Posterior Ring Injury

The posterior pelvic ring provides the issue of having bilateral injuries. On the right side the sacroiliac joint is wide anteriorly and mal-reduced. On the left side there is a zone two sacral fracture which extends into the S1 sacral body cranially. This fracture is also still gapped, and while there is some callus present at the sacral ala on CT scan, there are no signs of healing throughout the rest of the fracture. The risks

and benefits of each possible surgical strategy for each of the posterior injuries must be considered carefully. The left sided sacrum must have bone-to-bone contact and held with a stable construct for it to heal and the right sacroiliac joint must be reduced and held with sufficient fixation for it to heal. In this instance the sacrum was gapped and the whole construct only had one point of fixation with a right to left 6.5 mm partially threaded transiliac transsacral screw with 32 mm of threads placed initially. This screw had threads in the left ilium only and thus was trying to compress the right sacroiliac joint and the left sided sacral fracture. While a single screw may be able to compress the right sacroiliac joint, it will not provide sufficient compression across the left sacral fracture. A single screw is also likely not enough to control the flexion and extension of the right hemipelvis and vertical translation of the left hemipelvis [9, 16].The catastrophic anterior hardware failure and residual displacement in the posterior pelvic ring are likely due to lack of reduction and insufficient fixation construct posteriorly. Now the patient has an anteriorly gapped complete sacral fracture with broken hardware anteriorly, revision surgery was chosen as treatment for this patient.

Given the morbid obesity of our patient the potential complications of each intervention must be considered. Achieving an anatomic reduction of both the right SI joint and the left sacrum is paramount. For the sacrum to heal it must be reduced, compressed, and held with adequate stability. The most aggressive, but likely best means of obtaining an anatomic reduction for the sacral non-union would be to perform a prone open sacral reduction. Performing an open reduction would also allow for the fracture to be debrided of fibrinous tissue and allow for adjuvants such as allograft, autograft, or other factors to be added to the fracture site to help promote healing. However, an open posterior approach in a morbidly obese smoker has a high infection risk and wound complication rate, which could be more detrimental than the non-union [9].

Performing a supine open reduction of the right sacroiliac joint would again predispose the patient to infection and reaching the sacroiliac joint in a patient of this size would be very difficult given his massive body habitus. With this understanding, alternative means of improving the reduction were assessed. One way of adding extra-compression to the posterior pelvic ring would be the use of the c-clamp. This device could be placed either in the posterior aspect of the pelvis or onto the gluteal pillar to help compress the posterior pelvis. Again, because of the body habitus of the patient this would not work as the clamp points would not be long enough to reach the gluteal pillar. An alternative to these methods would be using multiple screws to preferentially squeeze the sacrum and provide additional points of fixation to stabilize the posterior ring. This could be achieved by using partially threated screws to provide compression. Review of the patients pre-operative CT scan showed the patient had large osseous sacral corridors that would be able to accommodate multiple screws. Given the residual displacement of the left sacral fracture and the right sacroiliac joint we felt that using multiple screws from both directions to help further reduction of the right and left posterior ring injuries would compress both and provide adequate stabilization to the posterior pelvic ring to heal.

Additionally, lumbopelvic fixation can be added to stabilize the posterior pelvis. In vitro studies have shown that ilio-sacral screw fixation combined with lumbopelvic fixation, effectively forming an osteosynthesis triangle, provides greater stiffness of the construct compared to ilio-sacral screws alone [17]. While triangular osteosynthesis has shown to increase construct stability it comes with its own set of complications and high need for removal [18]. Adding a lumbopelvic construct to our patient may increase the overall stability, but it increases the risk of infection as there is a high wound complication rate associated with morbidly obese patients undergoing spine fixation [19, 20]. After discussion with our spine colleagues the risk associated with performing lumbopelvic fixation, even percutaneously, would not outweigh the benefits given the high risk of infection and complications that can come with it.

After weighing all options, it was felt that a percutaneous reduction of the posterior ring with a combination of partially threaded ilio-sacral screws and transiliac-transsacral screws was the least invasive and most likely to obtain positive outcomes with relative low risk. The large osseous corridors would allow multiple ilio-sacral screws and transiliac-transsacral screws at both the S1 and S2 corridors. This would allow maximum compression and increase the stability of the fixation construct. Decision was made to forego adding lumbopelvic fixation given the increased morbidity of the procedure and because of the multiple points of fixation that the bony osseous corridors would allow. Furthermore, if the current plan was not successful, then the addition of lumbopelvic fixation could be used as a secondary plan.

As is customary in the treatment of nonunions, allograft, autograft, and other factors are frequently used to help obtain union. Autograft, allograft, and factors such as bone morphogenic protein, could potentially provide a benefit in the setting of sacral non-union [21, 22]. Autograft harvested from the posterior crest would provide ample graft, and it could be used in the fracture after debridement. Alternatively, case reports have shown bone morphogenetic protein (BMP) to potentially be beneficial in cases of refractory sacral non-union [21]. Performing percutaneous reduction and fixation would sacrifice the ability to use bone graft and other substitutes, but in this instance, the minimal gap could most likely be closed down with multiple large caliber lag screws.

Revision Surgery

To summarize there was an anterior symphysis injury with hardware failure, a partial right sacroiliac joint disruption with gapping anteriorly, and a left zone 2 sacral fracture with minimal signs of biological healing and persistent gapping. Plan for this patient was to start in the front with the removal of hardware and then revision fixation of the anterior symphysis followed by percutaneous posterior public ring fixation. By starting in the anterior portion of the pelvic ring we would be able to remove the broken hardware and then clamp down the symphysis to reduce it. As discussed, considerations to take into account for this surgery are the amount of scar tissue present which may preclude the dissection and freeing up the bladder. Preoperative CT scan showed that the bladder was near the symphysis and may even be partially incarcerated (Fig. 18.4). Given this a urology team member assisted with the dissection of the anterior pelvic ring and inspected the bladder for injury, once the anterior pelvic ring was dissected and the bladder was inspected. There was a small tear noted, which was repaired by the urology team. It was then protected, and the broken hardware was removed. Once the hardware was removed the symphysis was cleared of any scar tissue and the symphyseal cartilage was also removed to increase the construct stability by increasing the frictional forces through bone-to-bone contact [23]. This may also aid in fusion and healing of the symphysis. Attention was then turned to reducing the symphysis. There are multiple ways to approach this. One way to do this would be to apply 5.0 mm supracetabular Shanz pins and apply an external fixator device to help close the symphysis. This technique does not work as well when multiplanar correction is needed. Other considerations for reducing the anterior pelvic ring include the use of a point-to-point reduction clamps placed anteriorly. However, this relies on the quality of the bone and can be challenging to correct when deformity is present in multiple planes. Alternatively, a Jungbluth clamp can also be used, which allows for control in multiple planes. In this instance we used a Jungbluth clamp to aid in the reduction of the anterior surface (Fig. 18.5). This was performed by placing 3.5-mm screws anteriorly on each side of the symphysis and then

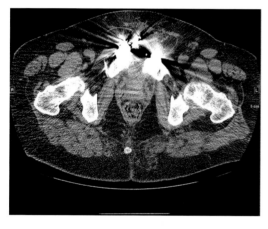

Fig. 18.4 CT scan showing bladder near the pubic symphysis

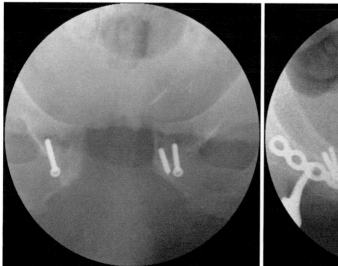
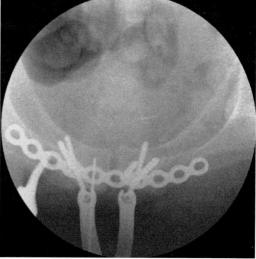

Fig. 18.5 Intra-op fluoroscopic images showing reduction of the anterior pelvis with a Jungbluth clamp

using the clamp to control the reduction. In most cases the following reduction steps can be useful when using a Jungbluth; reduce the pubic symphysis widening, reduce any flexion/extension deformity, and last correct anterior or posterior translation. After reduction was obtained, a 3.5-mm reconstruction plate was placed on the superior aspect of each parasymphysis to hold the reduction and keep the symphysis closed down. This plate was longer than the previous plate and had different hole spacing, which allowed for additional screws to be placed on each side of the symphysis in bone that had not been used at the initial surgery. These screws are placed in a cranial to caudal direction and placed bicortically to make sure that they have a greater purchase. Given the size of the patient and the fact that this was a revision case, a second plate was added anteriorly. This was a 2.7-mm plate placed on the anterior aspect of the symphysis and rami with multiple bicortical screws heading in the anterior to posterior direction. The cranial 1/3 of the rectus attachment site on the pubic body needs to be elevated to allow the placement of this plate. By performing symphysis reduction first, the right sacroiliac joint reduction improved.

Once the anterior pelvic ring was reduced and stabilized, attention was placed on the posterior pelvic ring. Again, given the patient body habitus it was felt that the best option to obtain a stable construct and minimize complications was to perform a percutaneous reduction using a combination of ilio-sacral and transiliac transsacral screws. First started by placing a partially threaded ilio-sacral screw across the right sacroiliac joint to compress this joint and reduce it. The start site started slightly posterior and aimed just cranial to the S1 foramina and directed a screw with a washer into the sacral body stopping just shy of midline, given the fact that he had a fracture line extending into the sacral body on the left side. Before final tightening, the previously placed right sided transiliac-transsacral screw was removed. With final tightening this screw further reduced and compressed the right sacroiliac joint. Then a guide wire was placed for a left to right transiliac-transsacral screw with partial threads inferior and slightly anterior to the right to left transiliac-transsacral screw going across

S1. This screw was also a transiliac-transsacral style because the maximum compressive force was desired, by having the threads across multiple cortices. Furthermore, potential screw compromise could occur if the screws were placed into the sacral body, secondary to the left sided sacral fracture extending into the sacral body. This screw also provides support to the right side of the posterior ring and had a force vector that was orthogonal to the fracture line. Prior to final tightening of the left to right transiliac-transsacral screw the right screw was removed to allow for compression across the left sided sacral fracture. Once this was placed another partially threaded transiliac-transsacral screw was placed across the original S1 corridor. Originally a 7.0-mm screw was used, this was upsized to a 7.5-mm screw, which provided excellent purchase and added additional compression across the left sided sacral fracture and again added additional stability to the right side of the posterior pelvic ring. After this screw was placed two partially threaded transiliac-transsacral screw in the S2 corridor to provide further compression to the left sided sacral fracture. Once this screw was final tightened, a fully threaded ilio-sacral screw anterior to the first left to right screw placed in the S1 corridor to reinforce the construct. This construct maximized the posterior pelvic ring stability and took advantage of the large osseous corridors. With revision open reduction and dual plating anteriorly, and six screws posteriorly, this treatment plan maximized construct stability while minimizing the potential risk to the patient.

Post-operative Course

Post-operatively the patient received 24 h of intravenous antibiotics. Immediate post-operative X-rays showed a reduced pelvic ring anteriorly with several screws placed in the posterior pelvis through the ilium and sacrum. All hardware appeared to be safe on imaging (Fig. 18.6). A post-operative CT scan was obtained to make sure all the screws were in a safe position and to evaluate the amount of compression across the posterior pelvic ring (Fig. 18.7). This showed that the technique used compressed the left sacral

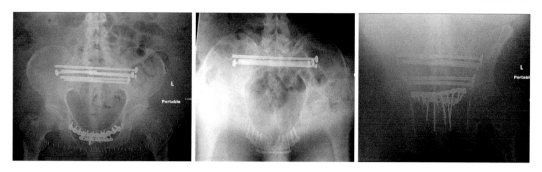

Fig. 18.6 Immediate post-op AP, inlet and outlet X-rays

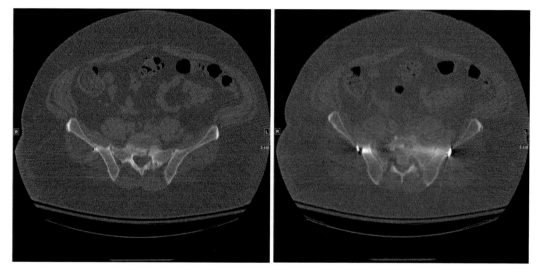

Fig. 18.7 Immediate post-op CT scan showing reduction of the right sacroiliac joint and decreased gap across the left sacral fracture

fracture and had improved the alignment of the right sacroiliac joint. The patient was placed on enoxaparin 40 mg BID for 6 weeks for deep venous thrombosis (DVT) prophylaxis. This was chosen given his BMI. Drains were placed anteriorly to help prevent the formation of a of a post-op hematoma. These were removed once the drainage was less than 10 cc per 12-h shift. He was kept non-weight bearing bilateral lower extremities and was slide board transfer only for 12 weeks. Due to the work of Brinker et al. vitamin D 25-hydroxy and calcium levels were checked. The patient was found to have a low vitamin D 25-hydroxy and was started on 2000 U daily for 6 weeks for repletion to maximize the patient's healing potential.

He was discharged from the hospital postoperative day 8. He was seen back at 2 weeks and staples were removed from his incisions without any issue. At 6 weeks the patient was seen in the clinic and was noted to be pain free. X-rays were obtained that showed maintenance of the alignment of the pelvic ring and without any signs of loosening of the hardware. The patient was seen back at 3 months post-operatively with pelvic X-rays that showed the pelvis had maintained alignment and there were no signs of loosening. He was allowed to be weight bearing as tolerated at this visit. Final follow-up at 2 years post-op showed that the patient had maintained reduction of his pelvic ring (Fig. 18.8) and was pain free and returned to his manual labor job.

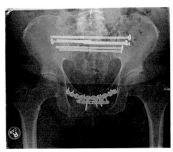 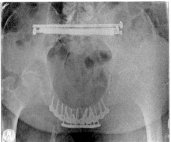 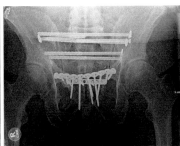

Fig. 18.8 2-year post-op AP, inlet and outlet X-rays

Summary: Lessons Learned

In summary this is a challenging case given the injury pattern and the patient's body habitus. The failure leading to non-union was likely the result of insufficient reduction and fixation posteriorly. This resulted in catastrophic failure of the anterior hardware resulting in a pelvic malunion. Initially, the patient was assessed at regular follow-up intervals. However, the treating team did not have the initial injury imaging. As a result, subtle findings of the right SI joint injury and the left zone 2 sacral fracture were underappreciated. Retrospectively, more effort should have been placed on obtaining the original imaging. Review of these images would have most likely led to an earlier surgical intervention. Even without the initial injury imaging the treatment team could have intervened earlier and added additional fixation to the posterior pelvic ring right when the patient first presented to clinic. However, he did not present until 6 weeks post-op and at this time he was already demonstrating signs of loosening and it is unknown whether additional posterior fixation would have prevented this catastrophic failure. Had the patient been seen immediately post-op with his initial imaging, the team would have likely leaned toward provided additional fixation. As a result, the patient required a significantly more complex revision surgery. However, an excellent outcome was obtained using the discussed treatment strategy.

References

1. Holdsworth FW. Dislocation and fracture-dislocation of the pelvis. J Bone Joint Surg Br. 1948;470(8):461–6. https://doi.org/10.1007/s11999-012-2422-4.
2. Tornetta P III, Matta J. Outcome of operatively treated unstable posterior pelvic ring disruptions. Clin Orthop Relat Res. 1996;329:186–93.
3. Taguchi T, Kawai S, Kaneko K, Yugue D. Surgical treatment of old pelvic fractures. Int Orthop. 2000;24:28–32.
4. Papakostidis C, Kanakaris NK, Kontakis G, Giannoudis P, v. Pelvic ring disruptions: treatment modalities and analysis of outcomes. Int Orthop. 2009;33(2):329–38. https://doi.org/10.1007/s00264-008-0555-6.
5. McLaren A, Rorabeck C, Halpenny J. Long-term pain and disability in relation to residual deformity after displaced pelvic ring fractures. Can J Surg. 1990;33(6):492–4.
6. Yin Y, Luo J, Zhang R, et al. Anterior subcutaneous internal fixator (INFIX) versus plate fixation for pelvic anterior ring fracture. Sci Rep. 2019;9(1):2578. https://doi.org/10.1038/s41598-019-39068-7.
7. Vigdorchik JM, Esquivel AO, Jin X, Yang KH, Onwudiwe NA, Vaidya R. Biomechanical stability of a supra-acetabular pedicle screw internal fixation device (INFIX) vs external fixation and plates for vertically unstable pelvic fractures. J Orthop Surg Res. 2012;7(1):31. https://doi.org/10.1186/1749-799X-7-31.
8. Bi C, Wang Q, Wu J, et al. Modified pedicle screw-rod fixation versus anterior pelvic external fixation for the management of anterior pelvic ring fractures: a comparative study. J Orthop Surg Res. 2017;12(1):185. https://doi.org/10.1186/s13018-017-0688-7.
9. Carson JT, Shah SG, Ortega G, Thamyongkit S, Hasenboehler EA, Shafiq B. Complications of pelvic and acetabular fractures in 1331 morbidly obese patients (BMI ≥ 40): a retrospective observational

study from the National Trauma Data Bank. Patient Saf Surg. 2018;12(1):26. https://doi.org/10.1186/s13037-018-0172-2.

10. Hupel TM, Mckee MD, Waddell J, Schemitsch EH. External fixation of rotationally unstable pelvic fractures in obese patients. J Trauma. 1998;45(1):111–5.

11. Dahill M, Mcarthur J, Roberts GL, et al. The use of an anterior pelvic internal fixator to treat disruptions of the anterior pelvic ring: a report of technique, indications and complications. Bone Joint J. 2017;99-B:1232. https://doi.org/10.1302/0301-620X.99B9.

12. Vaidya R, Colen R, Vigdorchik J, Tonnos F, Sethi A. Treatment of unstable pelvic ring injuries with an internal anterior fixator and posterior fixation: initial clinical series. J Orthop Trauma. 2012;26(1):1–8. www.jorthotrauma.com.

13. Fritz T, Mettelsiefen L, Strobel F, et al. A novel internal fixation method for open book injuries of the pubic symphysis—a biomechanical analysis. Clin Biomech. 2020;77:105009. https://doi.org/10.1016/j.clinbiomech.2020.105009.

14. Lange RH, Hansen ST. Pelvic ring disruptions with symphysis pubis diastasis indications, technique, and limitations of anterior internal fixation. Clin Orthop Relat Res. 1985;201:130–7. http://journals.lww.com/clinorthop.

15. Chip ML Jr, Ms RM. Evaluation of new plate designs for symphysis pubis internal fixation. Injury. 1996;41(3):498–502.

16. Lu Y, He Y, Li W, Yang Z, Peng R, Yu L. Comparison of biomechanical performance of five different treatment approaches for fixing posterior pelvic ring injury. J Healthc Eng. 2020;2020:5379593. https://doi.org/10.1155/2020/5379593.

17. Schildhauer TA, Ledoux R, Chapman JR, Bradford Henley M, Tencer F, Routt MLC. Triangular osteosynthesis and iliosacral screw fixation for unstable sacral fractures: a cadaveric and biomechanical evaluation under cyclic loads. J Orthop Trauma. 2003;17(1):22–31.

18. Sagi HC, Militano U, Caron T, Lindvall E. A comprehensive analysis with minimum 1-year follow-up of vertically unstable transforaminal sacral fractures treated with triangular osteosynthesis. J Orthop Trauma. 2009;23(5):313–21. www.jorthotrauma.com.

19. Marquez-Lara A, Nandyala SV, Sankaranarayanan S, Noureldin M, Singh K. Body mass index as a predictor of complications and mortality after lumbar spine surgery. Spine (Phila Pa 1976). 2014;39(10):798–804. https://doi.org/10.1097/BRS.0000000000000232.

20. Jiang J, Teng Y, Fan Z, Khan S, Xia Y. Does obesity affect the surgical outcome and complication rates of spinal surgery? A meta-analysis. Clin Orthop Relat Res. 2014;472(3):968–75. https://doi.org/10.1007/s11999-013-3346-3.

21. Nicodemo A, Capella M, Deregibus M, Massè A. Nonunion of a sacral fracture refractory to bone grafting: internal fixation and osteogenic protein-1 (BMP-7) application. Musculoskelet Surg. 2011;95(2):157–61. https://doi.org/10.1007/s12306-011-0131-x.

22. Giannoudis P, Psarakis S, Kanakaris NK, Pape HC. Biological enhancement of bone healing with bone morphogenetic protein-7 at the clinical setting of pelvic girdle non-unions. Injury. 2007;38S4:S43–8.

23. Lybrand K, Kurylo J, Gross J, Templeman D, Tornetta P. Does removal of the symphyseal cartilage in symphyseal dislocations have any effect on final alignment and implant failure? J Orthop Trauma. 2015;29(10):470–4.

Acetabulum Posterior Wall Fracture Failed Fixation

19

Amit A. Davidson, George D. Chloros, Nikolaos K. Kanakaris, and Peter V. Giannoudis

History of Previous Primary Failed Treatment

This is the case of a 58-year-old male accountant, otherwise fit and well who was a restrained driver during a road traffic accident at approximately 60 mph. At hospital presentation, he was alert and oriented and had the following closed injuries: Left acetabular posterior wall fracture dislocation (Fig. 19.1a), a right distal radius and ulna fracture, and a right ankle fracture. Further computed tomography (CT) scan imaging revealed an impaction of the superior acetabulum surface, multiple intra-articular small fragments and a minimally displaced transverse acetabular fracture (Fig. 19.1b, c).

A. A. Davidson · N. K. Kanakaris
Academic Department of Trauma and Orthopaedics, Leeds General Infirmary University Hospital, School of Medicine, University of Leeds, Leeds, UK
e-mail: n.kanakaris@nhs.net

G. D. Chloros
Academic Department of Trauma and Orthopaedics, School of Medicine, University of Leeds, Leeds, UK

Orthopedic Surgery Working Group, Society for Junior Doctors, Athens, Greece

P. V. Giannoudis (✉)
Academic Department of Trauma and Orthopaedics, School of Medicine, University of Leeds, Leeds, UK

NIHR Leeds Biomedical Research Center, Chapel Allerton Hospital, Leeds, UK

The patient was taken to the operating theatre within 4 hours of presentation and the dislocation of the head of the femur was reduced with the aid of a traction pin (Fig. 19.2).

Two days later, the patient was taken into the operating room for definite fixation. He was put in the prone position and his left acetabulum was approached via a standard Kocher-Langenbeck approach [1]. A two-level reconstruction was carried out: First, the impacted part of the posterior-superior dome of the acetabulum was elevated, reduced and fixed separately with the aid of two independent 2 mm screws [2]. Second, the posterior wall fragment (PWF) was reduced using two independent Lag screws and buttressed with a 10-hole reconstruction plate. The transverse fracture element was fixed using additional 5-hole reconstruction plate (Fig. 19.3).

Post-operative regimen included non-weight bearing of the left lower extremity for 10 weeks and discharge to a rehabilitation centre with regular clinic follow-ups. At the 4-week routine follow-up, the patient complained of persistent pain around the hip including the groin. Radiographs showed failure of the fixation with dislocation of the femoral head (Fig. 19.4). He was then referred to our unit for further management.

© The Author(s), under exclusive license to Springer Nature Switzerland AG 2024
P. V. Giannoudis, P. Tornetta III (eds.), *Failed Fracture Fixation*,
https://doi.org/10.1007/978-3-031-39692-2_19

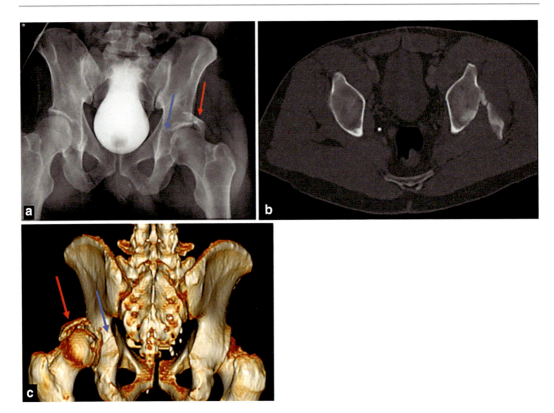

Fig. 19.1 (a) AP pelvic radiograph following the injury showing a left posterior wall fracture (red arrow) associated with a transverse nondisplaced acetabular fracture (blue arrow). (b) Computed tomography (CT) axial cuts showing the comminution and displacement of the left posterior wall fracture. (c) 3D CT reconstruction of the posterior left acetabulum demonstrating both the transverse fracture (blue arrow) and the posterior wall acetabular fracture dislocation (red arrow)

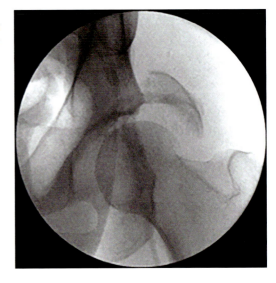

Fig. 19.2 Intra-operative oblique fluoroscopy view following application of a traction pin showing reduction of the dislocation of hip dislocation and a large posterior wall fracture 'sea gull sign'

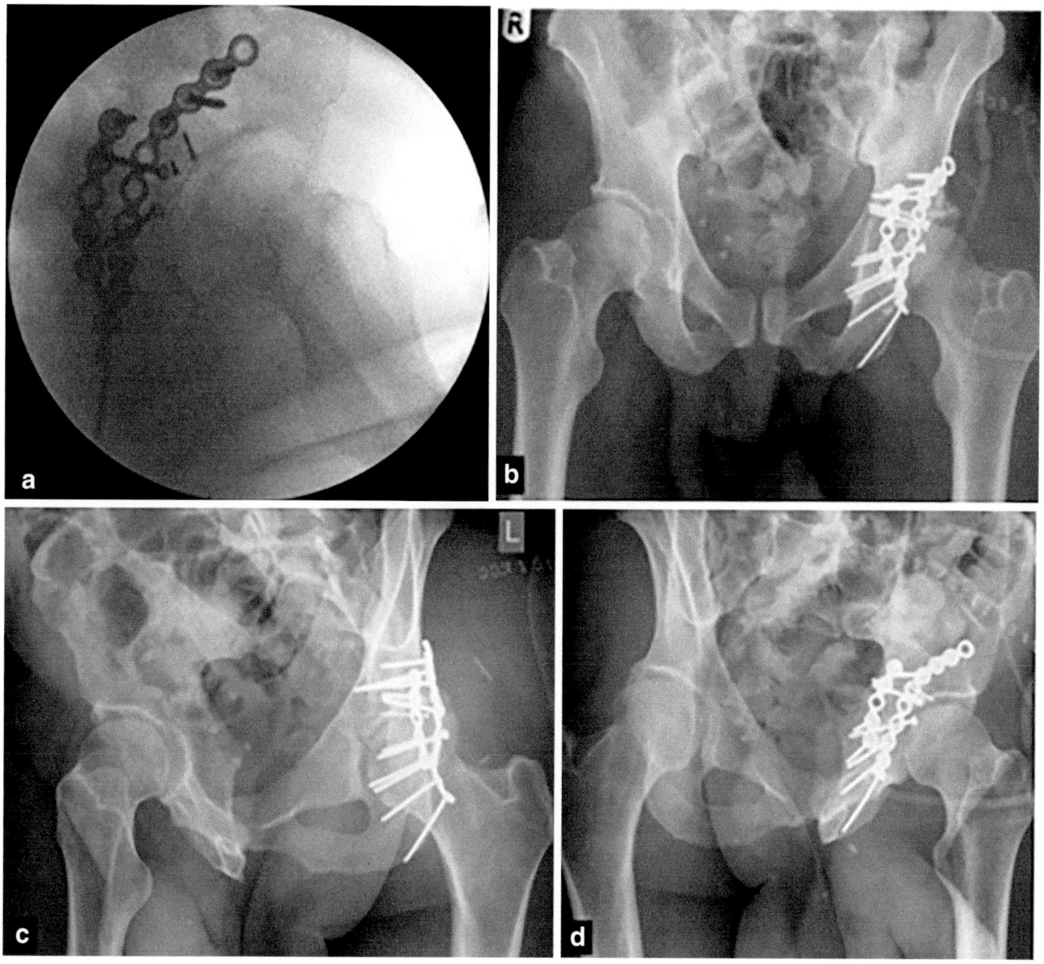

Fig. 19.3 (**a**) Intra-operative fluoroscopic oblique view showing reduction and fixation of the fracture, and the hip joint is now reduced. Two independent 2 mm screws hold the impacted dome fragment, which was elevated, and the joint line is congruent. A 10-hole reconstruction plate was applied in buttress mode. A 5-hole reconstruction plate was applied for fixation of the transverse fracture to prevent secondary displacement. (**b**) Post-operative AP pelvic radiograph. (**c**) Obturator oblique Judet view and (**d**) Iliac oblique Judet view showing adequate reduction and fixation of the fractures

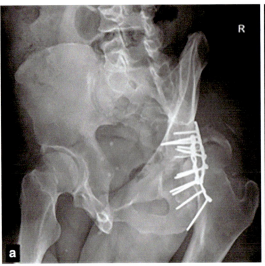 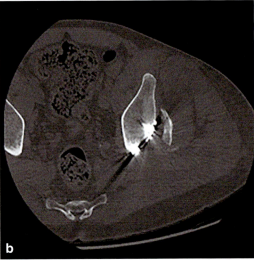

Fig. 19.4 (a) Obturator oblique view of the left acetabulum at 4 weeks post-operatively showing failure of fixation of the posterior acetabular wall fracture, associated with posterior dislocation of the femoral head. (b) Axial CT image showing the posterior wall fragment displaced anterolaterally

Evaluation of the Aetiology of Failure of Fixation

Several aetiologies may predispose to failure of treatment including trauma, infection, mechanical and biological factors. The patient did not recall any recurrent trauma and no clinical or laboratory test results supported infection as the cause for failure. Imaging revealed incorrect buttress positioning of the posterior wall fragment reconstruction plate as the reason for failure. Generally, after exposure of the fracture, reduction of the posterior wall is achieved by applying the lag screw technique. Buttressing the construct using a well-contoured reconstruction plate that closely follows the acetabular rim is essential to achieve stable fixation and to prevent secondary displacement. This reinforcement is necessary as strong forces are applied on this part of the acetabulum during flexion and the plate has to be applied close to the margins of the acetabulum. In this case, the anterior part of the buttress plate was positioned too superiorly and not on the edge of the acetabular wall. This positioning provided inadequate buttressing of the PWF which was the cause of failure (Fig. 19.5). A common contributor to insufficient reduction

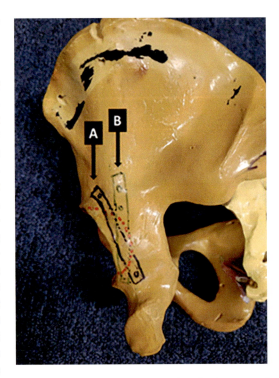

Fig. 19.5 Pelvic model demonstrating the fracture and plate position. Pelvic model in the lateral position (left acetabulum) indicating a posterior wall fracture (red dotted line). Plate placed in the correct position (shown by arrow A, illustrated in black). Green illustration of the plate representing erroneous placement of the plate as initially performed in this case (shown by arrow B) which led to loss of buttressing and failure of fixation

and fixation of PWF is when in marginal impaction injuries, subchondral bone is reinforced by bone graft but overstuffing of the void with bone graft can subsequently hinder successful reduction of the posterior wall fragment. However, in this case this doesn't seem to be the cause of failure as sufficient reduction was achieved during surgery [2–5].

Clinical Examination

This patient was evaluated 4 weeks after surgery and complained of increasing pain in the left hip. He denied fevers, chills or night sweats. The surgical wound was clean, dry and intact with no signs of infection. The left leg was slightly shortened, the hip mildly flexed and internally rotated. No neurological deficits were noted, and both active and passive movements of hip joint were restricted and painful.

Diagnostic-Biochemical and Radiological Investigations

In this case the main aetiology for failure was mechanical as stated above. The short interval between fixation and the failure didn't permit sufficient healing time of the fracture. Imaging evaluation included radiographs and a CT scan in order to evaluate the failure and plan the revision surgery. Blood tests were obtained in order to screen for the possibility of infection (white blood cells count (WBC) and C-reactive protein (CRP) levels were within normal limits.

Preoperative Planning

At this point, revision of fixation needs to be undertaken consisting of:

1. Removal of the independent lag screws and of the reconstruction buttress plate.
2. Reduction of the dislocated hip and fixation of the PWF.

Implants/Equipment Required:

- Bacterial cultures (routine practice to exclude infection as a cause of failure).
- Pelvic set reduction clamps.
- Two 3.5 mm independent lag screws.
- Matta pelvic reconstruction 3.5 mm plates (countered and fitted to be close to the rim of the acetabulum wall).

Pre-operative planning should not only include identifying failure of the fixation, but also how this issue would be addressed successfully and how potential complications can be avoided. It was expected that removal of hardware, reduction of the fracture and correct positioning of one buttress plate during the revision fixation will address the problem (plan A). However, in the scenario where the posterior wall fragment could be multifragmented/comminuted during reduction manoeuvres, additional rim plates might be necessary (plan B). As the cause of fixation is purely mechanical, no need for additional biological stimulation/bone graft enhancement is indicated in this case.

Revision Surgery

The procedure was performed with the patient under general anaesthesia, placed under traction in the prone position on a radiolucent flat-top fracture table under fluoroscopic guidance. The previous incision via the Kocher-Langenbeck approach [1] was utilized. Dissection of the soft tissue by layers was carried out: muscle and fascia were healthy looking; however, per protocol, soft tissue samples were sent for cultures. The posterior wall fracture was identified, and the PWF was displaced as one piece posteriorly while the femoral head was dislocated posteriorly. Removal of the posterior wall 10-hole Matta reconstruction plate was performed followed by a thorough washout. Reduction of the PWF was achieved with the aid of 1.6 mm K-wires and application of 2 independent 3.5 mm lag screws. A new Matta reconstruction plate was subse-

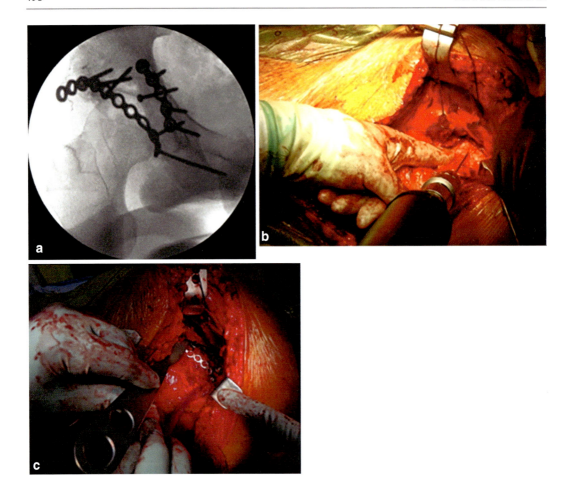

Fig. 19.6 Revision surgery. Intra-operative photography and fluoroscopy images. (**a**) Iliac oblique view of the left acetabulum showing adequate reduction and fixation of the fracture and the hip joint. The buttress plate now sits on the acetabular rim. (**b**) Intra-operative photography image demonstrating provisional fixation of the PWF with a 1.6 mm K wire. (**c**) Final position of the plate on the rim of the acetabulum

quently applied in buttress mode. The plate was now carefully contoured to fit on the edge of the anterosuperior part of the posterior acetabular wall, as shown in Fig. 19.5. Two screws anchored the plate in the inferior area to the ischium and two screws to the superior area. Intra-operative fluoroscopy confirmed adequate reduction and fixation (Fig. 19.6). At 4 months, the patient was pain-free with a full and symmetric range of motion of his hip. Radiographs confirmed adequate reduction and fixation of the fracture (Fig. 19.7).

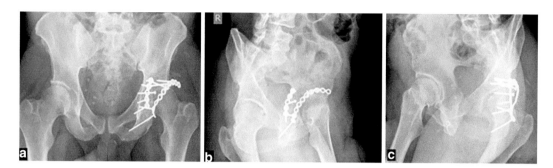

Fig. 19.7 Four-month post-operative radiographs. (**a**) AP pelvic radiograph, (**b**) iliac oblique Judet view and (**c**) obturator oblique Judet view showing adequate reduction and fixation of the PWF. There is some minor superolateral heterotopic ossification, while the transverse acetabular fracture has completely healed

Summary: Lessons Learned

Several factors must be considered when a posterior wall acetabular fracture fixation fails, including infection; however, by far the most frequent cause involves technical errors: Screw penetration in the joint and inadequate plate positioning are the most frequent. The latter was the case in this patient as inadequate positioning of the buttress plate did not capture the entirety of the posterior wall as it was not close to the acetabular rim and therefore predisposed to failure with dissociation of the PWF and re-dislocation of the hip joint.

References

1. Tosounidis TH, Giannoudis VP, Kanakaris NK, Giannoudis PV. The Kocher-Langenbeck approach: state of the art. JBJS Essent Surg Tech. 2018;8(2):e18.
2. Chloros GD, Ali A, Kanakaris NK, Giannoudis PV. Surgical treatment of marginal impaction injuries of the acetabulum associated with posterior wall fractures. JBJS Essent Surg Tech. 2022;12(1):e21.00004.
3. de Palma L, Santucci A, Verdenelli A, Bugatti MG, Meco L, Marinelli M. Outcome of unstable isolated fractures of the posterior acetabular wall associated with hip dislocation. Eur J Orthop Surg Traumatol. 2014;24(3):341–6.
4. Giannoudis P, Nikolaou V. Surgical techniques—how do I do it?: Open reduction and internal fixation of posterior wall fractures of the acetabulum. Injury. 2008;39(10):1113–8.
5. Giannoudis P, Tzioupis C, Moed B. Two-level reconstruction of comminuted posterior-wall fractures of the acetabulum. J Bone Joint Surg Br. 2007;89(4):503–9.

Intracapsular Proximal Femoral Fracture Failed Fixation

20

Paul L. Rodham, Vasileios Giannoudis, and Peter V. Giannoudis

History of Previous Primary Failed Treatment

A 37-year-old gentleman with a background of chronic hepatitis B infection initially presented as a trauma activation following an assault. He was received by a trauma team and found to be stable, having sustained injuries to his face, back and left hip. A trauma computed tomography (CT) was performed which demonstrated an undisplaced right L4 transverse process fracture, facial haematoma with no underlying fracture and a minimally displaced but comminuted left intracapsular neck of femur fracture (Fig. 20.1).

Once established to be physiologically stable with no other significant injuries, a decision was taken to perform an open reduction and internal fixation of the left sided neck of femur fracture. At 10 hours post-admission, he was taken to theatre and an open reduction was performed via an anterior approach achieving sagittal, coronal and rotational alignment. This was secured with three partially threaded 6.5 mm cannulated screws in an inverted triangle orientation (Fig. 20.2). He was discharged home 4 days post-fixation with a plan to toe touch weight-bear for a period of 12 weeks.

At his 3 months review his wounds had healed with no evidence of infection. He still complained of some occasional pain in the groin, discomfort during passive range of movement, and was unable to perform an active straight leg raise. Radiographs demonstrated no evidence of avascular necrosis, though the fracture was not yet healed. It was noted that at this point his fracture had begun to collapse and the screws were backing out (Fig. 20.3). He was counselled regarding his smoking and asked to continue with partial weight-bearing to protect his fixation. He was seen again at 4 months at which time he was able to perform a straight leg raise albeit with pain. Radiographs again demonstrated failure to progress towards union and therefore a CT scan was performed at 6 months post-operatively to assess fracture healing. This demonstrated no evidence of progression towards union of the femoral neck which had shortened and collapsed into varus (Fig. 20.4). A plan was therefore made at this stage for revision fixation at this time point.

P. L. Rodham · V. Giannoudis
Academic Department of Trauma and Orthopaedics, School of Medicine, University of Leeds, Leeds, UK
e-mail: p.rodham@nhs.net; vasileios.giannoudis@nhs.net

P. V. Giannoudis (✉)
Academic Department of Trauma and Orthopaedics, School of Medicine, University of Leeds, Leeds, UK

NIHR Leeds Biomedical Research Center, Chapel Allerton Hospital, Leeds, UK

© The Author(s), under exclusive license to Springer Nature Switzerland AG 2024
P. V. Giannoudis, P. Tornetta III (eds.), *Failed Fracture Fixation*,
https://doi.org/10.1007/978-3-031-39692-2_20

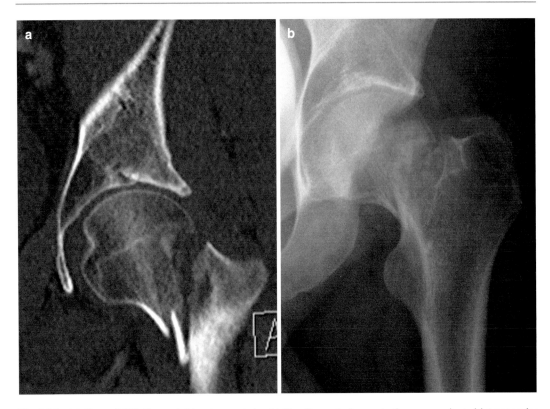

Fig. 20.1 (a) Coronal CT slice and (b) anteroposterior (AP) radiograph demonstrating a comminuted intracapsular neck of femur fracture (Pauwel type 3)

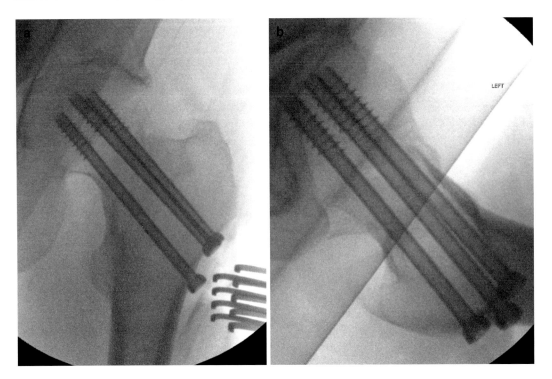

Fig. 20.2 (a) AP and (b) lateral intraoperative images demonstrating fixation with three partially threaded 6.5 mm cannulated screws in an inverted triangle configuration

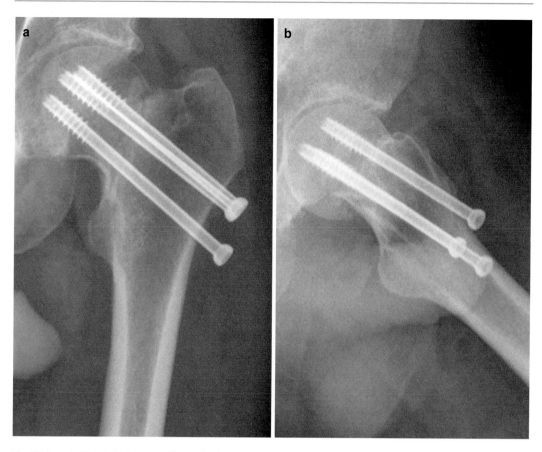

Fig. 20.3 (**a**) AP and (**b**) lateral radiograph taken at 3 months demonstrating collapse with shortening of the femoral neck, and backing out of the cannulated screws

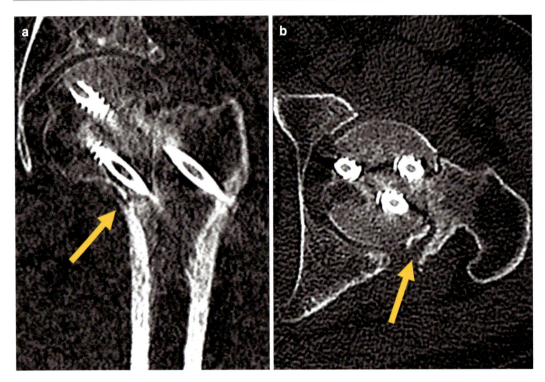

Fig. 20.4 (a) Coronal and (b) axial CT slices taken at 6 months post-operatively demonstrating non-union of the femoral neck which had shortened and collapsed into varus (see arrows)

Evaluation of the Aetiology of Failure of Fixation

From the initial images, it can be noted that this was a comminuted intracapsular neck of femur fracture which would be length unstable with a high degree of shear (Pauwel 3 type). Whilst a good reduction was achieved via an open approach, the aim to compress the fracture to maximize the chances of healing led to the use of three partially threaded screws which failed to maintain length as the fracture collapsed. This led to the development of varus angulation, further increasing the shear at the fracture site and predisposing to non-union. This may have been avoided through the use of a single fully threaded screw to maintain length, or a Pauwel screw perpendicular to the plane of the fracture to control shear (Fig. 20.5). Alternatively, a more secure fixation may have been achieved through the use of alternate implants such as a dynamic hip screw (DHS) with a complimentary de-rotation screw, or the use of a fixed angled construct such as the DePuy Synthes femoral neck system.

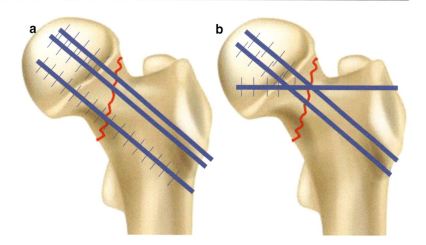

Fig. 20.5 Alternative screw constructs may have included the use of (**a**) a single fully threaded screw along the calcar, or (**b**) the use of a Pauwel screw perpendicular to the plane of the fracture

Clinical Examination

On assessment the patient continued to toe-touch weight-bear on the affected side. He had a well-healed operative scar with no evidence of localised infection. He experienced pain on all active and passive movements of the hip. There was a 1.2 cm leg length discrepancy.

Diagnostic-Biochemical and Radiological Investigations

In cases of fixation failure, particularly where an open reduction has been performed, it is pertinent to rule out fracture-related infection. Based on history and clinical examination, there was a low index of suspicion for this. Peri-operative blood tests demonstrated a WBC of 13,000 and a C-reactive protein (CRP) of 63. Infection could therefore not be ruled out and intraoperative sampling was performed to assess for infection. Blood investigations for bone health were also performed which demonstrated a low vitamin D level of 20 nmol/L; therefore, supplementation was provided in the perioperative period. For operative planning, a CT scan was performed which confirmed the presence of the non-union and also ruled out the possibility of avascular necrosis of the femoral head.

Preoperative Planning

Revision fixation was planned consisting of removal of the current implants, following which a subtrochanteric osteotomy would be performed to valgise the femoral neck. This would be secured with a dynamic hip screw, an anterior pate to control rotation and further biological stimulation would be provided through the implantation of bone marrow aspirate.

The following implants were selected:

- 5-hole 135-degree dynamic hip screw (DHS)
- 4-hole 3.5mm dynamic compression plate (DCP)

Revision Surgery

The patient was positioned supine on the operating fracture table with the image intensifier utilised throughout. Following appropriate preparation and draping, the lateral incision utilised to insert the cannulated screws was re-opened in order to gain access to the lateral femur. A 2.8 mm guide wire was introduced into each screw in sequence and utilised to guide screw removal. Once removed, the screw paths were curetted and samples taken for microbiological analysis.

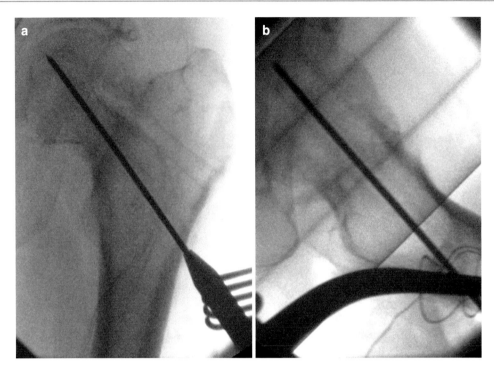

Fig. 20.6 (**a**) AP and (**b**) lateral intraoperative film demonstrating guide wire position at 130° to the femoral shaft, achieving a centre-centre position in the femoral head

At this point the 2.5 mm DHS guide wire was inserted at an angle of 130° with reference to the femoral shaft attaining a centre-centre position in the femoral head (Fig. 20.6). Once position was confirmed on the image intensifier, the appropriate length screw was selected. The femoral neck was prepared with a triple reamer to a length 5 mm below that of the screw, following which the screw was inserted (Fig. 20.7).

A closing wedge lateral cortex osteotomy is next marked, pre-drilled with a 3.5 mm drill bit and then completed with an osteotome (Fig. 20.8). At this point, a 5-hole plate was inserted and held to restore the natural neck shaft angle of 135°. Once the angle is recreated, the distal shaft was held to the femoral shaft with a Hargrove and secured with five cortical screws. To further provide rotational stability, the fixation was augmented with an anterior plate. The vastus was lifted with two Hohmann retractors to gain access to the anterior cortex, and the plate sited and secured with four cortical screws (Fig. 20.9).

To stimulate the biology at the osteotomy fracture site and facilitate healing, bone marrow

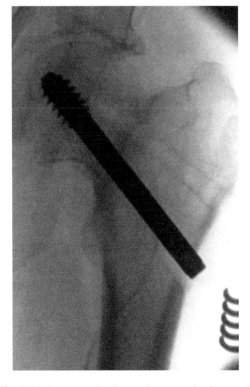

Fig. 20.7 Intraoperative image demonstrating lag screw position, sited prior to subtrochanteric osteotomy

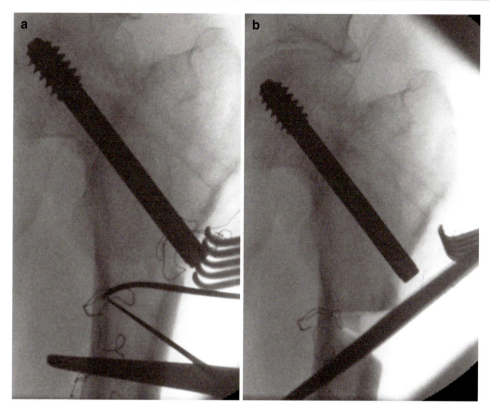

Fig. 20.8 (a) Intraoperative image demonstrating marking of osteotomy which was subsequently pre-drilled and (b) completed with an osteotome

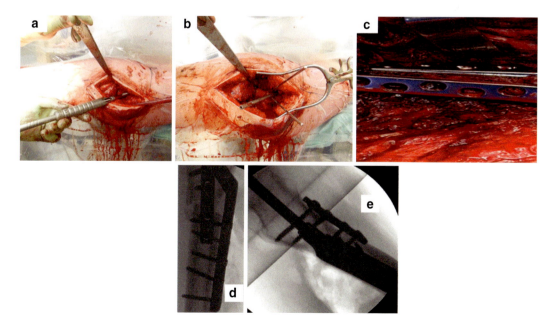

Fig. 20.9 Intraoperative pictures (a) showing insertion of dynamic hip screw, (b) the insertion of guide wires for planning of the subtrochanteric osteotomy; (c) the insertion of the anterior DCP plate (d) AP view; (e) Lateral view. Once an acceptable alignment was achieved, restoring the natural valgus, the osteotomy was secured with a 5-hole 135° DHS plate and augmented with an anterior 4-hole DCP

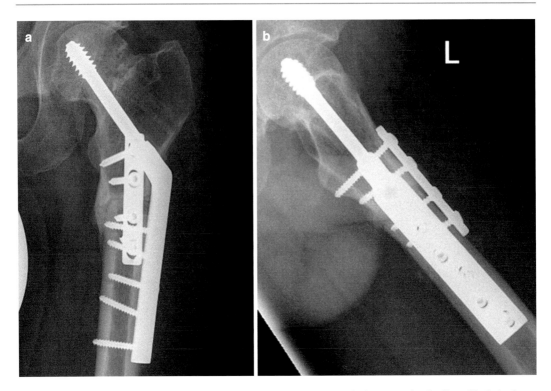

Fig. 20.10 (**a**) AP and (**b**) lateral radiographs taken 6 months post-operatively demonstrating healing of both the femoral neck and osteotomy sites

aspirate was taken from the iliac crest. A 1 cm incision was made 2 cm posterior to the anterior superior iliac crest, through which a trocar was introduced into the cancellous bone of the crest. Sixty millilitres of bone marrow aspirate were drawn into heparin prepared syringes in 20 mL aliquots. Bone marrow concentrate (7 mL) was then isolated via density gradient centrifugation and injected into the non-union site.

Post-operatively the patient was instructed to toe touch weight-bear for the first 3 months, following which weight-bearing was progressed as tolerated. At 6 months the patient was able to walk with a normal gait pattern, with his hip pain completely eradicated and demonstrable radiological union of both the subtrochanteric osteotomy and the femoral neck fracture (Fig. 20.10). He was discharged from the clinic at 2 years post-op with no residual symptoms arising from his left hip and no radiological evidence of femoral head avascular necrosis (AVN).

Summary: Lessons Learned

This case summarizes a young patient with known risk factors for non-union including smoking and hepatitis. He presented with early failure of fixation, likely due to failure to appropriately hold the fracture out to length in the presence of femoral neck comminution. As a result of poor hold, the femoral neck was able to shorted and collapse into varus. This may have been avoided through the use of a single fully threaded screw orientated perpendicular to the fracture line which would both maintain length and resist shear at the fracture site. This may also be prevented through the use of a fixed angle device. In this case, a successful outcome was achieved through a subtrochanteric osteotomy which was secured with orthogonal fixation via a DHS and DCP plate; biological stimulation through the addition of bone marrow aspirate concentrate also supported the local osteogenesis response. This technique could also be employed utilizing other implants such as a peri-articular proximal femoral plating system, a dynamic condylar screw or a blade plate.

Further Reading

Gavaskar AS, Chowdary NT. Valgus sliding subtrochanteric osteotomy for neglected fractures of the proximal femur; surgical technique and a retrospective case series. J Orthop Surg Res. 2013;8:4.

Hoshino CM, Christian MW, O'Toole RV, Manson TT. Fixation of displaced femoral neck fractures in young adults: fixed-angle devices or Pauwel screws? Injury. 2016;47(8):1676–84.

Mathews V, Cabanela ME. Femoral neck nonunion treatment. Clin Orthop Relat Res. 2004;419:57–64.

Xue G, Chen S, Zhou M, et al. Pauwels screw combined inverted triangle cannulated screws for the treatment of Pauwels type-III femoral neck fracture:- a new surgical method based on the morphology of the fracture. Research Square. 2020. https://doi.org/10.21203/rs.3.rs-38297/v1.

Extracapsular Proximal Femoral Fracture Intramedullary Nailing Failed Fixation

21

Paul L. Rodham, Vasileios Giannoudis, and Peter V. Giannoudis

History of Previous Primary Failed Treatment

A fit and well 31-year-old male initially presented to our institution following a fall from 40 ft. He was received as a trauma activation and presented in haemodynamic shock with significant head, chest and pelvic injuries. He was intubated on arrival and resuscitated with early blood products in a 1:1:1 ratio. His injuries included bilateral multi-level rib fractures with bilateral flail segments (bilateral chest drains inserted), L1–L4 transverse process fractures, a left both column acetabular fracture, a left scapular spine fracture, a left segmental humerus fracture, an open left both bone forearm fracture, and a comminuted left intertrochanteric fracture (Fig. 21.1).

He was taken to the critical care unit where he had ongoing resuscitation, associated with an improvement in both his physiological and bio-chemical parameters, and therefore a plan was made for early appropriate care for his injuries in a staged manner treating his open forearm and hip in one sitting, followed by a return to theatre 1–2 days later for treatment of his pelvis and left humerus. On the first day following injury he was taken to theatre where he underwent debridement and open reduction and internal fixation (ORIF) of his forearm fracture, and a long intramedullary nail for his intertrochanteric hip fracture (Fig. 21.2). This was uneventful, however, he unfortunately deteriorated with increased oxygenation requirement post-operatively whilst back in the intensive care unit, requiring ongoing cardiorespiratory and renal support. He subsequently underwent fixation of his pelvis on the 4th day post-admission, and fixation of his left humerus on the 20th day post-admission. He underwent a successful rehabilitation programme and was discharged home 49 days post-injury.

At 2 months the patient was reviewed in the clinic where he was able to walk with a single walking stick, and reported no pain in his left hip or groin. His wounds at this point were well healed with no clinical signs of infection and he had a full painless range of motion of the left hip. He was further seen at the 4-month mark at which point he had developed increasing pain, walked with a limp, and was noted to clinically be 2 cm shorter on his left side when compared to the right. Radiographs taken at this appoint-

P. L. Rodham · V. Giannoudis
Academic Department of Trauma and Orthopaedics, School of Medicine, University of Leeds, Leeds, UK
e-mail: p.rodham@nhs.net; vasileios.giannoudis@nhs.net

P. V. Giannoudis (✉)
Academic Department of Trauma and Orthopaedics, School of Medicine, University of Leeds, Leeds, UK

NIHR Leeds Biomedical Research Center, Chapel Allerton Hospital, Leeds, UK

© The Author(s), under exclusive license to Springer Nature Switzerland AG 2024
P. V. Giannoudis, P. Tornetta III (eds.), *Failed Fracture Fixation*,
https://doi.org/10.1007/978-3-031-39692-2_21

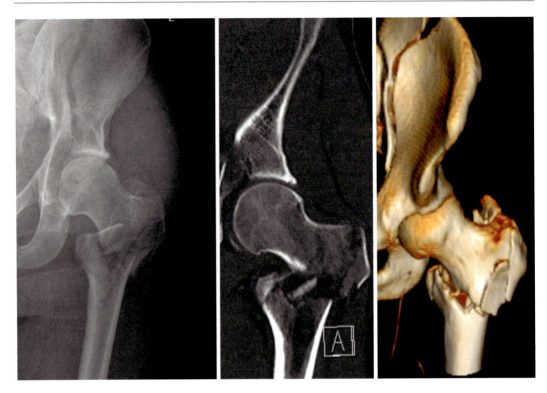

Fig. 21.1 AP plain radiograph, coronal CT slice and 3d reconstruction demonstrating a comminuted intertrochanteric neck of femur fracture and both column acetabular fracture

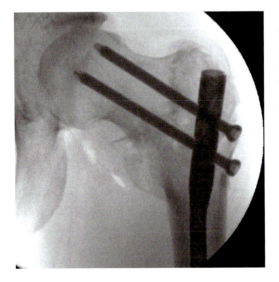

Fig. 21.2 The fracture was managed with a closed reamed intramedullary nail performed on post-injury day 1 (9 mm Versanail)

ment demonstrated that the fracture had collapsed into further varus, the most proximal of the proximal locking screws was cutting out, and the more distal of the proximal locking screws had broken (Fig. 21.3). A plan was therefore made for revision fixation at this time point.

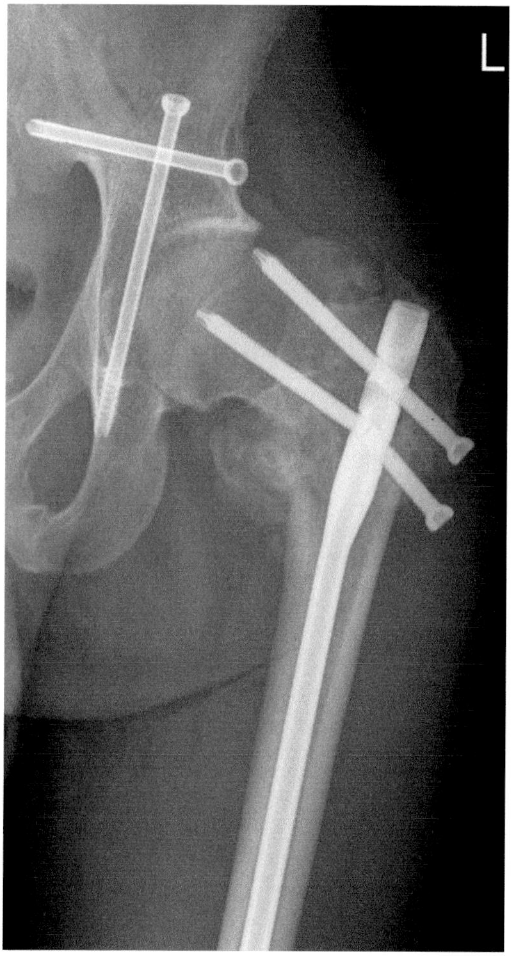

Fig. 21.3 AP radiograph of the left hip demonstrating collapse of the fracture into varus with breakage of the most distal proximal locking screw + cut out of the more proximal screw

made increasingly likely by the high tip-apex distance (40 mm), and the use of a device that wasn't proximally locked in the setting of femoral neck comminution.

Clinical Examination

On assessment this patient had an antalgic gait on the left-hand side, continuing to walk with a walking stick held in his right hand. He had shortening of the left limb by 2 cm. Passive movements of his left hip were comfortable; however, he had discomfort on active movements against resistance. All wounds from his original surgery were well healed with no clinical evidence of infection

Diagnostic-Biochemical and Radiological Investigations

Within this case the most pertinent diagnosis to rule out was fracture related infection. There was a low clinical index of suspicion however prior to proceeding to operative intervention blood investigations were sent to assess white cell count (WCC) (8.8), C-reactive protein (CRP) (31) and erythrocyte sedimentation rate (ESR) (60). Based on the biochemical markers, infection could not be excluded and consequently tissue samples would be needed to be sent to microbiology during the operative intervention. Computed tomography (CT) scan can assist in evaluating the degree of healing and the possibility of presence of avascular necrosis of the femoral head.

Evaluation of the Aetiology of Failure of Fixation

This was an early failure of an intramedullary device. From the initial images we note the comminution around the greater trochanter greater Trochanter (GT) which makes accurate entry difficult for this nail. The entry point on the intra-operative images was lateral to the greater trochanter, likely due to the guide wire falling into the split in the GT. This entry point predisposes to varus deformity which also explains the high position of the screws in the femoral head. Furthermore, cut out is

Preoperative Planning

Revision fixation would initially consist of removal of the current implants which was anticipated to be difficult given the broken screw. Following this the fracture non-union site would need to be mobilised and the proximal fragment valgised and secured appropriately. Following realignment, a defect was anticipated which would be filled with a combination of bone graft (autologous, allograft, xenograft).

The following implants were selected:

- 10-hole 95° angled blade plate
- 7-hole 3.5 mm dynamic compression plate (DCP)
- Demineralised bone matrix (DBM)
- Tutobone bovine xenograft

Revision Surgery

The patient was positioned supine on a fracture table with image intensifier utilised throughout. The distal locking screws were removed through the same stab incisions through which they had been inserted. Proximally the lateral incision utilised to insert the nail was re-opened, and extended distally to a point 10 cm below the lesser trochanter. Proximally a small split was made in the gluteal tendons to access the proximal end of the nail, whilst distally vastus lateralis was lifted to give access to the anterior and lateral surfaces of the femur.

Attention was then turned towards nail removal. The universal nail extractor was sited proximally following which the two proximal screws were removed. The most proximal screw was in continuity and therefore removed with ease; however, the distal screw was broken and was therefore over-drilled and extracted using the 'broken screw' removal set. Following screw removal, the nail was removed with ease. A curette was introduced through the entry point of the nail to take deep tissue specimens for microbiology.

The fracture was oblique, predominantly in the sagittal plane. This was marked and the non-union plane established through the use of two K-wires. These K-wires were subsequently utilised to guide the path of the osteotome which was utilised to mobilise the fracture (Fig. 21.4). Once the non-union was sufficiently mobilised the proximal fragment was manipulated using a Hargrove retractor, and drawn into a valgus orientation. At this point the guide wire for the blade plate is inserted at 95° to the anatomic axis of the femur running along the calcar under image intensifier guidance. Once in place a cannulated chisel is then introduced with care to ensure that the chisel is in line with the sagittal axis of the bone avoiding a flexion/extension deformity when the plate is secured to the bone (Fig. 21.5).

As the path was established, a 10-hole blade plate was introduced and secured to the femoral shaft using cortical screws. At this point the vastus was lifted forward using Hohmann retractors,

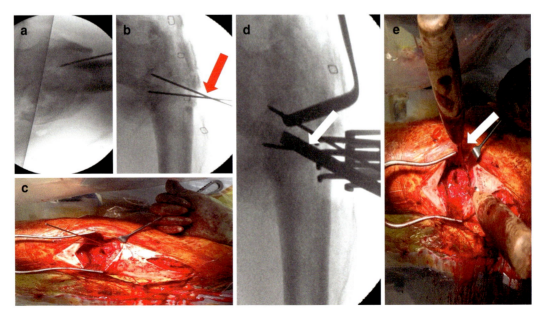

Fig. 21.4 (**a**, **b** and **c**) K-wires are initially utilised to define the plane of the non-union (red arrow) (**d** and **e**) Using an osteotome osteoclasis was performed

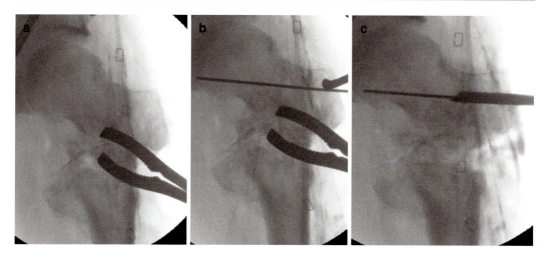

Fig. 21.5 (**a** and **b**) The proximal fragment is positioned using a Hargrove retractor following which the guidewire for the blade plate is inserted at 95° to the femoral anatomic axis (**c**) Care should be taken when inserting the chisel to ensure that this is perpendicular to the sagittal plane axis in order to minimise the risk of a flexion/extension deformity

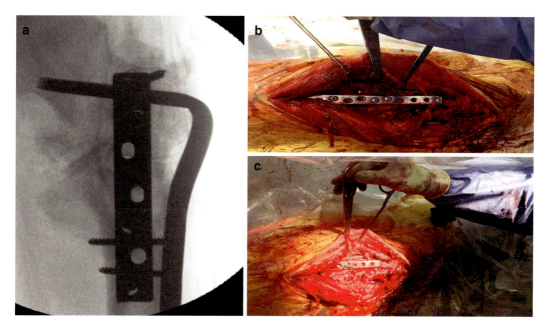

Fig. 21.6 (**a**, **b** and **c**) Once debrided the non-union was secured with a 10-hole 95° blade plate, and an orthogonal 7-hole DCP to provide additional rotational stability (AP hip fluoroscopic image and intra-operative images). The defect following debridement was managed with a combination of synthetic bone replacement (Tutobone) and demineralised bone matrix

and a 7-hole dynamic compression plate was placed anteriorly in order to achieve improved rotational stability. This was secured with 2 screws proximally, and 3 screws distally. Post-fixation there was a significant bone defect laterally. This was managed through the use of a structural bone substitute (xenograft, 'Tutobone'), whilst medially demineralised bone matrix was applied to provide additional osteoconductivity and osteoinductivity (Fig. 21.6).

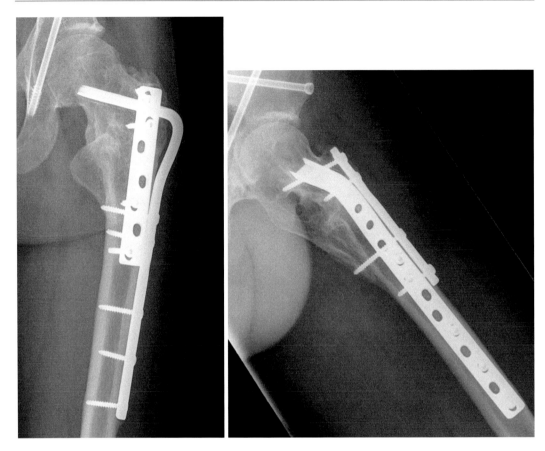

Fig. 21.7 Post-operative radiographs at a year follow-up showing full consolidation of the fracture

Post-operatively the patient was instructed to toe touch weight bear with crutches for 3 months, following which he progressed to full weight bearing as the graft consolidated. At one-year post-op his fracture had united both clinically and radiologically, and he was back to running distances of 3–6 miles. He developed some lateral thigh pain associated with the metalwork which resolved following removal of the metalwork 2 years post-revision fixation (Fig. 21.7).

Summary: Lessons Learned

This case summarises a young patient who presented with an early failure of an intramedullary device utilised in order to manage a comminuted intertrochanteric hip fracture. This was likely due to the initial varus reduction occurring due to a lateral entry point, and the long tip apex distance which meant that the screws had a poor hold in the femoral head. This was successfully managed with revision to an orthogonal blade plate/DCP construct, with an excellent clinical result. When managing these injuries, one should pay particular attention to the reduction achieved, focussing on avoiding varus and attaining good hold within the femoral head, controlling rotation. In these patients when using a trochanteric entry nail, often starting slightly medial to the tip of the trochanter will lead to an accurate entry point, as the patient's soft tissue mass and trajectory of the reamer will often push the operator laterally. Where comminution occurs, a static device should be used which will provide some protection against collapse of the fracture.

Further Reading

Baumgaertner MR, Curtin SL, Lindskog DM, Keggi JM. The value of the tip-apex distance in predicting failure of fixation of peritrochanteric fractures of the hip. J Bone Joint Surg Am. 1995;77:1058–64.

Haidukewych GJ. Intertrochanteric fractures: ten tips to improve results. J Bone Joint Surg. 2009;91(3):712–9.

Johnson NA, Uzoigwe C, Venkatesan M, Burgula V, Kulkarni A, Davison JN, Ashford RU. Risk factors for intramedullary nail breakage in proximal femoral fractures: a 10-year retrospective review. Ann R Coll Surg Engl. 2017;99(2):145–50.

Koyuncu Ş, Altay T, Kayalı C, Ozan F, Yamak K. Mechanical failures after fixation with proximal femoral nail and risk factors. Clin Interv Aging. 2015;17(10):1959–65.

Susbtrochanteric Femoral Fracture Failed Fixation

22

Vasileios P. Giannoudis, Paul L Rodham, Nikolaos K. Kanakaris, and Peter V. Giannoudis

History of Previous Primary Failed Treatment

A 72-year-old female with a background of rheumatoid arthritis, alcohol dependence and asthma presented to a district general hospital following a mechanical fall at home where she sustained a right subtrochanteric proximal femur fracture. This was a closed isolated injury (Fig. 22.1). She was medically optimised at the hospital overnight and underwent closed reamed intramedullary (IM) nailing 1 day following her admission (Fig. 22.2). She was mobilised full weight bearing following her original procedure and was discharged home approximately 2 weeks following orthogeriatric review, bone health optimisation and physiotherapy input.

At 6 weeks the patient was reviewed in the clinic where he was able to walk with a Zimmer frame; however, she reported pain in her right hip. Her wounds had healed with no clinical signs of infection. Radiographs taken at the time showed evidence of the fracture migrating into varus. She subsequently represented to the district general hospital 5 months later at which point she had developed increasing pain and inability to weight bear. Radiographs taken at this time demonstrated that the fracture had collapsed into further varus, with concern regarding the integrity of the IM nail metalwork (Fig. 22.3). One month afterward the patient was referred to our Tertiary Trauma Centre for revision surgery.

V. P. Giannoudis · P. L. Rodham · N. K. Kanakaris
Academic Department of Trauma and Orthopaedics,
School of Medicine, University of Leeds, Leeds, UK
e-mail: vasileios.giannoudis@nhs.net;
p.rodham@nhs.net; n.kanakaris@nhs.net

P. V. Giannoudis (✉)
Academic Department of Trauma and Orthopaedics,
School of Medicine, University of Leeds, Leeds, UK

NIHR Leeds Biomedical Research Center, Chapel
Allerton Hospital, Leeds, UK

© The Author(s), under exclusive license to Springer Nature Switzerland AG 2024
P. V. Giannoudis, P. Tornetta III (eds.), *Failed Fracture Fixation*,
https://doi.org/10.1007/978-3-031-39692-2_22

Fig. 22.1 AP pelvic radiograph demonstrating a right subtrochanteric proximal femur fracture

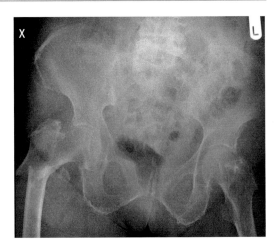

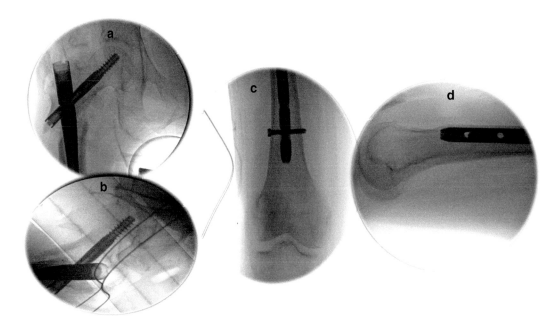

Fig. 22.2 (a–d) The fracture was managed with a closed reamed intramedullary nail

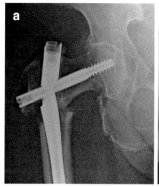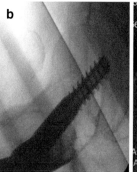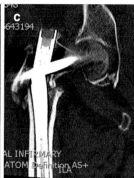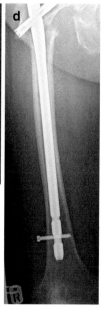

Fig. 22.3 (**a**) AP radiograph of the right hip demonstrating collapse of the fracture into varus with bending demonstrating of the proximal aspect of the nail (broken nail); (**b**) lateral radiograph; (**c**) CT coronal image showing the broken nail and the underlying non-union; (**d**) AP view femur showing the loose distal femoral screw

Evaluation of the Aetiology of Failure of Fixation

This was an early failure of an intramedullary device (Stryker Gamma-3 nail). From the initial images we note the inadequate fracture reduction. This entry point predisposes to varus deformity which also explains the high position of the screws in the femoral head. Furthermore, cut out is made increasingly likely by the suboptimal tip-apex distance.

Clinical Examination

The patient was unable to bear weight on the right extremity and the leg was painful on passive leg roll.

Diagnostic-Biochemical and Radiological Investigations

Within this case the most pertinent diagnosis to rule out was fracture-related infection. There was a low clinical index of suspicion; however, prior to proceeding to operative intervention blood investigations were sent to assess white cell count (WCC) (8.8) and C-reactive protein (CRP-10). Based on radiographic interpretation we were confident that this was a mechanical failure. A computed tomography (CT) was performed to confirm the non-union, the breaking of the metalwork and to provide further information in relation to the non-union local environment. In addition, it did not demonstrate any radiological features of avascular necrosis although for this specific point, a magnetic resonance imaging (MRI) scan would have been a better choice of investigation.

Preoperative Planning

Revision fixation would initially consist of removal of the current implant which was anticipated to be difficult given the broken nail. Following this, the non-union site would need to be mobilised and the proximal fragment valgised and secured appropriately. Following realignment, a defect was anticipated which would be filled with a combination of bone grafting (options considered were: autologous, allograft, xenograft and BMP-2). Distally 2 locking screws would be inserted instead of one which was the case previously.

The following implants were selected:

- AFFIXUS nail (130°)
- Bone-morphogenic protein-2 (BMP-2)
- Bone marrow aspirate
- Xenograft (tutobone cancellous chips)

Revision Surgery

The patient was positioned supine on a fracture table with image intensifier utilised throughout. The trunk was laterally flexed away from the operative site, with the contralateral leg flexed away from the operative site. The distal locking screws were removed through the same stab incisions through which they had been inserted. Proximally the lateral incision utilised to insert the nail was re-opened, and extended distally to a point 10 cm below the lesser trochanter. Proximally a small split was made in the gluteal tendons to access the proximal end of the nail, whilst distally vastus lateralis was lifted to give access to the anterior and lateral surfaces of the femur.

Attention was then turned towards nail removal. The universal nail extractor was sited proximally following which the broken tip of the nail was proximally removed. Then the cephalo-medullary screw was removed. Following the screw removal, the remaining of the broken nail was removed using hook from the Stryker nail extraction kit (Fig. 22.4). A curette was then introduced through the entry point of the nail where three deep tissue specimens as well as 2 bone samples were sent to microbiology for culture and sensitivity assessment.

The fracture was oblique, predominantly in the sagittal plane. This was marked and the non-union plane established through the use of a 'tru-

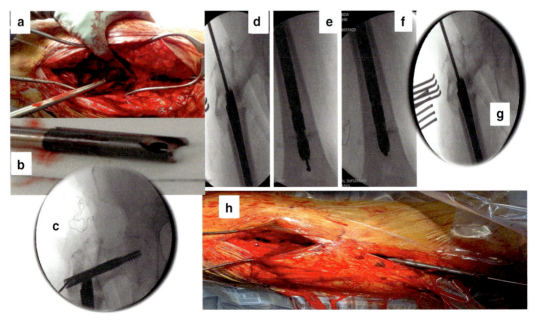

Fig. 22.4 Intraoperative imaging showing: (**a**) removal of broken proximal tip of the nail; (**b**) broken piece of nail; (**c**) insertion of guide wire for removal of cephalomedullary screw; (**d–g**) extraction of broken distal part of the nail with the hook rod; (**h**) removal of distal part of the nail

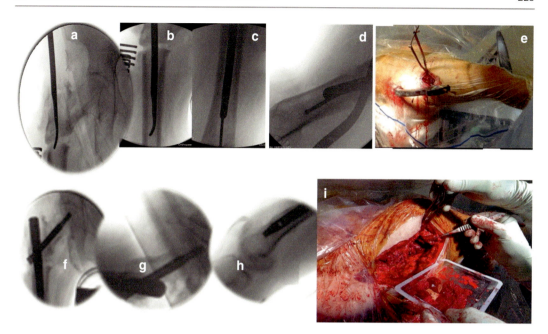

Fig. 22.5 (**a–d**) Insertion of the 'finger' reduction tool for accurate positioning of the guide wire within the intramedullary cavity of the femur; (**e**) insertion of lag screw using the jig after nail insertion; (**f–h**) AP, lateral and distal fluoroscopic view demonstrating fixation of the non-union with the Affixus nail; (**i**) Implantation of bone grafting to the lateral and medial non-union area

fuant'. Once the non-union was sufficiently mobilised using the 'finger' reduction instrument (Fig. 22.5a–d), the guide wire was inserted under image intensifier guidance and advanced in the midline of the distal femur in the AP and lateral x-ray plane in order to avoid the previous nail path, which was rather anteriorly close to the femoral cortex. Once the guidewire was in place, reaming of the intramedullary canal took place (1.5 mm above the selected nail diameter which was 13 mm), whereas Heygrove clamps were used around the subtrochanteric region allowing safe passage of the reamers and subsequently insertion of the nail.

The lag screw sheath assembly was inserted through the lag screw hole in the jig and using the previously sited skin incision the trocar was advanced until it made contact with the lateral femur (Fig. 22.5e). The 3.2 mm guide pin was inserted into 3.2 mm sleeve and drilled into position under image intensifier (assessing AP and lateral planes) so the pin was within 5 mm of the subchondral bone. The lag screw was measured and inserted at the appropriate length. Then the distal locking screws were inserted using a 4.3 mm graduated drill and the 4.3 mm drill measuring sleeve. The jig bolt that connects the insertion jig to the end of the nail using the jig bolt driver was removed in order to facilitate end cap insertion. There was a significant bone defect noted laterally and medially around the fracture site. This was managed through implantation of a structural bone substitute (xenograft, 'Tutobone') along with bone morphogenic protein-2 (BMP-2) and bone marrow aspirate (Fig. 22.5f–i).

Post-operatively the patient was instructed to toe touch weight bear with crutches for 4 weeks and subsequently to partial weight bearing progressing to full weight bearing by 12 weeks. Radiographs at 12 weeks were satisfactory (Fig. 22.6). At 9 months post-operatively her fracture had united both clinically and radiologically (Fig. 22.7), and she was able to mobilise pain free. Her rehabilitation was supported through the use of the physiotherapy services.

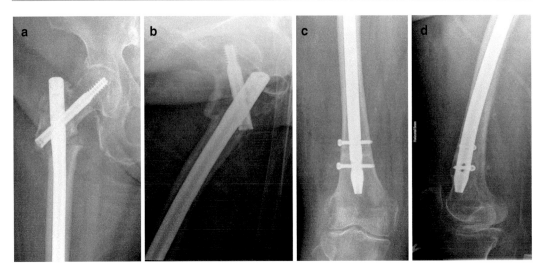

Fig. 22.6 (**a**) AP; (**b**) Lateral; (**c**) AP distal femur; (**d**) Lateral distal femur; 3 months post-operative imaging showing callous formation around non-union site

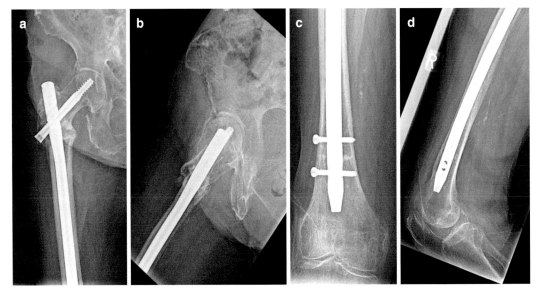

Fig. 22.7 (**a**) Ap view right hip; (**b**) Lateral view; (**c**) AP distal femur; (**d**) Lateral distal femur showing union of the fracture site at 9 months

Lessons Learned

This case summarises the difficulties that surgeons may face in treating patients who have risk factors for developing non-union including malnutrition/catabolic state and the use of disease modifying rheumatic drugs. As a result of a poorly reduced fracture (varus malignment) in the original operation and lack of medial cortical support this fracture failed in the relatively early stages. This may have been avoided through better pre-operative reduction under image intensifier, use of anti-rotation screw with the nail and insertion of a larger diameter nail to maximise stability within the fracture site.

Further Reading

Garrison I, Domingue G, Honeycutt MW. Subtrochanteric femur fractures: current review of management. EFORT Open Rev. 2021;6(2):145–51. https://doi.org/10.1302/2058-5241.6.200048. PMID: 33828858; PMCID: PMC8022017.

Giannoudis PV, Einhorn TA, Marsh D. Fracture healing: the diamond concept. Injury. 2007;38(Suppl 4):S3–6. https://doi.org/10.1016/s0020-1383(08)70003-2.

Krappinger D, Wolf B, Dammerer D, Thaler M, Schwendinger P, Lindtner RA. Risk factors for nonunion after intramedullary nailing of subtrochanteric femoral fractures. Arch Orthop Trauma Surg. 2019;139(6):769–77. https://doi.org/10.1007/s00402-019-03131-9. Epub 2019 Feb 7. PMID: 30729990; PMCID: PMC6514068.

Midshaft Femoral Plate Failed Fixation

23

Vasileios Giannoudis, Paul L. Rodham, and Peter V. Giannoudis

History of Previous Primary Treatment

A 75-year-old lady with a background of type II diabetes mellitus, atrial fibrillation, obesity and previous left total knee replacement presented following a twisting injury to left leg whilst undertaking gardening. Her injuries included an isolated closed neurovascularly intact left peri-prosthetic midshaft femoral fracture (Fig. 23.1a–c). Following review by the orthopaedic team she received a fascioiliaca block and was placed into a Thomas splint to improve the alignment of the fracture with repeated radiographs being taken. In order to assess the extent of the fracture and its relation to the total knee replacement a computed tomography (CT) was organised pre-operatively (Fig. 23.1d, e). She subsequently underwent open reduction and internal fixation of her femoral fracture on the 2nd day post-admission with a distal femoral polyaxial plate (Zimmer Biomet)

V. Giannoudis · P. L. Rodham
Academic Department of Trauma and Orthopaedics, School of Medicine, University of Leeds, Leeds, UK
e-mail: vasileios.giannoudis@nhs.net; p.rodham@nhs.net

P. V. Giannoudis (✉)
Academic Department of Trauma and Orthopaedics, School of Medicine, University of Leeds, Leeds, UK

NIHR Leeds Biomedical Research Center, Chapel Allerton Hospital, Leeds, UK

(Fig. 23.2). Post-operatively she was medically optimised (2* packed red blood cells, intravenous zolendronic acid infusion) and underwent rehabilitation with the physiotherapy team. She was discharged home 19 days post-admission.

At 1 month the patient was reviewed in the clinic where her wounds had healed nicely. She was further seen at 2 and 4 months post-operatively where she had a painless weight bearing. At 5 months post-operatively she was fully weight bearing and physiotherapy treatment improved her functional status. However, at 9 months, she had developed increasing pain, walking with an antalgic gait and was noted to clinically have a varus deformity on her left thigh when compared to the right. Radiographs taken at this appointment demonstrated that the poly-axial locking plate had broken and the proximal aspect of the fracture had not united [1] (Fig. 23.3). Her white blood cell (WBC) and C-reactive protein (CRP) levels (screening for infection) were within normal limits. She subsequently underwent revision surgery 2 weeks later (removal of broken polyaxial plate and debridement of left femur and 10-hole distal femur NCB plate (Zimmer Biomet) and 2 lag screws were applied to stabilise the femoral non-union. Tissue samples were sent to microbiology to investigate for low grade infection. The samples came back as negative of any microorganisms. Post-operatively she was advised to toe touch weight bear for 8 weeks before progressing to physio-

© The Author(s), under exclusive license to Springer Nature Switzerland AG 2024
P. V. Giannoudis, P. Tornetta III (eds.), *Failed Fracture Fixation*,
https://doi.org/10.1007/978-3-031-39692-2_23

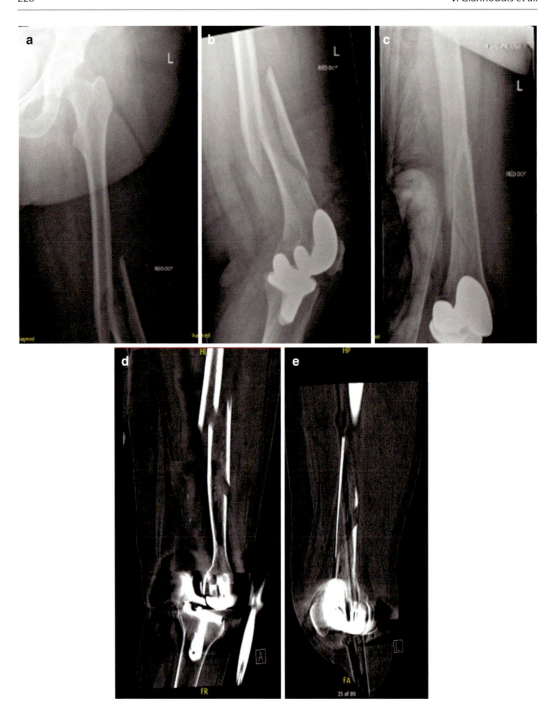

Fig. 23.1 Radiographs of left femur demonstrating a periprosthetic mid to distal 1/3 femoral fracture; (**a**) AP femur; (**b**) Lateral distal femur; (**c**) Lateral femur; (**d**) Coronal CT slice; (**e**) Sagittal CT slice

therapy assisted fully weight bearing (Fig. 23.4). Seven months following the revision surgery following a fairly innocuous stumble she reported inability to weight bear which again demonstrated that the NCB locking plate had broken (Fig. 23.5).

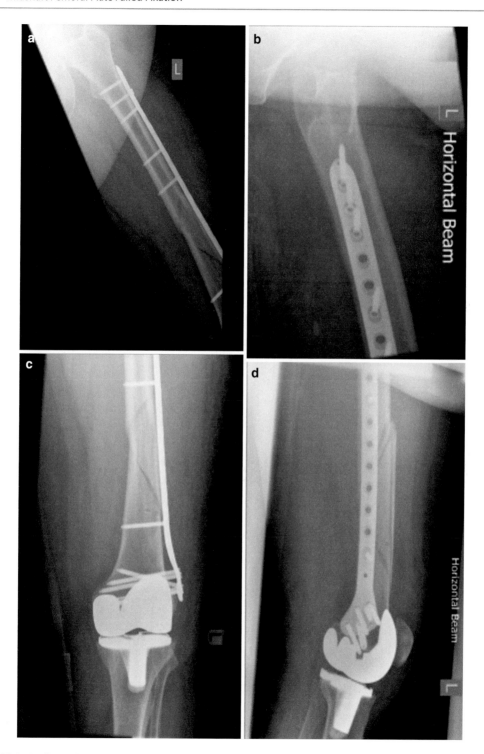

Fig. 23.2 Radiographs demonstrating that the left femoral fracture was managed with a distal femur polyaxial plating system on post-injury day 2; (**a**) AP proximal femur; (**b**) Lateral proximal femur; (**c**) AP distal femur; (**d**) Lateral distal femur

Fig. 23.3 Radiographs of left femur showing failure of the polyaxial distal femoral plate; (**a**) AP distal femur; (**b**) Lateral distal femur

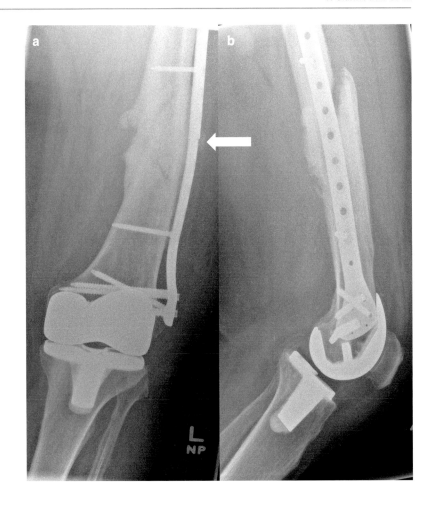

23 Midshaft Femoral Plate Failed Fixation

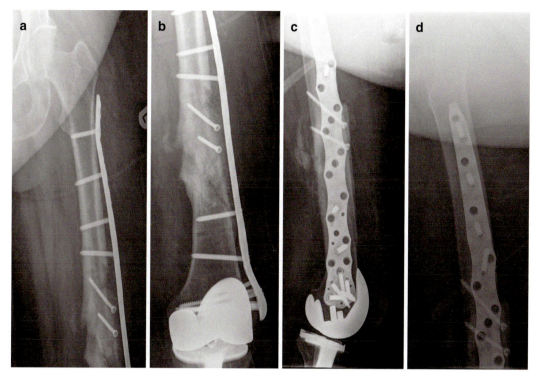

Fig. 23.4 Revision to NCB plate and lag screws; (**a**) AP proximal femur; (**b**) AP distal femur; (**c**) Lateral distal femur; (**d**) Lateral proximal femur

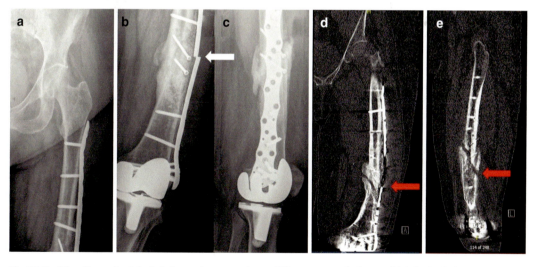

Fig. 23.5 AP radiograph of the left femur demonstrating breaking of the NCB locking plate; (**a**) AP proximal femur; (**b**) AP distal femur; (**c**) Lateral distal femur; (**d**) CT scan coronal view and (**e**) Sagittal view (red arrows) showing the femoral non-union

Evaluation of the Aetiology of Failure of Fixation

This was a failure of a polyaxial distal femur plate (Zimmer Biomet). From the initial images we note a 3-part femoral fracture. Subsequently, a NCB plate was used. Of note both locking system constructs failed. This is likely due to the underlying fracture fixation being too rigid a construct providing significant stress risers around the fracture site. This was attempted to be rectified by increasing the working length of the plate in the first revision surgery extending the plate from an 8 hole to 10 plate. Moreover, one has to consider a poor biological environment having the fracture been exposed surgically open on two occasions [2].

Clinical Examination

On assessment this patient was unable to mobilise. Shortening was noted to her left side by 3 cm. Her hip was externally rotated with the thigh being held in a flexed position. All wounds from his original surgery were well healed with no evidence of infection.

Diagnostic-Biochemical and Radiological Investigations

Within this case the most pertinent diagnosis to rule out was fracture-related infection. There was a low clinical index of suspicion; however, prior to proceeding to operative intervention blood investigations were sent to assess white cell count (WCC) (6.2), CRP (<5), both within normal limits. Intra-operative deep tissue samples were also taken which did not grow any organism. Based on radiographic interpretation we were confident that this was a mechanical failure and therefore no further imaging was sought prior to proceeding to revision fixation. In cases where doubt exists in the setting of implants, positron emission tomography-computed tomography (PET-CT) can be of value to evaluate for evidence of infection as well as tissue biopsy.

Pre-operative Planning

Revision fixation would initially consist of removal of the broken NCB locking plate. Since a plate had been used on two previous occasions (a load bearing device) a plan was made to stabilise the fracture non-union with a reamed intramedullary (IM) nail (a load sharing device). This was felt to be the most appropriate plan to provide a favourable mechanical environment. In addition, it was felt essential to provide an osteogenic stimulus at the non-union site with the application of autologous bone grafting in the form of reamer-irrigator aspirator harvesting device (RIA) in association with concentrated bone marrow aspirate (BMA) (loading of the RIA graft with autologous progenitor cells) harvested from the right pelvic iliac crest [3].

The following implants were selected

- 135° Affixus nail (long)
- RIA device (to harvest autologous bone graft from the contralateral femur)
- Bone marrow aspirate kit

Revision Surgery

The patient was positioned supine on a fracture table with image intensifier utilised throughout. The trunk was laterally flexed away from the operative site, with the contralateral leg prepared for RIA grafting. At induction 1 g of tranexamic acid was administered. A stab incision was made in the right iliac crest. A trocar was inserted and 60 mL of bone marrow aspirate was harvested. Using the BIoCue Zimmer Biomet system a 7 mL concentrated BMA was obtained. A standard procedure was used to harvest graft with the RIA device from the right femur (Fig. 23.6). A size 13 mm RIA reamer head was used. Following closure of the stab incision in the right buttock with 3/0 nylon stiches and application of a dressing, the right hip was placed in the flexed position for preparation of the revision surgery of the left femur.

After re-draping, the original incision on the left femur was utilised and the broken NCB plate with the two lag screws were removed. A curette was introduced through the non-union site of the midshaft of the femur where 5 deep tissue specimens (3 bone) were sent to microbiology for culture and sensitivity assessment. The non-union site was debrided adequately to bleeding bone.

The 3-part fracture was oblique both superiorly and inferiorly in the butterfly segment, predominantly in the sagittal plane. This was marked and the non-union plane established through the use of a 'trufuant'. At this point using the 'ball nose guide' the guide wire for the Affixus nail was inserted at under image intensifier guidance ensuring appropriate position on AP and lateral imaging. Once in place the proximal reamers were inserted in order to ensure that the position of the nail remained within the anatomical axis, Heygrove clamps were used around the midhsaft femoral region allowing safe passage of the reamers and insertion of the nail. The inserted nail was measured (380/11 mm) (Fig. 23.7).

The lag screw sheath assembly was inserted through the lag screw hole in the jig and using the previously sited skin incision the trocar was advanced until it made contact with the lateral femur. The 3.2 mm guide pin was inserted into 3.2 mm sleeve and drilled into position under image intensifier (assessing AP and lateral planes) so the pin was within 5 mm of the subchondral bone. The lag screw was measured at 95 mm and inserted after reaming. Subsequently the distal locking screws were inserted for locking of the nail. Using a screw driver, the set screw secures the lag screw in a static mode. The jig bolt that connects the insertion jig to the end of the nail using the jig bolt driver was removed in order to facilitate the nail end cap insertion.

Furthermore, the bone defect region around the midshaft of the femur was grafted with the combined RIA graft and concentrated bone marrow aspirate 7 mL. Post-operative radiographs are shown in Fig. 23.8.

The patient was instructed to partially weight bear with crutches for 4 weeks post-operatively, following which she progressed to full weight bearing. At 6 months post-operatively her fracture had united both clinically and radiologically (Fig. 23.9), and she was able to mobilise pain free. Her rehabilitation was supported through the use of the physiotherapy services.

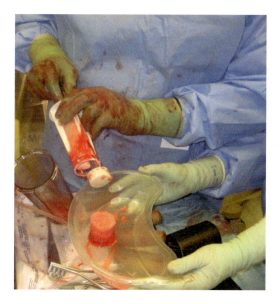

Fig. 23.6 RIA graft obtained from the right femoral shaft

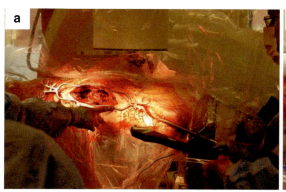 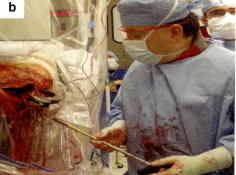

Fig. 23.7 (**a**) Insertion of Affixus nail; (**b**) insertion of lag screw

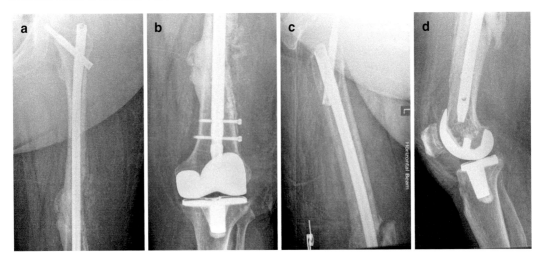

Fig. 23.8 Post-op radiographs of left femur; (**a**) AP left femur; (**b**) AP distal femur; (**c**) Lateral proximal femur; (**d**) Lateral distal femur

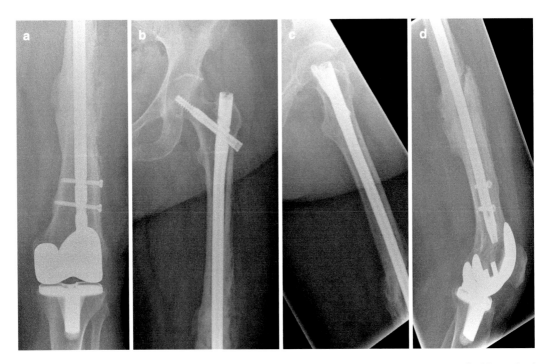

Fig. 23.9 Radiographs of left femur 9 months post-operatively showing union; (**a**) AP distal femur; (**b**) AP proximal femur; (**c**) Lateral proximal femur; (**d**) Lateral distal femur

Summary: Lessons Learned

This case summarises the difficulties that surgeons may face in treating patients who have periprosthetic midshaft femoral fracture. As a result of a poorly constructed biomechanical fixation the original operation using the polyaxial distal femoral plate and subsequently NCB plate failed likely to the significant stress risers that were occurring over the fracture site and a compromised biology. This may have been avoided using an intramedullary nail, a load sharing device and optimisation of the biological environment with RIA graft and concentrated bone marrow aspirate. This approach of optimum mechanics and biology facilitated a successful surgical outcome.

References

1. Kanakaris NK, Giannoudis PV. Locking plate systems and their inherent hitches. Injury. 2010;41(12):1213–9. https://doi.org/10.1016/j.injury.2010.09.038.
2. Giannoudis PV, Einhorn TA, Marsh D. Fracture healing: a harmony of optimal biology and optimal fixation? Injury. 2007;38(Suppl 4):S1–2. https://doi.org/10.1016/s0020-1383(08)70002-0.
3. Andrzejowski P, Giannoudis PV. The 'diamond concept' for long bone non-union management. J Orthop Traumatol. 2019;20(1):21. https://doi.org/10.1186/s10195-019-0528-0.

Distal Femur Plate Failed Fixation

24

Andrea Attenasio, Erick Heiman, Richard S. Yoon, and Frank A. Liporace

History of Previous Primary Failed Treatment

The patient in this case is a 75-year-old female who underwent open reduction and internal fixation (ORIF) of a closed, extra-articular, supracondylar distal femur fracture at an outside hospital 6 months prior to her presentation in our clinic. She initially presented with well healed incisions, limited mobility, distal thigh pain, and significantly decreased knee range of motion from 0° of extension to 70° of flexion. X-ray of the left femur from the time of presentation (Fig. 24.1) demonstrate use of a lateral distal femur locking plate with fracture lines still present and no signs of callus formation present. Infection was ruled out by obtaining erythrocyte sedimentation rate (ESR), c-reactive protein (CRP), and white blood cell (WBC) count, which were all within normal limits. A computed tomography (CT) scan (Fig. 24.2) confirmed the presence of a delayed union, demonstrating medial cortical consolidation at the fracture site, but no bridging callus of any

other cortex. At this time, she refused further operative intervention.

Over the next 3 months, she progressed in her ability to ambulate with minimal assistance, had no thigh pain, and regained functional knee range of motion. She completed a course of physical therapy, vitamin supplementation, and bone stimulation therapy; however, she continued to have limited radiographic evidence of bone healing. At 9 months status post original ORIF, a repeat CT scan was obtained, demonstrating no further healing. At this time, she was offered revision ORIF but due to her minimal pain and improved functional status, the patient elected to attempt further non-operative treatment.

At 11 months status post ORIF the patient had almost no pain at the fracture site and continued to be functional with activities of daily living. Despite having progressed well clinically, she presented to the emergency department with atraumatic thigh pain and inability to ambulate. Radiographic evaluation (Fig. 24.3) revealed a catastrophic failure of her previous fixation, and she subsequently underwent revision ORIF.

A. Attenasio · E. Heiman · R. S. Yoon
F. A. Liporace (✉)
Division of Orthopaedic Trauma & Adult
Reconstruction, Department of Orthopaedic Surgery,
Cooperman Barnabas Medical Center/Jersey City
Medical Center - RWJBarnabas Health, Livingston,
NJ/Jersey City, NJ, USA

© The Author(s), under exclusive license to Springer Nature Switzerland AG 2024
P. V. Giannoudis, P. Tornetta III (eds.), *Failed Fracture Fixation*,
https://doi.org/10.1007/978-3-031-39692-2_24

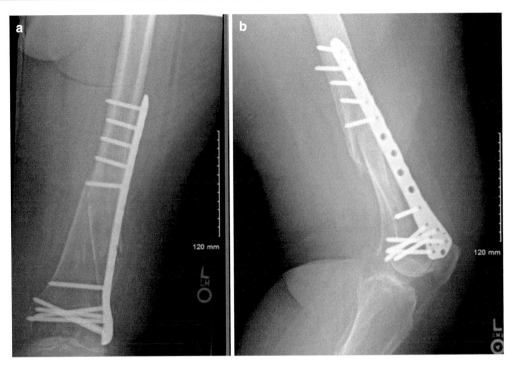

Fig. 24.1 AP (**a**) and lateral (**b**) radiographs of the left distal femur at time of initial presentation, 6 months status post ORIF. Demonstrates limited evidence of healing, fixed fracture gap, and recurvatum deformity

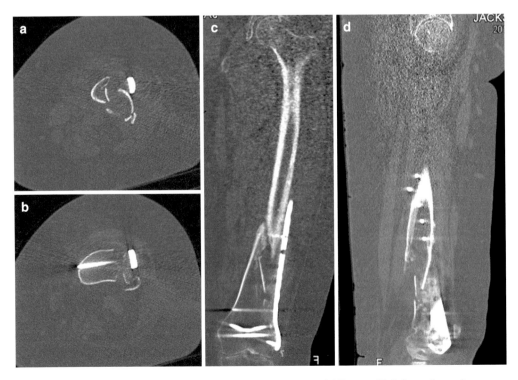

Fig. 24.2 Representative axial (**a**, **b**), coronal (**c**), and sagittal (**d**) cuts of CT scan of left femur 7 months status post ORIF demonstrating again, fixed fracture gap with no evidence of bridging callus across any or the four cortices

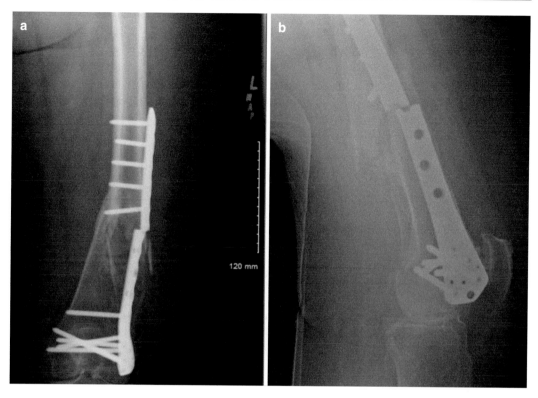

Fig. 24.3 AP (**a**) and lateral (**b**) radiographs of the left distal femur 11 months status post initial ORIF demonstrating catastrophic hardware failure of a broken plate and fracture through the site of the previous nonunion

Evaluation of the Etiology of Failure of Fixation

This patient's extra-articular distal femur fracture was initially treated with an ORIF using a lateral distal femur locking plate in bridge plating mode, the goal of which was to generate callus formation using only relative stability. The construct included the use of only locked screws in the distal and proximal segments, with a short working length. The use of all locked screws creates a very stiff construct. This, in combination with a fixed fracture gap and short segment fixation, led to late catastrophic hardware failure through the plate.

Distal femur fractures treated with lateral locked plating have a high incidence of nonunion. In a review of 15 articles, Henderson et al. noted healing complications in as few as 0% and as many as 32%. Implant failure typically occurred later in treatment, with a majority occurring at least 3 months post-operatively and half occurring greater than 6 months following initial ORIF [1]. Specifically, the treatment of geriatric, low-energy distal femur fractures with laterally based locked plating has a high complication rate. One-year mortality rates are reported as high as 25%, with early post-operative systemic complications of almost 40%, and an average hospital length of stay of 8 days. In the geriatric population, younger patients (aged 60–74) and those with surgical site infections were at a higher risk for nonunion [2].

The technique used for fixation of distal femur fractures greatly affects union rates. The use of a lateral locked plate with the use of only locked screws may create a construct that is too stiff. Under biomechanical testing, this type of construct does not allow enough motion (<0.1 mm) at the near cortex to induce callus formation [3].

When treating metaphyseal distal femur fractures with bridge plating, plate metallurgy, working length, screw density, and coronal alignment do not significantly affect union rates; however, the use of all locked screws in the diaphysis creates nearly a threefold increase in nonunion rate [4].

Clinical Examination

The patient was unable to bear weight on the affected extremity and the leg was painful on passive leg roll.

Diagnostic-Biochemical and Radiological Investigations

When working up a nonunion, it is important to have a stepwise approach at an appropriate time during the healing process. A nonunion is technically defined by the Centers for Disease Control and Prevention (CDC) as a fracture that is at least 9 months out from occurrence, is not healed, and has not shown any progression in healing over the previous 3 months [5]. However, this definition is not always pragmatic. A more practical definition hinges on the opinion of the treating provider to determine if a fracture has no potential to heal [6]. It is important to look at the patient as a whole and assess the biomechanics of fixation, host factors, and potential for infection.

Nonunions typically fall into one of four categories depending on the presence or absence of biology as well as the mechanics of fixation. Hypertrophic nonunions are characterized by an abundance of callus formation on plain radiographs. There is typically more than sufficient biology, but not enough mechanical stability. Oligotrophic nonunions are characterized by evidence of, but inadequate callus formation. Typically, vascularity is preserved but there is a combination of inadequate biology and/or mechanics for fracture healing. Atrophic nonunions are characterized by a complete lack of callus formation of plain radiographs. This is a situation where there is inadequate biology and potentially an overly rigid fixation construct.

When working up a fracture for any type of nonunion there are four factors that must be considered: motion, vascularity, fracture gap, and infection. The biomechanics of fixation can be evaluated on plain radiographs. It is important to understand the type of bone healing that was attempted to be achieved and understand if the construct appropriately addresses this goal. Does the fixation allow too much motion, or is it too rigid? Is there a fixed gap? Understanding and identifying the type of fixation utilized in the construct can help to delineate if there is either excess or not enough motion that may be contributing to the nonunion formation. It is important to attempt to assess the local biology of the fracture based on clinical and radiographic evaluation. Does it appear that excessive soft tissue stripping occurred either from the injury or surgical dissection? Systemic host factors are also important to assess. Is there an underlying endocrine disorder that may affect bone healing [7]? Poor nutritional status can also contribute to poor host biology and lack of bone formation. These factors can often be assessed via an appropriate laboratory workup. Finally, for all nonunions, infection should always be ruled out. This can often be achieved by obtaining blood work including WBC count, ESR, and CRP. If these are within normal limits, then there is low suspicion for underlying infection contributing to the formation of the nonunion. If these are elevated, it might be necessary to obtain either a CT-guided biopsy or an open biopsy and send the specimen for pathology and cultures.

The authors of this chapter recommend a thorough workup and evaluation as outlined in the case that is presented. At presentation to our office, approximately 6 months after initial ORIF there was little evidence of fracture healing and a nonunion workup was initiated consisting of advanced imaging and laboratory evaluation. A CT scan was ordered to investigate and define the amount of bony healing present. Blood work, including ESR, CRP, and WBC, was ordered to evaluate for underlying infection. A full endocrine panel was ordered to evaluate for underlying host factors that may impair bone healing. After a negative metabolic and infectious workup, it was determined that this case was an aseptic, atrophic nonunion of the distal femur with no underlying host factors contributing to the nonunion. Rigid short segment fixation along with a fixed fracture gap prevented appropriate biomechanics for secondary fracture healing to occur.

Pre-operative Planning

Pre-operative planning should include identification of the current implants, including both the type of implant and the manufacturing company, if possible. Accurate implant identification pre-operatively can help to facilitate removal by utilizing a company specific implant removal set. Having a universal broken screw removal set or universal nail extraction set available can also be useful in case the company of the original implant is unknown or as a backup set if removal becomes difficult. Tools such as conical extractors and trephines are valuable for extracting broken or stripped screws.

The pre-operative plan should also account for the revision construct, which can often depend on the etiology of the nonunion or fixation failure. In this case, we elected to revise to a nail-plate combination construct, and thus both sets of implants were readily available. Additionally, it is important to plan for possible use of bone graft and/or supplementation with bone marrow aspirate so that these products and harvest kits may also be available for use.

Implant Selection

When choosing a revision construct, understanding the etiology of nonunion is essential to successfully choosing the correct revision surgery. Various options include plate osteosynthesis, nail dynamization, exchange nailing, or use of a combination of constructs with or without the utilization of bone graft. For patients with distal femur nonunions after initial intramedullary nailing, the problem is often that the construct lacks enough stability for bone healing, and thus nail dynamization will likely worsen the problem. Exchange nailing with a larger diameter nail is often a reasonable revision construct for femoral shaft fractures, as it allows maintained stability due to achieving an isthmus fit while additionally offering osteogenic potential from reaming; however, in distal femurs, the wider canal diameter at the nonisthmal fracture location means that an intramedullary nail (IMN) alone will not provide adequate stability, and thus the construct is prone to failure. A study by Yang et al. found that exchange nailing with a larger diameter nail failed 50% of the time when the fracture location was nonisthmal compared to a 87% success rate for isthmal femoral nonunions [8]. Thus, the solution for distal femur nonunions after failed initial IMN is often to add stability via supplementation with plate osteosynthesis. In a study of distal femur nonunions that were initially fixed with IMN, revision of the nonunion via supplementation with a plate, and bone grafting over the nail, the nail/plate combination allowed for immediate weight bearing and a 100% consolidation rate [9].

Conversely, as discussed, initial treatment with a lateral locking plate often leads to a nonunion due to the construct being too rigid, especially if only locking screws are utilized. For these types of cases, such as the one presented here, a construct allowing for increased fracture motion is favorable to promote bony union. In the setting of this nonunion, the original fixation construct was too stiff with a short working length, and thus the decision was made to revise using a combination of fixation with a nail and a lateral locking plate. The use of the IMN in this construct allows for increased motion at the fracture site with the additional benefit of allowing immediate weight bearing with the use of a load sharing device. Additionally, using a plate in combination with the nail add needed stability to the nonisthmal fracture. Revising the plate construct to a longer working length that uses both locking and non-locking screws proximal to the fracture site in combination with the IMN creates a boxed construct with a smoother modulus of transition, resulting in a less rigid construct that allows for allowing for greater motion at the fracture site to promote fracture healing.

Biologic Considerations

In order to effectively treat a nonunion, revision constructs not only need to achieve sufficient stability and minimize fracture gaps, but it must also initiate osteogenic potential. While construct design will help to achieve adequate stability, the use of bone grafting can help to achieve the goals of minimizing fracture gaps and providing osteogenic stimulation. The decision to supplement fixation with bone graft often depends on the type of nonunion present. For hypertrophic nonunions caused by a lack of stability, the body has adequate biology for fracture healing, as indicated by the robust callus formation. These types of nonunions do not require biologic supplementation for adequate healing, and thus bone grafting may not be needed. In the setting of atrophic or oligotrophic nonunions, there is often a combination of factors leading to nonunion, and poor biologics can often contribute to lack of or poor callus formation, and thus supplementing fixation with bone graft may be beneficial for stimulating biology [10]. Additionally, nonunions with significant bone loss may require bone grafting in order to bridge the defects [6].

Different types of bone grafts may serve different functions. Bone marrow aspirate can be harvested from the anterior or posterior iliac crest and contains osteoprogenitor cells with osteogenic potential. The use of allogenic cancellous bone graft is primarily osteoconductive, which can be useful to compensate for bone loss; however, may be more beneficial when mixed with an autograft in order to enhance osteoinductive and osteogenic abilities [11]. Other bone graft substitutes such as calcium phosphate, calcium sulfate, or hydroxyapatite may also be useful in treating nonunions as they are both osteoconductive and thus good for filling defects. These types of bone graft also have the benefit of being able to be combined with antibiotics in the setting of infectious nonunions. Calcium phosphate in particular has the highest compressive strength as well as the slowest biodegradation time, allowing prolonged support for fracture healing [6].

In the presented case, a combination of types of bone graft was utilized to maximize benefits. Bone marrow aspirate concentrate was harvested from the iliac crest for its osteogenic and osteoinductive properties. It was combined with demineralized bone matrix and calcium phosphate for their osteoconductive properties and ability to fill residual bone defect.

Revision Surgery

The patient was positioned supine on a radiolucent table. A dual incision approach was used, ensuring an adequate skin bridge. The previous lateral incision was utilized and extended to expose the entire plate used for primary fixation as well as the nonunion site. A broken screw removal set was utilized to remove the plate and locking screws. The head had broken off of one of the proximal screws, and thus a trephine was used to remove the thread length of the screw.

Biopsy of the nonunion site was taken and set for pathology and cultures, all fibrinous tissue and non-bleeding bone were debrided from the nonunion site. The gram stain was negative. After keying in the medial spine of the fracture lines, a residual 4×2 cm defect was noted laterally. This preliminary reduction was held in place with a lobster reduction clamp (Fig. 24.4).

Next, insertion of a retrograde IMN was performed in standard fashion. Leaving the guide jig in place, an 18-hole lateral distal femur plate was then slid from distal to proximal through the distal incision, and an accessory incision was created proximally at the greater trochanter to place the plate at the vastus ridge. Part of vastus was taken down in order for the plate to sit directly on the lateral cortex, and the plate was contoured proximal with a slight bend to accommodate the greater trochanter. A drill bit was utilized proximally to maintain the position of the plate while distal fixation was achieved with locked screws around the knee. Using the distal jig aligned with the plate, locking screws were placed through both the nail and the plate. After distal locking fixation had been achieved, one screw was placed at the fracture site about the residual defect to act as a rebar for bone graft. Fixation was then

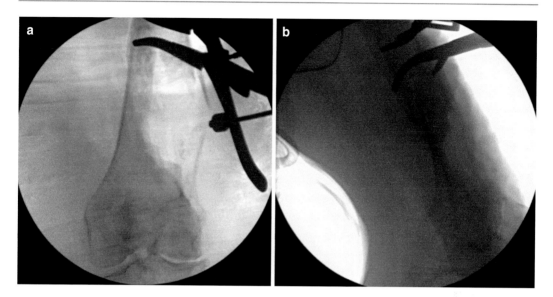

Fig. 24.4 AP (**a**) and lateral (**b**) intra-operative fluoroscopic images demonstrating the provisional reduction and defect after removal of broken hardware and debridement of nonunion

achieved proximally using nonlocking screws at the level of the lesser trochanter to compress the plate to the cortical surface of the bone. A screw was additionally directed up the femoral neck in order to provide additional protection, and a combination of locked and unlocked screws was used throughout the diaphysis of the femur, creating a smooth transition of stiffness. Finally, the proximal locking screws for the IMN were inserted.

Bone marrow aspirate concentrate was harvested from the iliac crest and inserted into the nonunion site in combination with demineralized bone matrix and calcium phosphate. Fracture alignment and fixation was confirmed with fluoroscopy, and the wound was copiously irrigated and closed.

Utilization of an IMN combined with the lateral plate was used to create a boxed construct with a transition of stiffness that allows for both secondary bone healing and immediate weight bearing, while spanning the length of the femur to protect from peri-implant fractures. The plate placement laterally was chosen to be proximal enough to allow for a total knee arthroplasty in the future without necessitating a removal of hardware (Fig. 24.5).

Post-operative Course

Post-operatively, the patient was made weight bearing as tolerated and allowed to perform knee range of motion and participate in physical therapy right away. She was discharged from the hospital post-operative day 1, after being cleared by physical therapy. At 2 weeks her knee range of motion was 0–90, and she was ambulating well with a walker. At 3 months she was ambulating with just a cane for assistance and had achieved full knee range of motion. She was overall experiencing minimal pain and was clinically nontender to palpation at the fracture site. At 6 months she continued to do well and was radiographically and clinically healed (Figs. 24.6 and 24.7). At 1-year follow-up, she continued to ambulate well without assistance and was able to perform all activities of daily living.

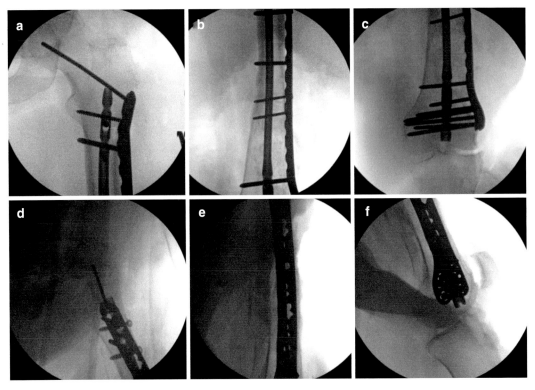

Fig. 24.5 AP (**a–c**) and lateral (**d–f**) intra-operative fluoroscopic images demonstrating the final nail/plate combination construct with bone graft in the defect

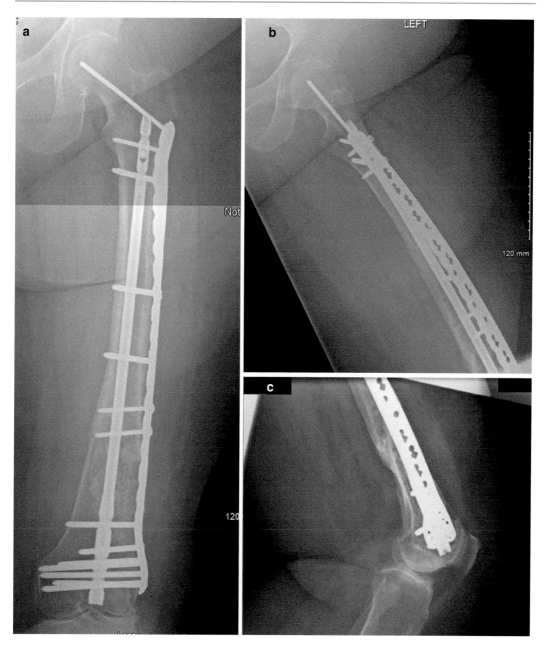

Fig. 24.6 AP (**a**) and lateral (**b**, **c**) post-operative radiographs of the femur 6 months status post revision ORIF to a nail plate combination construct demonstrating a well healed distal femur fracture

Fig. 24.7 Representative sagittal (**a**) and coronal (**b**) views of a CT scan obtained at 6 months follow-up demonstrating four cortex consolidation of fracture

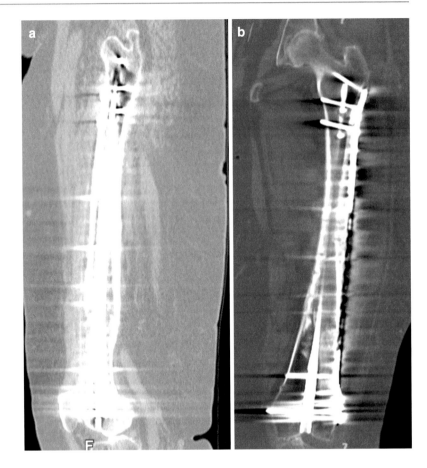

Lessons Learned

Surgical fixation of distal femur fractures, especially in the geriatric population, is not without complication and has a higher rate of nonunion. This can be largely dependent on the initial fixation strategy. Fixation that either lacks stability, such as use of an IMN, or that is too rigid, such as with a locking plate in the presented case, can subsequently lead to a nonunion. For this case, the rigid short segment fixation with residual fracture gap did not allow enough movement at the fracture site to stimulate biology and allow callus formation. Choice of initial construct for distal femur fractures should allow for flexible fixation for bridging construct to allow for secondary healing and allow for immediate weight bearing to minimize postoperative complications. Similarly, our revision construct sought to achieve these goals by utilizing a combination of IMN with the addition of a lateral plate.

References

1. Henderson CE, Kuhl LL, Fitzpatrick DC, Marsh JL. Locking plates for distal femur fractures: is there a problem with fracture healing? J Orthop Trauma. 2011b;25(Suppl. 1):S8–14.
2. Moloney GB, Pan T, Van Eck CF, Patel D, Tarkin I. Geriatric distal femur fracture: are we underestimating the rate of local and systemic complications? Injury. 2016;47(8):1732–6.
3. Bottlang M, Doornink J, Lujan TJ, Fitzpatrick DC, Marsh JL, Augat P, et al. Effects of construct stiffness on healing of fractures stabilized with locking plates. J Bone Jt Surg. 2010;92(Suppl. 2):12–22.

4. Harvin WH, Oladeji LO, Della Rocca GJ, Murtha YM, Volgas DA, Stannard JP, et al. Working length and proximal screw constructs in plate osteosynthesis of distal femur fractures. Injury. 2017;48(11):2597–601.
5. Brinker MR, O'Connor DP. Nonunions: Evaluation and Treatment. In: Browner BD, Jupiter JB, Krettek C, Anderson PA (eds) Skeletal Trauma: Basic Science, Management, and Reconstruction, 6th edn. vol 1. Elsevier, Amsterdam. 2020. pp 743–834.
6. Browner BD, editor. Skeletal trauma: fractures, dislocations, ligamentous injuries. Philadelphia: W. B. Saunders; 1992.
7. Brinker MR, O'Connor DP, Monla YT, Earthman TP. Metabolic and endocrine abnormalities in patients with nonunions. J Orthop Trauma. 2007;21(8):557–70.
8. Yang KH, Kim JR, Park J. Nonisthmal femoral shaft nonunion as a risk factor for exchange nailing failure. J Trauma Acute Care Surg. 2012;72(2):E60–4.
9. Hakeos WM, Richards JE, Obremskey WT. Plate fixation of femoral nonunions over an intramedullary nail with autogenous bone grafting. J Orthop Trauma. 2011;25(2):84–9.
10. Marsh J. Principles of bone grafting: non-union, delayed union. Surg Oxf. 2003;21(9):213–6.
11. Wu CC. Bone grafting techniques in treating fracture nonunion. Chang Gung Med J. 2000;23(6):319–30.

Distal Femur Periprosthetic Fracture Failed Fixation

25

Martin Gathen, Koroush Kabir, and Christof Burger

History of Previous Primary Failed Treatment

For distal femoral periprosthetic fractures, the most widely used classification system is the one proposed by Rorabeck and Lewis which describes three fracture types: type I refers to an undisplaced fracture and a well-fixed implant, type II refers to a displaced fracture and a well-fixed implant and type III refers to a displaced or non-displaced fracture and a loose implant. The most frequent complications are non-union/malunion, implant failure or infection, which can lead to high rates of failed fracture fixation and revision surgery [1]. The treatment gets even more challenging after failed fracture fixation due to possible bone defects or a devascularised bone stock. In addition, elderly patients are mostly affected and often present with multiple comorbidities and osteoporosis. The decision as to whether a re-do fixation or revision arthroplasty is to be performed depends on factors like fracture type, bone stock and the type of implant in situ. If the prosthesis is loose or if it is not possible to hold the distal fragment, revision arthroplasty should be considered [2]. The two most described fixa-

tion techniques in case the femoral component is well fixed (stable) are locked plating and retrograde intramedullary nailing. Below we present two examples of cases that failed and discuss the aetiology of failure and the strategy of revision surgery.

Case 1: Failed Internal Fixation

A 77-year-old female patient sustained a closed periprosthetic distal femur fracture, which corresponds to Rorabeck and Lewis's type II fracture type. The fracture line was located directly at the tip of the stem of the femoral component. The implanted prosthesis was a hinge revision system (EnduRo Hinge Knee System, B. Braun, Melsungen, Germany).

Primary treatment included open reduction and fixation via a large fragment LCP plate (DePuy Synthes, Raynham, Ma, USA). An additional locking attachment plate was inserted for further fixation (Fig. 25.1a, b). Five months later, the patient started experiencing pain in the right leg after normal weight bearing; the X-ray showed a failed fracture fixation with a broken plate and the non-union of the known femur fracture.

Case 2: Failed Internal Fixation

A 60-year-old female patient suffered a closed left periprosthetic distal femur fracture, which corresponds to Roraceck and Lewis's type II fracture type. In the local hospital, an open

M. Gathen · K. Kabir · C. Burger (✉)
Department of Orthopedics and Trauma Surgery,
University Hospital of Bonn, Bonn, Germany
e-mail: Martin.gathen@ukbonn.de;
Koroush.kabir@ukbonn.de;
christof.burger@ukbonn.de

© The Author(s), under exclusive license to Springer Nature Switzerland AG 2024
P. V. Giannoudis, P. Tornetta III (eds.), *Failed Fracture Fixation*,
https://doi.org/10.1007/978-3-031-39692-2_25

Fig. 25.1 (Case 1) (**a**) AP X-ray and (**b**) lateral X-ray of the right femur before revision surgery. The implant failure occurred directly on the level of the hypertrophic non-union between the first distal and the proximal screw from the former fracture zone

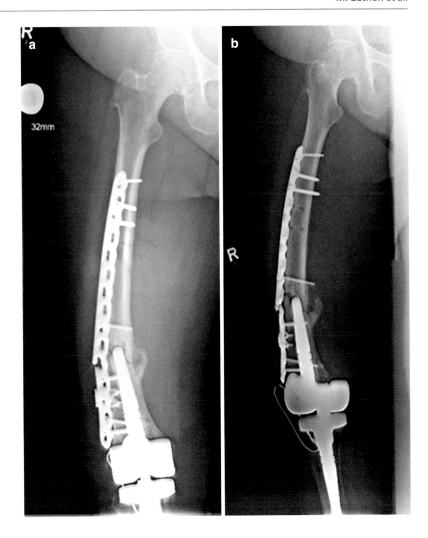

reduction and internal fixation using an NCB plate (non-contact bridging, Zimmer Biomet Holdings, Warsaw, IN, USA) was utilised for stabilisation. Unfortunately, the fracture failed to unite and at 6 months the second osteosynthesis took place with cancellous bone allograft (Fig. 25.2a, b). During the course of treatment, the wound showed clinical signs of infection, and multiple debridements were performed. The plate failed 8 months later (Fig. 25.3a, b) and the patient was transferred to a level I trauma centre.

Fig. 25.2 (Case 2) (**a**) AP X-ray; (**b**) lateral X-ray of the left distal femur after the first open reduction and internal fixation. There were no signs of loosening of the TKA. Fixation in a slightly extended position can be seen on the lateral view

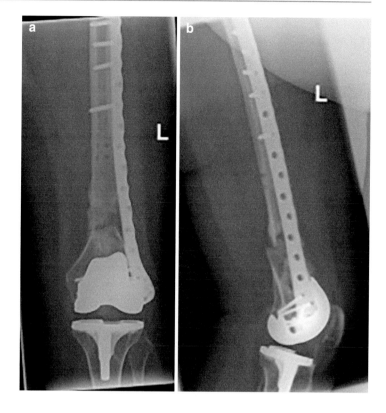

Fig. 25.3 (Case 2) (**a**) AP X-ray; (**b**) lateral X-ray of the left distal femur 8 months after first fracture fixation showing radiological signs of an atrophic non-union and failed plate fixation. No signs of prosthesis loosening can be seen

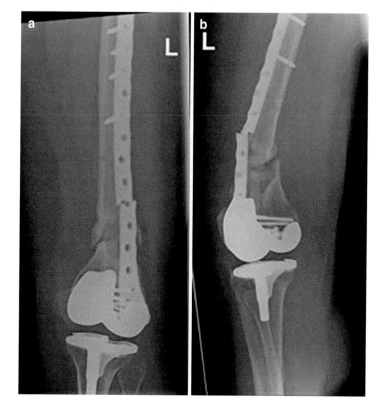

Evaluation of the Aetiology of Failure of Fixation

Case 1

Multiple factors led to the primary failure of the fixation (Fig. 25.1a, b). Firstly, a suboptimal plate was used for fixation. The design did not allow for the insertion of multiple distal locking screws and none of the distal screws had bicortical grips. Secondly, the first proximal screw was inserted directly proximal to the fracture zone and didn't facilitate the creation of an optimum working length, which led to the plate's failure. Furthermore, the osteoporotic bone stock led to inadequate fracture stabilisation.

Case 2

The main reason for the implant failure (Fig. 25.3a, b) was the development of an atrophic non-union and the subsequent surgical site infection. The persistent non-union and mechanical instability resulted in the fatigue failure of the plate [3]. Plate or screw failure reportedly occurs in 13–18% of cases. Biomechanical investigations suggest a failure rate when non-locking screws are used compared to locking screws, especially in osteoporotic bones [4].

Clinical Examination

Case 1

History of past illness: Hyperuricaemia and hyperlipidaemia were known past illnesses.

Clinical examination: The patient presented with isolated pain in the right upper leg for over 2 weeks. The leg was mildly swollen, and there were no clinical signs of hemarthrosis or infection.

Case 2

History of past illness: The patient suffered a stroke 6 years prior to the femur fracture. Furthermore, systemic lupus erythematosus disease was reported.

Clinical examination: The patient showed movement-dependent pain of the left distal femur. In addition, the patient described painful instability during weight bearing of the leg. After previous surgeries, the skin was compromised by scar tissue formation but showed no acute signs of infection and no neurological deficits.

Diagnostic—Biochemical and Radiological Investigations

Case 1

Besides the failed plate, the X-ray showed a hypertrophic non-union with a large medial osteophyte (Fig. 25.1a, b). At the time of admission, the C-reactive protein showed a normal blood concentration of 6.09 mg/L; leukocytes were also normal at 8.45 G/L. No other radiological investigations were felt to be necessary.

Case 2

X-rays (Fig. 25.3a, b) and a CT scan showed the implant breakage and the non-union of the distal femur. The previously implanted autologous cancellous bone showed no signs of integration. The knee prosthesis was not loosened. Blood investigations (CRP, FBC, ESR) and urine analyses were normal. Electrocardiogram, chest X-ray and arterial blood gas were also normal.

Preoperative Planning

Case 1

The implanted material was a standard plate. For potential problems due to broken screws, a special system should always be available. For those cases, our institution provides an intramedullary nail extraction set (Endocon, Wiesenbach, BW, Germany) and a screw removal set (Synthes, West Chester, PA, USA).

A 15-hole NCB plate (Zimmer Biomet Holdings, Warsaw, IN, USA) was templated for fracture fixation.

Autologous bone grafting was selected as the method of bone stimulation in this case.

Case 2

Due to the long duration of a low-grade infection, a two-stage revision surgery was decided. A custom-made fixed spacer was planned to be inserted after debridement to prevent the retraction of the joint capsule and shortening of the extensor mechanism. The cement spacer would be left in situ for 6 weeks.

Due to the devascularised bone stock and infection, a third plate fixation was not considered suitable and a distal femoral replacement procedure was chosen. The prosthesis selected was a rotating hinged revision system (MUTARS® GenuX®, Implantcast, Buxtehude, NI, Germany). The system allows for the reconstruction of tibial metaphyseal defects with artificial components [5]. Furthermore, long and uncemented stems can bridge the former fracture zone for intramedullary stability. The femoral condyles could be obtained, which could lead to a superiorly functional outcome when compared to a distal femoral replacement.

It was decided that if bone grafting in this case would be necessary for optimum stability of the prosthesis, a strut allograft could be used fixing it using two cable cerclage wires. The allograft can provide structural support while increasing the host bone stock without the possibility of harvesting complications [6].

Revision Surgery

Example 1
A true lateral approach was used as a standard approach suitable for most procedures. The primary implant was removed without any complications.

The fracture zone was debrided and tissues were sent to microbiology. The NCB plate was anatomically contoured and allowed for polyaxial screw placement with subsequent locking for stabilisation (Fig. 25.4 a–d). Divergent screw alignment increased the pull-out resistance and allowed for the fixation of the possible ventral and dorsal stems of the TKA. Some authors describe superior outcomes when using double-plate fixation for distal femur fractures [7]. Nevertheless, due to the less invasive approach, improved possibility for repositioning, and the high union rates, the standard procedure in our

institution remains to be single plate osteosynthesis.

The local environment was augmented using cancellous bone graft, which is often recommended in the literature [8]. For soft tissue coverage, the reconstruction of the Iliotibial tract is of utmost importance.

The patient was discharged home 5 days later. The wound healed without any problems.

Partial weight bearing with 15 kg for 6 weeks after surgery and free range of motion was allowed. Afterwards, full weight bearing was encouraged with the patient progressing uneventfully to healing 5 months later.

Example 2
During the first stage of surgery, the plate was removed using the original instruments of the NCB plate. Multiple specimens were taken and sent to microbiology laboratory during the debridement process. A custom-made fixed spacer was implanted to prevent the retraction of the joint capsule and shortening of the extensor mechanism. Therefore, 80 ml of antibiotic-loaded (Gentamicin and Vancomycin) bone cement was coated around two metal rods usually used for the dorsal stabilisation of the spine (Implantcast, Buxtehude, NI, Germany). The rods were connected, and the central defect area was filled with cement (Fig. 25.5a). The cement spacer was left in situ for 6 weeks. Further treatment consisted of regular laboratory controls and antibiotics based on an antibiogram.

For the second stage, the mediCAD v6.5 planning software was used (MediCAD, Altdorf, BY, Germany) (Fig. 25.5b). Digital templating has become a standard tool in total knee arthroplasty (TKA) in our institution and is useful in predicting implant size, necessary bone resection levels or the need for special implants [9].

Six weeks later, a left distal femur medial parapatellar arthrotomy approach was used. The cement spacer was removed. Another cycle of irrigation and debridement took place with samples sent to microbiology laboratory again. After debridement, the lateral aspect of the distal femur showed a bony defect zone. For supplementary stability, a strut allograft was inserted and fixed

Fig. 25.4 (Case 1) (**a**) AP X-ray of the right distal femur after removal of the broken plate and re-osteosynthesis via NCB plate. (**b**) Lateral X-ray of the right distal femur. (**c**) AP and (**d**) lateral X-ray of the right distal femur 6 months after revision surgery. The previous fracture zone shows bony consolidation

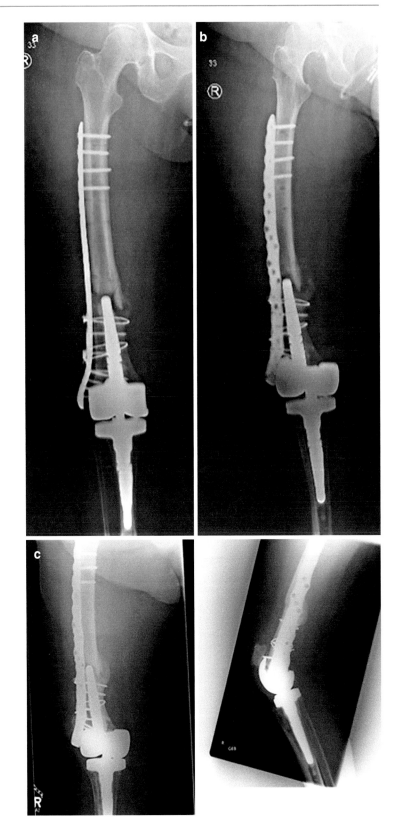

25 Distal Femur Periprosthetic Fracture Failed Fixation

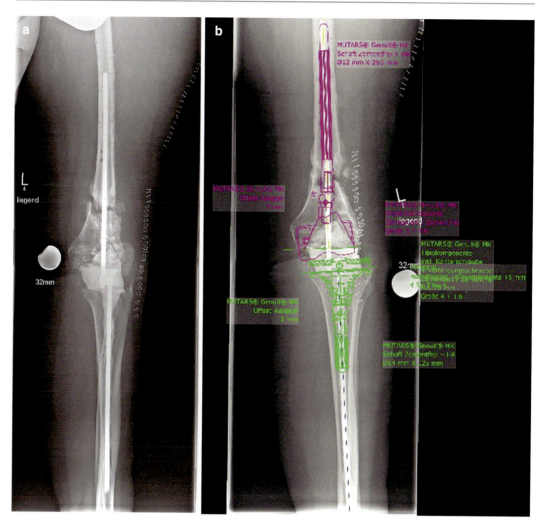

Fig. 25.5 (Case 2) (**a**) X-ray of the left knee joint after removal of the plate and the TKA and implantation of a custom-made static cement spacer. (**b**) Preoperative digital planning of the components was made using the mediCAD version 6.5 software

using two cable cerclage wires. The graft provided structural support while increasing the host bone stock without the possibility of bone graft harvesting complications [6].

Revision arthroplasty was performed using a rotating hinged revision system (MUTARS® GenuX®, Implantcast, Buxtehude, NI, Germany) (Fig. 25.6a, b).

The surgery took 183 min, and the intraoperative blood loss was 750 ml. No intra- or postoperative complications occurred. There were no restrictions concerning weight bearing or range of motion. Additional training of the range of motion was performed using a continuous passive motion machine. The patient was discharged home 12 days after surgery.

Fig. 25.6 (Case 2) (**a**) AP X-ray of the left knee joint after removal of the cement spacer and implantation of a revision knee arthroplasty. For further stability, a strut graft was utilised and fixated by two cable wires. (**b**) Lateral X-ray of the left knee joint after revision surgery

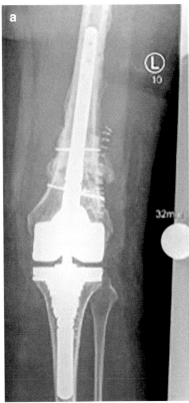 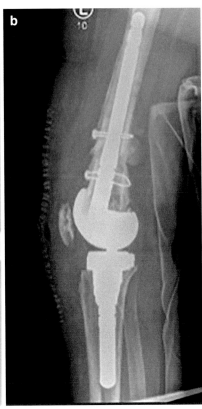

Summary of the Cases: Lessons Learned

Treatment of distal femur periprosthetic fractures remains a challenging task for orthopaedic and trauma surgeons. The described complication rates in the literature are very high (35–53%), often resulting in relevant costs and high first-year mortality rates for periprosthetic distal femur fractures of 27% of patients [10]. Questions pertaining to the optimal osteosynthesis techniques remain to be unanswered. Specialised centres and experienced surgeons with detailed knowledge of fracture fixation, revision arthroplasty and complication management are essential for a positive patient outcome. Besides the named surgical strategies, like re-ORIF or distal femoral replacement (DFR), surgeons need to take into account multiple patient-related factors, such as the state of soft tissue condition, bone stock or bone quality and the individual demands of each patient. The appropriate treatment option, especially after reinfection or massive soft tissue defects, and salvage procedures like knee arthrodesis or amputation could also be necessary [7, 11].

References

1. Ebraheim NA, Kelley LH, Liu X, Thomas IS, Steiner RB, Liu J. Periprosthetic distal femur fracture after total knee arthroplasty: a systematic review. Orthop Surg. 2015;7(4):297–305.
2. Johnston AT, Tsiridis E, Eyres KS, Toms AD. Periprosthetic fractures in the distal femur following total knee replacement: a review and guide to management. Knee. 2012;19(3):156–62.
3. Erhardt JB, Grob K, Roderer G, Hoffmann A, Forster TN, Kuster MS. Treatment of periprosthetic femur fractures with the non-contact bridging plate: a new angular stable implant. Arch Orthop Trauma Surg. 2008;128(4):409–16.
4. Ricci WM, Loftus T, Cox C, Borrelli J. Locked plates combined with minimally invasive insertion technique for the treatment of periprosthetic supracondylar femur fractures above a total knee arthroplasty. J Orthop Trauma. 2006;20(3):190–6.

5. Kohlhof H, Randau T, Kehrer M, Wirtz DC. Reconstruction of tibial metaphyseal defects with artificial components in revision arthroplasty (GenuX MK System). Oper Orthop Traumatol. 2020;32(4):284–97.

6. Hernández JT, Holck K. Periprosthetic femoral fractures: when I use strut grafts and why? Injury. 2015;46(Suppl. 5):S43–6.

7. Gathen M, Wimmer MD, Ploeger MM, Weinhold L, Schmid M, Wirtz DC, et al. Comparison of two-stage revision arthroplasty and intramedullary arthrodesis in patients with failed infected knee arthroplasty. Arch Orthop Trauma Surg. 2018;138(10):1443–52.

8. Buttaro MA, Farfalli G, Núñez MP, Comba F, Piccaluga F. Locking compression plate fixation of vancouver type-B1 periprosthetic femoral fractures. J Bone Joint Surg. 2007;89(9):1964–9.

9. Savov P, Windhagen H, Haasper C, Ettinger M. Digital templating of rotating hinge revision and primary total knee arthroplasty. Orthop Rev (Pavia). 2018;10(4):7811.

10. Streubel P. Mortality after periprosthetic femur fractures. J Knee Surg. 2013;26(01):27–30.

11. Wimmer MD, Hischebeth GTR, Randau TM, Gathen M, Schildberg FA, Fröschen FS, et al. Difficult-to-treat pathogens significantly reduce infection resolution in periprosthetic joint infections. Diagn Microbiol Infect Dis. 2020;98(2):115114.

Quadriceps Tendon Repair Failed Fixation

26

Patrick M. N. Joslin, Kristian Efremov, Robert L. Parisien, and Xinning Li

History of Previous Primary Failed Treatment

Rupture of the quadriceps tendon (QT) can be a devastating injury that, without timely management, can result in compromised knee function and the inability to effectively ambulate [1, 2]. Most ruptures are traumatic in nature, resulting from a sudden eccentric contraction on the outstretched leg [3, 4]. Partial or incomplete tears can be treated nonoperatively, while complete ruptures require operative intervention to regain the function of the extensor mechanism [5, 6].

With an incidence of only 1.37 patients per 100,000 persons/year, these injuries are relatively uncommon—males are affected four times more frequently than females (4.2:1), and the mean age of injury by sex is 50.5 and 51.7 years, respectively [3, 7]. QT injuries account for approximately 1.3% of all tendon and ligamentous injuries, with more than 94% of QT ruptures occurring in those aged 40 or older [3, 8]. When assessing any patient for a QT rupture, the clinician should maintain a high suspicion for any underlying or predisposing factors, particularly when the injury presents bilaterally or in the young patient [9–11].

This patient, who was employed in facilities as operating room cleaning staff, initially ruptured his right QT in a mechanical fall. After delays secondary to insurance issues, the patient was taken to the OR 3 months after the inciting injury. The primary, transosseous repair was conducted at an outside hospital. At the one-year follow-up appointment, the patient appeared to have no function of the extensor mechanism. He complained of weakness, difficulties getting up and down the stairs, and a persisting inability to ambulate without assistance.

On examination, he was unable to perform a straight leg raise, had a loss of active extension, and was markedly weak. There was obvious atrophy of the quadriceps. The subsequent MRI showed a complete rupture, with 5 cm of quadriceps tendon retraction, proximally. The patellar tendon was contracted distally by 1.5 cm. Using the contralateral tendon as a rough guide, this was about half the patient's anatomic length. The patient was referred to our institution for evaluation and treatment.

P. M. N. Joslin · K. Efremov
Department of Orthopaedic Surgery, Boston University School of Medicine, Boston, MA, USA

R. L. Parisien
Department of Orthopaedic Surgery & Sports Medicine, Icahn School of Medicine at Mount Sinai, New York, NY, USA

X. Li (✉)
Department of Orthopaedic Surgery, Boston University School of Medicine, Boston, MA, USA

Sports Medicine and Shoulder & Elbow Surgery, Boston University School of Medicine, Boston, MA, USA

© The Author(s), under exclusive license to Springer Nature Switzerland AG 2024
P. V. Giannoudis, P. Tornetta III (eds.), *Failed Fracture Fixation*,
https://doi.org/10.1007/978-3-031-39692-2_26

Evaluation of the Etiology of Failure of Fixation

After 3 weeks from injury, if a complete QT rupture has not been repaired, it is considered "chronic." This distinction is important, as it is a poor prognostic indicator for a successful repair, as after this timepoint tendon retraction and the deterioration of tissue quality influence the ease and strength of the repair. Chronic QT ruptures are most frequently seen in patients aged 40 or older [6]. Patients under 40 years of age most often sustain mid-tendinous ruptures, while those over 40 years of age tend to rupture at the bone-tendon insertion [4].

In the case of chronic ruptures, operative repair is necessary to restore function; despite surgery, many patients are unable to regain the function they had before injury [8, 12–15]. Further, we know that surgical repair following a failed primary repair results in worse functional and clinical outcomes as compared to acute primary repairs [12, 16]. In these settings, it can be unclear which surgical technique is optimal; ultimately, much of the success of the procedure depends on the quality of the remaining tendon and the degree of patellar and quadriceps tendon retraction.

The frequency of recurrent quadriceps tendon rupture or failed repair is hard to estimate. Few trials exist and data remains limited [17, 18]. By far the most important modifiable risk factor for rupture or failure is body mass index (BMI) [19]. Certain conditions including diabetes, SLE, RA, chronic renal disease, hyperparathyroidism, gout, and steroid and fluoroquinolone use are known to predispose to QT ruptures [15, 20–24]. Proven risk factors also include smoking, statin use, and any history of prior intraarticular injections [25]. Several studies have reported the presence of underlying degenerative changes in the ruptured quadriceps tendons of elderly patients, as well as 50% of those under the age of 55 [10, 21, 26, 27]. It is generally accepted that healthy, young tendons do not rupture.

The low-energy mechanism of injury that is common in QT ruptures in those over 40 years old suggests intrinsic weakness and degeneration of the tendon, which places the tendon at increased risk of injury. Some studies report the proportion of patients with a predisposing underlying condition prior to QT rupture to be as high as 76% [19]. Our patient had several underlying predisposing risk factors that likely initially weakened the tendon predisposing to the primary injury.

In our patient, failed fixation is likely secondary to the chronicity of the injury and the initial delay to primary repair—the patient was first taken to the OR for primary repair 3 months after the original injury. At that time, the quadriceps tendon was likely retracted, and the tissue quality was compromised. A primary repair technique was attempted which was insufficient to bring down the retracted tendon and resulted in a repair that was under tension. The patient never regained his extensor mechanism and most likely sustained an early failure of the repair. After the 1-year postoperative visit and following MRI, the patient was referred to the senior author for consultation of a revision reconstruction using an allograft implant.

Clinical Examination

A detailed history and comprehensive physical examination can often accurately diagnose a ruptured quadriceps tendon. Patients most often report an acute injury where the knee sustained a sudden, eccentric load [4]. This is classically followed by the triad of acute knee pain and tenderness at the site of the rupture, a lack of active knee extension against resistance or gravity, and a defect in the quadriceps tendon proximal to the superior pole of the patella [28, 29]. The latter is often referred to as the "suprapatellar gap sign" and is pathognomonic for a QT rupture. If a rupture is suspected, particular attention should be given to the medical history and a full assessment of any underlying intrinsic or extrinsic predisposing conditions or risk factors.

Patients may report an audible "pop" or sensation of a tear. On exam it is common to find knee swelling, effusion, ecchymosis, and difficulty or inability to bear weight. Patients with complete

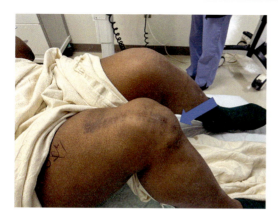

Fig. 26.1 Patient with a chronic, right quadriceps tendon tear, with a previous failed repair on the ipsilateral side. *Patella baja* is clearly observed on the affected side, immediately obvious when compared to the contralateral side

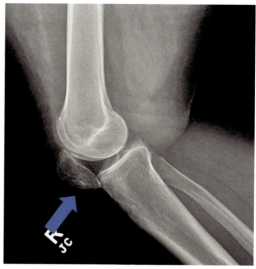

Fig. 26.2 Lateral X-ray of the knee, arrow (blue) showing patella baja

QT ruptures will have a complete loss of the extensor mechanism with the inability to actively extend the knee against gravity or resistance, in addition to an appreciable extensor lag sign. With incomplete tears, knee extension may only be somewhat impaired, while complete tears typically result in the loss of all active knee extension. In the chronic setting, the patella tendon may contract and shorten with severe patella baja on clinical presentation (Fig. 26.1).

It is important to obtain a reliable assessment of both passive and active knee range of motion. This may present a challenge as observed deficiencies may be secondary to pain or a true failure of the extensor mechanism. An aspiration and intraarticular anesthetic injection may improve the exam by relieving the pain.

Diagnostic-Biochemical and Radiological Investigations

Plain anteroposterior and lateral radiographs of the knee are the recommended initial imaging modality in the diagnostic workup of a QT rupture. The plain film is useful for ruling out any associated osseous disruptions and frequently has findings indicative of a QT rupture including patella baja (Fig. 26.2), the presence of a suprapatellar mass, and/or forward tilting of the patella [8, 30]. A radiograph of the contralateral knee is fundamental to determine the length of the native patella tendon and patella height. This is done via the Insall-Salvati, Caton-Deschamps, or Blackburne-Peel ratios. This is compared to the injured side and informs the degree of tensioning during repair.

A good history and physical exam with plain films are often enough to accurately diagnose a QT rupture [30, 31]. If the diagnosis remains unclear after these examinations are complete, ultrasound and magnetic resonance imaging are useful. While ultrasound is almost universally available, inexpensive, and able to reliably diagnose a tear, technician skill and experience are paramount for accurate diagnosis; this becomes particularly relevant when there is associated swelling and effusion or hematoma formation [13, 32, 33].

In assessing a chronic tear, MRI is the gold standard [34]. MRI allows for the evaluation of tendon length, quadriceps muscle quality, and the degree of retraction (Fig. 26.3). This assessment is critical when considering a revision QT rupture repair and/or reconstruction. Surgical planning for graft and tendon lengths will include measurements obtained from this MRI. Outcomes in patients with significant muscle atrophy and sig-

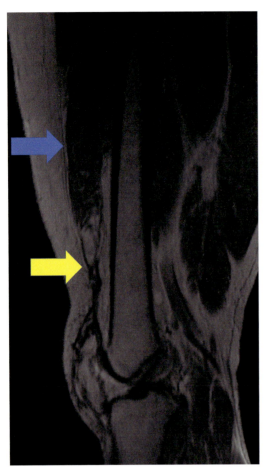

Fig. 26.3 Sagittal T1 weighted MRI view of thigh. Arrow (yellow, inferior) shows the chronic quadriceps tendon tear and degree of retraction. Arrow (blue, superior) shows the quadriceps muscle with significant atrophy

nificant retraction may not reach acceptable levels. As such, comprehensive preoperative discussions with, and evaluations of, the patient are imperative for a successful surgery.

Preoperative Planning

Revision QT repair/reconstructive surgery requires a similar setup as acute repair. Drapes, stockinette, and Coban (3M Company, St. Paul, MN) are needed to drape the knee and surrounding field. A pair of each of the following types of retractors is also required: Weitlander, Volkman, and Army-Navy. A pneumatic tourniquet is used for this procedure.

Primary repair is typically performed via trans-osseous (TO) tunnels or suture anchor (SA) fixation, requiring no special equipment to remove the previous fixation. A bovie, rongeurs, and scissors are usually sufficient to remove any interfering scar tissue and prior fixation material. Triangles of different sizes should be available to bring the knee into semi-flexion as required.

For revision fixation, titanium metal anchors are preferred (Corkscrew FT II Suture Anchor, 5.5 mm × 16.3 mm, Titanium) loaded with #2 FiberWire (Arthrex). In the following technique, an Achilles allograft with a bone block was utilized with lag screw fixation of the bone block. A saw and osteotomes are required to prepare the bone plug and the implant docking site on the tibia, as well as a drill and K-wires to provisionally fix the bone block.

In terms of implant selection, the two most common surgical techniques to repair the quadriceps tendon are the transosseous (TO) and suture anchor (SA) methods. TO is the traditional and most well-described repair technique, which involves drilling tunnels through the long axis of the patella in line with the quadriceps tendon, through which nonabsorbable sutures are passed and tied over a bone bridge to fixate the tendon. The TO technique has a reliable record of good clinical predictability and low costs [5, 13, 35].

The SA repair technique involves fixation of the quadriceps tendon via suture anchors placed in the proximal aspect of the patella and has demonstrated favorable biomechanical and clinical results [36–38]. Advances in suture anchor technology with the advent of suture tape and knotless fixation have also demonstrated promising results; this technique may increase overall construct stiffness with greater ultimate load-to-failure tolerances [39, 40]. While the TO approach to QT rupture repair has a proven track record, there is currently no clear consensus on superiority with postoperative outcomes of TO failing to show consistently desirable results [16, 20, 41, 42]. Currently, it remains unclear which technique offers the best outcomes [43]. However, in the setting of revision chronic quadriceps tendon repair, where previous tunnels have been drilled, SA fixation of the rupture is preferred over TO.

A fresh Achilles tendon allograft with bone block is used to help reconstruct the patella tendon. However, no additional bone grafting is necessary.

Revision Surgery

The patient is positioned supine on the operating table, and the range of motion is evaluated under anesthesia. A tourniquet is placed above the incision site on the operative extremity, as high on the thigh as possible. The operative extremity is prepped and draped in a standard sterile fashion, and the incision is marked overlying the previous incision. The tourniquet is then inflated, and the leg is placed on the triangle (Fig. 26.4a). A large incision is then made over the previous scar which extends from the insertion of the quadriceps tendon on the proximal patella to below the tibial tubercle. It is very important to have a large anterior midline incision in the case of chronic ruptures, as identification and mobilization of the tendon, as well as any scar removal, requires adequate exposure. The length of the patellar tendon is next measured from the bottom of the patella to the insertion on the tibial tubercle (Fig. 26.4b). This should be compared to the contralateral patella tendon length, which should be known from MRI and verified during preoperative planning.

In this case, the patellar tendon was retracted and required a Z-plasty to bring it back to the length of the contralateral side which was 4 cm (Fig. 26.5). Both ends of the tendon were then stitched using a Krakow stitch. The Achilles graft tendon is then prepared on the back table, with the bone block measuring 3 × 1.5 cm with a triangular shape (Fig. 26.6). Just distally to the tibial tubercle, a bone block is removed in

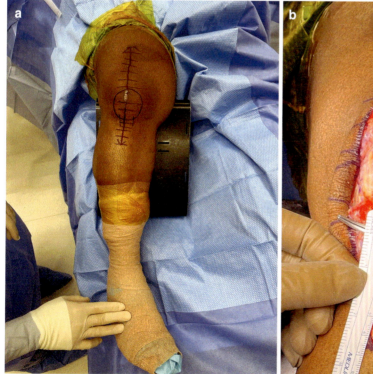
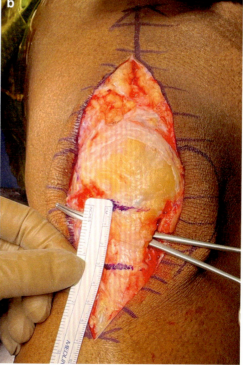

Fig. 26.4 (**a**) Patient is positioned supine, prepped, and draped in the standard sterile fashion. The knee is placed on a triangle and the patella and incision are marked. (**b**) The length of the patellar tendon is measured from its origin on the inferior pole of the patella to the tibial tubercle

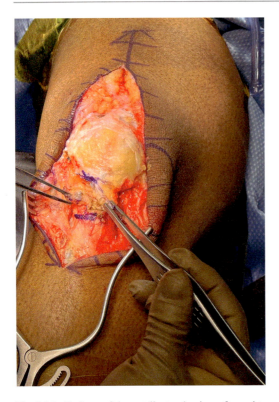

Fig. 26.5 Z-plasty of the patellar tendon is performed to lengthen the tendon to anatomic length

the same shape and size for the allograft using a sawblade and osteotomes (Fig. 26.7). The allograft is then placed and fixated using a single bicortical lag screw (Fig. 26.8). Focus is then shifted to the quadriceps tendon. Careful dissection of all tissue is required, with resection and removal of any interfering scar tissue. The quadriceps muscle is identified, cleared of adhesions, and made sure that the muscle has good excursion. Sutures are placed on the remaining quad tendon tissue for traction (Fig. 26.9a, b).

The inferior pole of the patella is then prepared and two 5.5 mm metal suture anchors are inserted on each side of the patellar tendon (Fig. 26.10a). The desired length of the patella tendon is then marked on the allograft (Fig. 26.10b) and the sutures from the anchors are used to fix the allograft to the patella tendon (Fig. 26.11a, b).

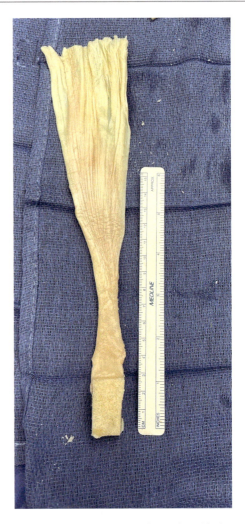

Fig. 26.6 Achilles tendon allograft with bone block, used to augment this revision. In this case, the bone block is prepared on the back table to 3 × 1.5 cm, with a triangular shape

Three metal anchors are then inserted at the 11, 12, and 1 o'clock positions on the proximal patella, at the insertion of the quadriceps tendon (Fig. 26.12a). The anchor sutures are then passed into the medial, central, and lateral sections of the quadriceps tendon using Krakow sutures and tied down in extension (Fig. 26.12b, c). Once this part of the repair is achieved, the remaining allograft is placed over the patella (Fig. 26.13) and quadriceps tendon as reinforcement and sutured using interrupted #2 Ethibond

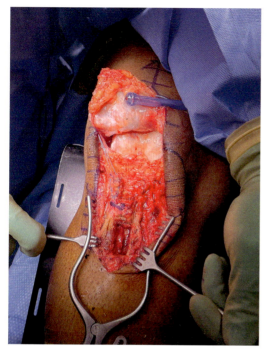

Fig. 26.7 Preparation of the graft docking site, distal to the tibial tubercle

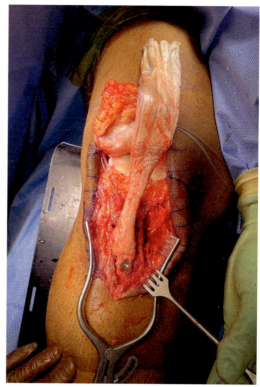

Fig. 26.8 Placement of the graft and fixation with a lag screw

sutures (Fig. 26.14). The retinaculum was then closed using #2 sutures. The range of motion is tested from 0 to 60°. The joint is irrigated, and the skin is closed with 2-0 Monocryl and a running 2-0 Nylon.

The incision is then dressed with Bacitracin, 4 × 4, ABDs, and Webril and placed in a well-padded cylindrical cast in full extension. Revision repair and augmentation can be performed as a same day surgery. The patient is made partial weight-bearing with bilateral axillary crutches.

The first follow-up is at 2 weeks for suture removal. The patient is placed in a cast for another 2 weeks. The patient is then transitioned to a hinged-knee brace at 4 weeks after surgery, at which point the patient is started on physical therapy with 0–60° of active and passive range of motion. Full recovery is between 6 and 9 months depending on the patient.

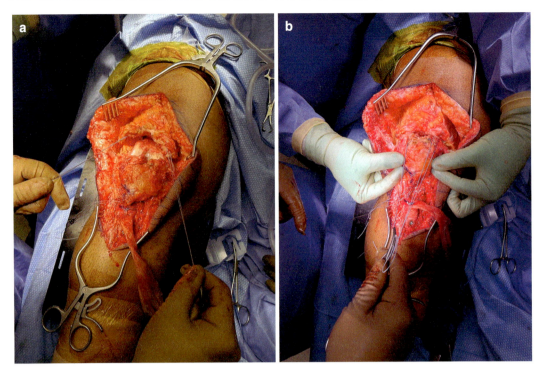

Fig. 26.9 (**a**) Sutures are placed on the quadriceps tendon after it is cleared from adhesion. (**b**) Excursion of the quadriceps is checked to make sure it can be brought to the level of the patella

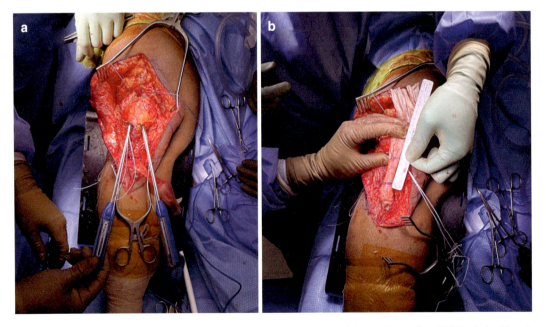

Fig. 26.10 (**a**) Two 5.5 mm metal suture anchors are inserted on each side of the patellar tendon. (**b**) The desired length of the patellar is marked at the spot where it will be fixed to the patella

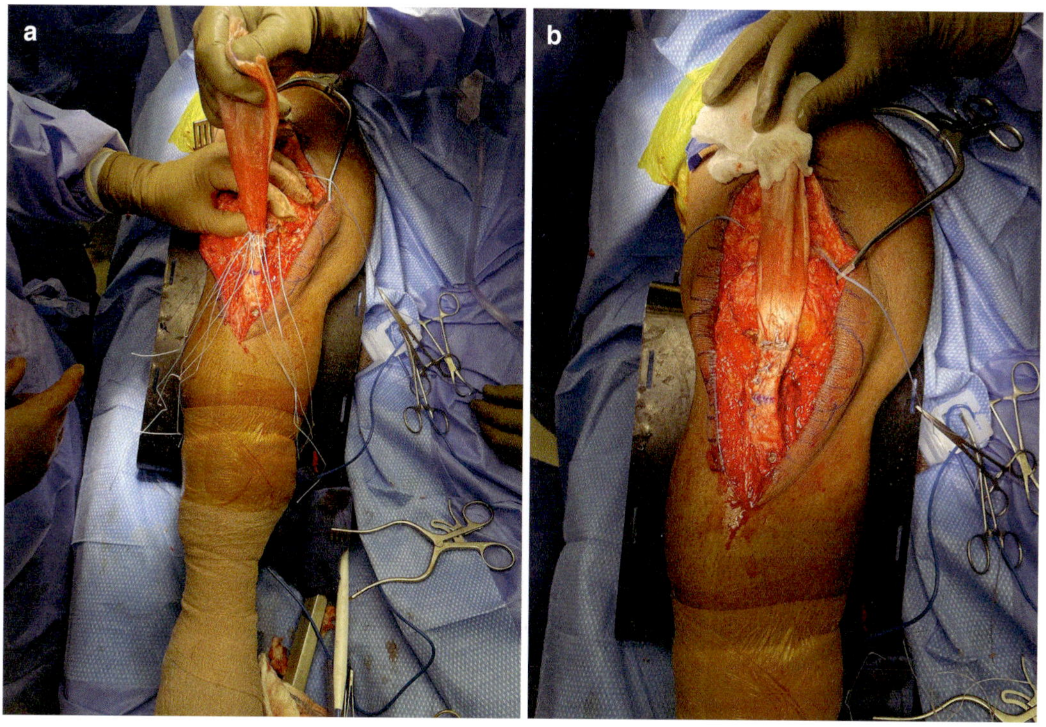

Fig. 26.11 (a) The sutures from the anchors are passed through the Achilles tendon allograft. (b) View of the tendon after completion of the suture

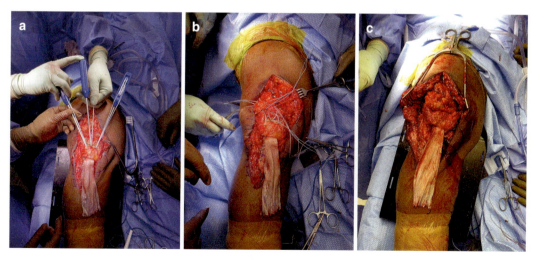

Fig. 26.12 (a) Three 5.5 mm metal anchors are inserted at the 11, 12, and 1 o'clock positions on the proximal patella, at the insertion of the quadriceps tendon. (b) The sutures from the anchors are passed through the quadriceps tendon with a Krakow technique. (c) View of the knee after the quadriceps repair is performed

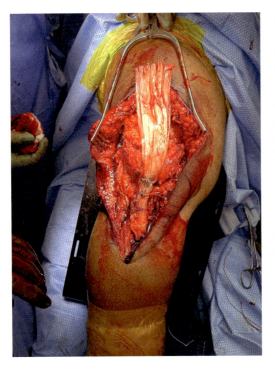

Fig. 26.13 The Achilles allograft is passed over the native patellar and quadriceps tendons

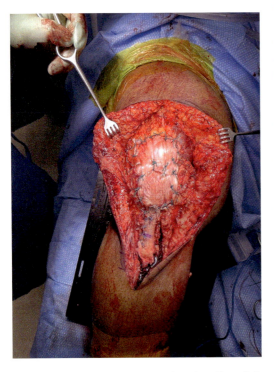

Fig. 26.14 The final construct, after the allograft is sutured with #2 Ethibond, anchoring it to the remaining quadriceps and patellar tendons

Summary: Lessons Learned

Delay in surgical treatment of QT ruptures can lead to compromised outcomes and chronic failure, turning a relatively straightforward primary surgery into a major reconstructive procedure. In repairing these failed repairs or chronic ruptures, it is critical the quadriceps tendon is fixed to the patella tension free. For this to be achieved, the length of the contralateral patellar tendon needs to be measured so that the ipsilateral side can be appropriately lengthened, if there is a side-to-side difference. In addition, excessive scar tissue forms at the site of a chronic rupture, requiring meticulous, and often time-consuming, debridement and release. When the quadriceps tendon is retracted, lengthening techniques, to include V-Y, or scar tissue release, must be performed to allow the QT to reach the patella in a tension-free state.

As the quality of this tissue is inevitably poor, an Achilles tendon allograft provides an excellent, and relatively simple, way to reinforce both the patellar tendon lengthening and the quadriceps tendon repair constructs. Suture anchor fixation of the patella and QT provide reliable repair strength and good clinical outcomes for these complex, chronic ruptures. After the repair is completed in the OR, knee flexion should be tested to 60 degrees, ensuring that an adequate and tension-free repair has been achieved. If this is not done correctly, the chances of repeated failure are high.

In contrast to primary repairs, when it may be advisable to start early range of motion, as with most revision surgeries, more clinical caution and patience are required. The patient should be encased in a circular cast in the OR in extension, checked at 2 weeks for a wound check and suture removal, and then re-casted for 2 weeks. At 4 weeks postoperatively, the final cast is removed and replaced with a hinged brace; at this time formal PT is also initiated. In the first 4 weeks, ROM should be limited to zero to 60°, with a 10° increase every week thereafter. Strengthening starts at 3 months after surgery, with formal PT two to three times, in person, per week. The patient should be counseled that a full recovery will take, at minimum, 6–9 months. Furthermore, after this type of complex reconstruction and a prior failed repair, it is important to talk frankly with patients regarding realistic expectations for final outcomes. In the senior author's experience, most patients will have a 20–30° decrease in overall flexion, and usually a residual 5° of extensor lag. There may also be varying degrees of residual weakness, depending on the degree of atrophy and viable muscle left at the time of repair.

References

1. Boudissa M, Roudet A, Rubens-Duval B, Chaussard C, Saragaglia D. Acute quadriceps tendon ruptures: a series of 50 knees with an average follow-up of more than 6 years. Orthop Traumatol Surg Res. 2014;100(2):213–6.
2. Boublik M, Schlegel TF, Koonce RC, Genuario JW, Kinkartz JD. Quadriceps tendon injuries in national football league players. Am J Sports Med. 2013;41(8):1841–6.
3. Clayton RA, Court-Brown CM. The epidemiology of musculoskeletal tendinous and ligamentous injuries. Injury. 2008;39(12):1338–44.
4. Rasul AT Jr, Fischer DA. Primary repair of quadriceps tendon ruptures. Results of treatment. Clin Orthop Relat Res. 1993;289:205–7.
5. Ramseier LE, Werner CM, Heinzelmann M. Quadriceps and patellar tendon rupture. Injury. 2006;37(6):516–9.
6. Elattar O, McBeth Z, Curry EJ, Parisien RL, Galvin JW, Li X. Management of chronic quadriceps tendon rupture: a critical analysis review. JBJS Rev. 2021;9(5):e20. https://doi.org/10.2106/JBJS. RVW.20.00096.
7. Garner MR, Gausden E, Berkes MB, Nguyen JT, Lorich DG. Extensor mechanism injuries of the knee: demographic characteristics and comorbidities from a review of 726 patient records. J Bone Joint Surg Am. 2015;97(19):1592–6.
8. Siwek CW, Rao JP. Ruptures of the extensor mechanism of the knee joint. J Bone Joint Surg Am. 1981;63(6):932–7.
9. Hak DJ, Sanchez A, Trobisch P. Quadriceps tendon injuries. Orthopedics. 2010;33(1):40–6.
10. Trobisch PD, Baumann M, Weise K, Fischer R. Rupture of the quadriceps tendon after lateral retinaculum release by arthroscopy. Unfallchirurg. 2010;113(6):501–3.
11. Meester S, Lee S. Spontaneous bilateral quadriceps tendon rupture. Am J Emerg Med. 2018;36(6):1123. e5–7.
12. Scuderi C. Ruptures of the quadriceps tendon; study of twenty tendon ruptures. Am J Surg. 1958;95(4):626–34.
13. Ilan DI, Tejwani N, Keschner M, Leibman M. Quadriceps tendon rupture. J Am Acad Orthop Surg. 2003;11(3):192–200.
14. Yilmaz C, Binnet MS, Narman S. Tendon lengthening repair and early mobilization in treatment of neglected bilateral simultaneous traumatic rupture of the quadriceps tendon. Knee Surg Sports Traumatol Arthrosc. 2001;9(3):163–6.
15. Ciriello V, Gudipati S, Tosounidis T, Soucacos P, Giannoudis PV. Clinical outcomes after repair of quadriceps tendon rupture: a systematic review. Injury. 2012;43(11):1931–8.
16. Rougraff BT, Reeck CC, Essenmacher J. Complete quadriceps tendon ruptures. Orthopedics. 1996;19(6):509–14.
17. Oliva F, Marsilio E, Migliorini F, Maffulli N. Complex ruptures of the quadriceps tendon: a systematic review of surgical procedures and outcomes. J Orthop Surg Res. 2021;16(1):547.
18. Leciejewski M, Królikowska A, Reichert P. Polyethylene terephthalate tape augmentation as a solution in recurrent quadriceps tendon ruptures. Polim Med. 2018;48(1):53–6.
19. Shah MK. Simultaneous bilateral rupture of quadriceps tendons: analysis of risk factors and associations. Southern Med J. 2002;95(8):860–7.
20. Konrath GA, Chen D, Lock T, et al. Outcomes following repair of quadriceps tendon ruptures. J Orthop Trauma. 1998;12(4):273–9.
21. Vidil A, Ouaknine M, Anract P, Tomeno B. Trauma-induced tears of the quadriceps tendon: 47 cases. Revue de chirurgie orthopedique et reparatrice de l'appareil moteur. 2004;90(1):40–8.
22. Stern RE, Harwin SF. Spontaneous and simultaneous rupture of both quadriceps tendons. Clin Orthop Relat Res. 1980;147:188–9.
23. Levy M, Goldstein J, Rosner M. A method of repair for quadriceps tendon or patellar ligament (tendon) ruptures without cast immobilization. Preliminary report. Clin Orthop Relat Res. 1987;218:297–301.
24. Razzano CD, Wilde AH, Phalen GS. Bilateral rupture of the infrapatellar tendon in rheumatoid arthritis. Clin Orthop Relat Res. 1973;91:158–61.
25. Deren ME, Klinge SA, Mukand NH, Mukand JA. Tendinopathy and tendon rupture associated with statins. JBJS Rev. 2016;4(5):e4.
26. Kannus P, Jozsa L. Histopathological changes preceding spontaneous rupture of a tendon. A controlled study of 891 patients. J Bone Joint Surg Am Vol. 1991;73(10):1507–25.
27. Yepes H, Tang M, Morris SF, Stanish WD. Relationship between hypovascular zones and patterns of ruptures of the quadriceps tendon. JBJS. 2008;90(10):2135–41.
28. Pope JD, El Bitar Y, Plexousakis MP. Quadriceps tendon rupture. In: StatPearls. Treasure Island, FL: StatPearls Publishing; 2022.
29. Nori S. Quadriceps tendon rupture. J Family Med Prim Care. 2018;7(1):257–60.

30. Kaneko K, DeMouy EH, Brunet ME, Benzian J. Radiographic diagnosis of quadriceps tendon rupture: analysis of diagnostic failure. J Emerg Med. 1994;12(2):225–9.

31. Spector ED, DiMarcangelo MT, Jacoby JH. The radiologic diagnosis of quadriceps tendon rupture. N J Med. 1995;92(9):590–2.

32. O'shea K, Kenny P, Donovan J, Condon F, McElwain J. Outcomes following quadriceps tendon ruptures. Injury. 2002;33(3):257–60.

33. Rizio L, Jarmon N. Chronic quadriceps rupture: treatment with lengthening and early mobilization without cerclage augmentation and a report of three cases. J Knee Surg. 2008;21(1):34–8.

34. Volk WR, Yagnik GP, Uribe JW. Complications in brief: Quadriceps and patellar tendon tears. Clin Orthop Relat Res. 2014;472(3):1050–7.

35. Belk JW, Lindsay A, Houck DA, et al. Biomechanical testing of suture anchor versus transosseous tunnel technique for quadriceps tendon repair yields similar outcomes: a systematic review. Arthrosc Sports Med Rehabil. 2021;3(6):e2059–66.

36. Lighthart WA, Cohen DA, Levine RG, Boucher HR. Suture anchor versus suture through tunnel fixation for quadriceps tendon rupture: a biomechanical study. Orthopedics. 2008;31(5):441.

37. Hart ND, Wallace MK, Scovell JF, Krupp RJ, Cook C, Wyland DJ. Quadriceps tendon rupture: a biomechanical comparison of transosseous equivalent double-row suture anchor versus transosseous tunnel repair. J Knee Surg. 2012;25(04):335–40.

38. Bushnell BD, Whitener GB, Rubright JH, Creighton RA, Logel KJ, Wood ML. The use of suture anchors to repair the ruptured quadriceps tendon. J Orthop Trauma. 2007;21(6):407–13.

39. Kindya MC, Konicek J, Rizzi A, Komatsu DE, Paci JM. Knotless suture anchor with suture tape quadriceps tendon repair is biomechanically superior to transosseous and traditional suture anchor–based repairs in a cadaveric model. Arthroscopy. 2017;33(1):190–8.

40. Richards DP, Barber FA. Repair of quadriceps tendon ruptures using suture anchors. Arthroscopy. 2002;18(5):556–9.

41. West JL, Keene JS, Kaplan LD. Early motion after quadriceps and patellar tendon repairs: outcomes with single-suture augmentation. Am J Sports Med. 2008;36(2):316–23.

42. De Baere T, Geulette B, Manche E, Barras L. Functional results after surgical repair of quadriceps tendon rupture. Acta Orthop Belg. 2002;68(2):146–9.

43. Corÿdon Hochheim M, Bartels E, Vestergård IJ. Quadriceps tendon rupture. Anchor or transosseous suture? A systematic review. Muscles Ligaments Tendons J (MLTJ). 2019;9(3):356.

Patella Tendon Repair Reconstruction for Failed Fixation

27

Patrick M. N. Joslin, Kristian Efremov, Robert L. Parisien, and Xinning Li

History of Previous Primary Failed Treatment

While patellar tendon (PT) ruptures only occur half as commonly as quadriceps tendon ruptures, they have the same potentially devastating effect [1]. Without repair, a ruptured PT will prevent normal functioning of the extensor mechanism and compromise the ability to ambulate normally. In contrast to ruptures of the quadriceps tendon, which occur most often in those over age 40, PT ruptures occur far more commonly in those under 40 and frequently result from direct trauma during activity [2, 3]. Generally, the injury is sustained when there is a sudden contraction of the quadriceps muscle against a partially flexed knee or there is an applied downward force on the knee when it is flexed greater than 60°, the point at which the greatest forces are acting on the tendon [4].

P. M. N. Joslin · K. Efremov
Department of Orthopaedic Surgery, Boston University School of Medicine, Boston, MA, USA

R. L. Parisien
Department of Orthopaedic Surgery & Sports Medicine, Icahn School of Medicine at Mount Sinai, New York, NY, USA

X. Li (✉)
Department of Orthopaedic Surgery, Boston University School of Medicine, Boston, MA, USA

Sports Medicine and Shoulder & Elbow Surgery, Boston University School of Medicine, Boston, MA, USA

Rupture of the PT is the third most common cause of extensor mechanism disruption after patellar fractures and quadriceps ruptures [5]. Biomechanical studies suggest that it takes about 17.5 times a person's body mass to rupture a healthy PT. [6] Acute rupture most often affects men and is usually treated with primary surgical repair [3]. A chronic or neglected PT rupture that presents beyond 6 weeks can result from missed diagnoses, neglect, or failed "native" treatment and complicates future revision surgery if repair is desired [7, 8]. When a primary repair fails or is reinjured, a chronic injury results.

Prior studies have shown that for acute ruptures, early repair can reliably produce acceptable outcomes for patients [9]. Chronic repairs are less predictable as a result of several factors. Most acute ruptures can be repaired primarily, while chronic repairs often require tendon reconstruction. The repetitive nature of these chronic injuries often results in substantial tendon degeneration, loss of fibers, thinning and weakening, in addition to retraction. For a neglected or chronic rupture, the quality of the tendons and the degree of retraction, in addition to atrophy of the quadriceps, make functional outcomes uncertain. Additionally, any scar tissue, wires, implants, or sutures remaining from prior failed fixation add complexity. If there is tendon retraction, tendon reconstruction may require grafting and lengthening procedures.

© The Author(s), under exclusive license to Springer Nature Switzerland AG 2024
P. V. Giannoudis, P. Tornetta III (eds.), *Failed Fracture Fixation*,
https://doi.org/10.1007/978-3-031-39692-2_27

For complete tears, non-surgical management is not effective, and surgical repair of the PT should be attempted as soon as possible after injury and ideally within 3 weeks [3]. Techniques for repair include reinsertion of the ruptured tendon stump and end-to-end suture fixation, often reinforced with cerclage [10–12]. For an acute primary repair, several approaches can used with end-to-end repair and transosseous (TO) techniques using sutures for fixation being common [3, 13–16].

Additional techniques for the reconstruction involve both allo- and autografts [11, 17, 18]. Synthetic materials have also been used for repair, including carbon fiber, Dacron, and Ligament Augmentation Reconstruction System (LARS) [19, 20]. Graft techniques are most often used in repairing a chronic injury, as augmentation is needed to reconstruct tendon length that is lost secondary to degeneration and retraction. Techniques using allograft Achilles tendon augmentation have shown consistent success in the repair of chronic PT ruptures and are the authors' preferred graft type for chronic repairs [18, 21–23].

Our patient was a 32-year-old male who initially sustained a right patellar tendon rupture while playing basketball. This was repaired in a primary fashion. Two years later, the patient suffered a second injury (accidental fall) that resulted in a re-ruptured PT. He presented 8 years later. The patient complained of a persistent inability to run, difficulty in climbing stairs, and a disabling limp.

Evaluation of the Etiology of Failure of Fixation

In the herein case, the etiology of rupture was a secondary injury. The incidence of PT ruptures is highest for men in their third and fourth decades of life and affects women about half as often [24]. It is hypothesized that, at least in part, a male's larger size and strength confers the greater forces on the tendon needed to cause failure; for females, the ability of their sex hormones to cause ligament laxity during the menstrual cycle is hypothesized to be protective [5].

In most injuries, the patellar tendon is avulsed from its insertion on the distal pole of the patella—tears in the body of the tendon can suggest the presence of underlying predisposing conditions [25, 26]. It is generally accepted that PT ruptures occur in tendons that are weakened secondary to degeneration and that healthy tendons are not prone to failure [14]. In the young athlete, this may be through repetitive microtrauma, which over time weakens the tendon [27].

Obesity is a central, and highly modifiable, risk factor [5, 28]. Several preexisting chronic conditions are also known to predispose to PT rupture, often seen in older patients who sustained the injury during nonstrenuous activity. These include rheumatoid arthritis, lupus, steroid and fluoroquinolone use, kidney disease, and diabetes mellitus [1, 7, 25, 29]. In the elderly population, the main causal factor contributing to the injury is intrinsic weakness from chronic degeneration; to date, several studies have shown that structural changes that accumulate in the tendon over time lead to weakness and ultimate failure [14, 30, 31]. It is important to evaluate the patient's medical history prior to planned complex reconstruction. Finally, PT ruptures can be a rare iatrogenic injury, as a complication of total knee arthroplasty or any operation that encounters the tendon throughout its course [13, 24].

Clinical Examination

A detailed history and comprehensive physical examination can be enough to diagnose a patellar tendon rupture. Patients will most often report an acute injury to the knee, associated with immediate infrapatellar pain and swelling. They may not be able to weight bear or ambulate. Some patients will report hearing a "pop" or that the knee gave way [7]. This will usually result from an event where the quadriceps contracted strongly against a partially flexed knee, such as seen in jumping sports or missing a step descending the stairs [9].

On inspection, the knee may show abrasions or lacerations if there is a direct trauma. There is often associated ecchymosis, swelling, and a high-riding patella. It is helpful to measure the patellar height and compare it to the contralateral side. Significant hematomas are also not uncommon findings.

It is important to palpate the joint lines, patella, and popliteal fossa to assess for any direct trauma. A PT rupture will also present with a palpable defect below the level of the inferior pole of the patella associated with infrapatellar pain. It is important to assess the degree of swelling and/or effusion if it is present. These complicating factors can make the clinical examination of the extensor mechanism difficult to interpret.

Range of motion will be decreased, and in the case of a complete rupture, active knee extension will be lost [30]. If the quadriceps tendon and retinacula are intact, some active extension may be preserved but will show an extensor lag [32]. Patients with a PT rupture will be unable to hold a passively extended knee or actively straighten the leg in a resting flexion position.

When there is concern for a PT injury, the ability to perform these physical exam maneuvers holds significant clinical value. Thus, it is important that the assessment of the limitations in function and ROM is accurate. As such, aspiration of any suprapatellar hematoma or effusion, and the injection of an intraarticular anesthetic prior to physical examination, may improve clinical interpretation.

In this case, the patient had a high riding patella and quadriceps atrophy. The patella could be manually reduced only 2 cm inferiorly indicating substantial retraction.

Diagnostic-Biochemical and Radiological Investigations

Plain anteroposterior and lateral X-rays of the knee will help in the diagnosis of a PT rupture and should be initial imaging. Plain films are useful for ruling out any associated bony disruptions and frequently show *patella alta* and an Insall-Salvati ratio greater than 1.2 [33]. This ratio is measured as length from the tibial tubercle to the inferior patellar pole, over the length of the patella [34]. Avulsion fractures are also commonly seen. A radiograph of the contralateral knee is also fundamental to measure the normal length of the patellar tendon, from the distal pole of the patella to the insertion on the tibial tuberosity. Knowing the normal patella tendon length will also help to plan for the revision reconstruction surgery.

A thorough history and physical exam with plain radiographs can often suffice in diagnosing a PT rupture. If there is still uncertainty, ultrasound and magnetic resonance imaging are useful. In assessing a chronic tear, an MRI will likely be critical. Before surgery, the length of tendons and the presence and degree of retraction need to be assessed. Atrophy and fatty infiltration are also important considerations and will aid in surgical planning. In this case, the diagnosis was clear from the history and examination. Additionally, an MRI scan was obtained which showed a complete rupture of the patellar tendon with 6 cm of retraction inferiorly (Fig. 27.1). MRI was obtained to evaluate for tendon length and retraction prior to planned reconstruction.

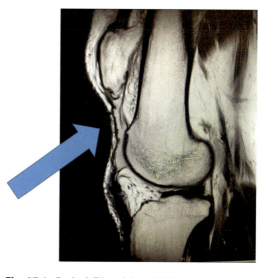

Fig. 27.1 Sagittal T1 weighted MRI of the knee. Blue arrow indicates tear of the patellar tendon at the proximal insertion site. *Patella alta* is clearly observed

Preoperative Planning

Revision patellar tendon reconstruction surgery poses two issues: how to bring the patella down to its anatomic position and what to use to reconstruct or augment the patellar tendon. To reduce the patella, several methods have been proposed including traction and external fixation [3, 35]. Both of these, however, require long treatment times before the surgical procedure. Lengthening of the quadriceps tendon allows for a one-stage procedure [36]. For tendon reconstruction, Achilles allografts are commonly used. If these are not available, an ipsilateral hamstring autograft can be used [36, 37].

Many primary repairs are performed with transosseous sutures or anchors. In those cases, no special equipment is needed for the removal of previous sutures. If a cerclage wire was used in the original repair, a wire cutter will be required. Bovie, blades, rongeurs, and scissors are necessary for removal of any prior fixation, interfering scar tissue, and performing tendon lengthening. The following are the materials needed in the operating theatre for a patellar tendon reconstruction using an Achilles allograft with lengthening of the quadriceps tendon. For a sterile surgical field, drapes, Stockinette, and coban are required. A pneumatic tourniquet of appropriate size and knee triangles, to place the knee in semi-flexion, will be used. Autostatic or manual retractors can be used, depending on surgeon preference; we recommend having at least one pair of Weitlander, Volkman, and Army-Navy retractors on hand. The Achilles allograft with a bone block of adequate size is required for the following technique. A lag screw for fixation of the bone block to the tibia is also required. Titanium metal anchors loaded with sutures (Corkscrew FT II Suture Anchor, 5.5 mm × 16.3 mm, Titanium, with three #2 FiberWire (Arhtrex) and their Punch/Tap) are needed for securing the graft tendon to the patella. Saw and osteotomes are required to both size the bone plug and complete the tibial osteotomy. Ethibond #2 sutures are needed for the closure of the quadriceps lengthening. An acellular allograft dermal matrix can also be used after lengthening to reinforce the insertion site of the tendon. The materials for a plaster fiberglass circular cast will also be needed at the end of the procedure.

In terms of implant selection, similar to the repair of the quadriceps tendon discussed in the previous chapter, the two most common surgical techniques to repair the patellar tendon are the transosseous (TO) and suture anchor (SA) methods. TO is the original and most used technique, which involves tunnel drilling through the patella in line with the patellar tendon. Through these tunnels, nonabsorbable sutures are shuttled and tied over a bone-bridge to fixate the tendon. This technique has low costs and requires little additional material.

The SA repair method of fixation of the patellar tendon via suture anchors placed in the distal pole of the patella has demonstrated favorable biomechanical and clinical results. Advances in suture anchor technology with the advent of suture tape and knotless fixation have also demonstrated promising results; this technique may increase overall construct stiffness with greater ultimate load-to-failure tolerances [20–22]. While the TO approach to QT rupture repair has a proven track record, there is currently no clear consensus on superiority with postoperative outcomes of TO failing to show consistently desirable results [15, 23–25]. A recent review showed less gap formation with this technique compared to TO [33].

There is no need for bone grafting in this soft tissue injury. An Achilles tendon allograft is used for the repair.

Revision Surgery

The patient is positioned supine on the operating table and a tourniquet is placed at the base of the thigh (Fig. 27.2a). The length of the contralateral patellar tendon should be measured before draping (Fig. 27.2b). The operative limb is then prepped and draped in a sterile fashion with the knee placed on a triangle to bring it into semi-flexion. The incision site is then marked; this should be centered over the previous incision,

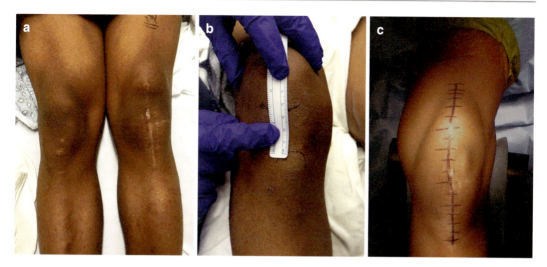

Fig. 27.2 (a) Patient with a chronic, right patellar tendon tear, with a previous failed repair on the ipsilateral side. *Patella alta* is seen on the affected side. (b) Measurement of the distance between the inferior pole of the patella and the tibial tubercle. (c) After the knee is prepped and draped, the skin incision is marked over the previous surgical scar

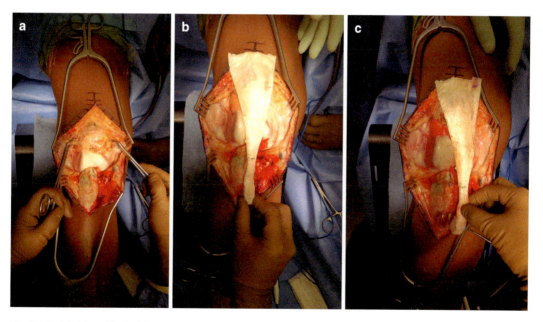

Fig. 27.3 (a) After skin incision and a full exposure is carried out, a complete tear of the patellar tendon is seen. (b) An Achilles tendon allograft is superimposed over the patella that will be used to reinforce the repair. (c) A trough is created at the level of the tibial tubercle. It should measure about 15–25 mm in length and about 10 mm in depth. This is the docking site for the autograft bone block placement

beginning at the most proximal portion of the retracted patellar tendon, to just distal to the tibial tubercle (Fig. 27.2c).

The remnant of the patellar tendon is then identified, and the maximal distal excursion of the patella is tested (Fig. 27.3a). Next the Achilles

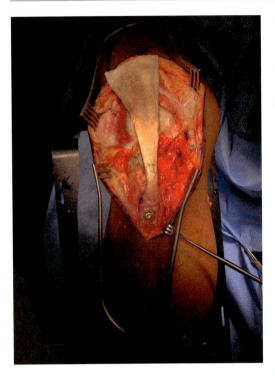

Fig. 27.4 Placement of the graft and fixation with a lag screw

tendon allograft is thawed to allow for preparation on the back table. Beginning at the osteotendinous junction of the Achilles graft, the length of the graft is measured and marked to match the contralateral PT length (Fig. 27.3b). A trough is made at the proximal tibia at the level of the tibial tubercle, 2 cm in sagittal length, with a depth of 10 mm (Fig. 27.3c). On the back table the bone plug is prepped and shaped to fit into the trough. When the plug is inserted and seated snugly into the tibial docking site, it is then impacted with a tamp and synthesized with a 4.5 cortical screw (Fig. 27.4).

Focus is next turned to the quadriceps tendon, which, along with the medial and lateral retinacula, is released and cleared of adhesions. The quadriceps tendon is then marked, and a V-Y tendon lengthening is performed with the V centered over the patella (Fig. 27.5a). Based on preoperative planning, the required quadriceps tendon lengthening is achieved by closing the apex part of the V in a side-to-side fashion (Fig. 27.5b). The proximal portion of the remaining patellar tendon is then brought together with the rectus femoris and fixed using a Krackower suture (Fig. 27.6a). To reinforce the lengthening, an acellular allograft dermal matrix is then placed on top and sutured in place using figure-eight stitches (Fig. 27.6b).

The distal pole of the patella is then cleared, and three suture-loaded metal anchors are inserted at the 5, 6, and 7 o'clock positions (Fig. 27.7a). The sutures from the anchors are then passed through the Achilles tendon graft at a level that allows for good tension between full extension and 90 degrees of flexion (Fig. 27.7b). The proximal fan of the graft is then passed over the patella and sutured over the top of the quadriceps tendon (Fig. 27.7c). The medial and lateral retinacula are next closed onto the dermal matrix and tendon graft construct (Fig. 27.8a).

After the irrigation, the skin is closed in a layered fashion. It is this author's preference to close the skin with Nylon 2.0 for all revision surgeries (Fig. 27.8b). After sterile dressing, the leg is then placed in a circular long leg cast in 20 degrees of flexion for 6 weeks.

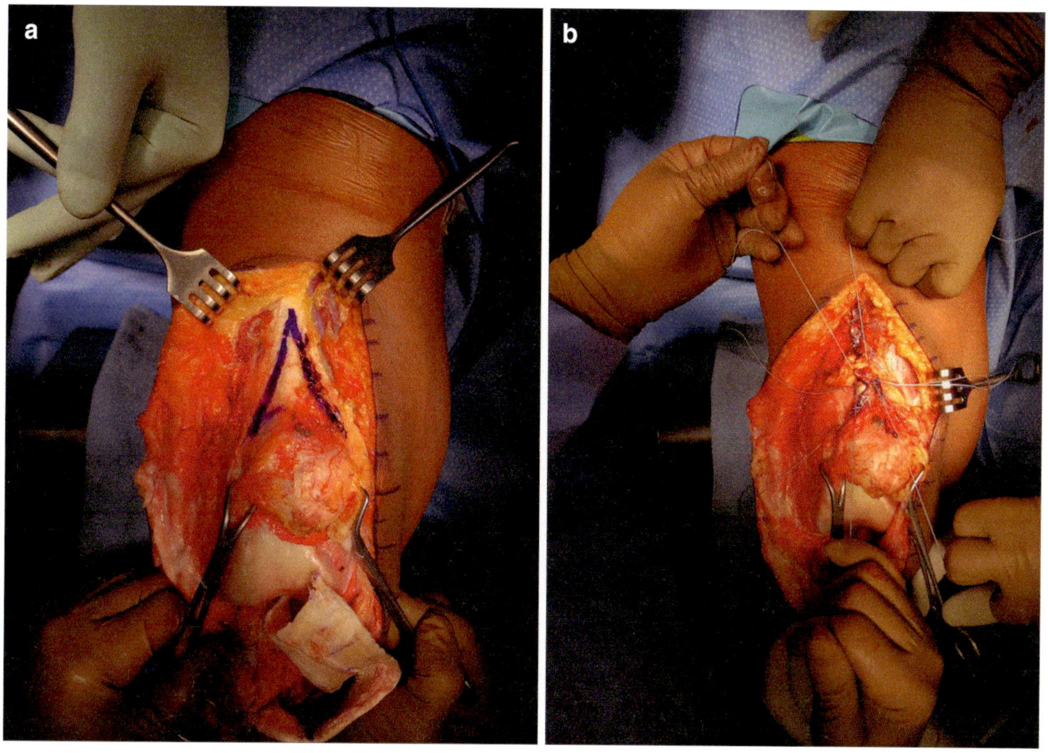

27 Patella Tendon Repair Reconstruction for Failed Fixation

Fig. 27.5 (**a**) Marking at the level of the quadriceps tendon for the V-Y lengthening. (**b**) After the desired lengthening was obtained, the apex part of the V is closed in a side-to-side manner

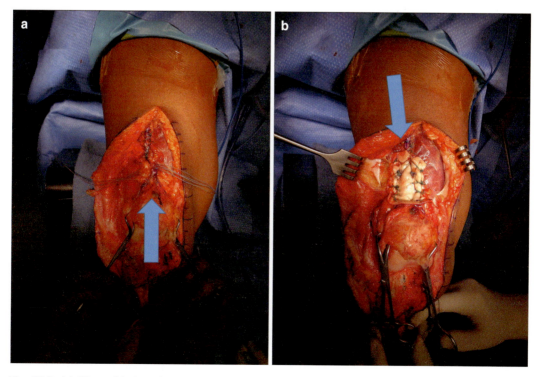

Fig. 27.6 (**a**) The residual tendon over the proximal patella and the rectus femoris is then krackowed and brought together. (**b**) A synthetic graft jacket is then placed on top of the quadriceps tendon over the lengthening to reinforce the tissue using figure-of-eight stitches

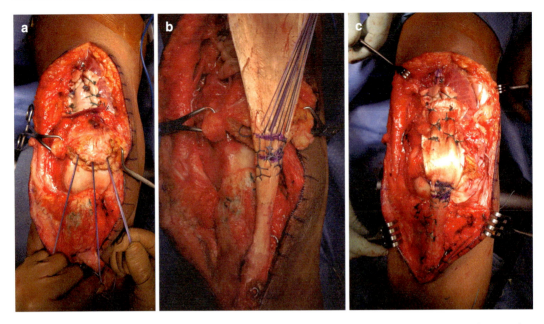

Fig. 27.7 (**a**) Three 5.5 mm metal anchors are placed on the inferior margin of the patella anteriorly at the 5, 6, and 7 o'clock position. (**b**) The Achilles tendon graft is marked at the level that gives the patient the best extension and 90 degrees of flexion. The sutures from the anchors are then passed through the tendon at that level. (**c**) The proximal fan-like part of the graft is then sutured over the quadriceps

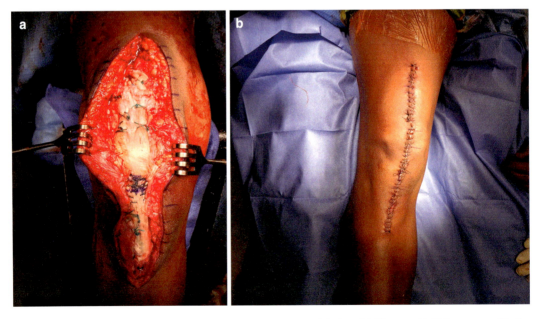

Fig. 27.8 (**a**) The medial and lateral retinacula are closed onto the graft jacket. (**b**) Closure with Nylon sutures. The leg is then placed in cylindrical long leg cast in 20 degree of flexion

Lessons Learned

This case highlights several particularly high-yield elements of surgical reconstruction that an orthopedic surgeon will be comfortable with when encountering revisions for failed primary repair or chronic patellar tendon injuries. As with most revision surgeries and chronic injuries, the repair will be complicated by a large amount of scar formation, especially around the original insertion of the patellar tendon. This needs to be carefully removed and debrided. The quadriceps tendon will also have undergone significant retraction, which needs to be lengthened to achieve an adequate and tension-free repair. Without this, there is a high-risk recurrent rupture, patella alta, loss of flexion, and ultimately a compromised gait or extensor lag. Finally, there may not be adequate tissue to facilitate the repair. In these cases, one should have available a graft to reinforce/reconstruct the patellar tendon. An Achilles tendon allograft with a bone block is an excellent choice, as it provides a relatively simple yet reliable method of fixation on the tibia, while also reinforcing the overall construct. Before closure, it is imperative the surgeon test the range of motion to ensure a tension-free repair between 0° and 60°.

As with revision quadriceps tendon repairs, after a complex knee reconstruction, the patient should be placed in a cast for the initial post-operative period as this offers better protection than a hinged brace. The cast should be removed at 2 weeks for a wound check and replaced with a new one for another 4 weeks, at which time it can be substituted with a brace and formal PT can be initiated. Full recovery should be expected around 9 months after surgery; this can vary based on the degree of muscle atrophy present before reconstruction. Furthermore, it is essential to discuss post-operative expectations with the patient. Failed primary patella tendon repair that requires extensive complex reconstruction will take a long time to recover. Additionally, the patient may still have a 5–10° extensor lag given the complexity of the recon-

struction. Also, if there is preexisting arthritis underneath the patella, doing this reconstruction, the patient may experience residual pain due to the arthritis.

References

1. Matava MJ. Patellar Tendon ruptures. J Am Acad Orthop Surg. 1996;4(6):287–96.
2. Ramsey RH, Muller GE. Quadriceps tendon rupture: a diagnostic trap. Clin Orthop Relat Res. 1970;70:161–4.
3. Siwek CW, Rao J. Ruptures of the extensor mechanism of the knee joint. J Bone Joint Surg Am. 1981;63(6):932–7.
4. Miller RH. Knee injuries. Campbell's Oper Orthop. 2003;3:2182–99.
5. Pires EAR, Prado J, Hara R, et al. Epidemiological study on tendon ruptures of the knee extensor mechanism at a level 1 hospital. Rev Bras Ortop. 2012;47(6):719–23.
6. Zernicke RF, Garhammer J, Jobe FW. Human patellar-tendon rupture. J Bone Joint Surg Am. 1977;59(2):179–83.
7. Steele R, Hayden SR, Ward N, Macias M. Patellar Tendon Rupture Bedside Diagnosis. J Emerg Med. 2021;60(3):384–6.
8. Sundararajan SR, Srikanth KP, Rajasekaran S. Neglected patellar tendon ruptures: a simple modified reconstruction using hamstrings tendon graft. Int Orthop. 2013;37(11):2159–64.
9. Schenck RC Jr, Heckman JD. Injuries of the knee. In: Paper presented at: Clinical symposia (Summit, NJ: 1957); 1993.
10. Greis PE, Lahav A, Holmstrom MC. Surgical treatment options for patella tendon rupture, part II: chronic. Orthopedics. 2005;28(8):765–9. quiz 770–761
11. Van der Zwaal P, Van Arkel ER. Recurrent patellar tendon rupture: reconstruction using ipsilateral gracilis and semitendinosus tendon autografts. Injury. 2007;38(09):320–3.
12. Ong BC, Sherman O. Acute patellar tendon rupture: a new surgical technique. Arthroscopy. 2000;16(8):869–70.
13. Garner MR, Gausden E, Berkes MB, Nguyen JT, Lorich DG. Extensor mechanism injuries of the knee: demographic characteristics and comorbidities from a review of 726 patient records. JBJS. 2015;97(19):1592–6.
14. Kelly DW, Carter VS, Jobe FW, Kerlan RK. Patellar and quadriceps tendon ru p tures—jumper's knee. Am J Sports Med. 1984;12(5):375–80.
15. Matava MJ. Patellar tendon ruptures. JAAOS-J Am Acad Orthop Surg. 1996;4(6):287–96.

16. Wang C, Nastasi A. Neglected rupture of bilateral patellar ligaments. N Y State J Med. 1974;74(1):85–6.
17. Dejour H, Denjean S, Neyret P. Treatment of old or recurrent ruptures of the patellar ligament by contralateral autograft. Rev Chir Orthop Reparatrice Appar Mot. 1992;78(1):58–62.
18. Casey MT Jr, Tietjens BR. Neglected ruptures of the patellar tendon. A case series of four patients. Am J Sports Med. 2001;29(4):457–60.
19. Evans PD, Pritchard GA, Jenkins DH. Carbon fibre used in the late reconstruction of rupture of the extensor mechanism of the knee. Injury. 1987;18(1):57–60.
20. Levin PD. Reconstruction of the patellar tendon using a dacron graft: a case report. Clin Orthop Relat Res. 1976;118:70–2.
21. Wascher DC, Summa CD. Reconstruction of chronic rupture of the extensor mechanism after patellectomy. Clin Orthop Rel Res. 1998;357:135–40.
22. McNally PD, Marcelli EA. Achilles allograft reconstruction of a chronic patellar tendon rupture. Arthroscopy. 1998;14(3):340–4.
23. Falconiero RP, Pallis MP. Chronic rupture of a patellar tendon: a technique for reconstruction with Achilles allograft. Arthroscopy. 1996;12(5):623–6.
24. Abril J, Alvarez L, Vallejo J. Patellar tendon avulsion after total knee arthroplasty: a new technique. J Arthroplast. 1995;10(3):275–9.
25. Rosa B, Campos P, Barros A, Karmali S, Gonçalves R. Spontaneous bilateral patellar tendon rupture: case report and review of fluoroquinolone-induced tendinopathy. Clin Case Rep. 2016;4(7):678.
26. Mencia M, Edwards A, Ali T. Spontaneous bilateral patellar tendon ruptures in a patient with chronic renal failure: a case report. Internet. J Emerg Med. 2012;7(2)
27. Kellersmann R, Blattert TR, Weckbach A. Bilateral patellar tendon rupture without predisposing systemic disease or steroid use: a case report and review of the literature. Arch Orthop Trauma Surg. 2005;125(2):127–33.
28. Webb LX, Toby EB. Bilateral rupture of the patella tendon in an otherwise healthy male patient following minor trauma. J Trauma. 1986;26(11):1045–8.
29. Enad JG. Patellar tendon ruptures. South Med J. 1999;92(6):563–6.
30. Rosenberg JM, Whitaker JH. Bilateral infrapatellar tendon rupture in a patient with jumper's knee. Am J Sports Med. 1991;19(1):94–5.
31. Kannus P, Józsa L. Histopathological changes preceding spontaneous rupture of a tendon. A controlled study of 891 patients. J Bone Joint Surg Am. 1991;73(10):1507–25.
32. Hsu H, Siwiec RM. Patellar tendon rupture. In: StatPearls. StatPearls Publishing; 2021.
33. Verhulst FV, van Sambeeck JDP, Olthuis GS, van der Ree J, Koëter S. Patellar height measurements: Insall-Salvati ratio is most reliable method. Knee Surg Sports Traumatol Arthrosc. 2020;28(3):869–75.
34. Biedert RM, Tscholl PM. Patella Alta: a comprehensive review of current knowledge. Am J Orthop (Belle Mead NJ). 2017;46(6):290–300.
35. Elattar O, Coleman SH, Warren RF, Rozbruch SR. neglected patellar tendon rupture with massive proximal patellar migration treated with patellar transport and staged allograft reconstruction: a report of 2 cases. Orthop J Sports Med. 2016;4(11):2325967116672175.
36. Mandelbaum BR, Bartolozzi A, Carney B. A systematic approach to reconstruction of neglected tears of the patellar tendon. A case report. Clin Orthop Relat Res. 1988;235:268–71.
37. Maffulli N, Del Buono A, Loppini M, Denaro V. Ipsilateral hamstring tendon graft reconstruction for chronic patellar tendon ruptures: average 5.8-year follow-up. J Bone Joint Surg Am. 2013;95(17):e1231–6.

Patella Fracture Failed Fixation

28

Daniel Scott Horwitz
and Taikhoom M. Dahodwala

History of Previous Primary Failed Treatment

Revisiting the anatomical characteristics of the patella is an essential step to understand issues surrounding fixation failures. The patella is the largest sesamoid bone in the human body, and it forms the anterior aspect of the knee joint. The patella bridges the quadriceps muscle and the patellar tendon on the superior and inferior aspects, respectively. The patellar ligament attaches the inferior pole of the patella to the tibial tubercle. On the lateral and medial borders, the retinacula are attached, providing stability in the coronal plane to the patella. The lateral and medial retinacula are formed from various muscles; these are the vastus lateralis, the iliotibial band, quadriceps aponeurosis, and the vastus medialis [1]. Posteriorly there is a bare articulating surface, with a vertical ridge that separates the medial and lateral facets of the patella. The patellofemoral joint is formed by the articulation of the femoral trochlea with the patella [2], and the percentage of contact between the two surfaces varies depending on the flexion of the knee [3]. Hence, it is important to keep in mind that the patella is anchored from all sides with soft tissues, including muscles and tendons constantly trying to pull it out of position and minor surgical deficiencies may result in complete failure of the construct.

We wish to discuss a 72-year-old male, non-smoker, with a history of falls on the sidewalk with direct impact to the anterior aspect of the left knee, consistent with a moderate to high energy mechanism. On inspection, the knee was swollen on the anterior aspect with a peripatellar hematoma visible. A thorough inspection of the skin was carried out to rule out an open fracture and any skin compromise that would affect surgical exposure. Palpation revealed edema and tenderness of the knee joint and a bony gap with a nonfunctional extensor mechanism. Joint aspiration was deemed unnecessary for hemarthrosis.

For radiographic examination, anteroposterior, lateral and axial X-ray views of the knee were taken to help clarify the type of fracture and exclude any associated injury to the knee. On review of these radiographs, a comminuted patella fracture classified as an AO 34-C3.3 along with a nondisplaced proximal fibula fracture was noted (Fig. 28.1). Computed tomography (CT) scan was deemed to be unnecessary as the radiographs showed a transverse fracture with two additional sagittal fractures.

The treatment chosen for this fracture was interfragmentary screw fixation of the transverse fracture and further sagittal fragment fixation using additional screws based on the comminution and the fracture displacement.

D. S. Horwitz (✉) · T. M. Dahodwala
Department of Orthopaedics, Geisinger Health System, Danville, PA, USA
e-mail: dshorwitz@geisinger.edu

© The Author(s), under exclusive license to Springer Nature Switzerland AG 2024
P. V. Giannoudis, P. Tornetta III (eds.), *Failed Fracture Fixation*,
https://doi.org/10.1007/978-3-031-39692-2_28

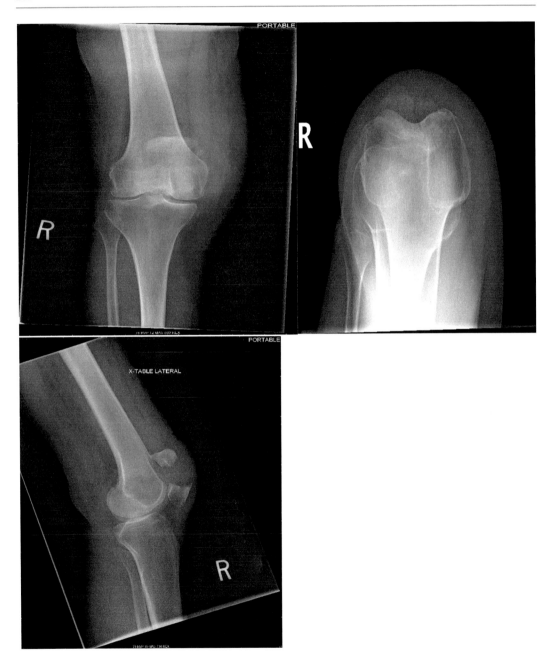

Fig. 28.1 Right patella preoperative radiographs

A midline incision was made directly over the patella fracture down through the skin and subcutaneous tissue, and at this point of time, we were able to directly visualize the knee joint. There was a proximal and a distal fracture component, and comminution medially on the proximal and distal segments. The fracture edges were thoroughly debrided using rongeur, curettes, bulb syringe, and a knife. The medial comminuted piece proximally and distally were both reduced using a small pointed tenaculum and then held in place with 0.062 K-wires. Next, 0.062 K-wires were used for joysticks to reduce the proximal and distal fracture fragments, and a reduction clamp was placed. Wires for cannulated 3.5mm fully threaded screws were placed across the transverse fracture segments; alignment was confirmed and fully threaded screws were placed after using a cannulated drill. The smaller medial fracture fragments were secured with solid 2.4 mm screws, and a suture passer was used to pass #5 Fiberwire through the cannulated screws, securing it in a figure-of-eight fashion. Final fluoroscopic images can be seen in Fig. 28.2 whereas post-operative radiographs showed anatomic reduction of the joint line (Fig. 28.3). The wound was then copiously irrigated, and the wound was closed in a standard layered fashion.

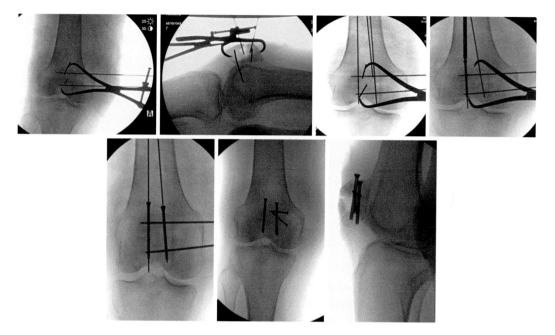

Fig. 28.2 Intraoperative primary surgery images showing reduction steps and final reconstruction of the right patella fracture

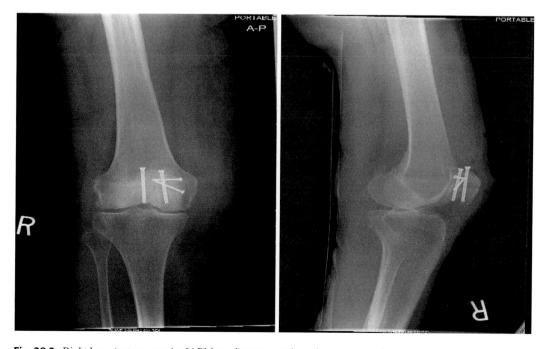

Fig. 28.3 Right knee (anteroposterior [AP]-lateral) postoperative primary surgery films

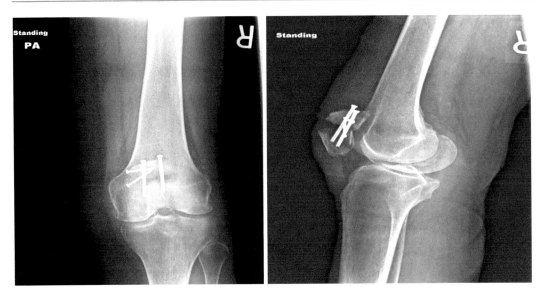

Fig. 28.4 Right patella AP-lateral radiographs showing fixation failure

The patient returned at 2 weeks for suture removal and was weight-bearing in a brace maintaining full extension of the knee. New radiographs obtained revealed a catastrophic failure of fixation with clear coronal fragmentation of the inferior patellar pole. Displacement of the articular surface was felt to be unacceptable in this otherwise active patient (Fig. 28.4).

Evaluation of the Etiology of Failure of Fixation

Ultimately, the failure of fixation, in this case, was related to an underestimation of the comminution of the major distal fragment in the coronal plane. Despite a careful intraoperative assessment, it was not appreciated that there was a pre-existing coronal defect distally that would lead to a split and catastrophic failure of reduction. Despite the use of suture augmentation, the primary mode of fixation initially relied on the vertically oriented cannulated screws, and once the distal pole split, they were no longer contained.

The coronal plane fractures would likely have been visualized on a fine-cut CT scan, a study not obtained in this case. The senior author typically obtains these studies with 3D reconstruction to aid in operative planning, with the idea that too much information is better than not enough information. Due to the distance the patient lived from the medical center and travel issues, the decision was made to proceed in this case without advanced imaging. That was clearly, in retrospect, an error.

Clinical Examination

The patient was weight-bearing in a brace maintaining full extension of the knee. No wound complications were noted. There was no distal neurovascular deficit. Flexion movement was associated with painful stimuli.

Diagnostic-Biochemical and Radiological Investigations

As the patient was followed regularly and had no signs of Infection and there was no concern for metabolic abnormalities, the assumption was that an underestimation of fracture comminution was the principal cause of failure. This can occur in any setting but, based on our experience, it is more likely in the elderly patient with overall poorer bone quality, where small nondisplaced fractures are often more difficult to appreciate visually. In other cases, infection and metabolic issues should be ruled out. A CT scan demonstrated in more detail the coronal plane fractures and the gap that developed between the implants the failure of fixation.

Preoperative Planning

Our standard treatment for highly comminuted patella fractures is anterior plating using mini fragment or mesh-type plates at the index procedure, and we felt that this technique would still provide the best option for stable fixation [4]. In evaluating whether the cannulated and the interfragmentary screws would need to be removed, we considered the role they might play in assisting in obtaining the reduction we had previously been very satisfied with. Appreciating that the screws appeared to be stable in the proximal patellar fragment and the medial to lateral mini fragment screws appeared nondisplaced, we formulated the plan of retaining these screws, reducing the inferior pole "split" fragments to those screws and then placing a locking anterior plate with unicortical screws.

Revision Surgery

The old incision was utilized and carried down through deep subcutaneous tissues. The previous figure-of-eight suture was identified; it was cut and then removed. We then removed large quantities of fibrinous tissue from the fracture from dorsally to the articular surface. Great care was taken to preserve the medial and lateral retinaculum. A large bone-holding tenaculum was used and placed proximally and distally and we were able to bring both the dorsal and the articular surface distally into near anatomic alignment.

A titanium mesh plate was cut and contoured to fit the dorsal aspect of the patella. It was positioned and secured proximally and distally with 2.7 mm nonlocked screws. Multiple locked screws were then placed proximally and distally to provide a dorsal tension band to the entire patella. A #2 Fiberwire was then brought through the origin of the patellar tendon, and this was sutured to the mesh plate for augmented fixation of the inferior pole.

Flouroscopy was used in anteriorposterior, lateral, and internal and external rotational views to confirm that excellent overall alignment had been achieved (Fig. 28.5).

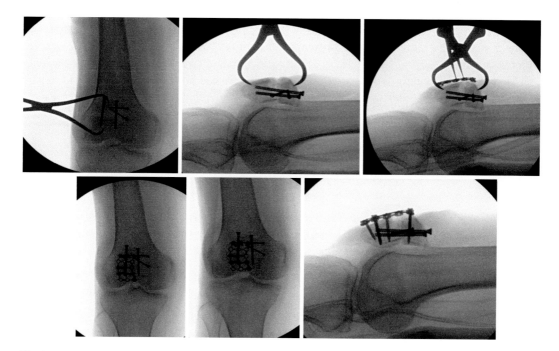

Fig. 28.5 Intraoperative images showing revision surgery steps

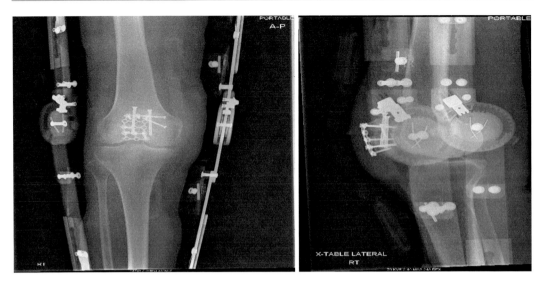

Fig. 28.6 Right patella AP and lateral post-revision surgery radiographs

The knee was brought through a range of motion of 0–60° and the fixation was noted to be extremely stable. Because of the poor bone quality and nature of the revision surgery, full flexion was not attempted in the OR. The wounds were copiously irrigated. Subcutaneous flaps were developed in the preexisting scar tissue medially and laterally. The skin was then closed in a standard layered fashion. The patient was placed in a hinged knee brace locked in full extension. Figure 28.6 shows the post-operative radiographs with fracture reduction.

The patient returned for a wound check in approximately 2 weeks and the sutures were removed. No wound issues were noted. Full weight-bearing in locked extension was allowed but no formal physical therapy was initiated until 6 weeks. Radiographs at 6 weeks (Fig. 28.7) confirmed maintenance of reduction, and physical therapy was now initiated with active flexion and passive extension only, under supervision.

At 3 months, flexion of 110–115° was noted and aerobic conditioning and extension strengthening exercises were initiated. At 6 months, the patient had returned to almost preinjury activity levels and had minimal complaints of knee pain or hardware prominence (Fig. 28.8).

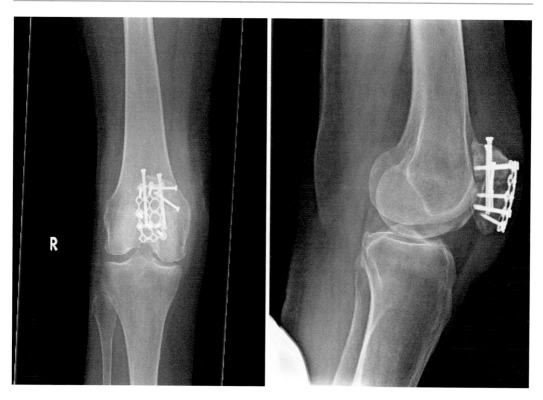

Fig. 28.7 Right patella AP and lateral 6 weeks post-revision surgery radiographs

Fig. 28.8 Right patella AP and lateral 6 months post-revision surgery radiographs showing maintenance of reduction and fracture healing

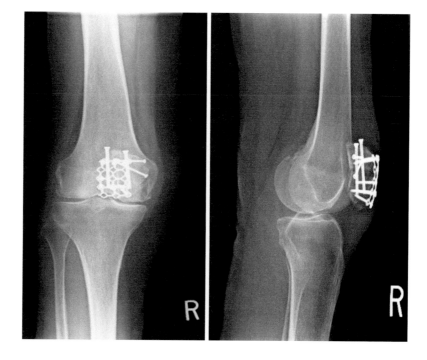

Lessons Learned

This case is a clear demonstration that comminuted patella fractures may be difficult to fully assess on plain films, and coronal plane elements can be easily missed. For this reason, the authors strongly suggest obtaining high-quality CT scans, when possible, to better evaluate comminuted fractures [5]. That being said, there may be times when this is impossible due to the logistics, timing, or other factors beyond the surgeon's control. In those cases, we suggest a low threshold for a combined fixation. Augmentation using a plate in cases of multiple fracture fragments, especially in the older patient, should be considered [6]. Reduction and fixation can proceed using whatever type of pin/screw/tension band construct the surgeon is comfortable with, and this can then be augmented easily with a low profile anterior "tension band plate" with 4–6 locked screws. Alternatively, if coronal plane elements are appreciated after a CT scan or intraoperatively, we would urge primary fixation with an anterior plate and suture augmentation as needed.

Fortunately, this case also represents a good outcome that can be achieved with early (6 weeks) recognition of failure and revision surgery. A "watch and wait" approach is not recommended in an otherwise functional patient as a poorly functioning knee extensor mechanism will likely be a major disability. In addition, by choosing an alternate method of primary fixation (i.e., anterior tension band plating vs interfragmentary screws), it is possible to achieve stable, reliable fixation even in the geriatric population.

References

1. Andrikoula S, Tokis A, Vasiliadis HS, Georgoulis A. The extensor mechanism of the knee joint: an anatomical study. Knee Surg Sports Traumatol Arthrosc. 2006;14(3):214–20. https://doi.org/10.1007/s00167-005-0680-3.
2. Melvin JS, Mehta S. Patellar fractures in adults. J Am Acad Orthop Surg. 2011;19(4):198–207. https://doi.org/10.5435/00124635-201104000-00004.
3. Loudon JK. Biomechanics and pathomechanics of the patellofemoral joint. Int J Sports Phys Ther. 2016;11(6):820–30.
4. Hargett D, Sanderson B, Little M. Patella fractures: approach to treatment. J Am Acad Orthop Surg. 2021;29(6):244–53. https://doi.org/10.5435/JAAOS-D-20-00591.
5. Sim JA, Joo YB, Choi W, Byun SE, Na YG, Shon OJ, Kim JW. Patellar fractures in elderly patients: a multicenter computed tomography-based analysis. Arch Orthop Trauma Surg. 2021;141(9):1439–45. https://doi.org/10.1007/s00402-020-03526-z.
6. Fehske K, Berninger MT, Alm L, Hoffmann R, Zellner J, Kösters C, Barzen S, Raschke MJ, Izadpanah K, Herbst E, Domnick C, Schüttrumpf JP, Krause M, Komitee Frakturen der Deutschen Kniegesellschaft (DKG). Aktueller Versorgungsstandard von Patellafrakturen in Deutschland [Current treatment standard for patella fractures in Germany]. Unfallchirurg. 2021;124(10):832–8. https://doi.org/10.1007/s00113-020-00939-8.

Tibial Plateau Plating Failed Fixation

29

Chang-Wug Oh and Peter V. Giannoudis

History of Previous Primary Failed Treatment

A 47-year-old male was admitted to the local hospital after stepping into a pothole whilst jogging and sustaining a right knee twisting injury. He had a past medical history of asthma. He was a keen sportsman, exercising at least three times a week.

On admission, trauma primary and secondary surveys revealed an isolated right tibial plateau fracture (Fig. 29.1).

He had preserved sensation and limb distal pulses were unremarkable. He was placed in an above knee backslap in the Emergency Department, and he was admitted for further management of the fracture. The following day, he underwent a CT scan of the right knee. The 3D scan reconstruction is shown in Fig. 29.2.

The right leg was kept elevated, and he was prescribed chemical thromboprophylaxis (tinzaparin) treatment. Five days later, he was taken to theatre by the local team and through a posterior medial approach, the fracture was exposed and stabilised. Immediate post-operative radiographs are shown in Fig. 29.3.

The radiographs were deemed to be satisfactory. The patient was discharged home with the advice to toe touch weight bearing and to start early range of motion 0–45 degrees initial first 3 weeks.

He was subsequently seen in the outpatient clinic 4 weeks later when he was complaining of increasing pain during movement. Radiographs taken revealed loss of reduction and loosening of the metal work (screws backing out) (Fig. 29.4).

C.-W. Oh (✉)
Department of Trauma & Orthopaedic Surgery, School of Medicine, Kyungpook National University Hospital, Daegu, South Korea

P. V. Giannoudis
Academic Department of Trauma and Orthopaedics, School of Medicine, University of Leeds, Leeds, UK

NIHR Leeds Biomedical Research Center, Chapel Allerton Hospital, Leeds, UK

© The Author(s), under exclusive license to Springer Nature Switzerland AG 2024
P. V. Giannoudis, P. Tornetta III (eds.), *Failed Fracture Fixation*,
https://doi.org/10.1007/978-3-031-39692-2_29

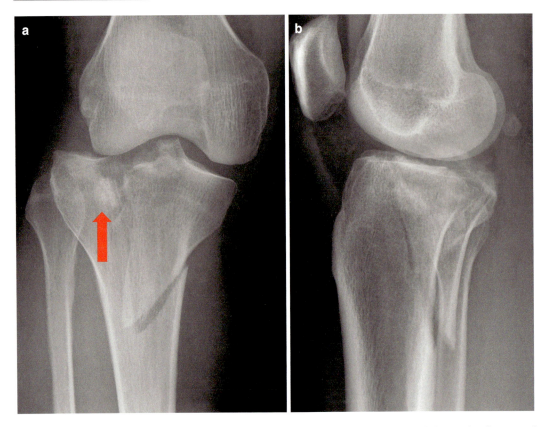

Fig. 29.1 Radiographs of the right knee: (**a**) AP; (**b**) lateral demonstrating a posteriomedial plateau shearing type of injury. They also show a depressed intra-articular posterior lateral margin fragment (red arrow)

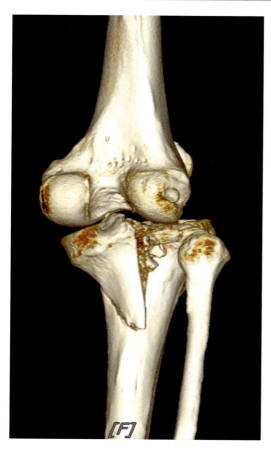

Fig. 29.2 3D right knee reconstruction showing the posterior medial injury pattern as well as the posterior rim comminution

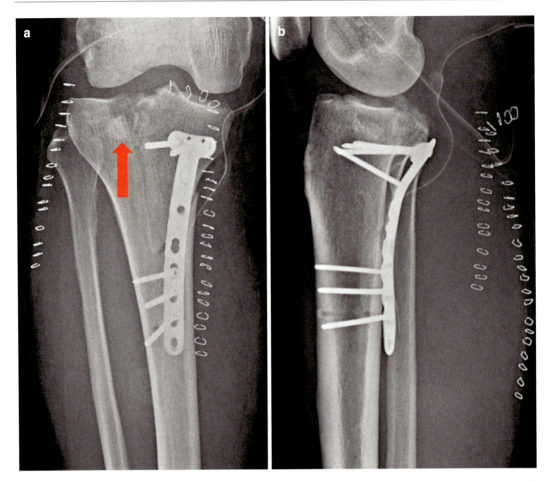

Fig. 29.3 Immediate post-operative (**a**) AP and (**b**) lateral radiographs of right knee show stabilisation of the tibial plateau fracture with a posterior medial buttress plate

Fig. 29.4 Radiographs at 4 weeks (**a**) AP and (**b**) lateral right knee showing loss of reduction and loosening of the metal work. There is diastasis of the posterior medial tibial fragment and varus deformity

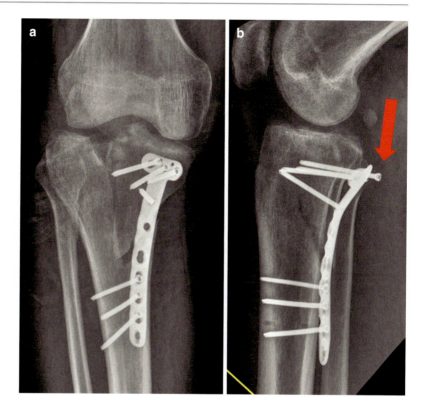

Evaluation of the Aetiology of Failure of Fixation

The post-operative radiographs (Fig. 29.3) demonstrate that the fracture was never reduced anatomically, and there was residual varus deformity. Moreover, the posterior lateral impacted segment was never reduced. Consequently, the abnormal biomechanical loading and inherent fracture instability led to further displacement and loosening of the metal work.

In this case, the so-called 'split wedge fragment' characterised by 1, 2, and 3 points represents the area where the shearing force bisected the rim of the plateau in two places (**1 posterior; 2 medial**) and then the force exited the metaphysis at **point 3** (third place) (Fig. 29.5).

The split wedge fragment and the continuity of the rim are the major determinants of joint stability. Anatomical reduction of the split wedge restores rim continuity. Maintenance of reduction by buttressing the split wedge fragment leads to restoration of stability and axial alignment but in this case, there was a failure to address this principle for a successful reconstruction and outcome.

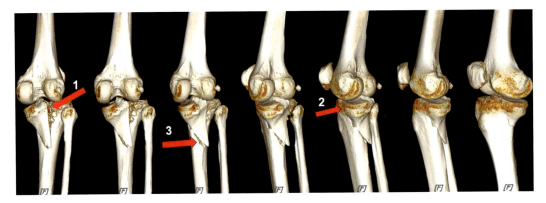

Fig. 29.5 Different views of the 3D coronal views of the right knee. Points 1,2,3 demonstrate the areas where the shearing forces bisected the rim of the posterior medial plateau segment (1 posterior; 2 medial; 3 metaphyseal points)

Clinical Examination

At the 4-week follow-up, on clinical assessment the wound had healed without any complications (Fig. 29.6). There was no redness, soft tissue swelling or erythema.

There was no distal neurovascular deficit. The patient remained systemically well. Passive and active movement was possible from −20 degrees of extension to about 45 degrees of flexion and this arc of movement was associated with pain (Fig.29.7).

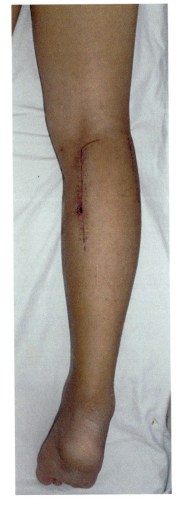

Fig. 29.6 Clinical photo in the clinic demonstrating a health scar over the posterior medial area of the right knee and an obvious varus deformity

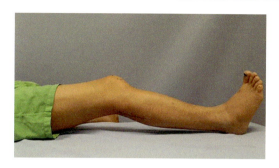

Fig. 29.7 Lateral view of the right knee demonstrating a 20 degrees fixed flexion deformity

Diagnostic-Biochemical and Radiological Investigations

In this case, it was important to exclude underlying low-grade infection. Haematological and biochemical investigations were requested which revealed a normal white blood count, ESR and CRP. From both the clinical examination and the biochemical and haematological screening, there was no evidence of infection.

The plain radiographs taken were complemented with a new computed tomography scan to allow a more detailed evaluation of the problem (Fig. 29.8).

Fig. 29.8 (**a**) 3D – axial view; (**b**) 3D – coronal posterior knee view showing the failure of fixation in more detail. Red arrow shows loosening of screws and plate; white arrow shows depressed impacted intra-articular bone segment, which was not reduced at the time of reconstruction

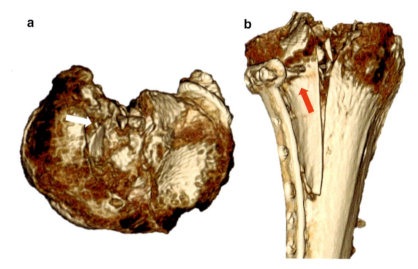

Preoperative Planning

Following the analysis of the failure of the fixation, the preoperative plan implemented included the following:

1. Utilised the same incision to remove the plate used and clean the previous fracture planes for reduction of the posterior medial fragment.
2. Osteosynthesis of the posterior medial fragment with a posterior buttress plate and a medial plate to provide optimum stability.
3. Anterior lateral incision and sub-meniscal elevation for visualisation of the joint.
4. Osteotomy of the lateral plateau for getting access to the central depressed segment.
5. Elevation, reduction and fixation of the depressed fragment with lag screws using the rafting fixation technique.
6. Fixation of the osteotomised fragment with a lateral buttress plate.

Choices Behind Implant Selection

The small fragment set and 3.5 mm screws would be adequate to address the depressed central-based posterior lateral impacted fragment. Small fragment 3.5 plates were selected for fixation of the posterior medial plateau fragment. For the osteotomised lateral tibial plateau, a T-plate was selected.

Which Bone Grafts Are Needed and Why?

In case following elevation and reduction of the fragments residual bone voids were present, then a bone cement (bone substitute) (Hydroset, Stryker, USA) would be used for maintenance of reduction. This biological material has good resistant compressive forces and interdigitates and integrates well with the local host environment.

Revision Surgery

Under general anaesthesia, the patient was positioned prone on a radiolucent table (OSI). A foley urinary catheter was inserted and a tourniquet. A soft bolster was placed under the contralateral hip to provide rotation to the affected knee. Moreover, a stuck of towels or soft bolsters can be used to flex the knee to be operated (Fig. 29.9). The surgeon stands on the contralateral side and the fluoroscopy unit is placed on the side of the affected knee.

The old incision was reopened with the vertical limp of the incision directly over the dorsal medial margin of the medial gastrocnemius. Full fasciocutaneous flaps were created and the lesser saphenous and nervous suralis were identified and protected. The soleus muscle was pilled off and more proximally elevation of the popliteus muscle was carried out. Hommans retractor was placed at the lateral tibial crest (proximal placement is avoided to prevent injury of the posterior tibial recurrent artery). The previous plate was removed. The fracture was mobilised with an osteotome as shown in Fig. 29.10.

Using pointing reduction forceps, the fracture was reduced (Fig. 29.11).

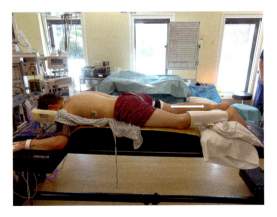

Fig. 29.9 Patient is positioned prone on the OSI table as shown. The white arrow indicates the side of the incision

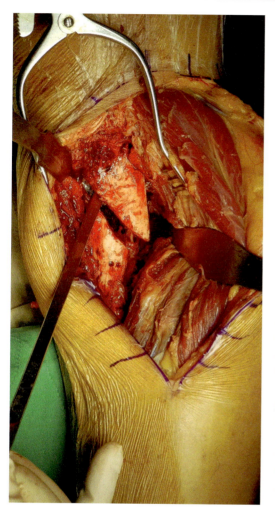

Fig. 29.10 Intraoperative picture showing mobilisation of the posterior medial fragment with an osteotome

Subsequently, the fracture was stabilised with 2 × 3.5 mm small LCP plates, one placed posteriorly and one posterior medially (Fig. 29.12).

Then the medial wound was closed in layers over one drain and attention was given to the central posteriorly laterally depressed fragment (Fig. 29.13).

The tourniquet was deflated after the closure of the medial incision. The patient was repositioned in the supine approach. A sandbag was placed under the affected hip for maintenance of the neutral position of the leg. The tourniquet was re-inflated. After sterilisation of the surgical field, an anterior lateral approach was then carried out. A bolster was used to flex the knee at 30 degrees.

An incision was made starting 4 cm proximal to the knee joint line along with midline of the lateral side and then towards Gerdy's tubercle and down to the lateral side of the tibial tuberosity. Using a blade, the iliotibial band was incised and a sharp dissection was carried out in Gerdy's tubercle.

An external fixator was applied to span the joint. A capsulotomy was performed by incising the tibial meniscal ligament and after tagging the meniscus and elevating, the articular surface was visualised. Then using an osteotome, the lateral tibial condyle was osteotomised in order to get access to the posterior lateral central depression area (Fig. 29.14).

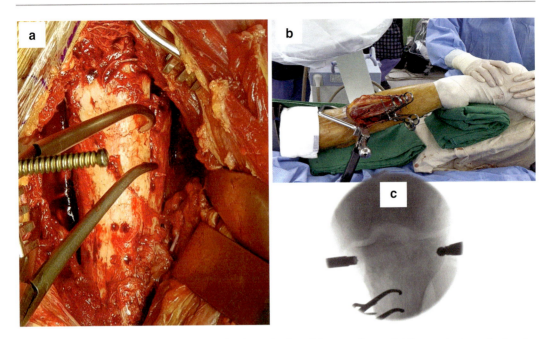

Fig. 29.11 (**a**) and (**b**) Intraoperative images showing reduction of the posterior medial fragment using reduction forceps. (**c**) Fluoroscopic image showing fracture reduction

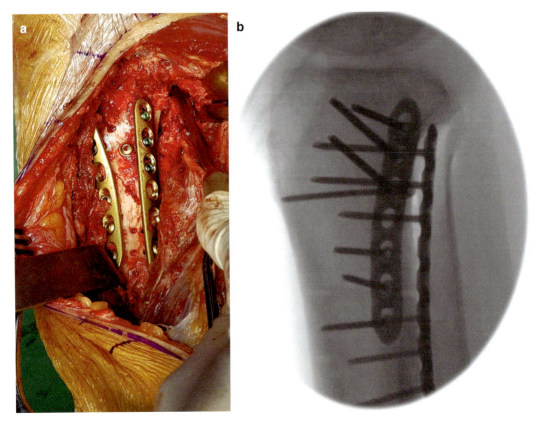

Fig. 29.12 (**a**) Intraoperative image showing fixation of the posterior medial plate with two plates. (**b**) Intraoperative fluoroscopic image showing fixation

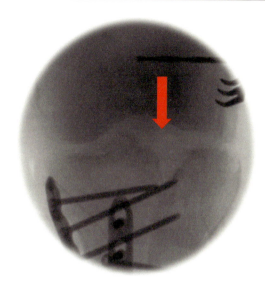

Fig. 29.13 AP right knee fluoroscopic view demonstrating the posterior lateral centrally based depressed fragment

The depressed fragment was identified, mobilised and reduced to its anatomical position and stabilised with 2 × 3.5 mm screws (Fig. 29.15).

The osteotomised fragment was then reduced and stabilised with 3 × 3.5 mm screws. Then a T-plate was applied for buttressing of the lateral tibial plateau (Fig. 29.16). On this occasion, no bone graft was felt to be necessary to be implanted.

Following the completion of the lateral plateau reconstruction, the meniscus tagged suture was removed. The capsule was repaired, and the wound was closed in layers with 2/0 Vicryl and 3/0 subcuticular sutures. The drain was removed after 48 hours. Post-operative images are shown in Fig. 29.17.

The patient was advised to mobilise toe touch weight bearing for 4 weeks, then partial weight bearing and by 3 months full weight bearing. Physiotherapy was initiated 2 weeks after revision surgery when the wounds had fully healed. Thromboprophylaxis was prescribed for 8 weeks. At 2 years follow-up, the patient had an excellent radiological and clinical outcome with a full range of motion of the right knee and no radiological signs of osteoarthritis (Fig. 29.18).

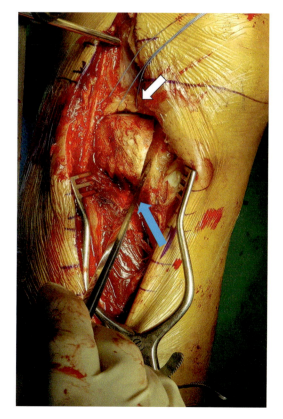

Fig. 29.14 Intraoperative picture showing the mobilisation of the lateral meniscus (white arrow) and the osteotomy of the lateral tibial plateau (blue arrow)

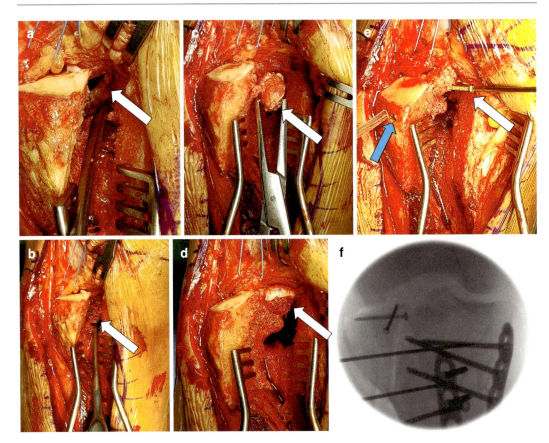

Fig. 29.15 Intraoperative images showing: (**a**) after pulling apart the osteotomised anterior plateau segment identification of the depressed fragment; (**b**) elevation of the fragment with an osteotome; (**c**) complete mobilisation of the fragment prior to anatomical reduction; (**d**) anatomical fragment reduction; e) fixation with two 3.5 mm screws; and (**f**) fluoroscopic image showing reduction of the fragment

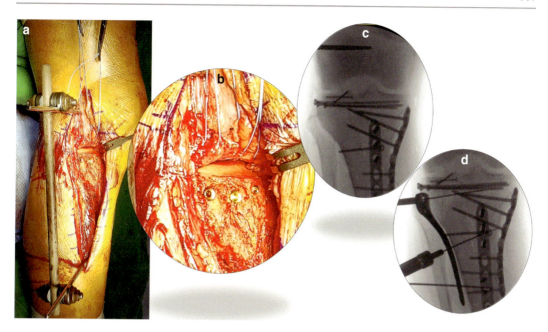

Fig. 29.16 (**a**) Intraoperative image showing anterior lateral incision and the right knee joint spanned with an external fixator; (**b**) the osteotomised fragment stabilised with three screws; (**c**) fluoroscopic AP right knee image showing fixation of the joint anatomically reduced; (**d**) application of the T-shape plate on the lateral tibial plateau area

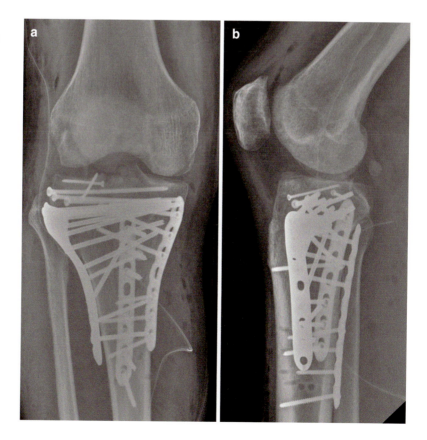

Fig. 29.17 (**a**) AP and (**b**) lateral post-operative radiographs of the right knee following revision surgery

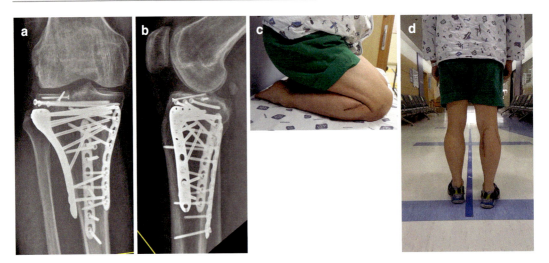

Fig. 29.18 (**a**) AP; (**b**) lateral right knee radiographs at 2 years follow-up; (**c**) and (**d**) clinical pictures showing full knee flexion and no deformity of the joint

Lessons Learned

Management of tibial plateau fractures remains challenging as seen in the herein case. The goals of treatment remain restoration of the mechanical axis, anatomical joint reduction, preservation of the meniscus and early knee range of motion to restore the function. An initial detailed evaluation of the patient profile and injury characteristics is essential for a successful outcome. Acquisition of computed tomography is essential for accurate evaluation of the fracture lines and identification of marginal impaction lesions. The timing of reconstruction is dependent on the states of the soft tissues.

The medial compartment carries more load than the lateral one and that is the reason of being more dense and needs more force to be fractured. The uneven axial load distribution between the medial and lateral tibial plateaus (more loads being transmitted through the medial compartment) is the reason why persisting posteromedial displacement is not tolerated and is vital to provide anatomical reduction and stable fixation. This was not achieved in the case presented and thus the reason for failure (not optimal reduction and poor osteosynthesis). For the impacted posterior lateral fragment, a different incision was necessary to allow access and optimum conditions for reconstruction.

Overall, this case summarises the aetiology of failure of a tibial plateau fracture that was managed with open reduction and internal fixation. Due to poor reduction, malalignment (varus) and abnormal loading failure of fixation was quite early. The subsequent revision carried out allowed the opportunity to also address the reduction and fixation of the posterior lateral depressed fragment. Such a strategy can be considered by surgeons when they are dealing with similar situations of failure of fixation of tibial plateau fractures.

Further Reading

1. Yang X, Pan M, He H, Jiang W. Feasibility of the modified inverted L-shaped approach for posterolateral tibial plateau fracture: a retrospective study. Medicine (Baltimore). 2022;101(40):e31057. https://doi.org/10.1097/MD.0000000000031057.
2. Zhu F, Jiao J, Huang Y, Xiao F, Zuo W, Chen M, Wang X, Wang J. A preliminary study of the surgical approach for posterior tibial plateau fractures: based on posterior fragment segment classification. Injury. 2022;53(11):3820–7. https://doi.org/10.1016/j.injury.2022.09.009.
3. Gálvez-Sirvent E, Ibarzábal-Gil A, Rodríguez-Merchán EC. Complications of the surgical treatment

of fractures of the tibial plateau: prevalence, causes, and management. EFORT Open Rev. 2022;7(8):554–68. https://doi.org/10.1530/EOR-22-0004.

4. Akdemir M, Türken MA, Turan AC, Biçen AÇ, Kılıç Aİ. Clinical and radiological significance of posteromedial fragment in tibial plateau fractures. J Orthop. 2022;31:110–6. https://doi.org/10.1016/j.jor.2022.04.012.

5. Schatzker J, Kfuri M. Revisiting the management of tibial plateau fractures. Injury. 2022;53(6):2207–18. https://doi.org/10.1016/j.injury.2022.04.006.

6. Rosteius T, Rausch V, Pätzholz S, Lotzien S, Königshausen M, Schildhauer TA, Geßmann J. Factors influencing the outcome after surgical reconstruction of OTA type B and C tibial plateau fractures: how crucial is the restoration of articular congruity? Arch Orthop Trauma Surg. 2023;143(4):1973–80. https://doi.org/10.1007/s00402-022-04405-5.

7. Giordano V, Pires RE, Pimenta FS, Campos TVO, Andrade MAP, Giannoudis PV. Posterolateral fractures of the tibial plateau revisited: a simplified treatment algorithm. J Knee Surg. 2022;35(9):959–70. https://doi.org/10.1055/s-0040-1721026.

8. Goff T, Kanakaris NK, Giannoudis PV. Use of bone graft substitutes in the management of tibial plateau fractures. Injury. 2013;44(Suppl. 1):S86–94. https://doi.org/10.1016/S0020-1383(13)70019-6.

Proximal Tibial Intramedullary Nailing Failed Fixation

30

Sushrut Babhulkar, Sunil Kulkarni, and Sangeet Gawhale

History of Previous Primary Failed Treatment

A 45-year-old man sustained an isolated closed right proximal tibial fracture (segmental AO 42-C3) following a motorcycle accident. He was initially seen, examined and managed at the local hospital where his right tibia was placed in a back slab and was admitted for further management. There was no neurovascular deficit present. Two days later he underwent reamed intramedullary nailing fixation through a transpatellar approach. He was discharged home, advised to mobilise partial weight bearing and prescribed chemical thromboprophylaxis for a period of 4 weeks.

However, 5 weeks later he was referred to our institution as he continued to experience painful stimuli on weight bearing.

S. Babhulkar (✉)
Orthopedics & Traumatology,
D M Medical College, Centre for Joint Reconstruction Surgery, Sushrut Institute of Medical Sciences, Research Centre & Post-Graduate Institute of Orthopedics, Nagpur, Ramdaspeth, India

S. Kulkarni
Miraj, Maharashtra, India

S. Gawhale
Mumbai, India

Evaluation of Aetiology of Failure of Fixation

Radiographs taken on initial assessment (Fig. 30.1) revealed a malaligned fixation (valgus and apex anterior deformity). This can be attributed to the following reasons:

1. The mismatch that exists between the diameter of the bone and the diameter of the nail at the proximal tibial area prevents intimate contact between the nail and the endosteal surface; thus, the nail does not aid in reduction of fracture.
2. The natural bony anatomy and muscular attachments of the proximal tibia contribute to common deformities after fracture with subsequent malalignment during intramedullary nailing (IMN) placement [1]. The dynamic forces via the patellar tendon pull the proximal fragment into an apex anterior angulation, whereas the attachment of the pes anserinus commonly causes valgus stress on the same fragment. Before operative fixation, these forces create the potential for improper reduction and difficult reaming and suboptimal nail placement. During operative nailing of proximal fractures with the knee in hyperflexion, the patellar tendon draws the proximal fragment into a procurvatum deformity.

© The Author(s), under exclusive license to Springer Nature Switzerland AG 2024
P. V. Giannoudis, P. Tornetta III (eds.), *Failed Fracture Fixation*,
https://doi.org/10.1007/978-3-031-39692-2_30

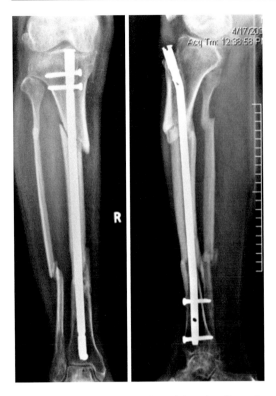

Fig. 30.1 Anteroposterior (AP) and lateral radiographs of the right tibia stabilised with intramedullary (IM) nailing showing loss of reduction and malalignment

3. More distal bends in the nail, particularly older designs, cause malreduction at the fracture site.
4. Older design of nails like the one used in this occasion with the proximal transverse locking option cannot control valgus/varus in fractures.

Clinical Examination

On inspection of the right tibia, there was no erythema present around the proximal and distal scars. On palpation the anterior apex tibia deformity was palpable as well as the tip of the nail proximally. There was some residual swelling around the ankle joint. However, there was no knee joint effusion. The range of motion of the knee was flexion to 85° associated with pain and full extension recovery. There was no ligamentous instability present on varus/valgus strain. The anterior and posterior drawer test was unremarkable. Right hip and right ankle movements were full and pain free. There was no distal neurovascular deficit present. No muscular wasting was apparent.

Diagnostic Biomechanical and Radiological Investigations

In this case despite the healthy state of the soft tissues, one cannot exclude the possibility of low-grade infection. Baseline blood investigations to screen for infection were requested including full blood count (FBC), C-reactive protein (CRP), erythrocyte sedimentation rate (ESR), liver function test, thyroid function, vitamins D and U/E. As there was a positive history of diabetes in the family, screening for diabetes was also carried out. Further diagnostics in the form of computed tomography (CT) can provide further information in terms of the state of fracture healing, presence of infection and loosening of the implant.

Preoperative Planning

The steps of the revision surgery consist of:

(a) Removal of the previous implant

For this step the same incisions would be utilised. After implant removal, tissue (bone fragments) cultures can be sent to microbiology to exclude low-grade infection. Reaming of the medullary canal would allow a nail of greater diameter to be inserted. It will also generate reaming debris, which can support the healing of the fracture.

(b) Fracture reduction

There are different techniques to facilitate fracture reduction including (Figs. 30.2 and 30.3):

- Plate fixation with anterior placed screws to allow insertion of the nail
- Insertion of one screw in each fragment and maintenance of reduction with a Farabeuf clamp

Fig. 30.2 (**a**) Intraoperative image showing a proximal tibial fracture reduced with the application of two cortical screws and the Farabeuf clamp. (**b**) Image intensifier image showing fracture reduction

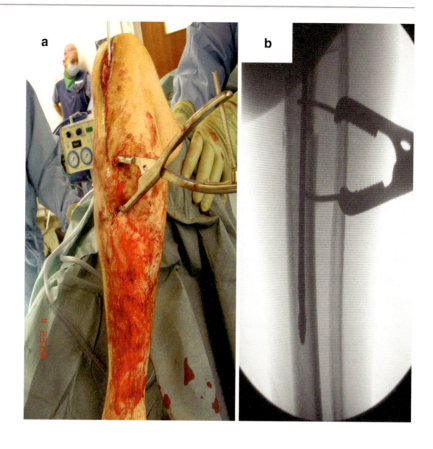

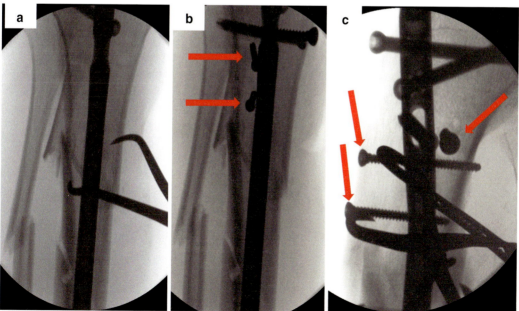

Fig. 30.3 Reduction techniques for proximal tibial fractures: (**a**) Application of pointed reduction forceps; (**b**) AP and (**c**) lateral fluoroscopic images showing the application of Poller screws (red arrows)

- Use of a reduction forceps
- Insertion of Poller screws

In addition, one can use the option of suprapatellar nailing (nailing in semi-extension) allowing better control of the fracture and reduction. In this case due to the previous incision and the entry point has already been made, this option was not considered.

(c) Insertion of a new implant for fixation (IM nail)
   Alternatively the nail implant can be revised to a proximal locking plate.
(d) Proximal and distal locking of the nail
(e) Consideration of bone grafting
   For bone grafting different options can be considered such as:
   (i) Autologous bone graft harvested from the anterior or posterior iliac crest
   (ii) Demineralised bone matrix (DBM)
   (iii) Bone morphogenetic protein 2
   (iv) iv: Allograft

Implants Required

- Nail extraction kit
- New nail kit (Synthes Expert tibial nail)
- Osteotomes and curettage for autologous graft harvesting from the pelvic iliac crest should a decision is taken to proceed with bone grafting

Revision Surgery

The patient is positioned supine on a fracture table [2]. Bolsters can be used to flex the knee joint as indicated to facilitate easy extraction of the previous implant. No tourniquet was used (Fig. 30.4).

Old incisions were utilised [3]. Proximally the patellar tendon was protected, and the tip of the nailing was identified. In this case there was no end cap, but if there is one it must be removed.

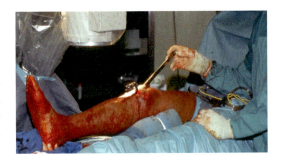

Fig. 30.4 Intraoperative image with the patient in the supine position (a bolster is placed behind the knee joint)

The extraction rod is engaged in the nail and after secure attachment the proximal and distal locking screws were removed. The nail was removed easily. A guidewire was inserted after the fracture was reduced with a reduction forceps. Using a ruler, the length of the new nail was determined. Reaming was carried out up to 12.5 mm. Tissues from reaming were also sent to microbiology for culture and sensitivity.

Subsequently, taking into consideration the previous fracture displacement and the original entry point [4], Poller screws were inserted to facilitate easy advancement of the nail whilst maintaining reduction (Fig. 30.5). Proximal and distal locking screws were then inserted.

As there was good fracture alignment and contact and no bone grafting was felt to be necessary. The wounds were closed in layers with 1 polydioxanone suture (PDS), 2/0 Vicryl and 3/0 nylon for the skin. The patient was discharged home 3 days later with a prescription of tinzaparin (4500 IU) for a period of 6 weeks for thromboprophylaxis. Tissue cultures were negative.

The patient was advised to mobilise toe-touch weight bearing the first 3 weeks, progressing thereafter to partial weight bearing (PWB) and full weight bearing at the 8-week time point. He was followed up in the outpatient clinic at regular intervals (4, 8 and 12 weeks and then at 6, 9 and 12 months). At 8 weeks, his radiographs showed progression of healing proximally (Fig. 30.6).

He progressed uneventfully to healing without any postoperative complications.

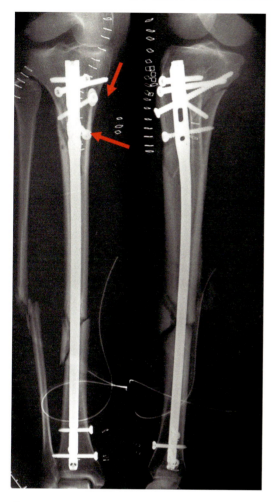

Fig. 30.5 AP and lateral radiographs postoperatively showing the application of Poller screws

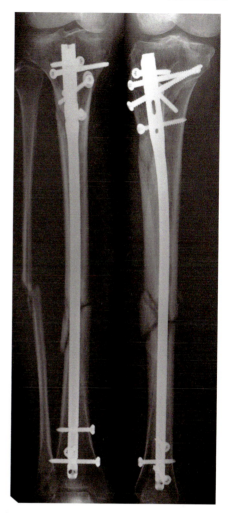

Fig. 30.6 AP and lateral radiographs showing at 8 weeks healing of the fracture proximally with good overall alignment, no loss of reduction and progressive evolution of healing distally

Summary: Lessons Learned

Proximal one-third tibial fractures have an alarming high rate of malalignment. The malalignment is usually valgus and apex anterior angulation [5]; posterior translation of the tibial shaft relative to the proximal fragment can also occur. This displacement is exacerbated in the older nail designs with a more digital Herzog bent by creating a wedge effect of the fracture.

Anatomic knowledge of the tibial intramedullary canal is important for proper nail placement. The canal of the tibia is widest in diameter in the metadiaphysis offering the least purchase for fracture reduction with IM nails.

Selection of the appropriate entry point to avoid malalignment is crucial when nailing these fractures. Numerically, this turns out to be 9 mm lateral to midline, and a mere 23 mm wide. In essence, a proper starting point for tibial IMN lies lateral to the midline and anterior to the joint surface, near the medial border of the lateral tibial spine on the anteroposterior (AP) radiograph and at the anterior border of the juncture of the anterior surface of the tibia and the articular surface on the lateral radiograph. Any deviation from this safe zone is likely to increase the difficulty of nail insertion and contribute to translational and angular deformities. Nail start hole penetration below this zone is risky for posterior cortical penetration and may contribute to further eccentric reaming that can put the extensor mechanism at jeopardy. Nail insertion above this area will cause damage to articular surfaces, anterior horn of the menisci, or intermeniscal ligament.

In summary, in order to avoid complications in proximal third fractures related to loss of reduction and implant failure, the following points seem to be of paramount importance:

1. Preoperative planning: Proper preoperative planning is essential for successful intramedullary nailing of proximal tibia fractures. The surgeon should carefully evaluate the fracture pattern, intra-articular extension if any and the degree of comminution to determine the appropriate size and type of implant.

2. Adequate reduction and fixation: Adequate reduction and fixation of the fracture are crucial in preventing failure of the implant. The surgeon should aim for anatomical reduction and proper alignment of the fracture to avoid malunion, nonunion or implant failure.

3. Proper implant placement: Proper placement of the implant is essential to avoid complications such as intra-articular penetration, cortical perforation or malalignment. The surgeon should carefully assess the entry point and the trajectory of the implant to avoid these complications. The newer trend of the suprapatellar approach seems to be helping in proper nail placement without losing initial reduction and also ease of achieving reduction of the hyperextended proximal fragment.

4. Supplemental fixation: In some cases, supplemental fixation may be necessary to improve the stability of the implant and prevent failure. This may include the use of Poller screws, plates to achieve reduction or external fixation.

References

1. Dunbar RP, Egol KA, Jones CB, Ostrum RF, Humphrey CA, Ricci WM, Phieffer LS, Teague DC, Sagi HC, Pollak AN, Schmidt AH, Sems A, Pape HC, Morshed S, Perez EA, Tornetta P 3rd. Locked plating versus nailing for proximal tibia fractures: a multicenter RCT. J Orthop Trauma. 2023;37(4):155–60. https://doi.org/10.1097/BOT.0000000000002537.

2. Rayes J, Willms S, Buckley R. Proximal to midshaft closed tibial fracture—infra or supra-patellar nailing? Injury. 2022;53(10):3067–9. https://doi.org/10.1016/j.injury.2022.08.001.

3. Patel AH, Wilder JH, Lee OC, Ross AJ, Vemulapalli KC, Gladden PB, Martin MP 3rd, Sherman WF. A review of proximal tibia entry points for intramedullary nailing and validation of the lateral parapatellar approach as extra-articular. Orthop Rev (Pavia). 2022;14(1):31909. https://doi.org/10.52965/001c.31909.

4. Abdalaziz H, Bates P, Iliadis A, Vris A. Clamped percutaneous Poller screws to assist intramedullary nailing of proximal third tibia shaft fractures. Ann R Coll Surg Engl. 2022;104(1):74–5. https://doi.org/10.1308/rcsann.2021.0098.

5. Padubidri A, Sorkin AT, Gudeman A, Natoli RM, Gaski GE. Intramedullary nail fixation of intra-articular and extra-articular proximal tibia fractures. J Surg Orthop Adv. 2021;30(1):55–60.

Proximal Tibia Plating Failed Fixation

31

Heather A. Vallier

History of Previous Primary Failed Treatment

Proximal tibia fractures of the metaphysis, meta-diaphysis and diaphysis occur commonly, with a bimodal age distribution, associated with lower energy mechanisms in elder patients and higher energy mechanisms, generally in younger and middle-aged patients. The majority of these fractures are extra-articular or with a nondisplaced extension of the fracture within the sagittal plane into the tibial plateau [1]. The surrounding soft tissue envelope includes minimal anterolateral musculature, more robust posterior musculature and the subcutaneous border of the anteromedial proximal tibia. Underlying knee arthrosis with associated stiffness and subchondral sclerosis may increase the risk for fracture and displacement in this location. Concurrent knee ligament injuries are common and may require repair or reconstruction.

Our case example includes a 52-year-old man who had multiple injuries in a high-speed motorcycle crash. He sustained a brief loss of consciousness, several left rib fractures with pneumothorax, left open radius and ulna shaft fractures and a fracture of the left proximal tibia (Fig. 31.1). Following resuscitation and administration of intravenous antibiotics, he went to the operating room for debridement and open reduction and internal fixation (ORIF) of his forearm, as well as closed reduction and spanning external fixation of the knee for the left tibia fracture (Fig. 31.2). Due to severity of soft tissue swelling about the left tibia, definitive surgery was deferred. The patient's history was significant for alcohol and recreational drug abuse and tobacco abuse (45 pack-years). He returned to the operating room 12 days later for open reduction and internal fixation of the proximal tibia with a locking plate and a combination of standard and locking small fragment screws (Fig. 31.3). Non-weight-bearing was anticipated for 2–3 months postoperatively, depending on fracture healing. He discharged from the hospital on postoperative day 2 and returned to the outpatient clinic 2 weeks later, where his tibia surgical wounds had healed, and knee range of motion was recommended. He did not return 6 weeks later as he had been advised. One year later he returned to the clinic complaining of persistent pain and activity-related swelling. His history, physical examination and radiography suggested nonunion of the tibia, and revision surgery was

H. A. Vallier (✉)
Department of Orthopaedic Surgery, Case Western Reserve University, Cleveland, OH, USA

© The Author(s), under exclusive license to Springer Nature Switzerland AG 2024
P. V. Giannoudis, P. Tornetta III (eds.), *Failed Fracture Fixation*,
https://doi.org/10.1007/978-3-031-39692-2_31

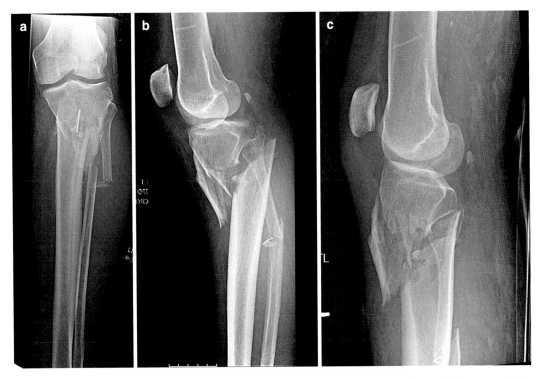

Fig. 31.1 Anteroposterior (**a**) and lateral (**b**, **c**) views of the left tibia obtained on presentation to the emergency department show comminuted displaced proximal tibia shaft fracture, including displaced fractures of the proximal fibula and of the tibia tuberosity. Nondisplaced fracture extension into the tibia plateau is present

advised (Fig. 31.4). Laboratory tests and a computed tomography (CT) scan were ordered; however, he did not obtain these, rather did not return to the clinic for 15 more months, after he had been arrested and sent to jail, followed by an inpatient program for substance abuse. Workup in anticipation of revision surgery was advised but denied by authorities until the patient had completed his rehabilitation program. He returned to the outpatient orthopaedic clinic, then 2.5 years after the initial surgery, with a nonunion and failed fixation (Fig. 31.5).

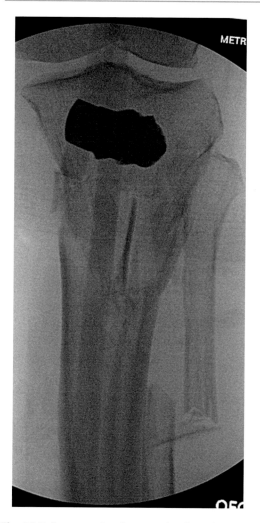

Fig. 31.2 Intraoperative fluoroscopic views following closed reduction and spanning external fixation of the proximal tibia fracture

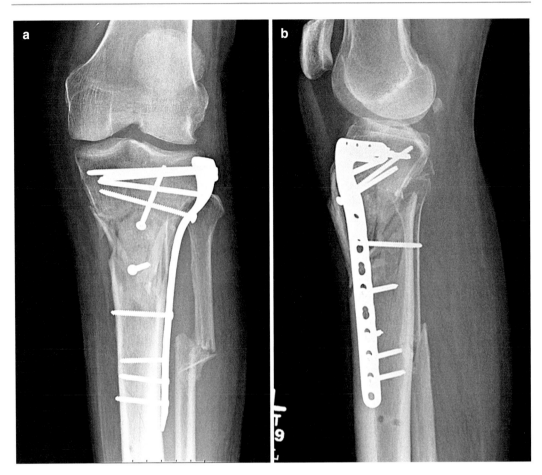

Fig. 31.3 Postoperative anteroposterior (**a**) and lateral (**b**) views showing open reduction and internal fixation of the proximal tibia with a small fragment proximal tibia locking plate and a combination of standard and locking screws

Fig. 31.4 Anteroposterior (**a**) and lateral (**b**) vies of the left tibia obtained 1 year after the index procedure demonstrate the articular surface and the tibial tubercle fractures to be united, while a primary fracture line, best visualized on the lateral view, has not united

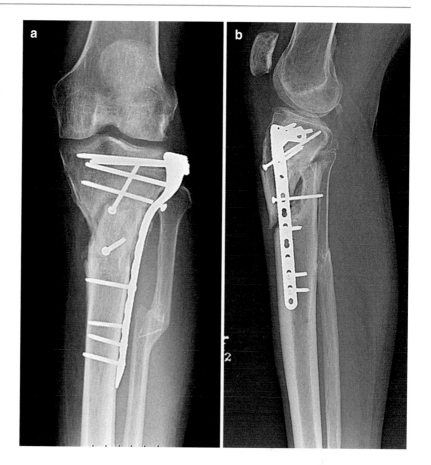

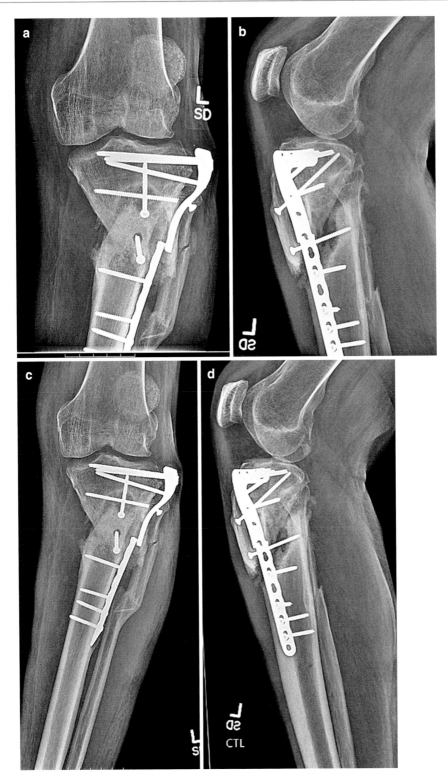

Fig. 31.5 Anteroposterior (**a**, **c**) and lateral (**b**, **d**) views of the tibia obtained 15 months later show persistent nonunion of the tibia, with fracture of the plate and gross malalignment. The initial fibula fracture had united, then refractured slightly proximally

Evaluation of the Aetiology of Failure of Fixation

The patient developed a nonunion of the proximal tibia with failed plate fixation. Although one small fragment screw had been placed across that fracture site to achieve compression during the initial surgery, insufficient stability was present there over time, in conjunction with poor local biology, resulting in an atrophic appearing nonunion. The poor healing capability was likely a combination of the injury and patient factors. A high-energy mechanism of injury with surrounding soft tissue damage, coupled with local surgery, generated an environment expected to have prolonged healing time. The additional detriments of chronic poor vascularity due to extensive tobacco use and underlying malnutrition likely contributed to minimal healing response [2–6]. Nonadherence to initial non-weight-bearing recommendations probably accelerated the loosening of the fixation, especially at the area of the eventual nonunion. Over time, the plate fractured at the site of nonunion due to implant fatigue.

Clinical Examination

In addition to obtaining a thorough medical history, including medical and social risk factors for poor healing, awareness of the patient's vocational and recreational goals is important to achieving mutual understanding regarding likely benefits of surgery. Clinical examination should entail assessment of gait, focused on mobility, alignment and strength of the affected limb, and evaluation of adjacent knee and ankle joints for associated contractures. Contractures can impair osseous correction and may require procedures for soft tissue release or lengthening. Assessment of other areas of prior injury on the ipsilateral and contralateral limb must be made, and evaluation of underlying musculoskeletal variations at baseline should also be undertaken. Leg length discrepancy, and potential angular and rotational malalignment of the tibia and other parts of the legs should be identified [5]. Soft tissue surrounding the proximal tibia should be assessed for old traumatic and surgical scars, which may direct removal of prior implants and revision fixation. Soft tissues should be assessed for integrity and healing capability, presence of sinus tracts (active or remote) and pliability if drastic changes in limb alignment are anticipated [3, 4]. Involvement of a plastic surgeon to assist with elevation and management of old soft tissue flaps for coverage and/or augmentation of existing soft tissue coverage is often worthwhile. A thorough motor and sensory neurological examination and pulse examination should be documented.

Our patient from the case example had well-healed scars overlying the proximal and distal portions of the lateral plate. Small scars corresponding to the fixation for the tibial tubercle and for the primary oblique fracture line were also well-healed. Gross deformity and some mobility and pain were present at the site of the nonunion and failed fixation. Minimal swelling was noted. No sinus tracts or active wounds were present. The patient was using a cane to ambulate, not able to place weight on the affected left leg. Mild stiffness of the left knee and ankle were present and all muscle groups of the left leg appeared atrophic, consistent with disuse. Distal sensation and motor function were intact, and his dorsalis pedis and posterior tibial pulses were normal, symmetrical with the contralateral side.

Diagnostic-Biochemical and Radiological Investigations

Laboratory evaluation at a minimum should include complete cell count with differential, platelets, international normalized ratio (INR), albumin, C-reactive protein (CRP) and erythrocyte sedimentation rate (ESR). Tobacco cessation in longstanding tobacco users is a prerequisite to undertaking surgical treatment of nonunion for many practitioners. Urine cotinine testing is inexpensive, sensitive and easy to do. Optimization of protein malnutrition and correction of vitamin D deficiency should be encouraged preoperatively [2–4].

The patient in our case example had recently relocated to a group home, where he was getting regular meals, and he had been sober (of alcohol and recreational drugs) for approximately 3 months preoperatively. His total lymphocyte count was 2000 and his albumin was 4.2, suggesting ample protein stores to proceed with surgery. His ESR and CRP were normal, which, along with no history of prolonged wound drainage or sinus tracts, suggested the possibility of aseptic nonunion [3, 6].

Radiographic evaluation should include biplanar views of the entire tibia, including the knee and ankle. Pathology such as arthrosis, other remote fractures and retained implants must be thoroughly investigated. Full-length standing radiographs of the legs may be beneficial [5]. Computerized tomography to assess alignment, healing and/or to discern bone quality, and possible presence of infection is generally indicated. Consultation with the radiologist regarding specific planes and dimensions for image reformatting may be helpful; adjustment of the technique to minimize implant artefact may also be performed to enhance the utility of advanced imaging studies.

Plain radiography often suggests atrophic or hypertrophic nonunion. While a hypertrophic nonunion reflects insufficient fracture stability, an atrophic nonunion reflects poor local biology, but may also reflect insufficient stability of fixation [1, 6]. Our case example demonstrated healing of the articular surface, tibial tuberosity and other secondary fractures; however, the primary area of fracture displacement on the initial injury radiographs (Fig. 31.1) had not united (Figs. 31.4 and 31.5). Although it is somewhat atrophic, the nonunion was likely due to insufficient stability in that area. This fracture pattern and orientation is relatively common, and attention to accurate reduction and interfragmentary compression of that fracture in the initial setting will mitigate the risk of nonunion.

Preoperative Planning

Preoperative planning includes implant removal, specific screwdrivers or other tools, which may be needed depending on the types of implants to be removed. Consultation with industry vendors may aid in identification of implants and specific instruments and instructions to facilitate removal. In the case example, small fragment hexagonal and locking screwdrivers were necessary. Broken screw removal tools should also be available, in case retention of screw fragments prevents sufficient reduction or fixation during the revision procedure. Osteotomes and rongeurs to remove bone adjacent to and overlying implants may be required. Once implants have been removed, curettes are needed to remove fibrinous material from old screw tracts. Intraoperative cultures should always be taken. I prefer to take at least two or three cultures from the nonunion and adjacent implants. Antibiotic prophylaxis should be deferred until cultures have been obtained [6].

Implant selection should be based on the location and orientation of the nonunion, the size of the proximal fragment, the presence (or absence) of intact extensor mechanism of the knee and the mechanical environment needed to optimize fracture healing. In other words, the malalignment should be corrected, nonunions compressed and nonunions stabilized in a mechanically sound way, ideally to promote early weight-bearing [5, 7, 8]. While intramedullary nails often afford earlier return to weight-bearing, nails may not provide adequate purchase of the proximal segment, particularly in osteoporotic bone and/or small fracture fragments [9, 10]. Another consideration is that when surgical exposure to remove plates will be extensive, the local biology is already disrupted by surgery in that area, whereas the intramedullary biology has not yet been disrupted, as in our case example [10–14]. While intramedullary nail fixation would be possible, it would also produce some initial, though temporary, disruption of the medullary blood supply, limiting the early healing in that area.

Our case example warranted interfragmentary compression of the nonunion, using large fragment screws, followed by protection with revision lateral plating. Lateral plating, with a large fragment plate, was chosen to minimize additional surgical dissection, to provide a different shape of implant, with new screw configurations in fresh locations, and to permit a combination of locking and standard screws, based on intraoperative assessment of bone quality. A second plate placed medially could be considered, but was not thought to be mechanically necessary, and would create more disruption of the surrounding soft tissue envelope and periosteum, to the detriment of healing of the nonunion [12].

The mainstay of adjuncts to healing of atrophic nonunions is iliac crest bone graft. Although a plethora of products exist as bone graft substitutes, some osteoconductive and some osteoinductive, the evidence-based assessment of each category is beyond the scope of this chapter [15]. In a young or middle-aged person, my preferred method is to harvest iliac crest autograft. Reamer/irrigator/aspirator (RIA) intramedullary harvest could also be considered [16]. However, variability in osteogenic potential has been noted, depending on the RIA technique.

Revision Surgery

The patient was taken to the operating room where he received general anaesthesia. He was positioned supine on a radiolucent table, with a small bump beneath the left hip. This provided slight internal rotation of the left leg to facilitate surgical access and imaging. The bump also facilitated access to the left anterior iliac crest for bone graft harvest. The entire left lower extremity and hemipelvis were sterilely prepped and draped.

The old lateral scars overlying the proximal and distal portions of the tibia plate were incised and connected with an extensile exposure. Tourniquet was not used, so that the soft tissue and bony vascularity could be readily assessed. Locked screws within the proximal portion of the plate were still locked to the plate. Implants were removed from the proximal segment. The distal screws in the plate had also maintained some purchase in the bone. All screws and the plate fragment were removed from that area. No gross evidence of infection was present. Anterior dissection was performed to access the two screws outside of the plate, and each was removed. Cultures were obtained from fibrinous tissue around the implants near the nonunion and from tissue within the nonunion. Intravenous antibiotics were administered.

Using fresh gloves and instruments, cancellous bone graft was harvested from the anterior iliac crest, via a cortical window. Haemostasis was achieved at that site, and layered closure was performed. The nonunion site was debrided of intervening fibrous tissue, and it was mobilized using osteotomes (Fig. 31.6a–d). The nonunion site appeared to have viable bone margins. Iliac crest bone graft was then placed within the nonunion and the nonunion was reduced and clamped, re-establishing appropriate sagittal and coronal plane alignment (Fig. 31.6e, f).

Interfragmentary compression across the nonunion was achieved with large fragment screws (Fig. 31.6f–h). A large fragment proximal tibia locking plate was then applied to the lateral cortex. A standard screw was inserted within the proximal portion of the distal fragment to secure the plate to the bone. Purchase was moderately good. Locked screws and standard screws were inserted within the proximal fragment. Due to the retained screw fragment, two of the locking screw trajectories could not be used, so standard screws were placed. The construct was completed with three additional bicortical standard screws distally (Fig. 31.6i, m).

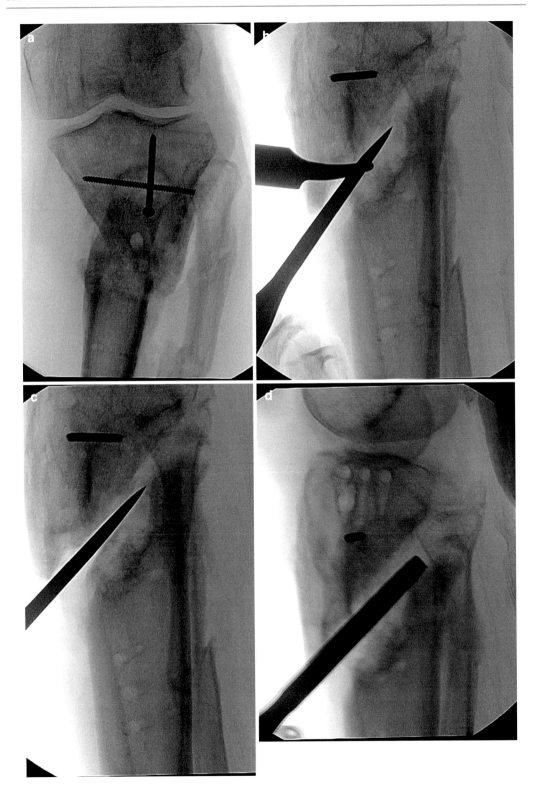

Fig. 31.6 Intraoperative fluoroscopic views show removal of the prior implants (**a**), and debridement and mobilization of the nonunion (**b–d**). The nonunion was reduced (**e, f**) and interfragmentary compression was achieved across the nonunion (**g, h**). Lateral plate fixation was performed (**i, m**)

31 Proximal Tibia Plating Failed Fixation

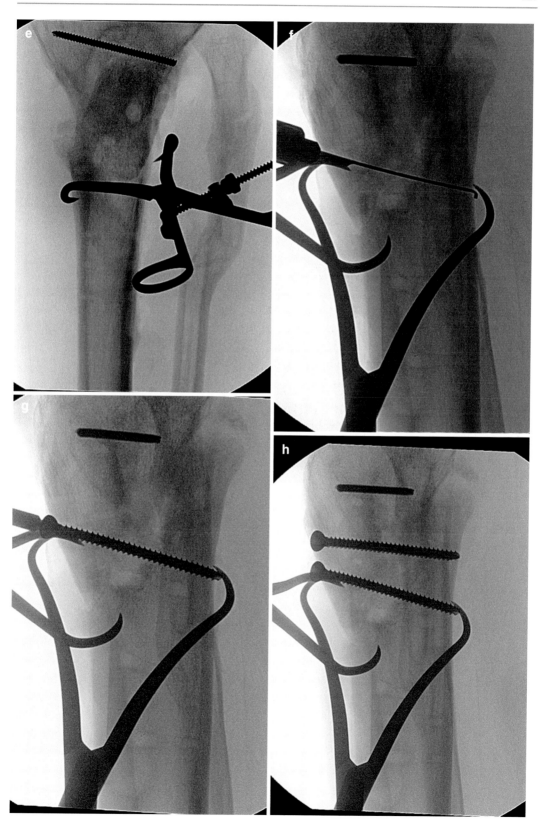

Fig. 31.6 (continued)

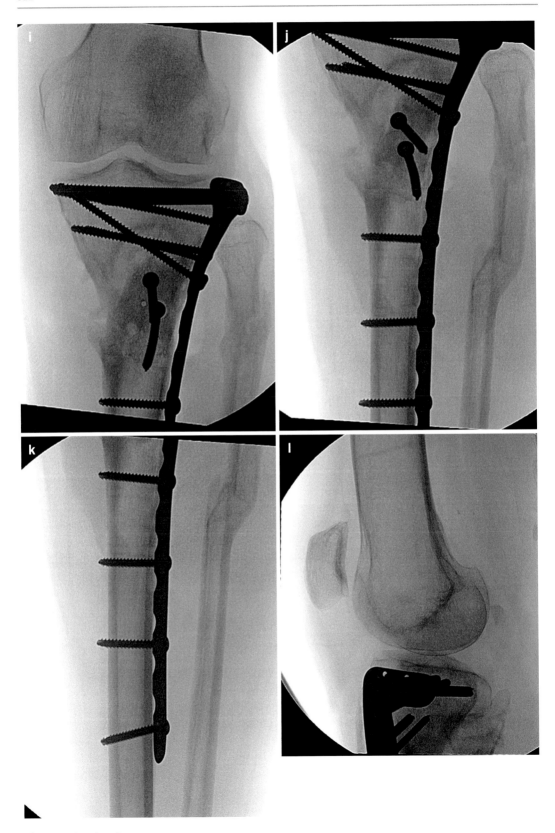

Fig. 31.6 (continued)

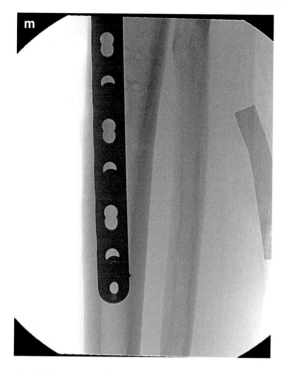

Fig. 31.6 (continued)

The wound was copiously irrigated. One gram of vancomycin powder and 1.2 g of tobramycin powder were mixed with a few drops of normal saline to develop a thick paste, which was applied throughout the wound bed. Layered closure was then performed. The patient was placed into a long leg posterior splint to encourage soft tissue rest. He was admitted to the hospital overnight for pain control and for intravenous antibiotics. He was discharged home the following day maintaining a non-weight-bearing status on the left leg. At the 3-week postoperative period, the wounds had healed and knee range of motion was initiated, but non-weight-bearing was recommended for 1 month.

Summary: Lessons Learned

Thoughtful assessment of patient and injury features will result in the most effective treatment plans. This high-energy proximal tibia fracture was treated with staged internal fixation. Suitable fracture alignment was achieved, and soft tissues healed without incident. However, more interfragmentary compression and larger initial implants may have afforded a better mechanical environment to achieve primary fracture union. More aggressive perioperative interventions to address underlying tobacco, alcohol and drug abuse may have been successful long-term, which could have provided a more vascular and better nourished healing environment. Patient engagement in those activities would also have likely coincided with his adherence to weight-bearing restrictions, and attendance at scheduled clinic visits.

References

1. Schmidt AH, Finkemeier CG, Tornetta P III. Treatment of closed tibial fractures. J Bone Joint Surg Am. 2003;85A:352–68.
2. Brinker MR, O'Connor DP, Monla YT, Earthman TP. Metabolic and endocrine abnormalities in patients with nonunions. J Orthop Trauma. 2007;21:557–70.
3. Brinker MR, Macek J, Laughlin M, Dunn WR. Utility of common biomarkers for diagnosing infection in nonunion. J Orthop Trauma. 2021;35:121–7.

4. Chan DB, Jeffcoat DM, Lorich DG, Helfet DL. Nonunions around the knee joint. Int Orthop. 2010 Feb;34(2):271–81.
5. Green SA, Gibbs P. The relationship of angulation to translation in fracture deformities. J Bone Joint Surg Am. 1994;76A:390–7.
6. Nauth A, Lee M, Gardner MJ, Brinker MR, Warner SJ, Tornetta P 3rd, Leucht P. Principles of nonunion management: state of the art. J Orthop Trauma. 2018;32(Suppl. 1):S52–7.
7. Güven M, Ceviz E, Demirel M, Ozler T, Kocadal O, Onal A. Minimally invasive osteosynthesis of adult tibia fractures by means of rigid fixation with anatomic locked plates. Strategies Trauma Limb Reconstr. 2013;8:103–9.
8. Presutti M, Goderecci R, Palumbo P, Giannetti A, Mazzoleni MG, Randelli FMN, Angelozzi M, Calvisi V, Fidanza A. A novel biplanar medial opening-wedge high tibial osteotomy: the Z-shaped technique. A case series at 7.2 years follow-up. J Orthop Traumatol. 2021;22:53.
9. Aldemir C, Duygun F. Outcome of locked compressive nailing in aseptic tibial diaphyseal nonunions without bone defect. Indian J Orthop. 2019;53(2):251–6.
10. Lindvall E, Sanders R, Dipasquale T, Herscovici D, Haidukewych G, Sagi C. Intramedullary nailing versus percutaneous locked plating of extra-articular proximal tibial fractures: comparison of 56 cases. J Orthop Trauma. 2009;23:485–92.
11. Berven H, Brix M, Izadpanah K, Kubosch EJ, Schmal H. Comparing case-control study for treatment of proximal tibia fractures with a complete metaphyseal component in two centers with different distinct strategies: fixation with Ilizarov frame or locking plates. J Orthop Surg Res. 2018;13:121.
12. Morwood MP, Gebhart SS, Zamith N, Mir HR. Outcomes of fixation for periprosthetic tibia fractures around and below total knee arthroplasty. Injury. 2019;50:978–82.
13. Naik MA, Arora G, Tripathy SK, Sujir P, Rao SK. Clinical and radiological outcome of percutaneous plating in extra-articular proximal tibia fractures: a prospective study. Injury. 2013;44:1081–6.
14. Palmer SH, Handley R, Willet K. The use of interlocked 'customized' blade plates in the treatment of metaphyseal fractures in patients with poor bone stock. Injury. 2000;31:187–91.
15. Watson JT, Anders M, Moed BR. Management strategies for bone loss in tibial shaft fractures. Clin Orthop Rel Res. 1995;315:138–52.
16. Martella A, Schumaier AP, Sirignano MN, Sagi HC, Wyrick JD, Archdeacon MT. Reamer irrigator aspirator (RIA) versus iliac crest bone grafting (ICBG) and proximal tibial curettage (PTC): is there a difference in blood loss and transfusion rates? J Orthop Trauma. 2022;36(4):163–6.

Extra-Articular Tibial Shaft Ilizarov Failed Fixation

32

Paul Nesbitt, Chris West, Waseem Bhat, Martin Taylor, Patrick Foster, and Paul Harwood

History of Previous Failed Primary Treatment

A young male patient, who was previously fit and well, presented to our department following a workplace accident where a heavy weight fell on his leg. This was an isolated, closed injury and there was no sign of compartment syndrome. Plain radiographs revealed that the patient had suffered a minimally displaced fracture of the distal tibial metadiaphysis (Fig. 32.1). A deformity of the tibia was present, and the patient was aware of this and thought it was related to a childhood injury, though he could not remember this. The fracture was well aligned and therefore the injury was managed non-operatively, initially in a long leg plaster, which was converted to a Sarmiento cast at 6 weeks post-injury and the patient allowed to weight-bear (Fig. 32.2a). It was noted that due to the pre-existing deformity there may be a propensity for the fracture to dis-

P. Nesbitt · C. West · W. Bhat · M. Taylor · P. Foster
Leeds Major Trauma Center, Leeds Teaching Hospitals, NHS, Trusts, Leeds, UK
e-mail: christopherwest@nhs.net; w.bhat@nhs.net; martin.taylor13@nhs.net; patrick.foster@nhs.net

P. Harwood (✉)
Major Trauma Centre, Leeds Teaching Hospitals NHS Trust, Leeds, UK

Department of Trauma and Orthopaedics, Clarendon Wing, Leeds General Infirmary, Leeds, UK
e-mail: paulharwood@nhs.net

place on loading and careful monitoring would be required. After 16 weeks of non-operative management, there was little evidence of fracture healing and the fracture had displaced into varus and apex posterior angulation. The position was deemed unacceptable and surgical intervention planned.

The patient was referred to the limb reconstruction service for an opinion on further management. Though there was little callus formation at the fracture, computed tomography (CT) scanning suggested there was some biological activity present. Blood tests were undertaken, including for bone biology, which were all normal. The patient again denied any significant medical history and there was nothing to suggest a pathological fracture or infection at this point. The pre-existing deformity of the tibia along with a narrow medullary canal made nailing challenging and therefore it was decided that external ring fixation would be used. This would allow correction of both the fracture displacement and pre-existing deformity, afford stability and allow fracture stimulation by distraction or compression. A Hexapod ring fixator (Smith and Nephew Taylor Spatial Frame) was applied (Fig. 32.3), and the axis gradually corrected with slight distraction, over 8 weeks (Fig. 32.4a). Standing alignment radiographs showed good restoration of the mechanical axis of the limb, but a leg length discrepancy of approximately 2.5 cm noted (Fig. 32.4b). It was felt that this was likely related

© The Author(s), under exclusive license to Springer Nature Switzerland AG 2024
P. V. Giannoudis, P. Tornetta III (eds.), *Failed Fracture Fixation*,
https://doi.org/10.1007/978-3-031-39692-2_32

Fig. 32.1 Anteroposterior (AP) and lateral radiographs of the injury at presentation

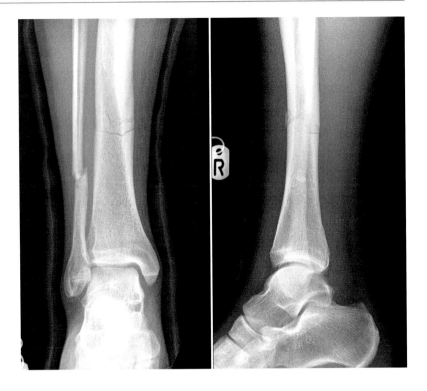

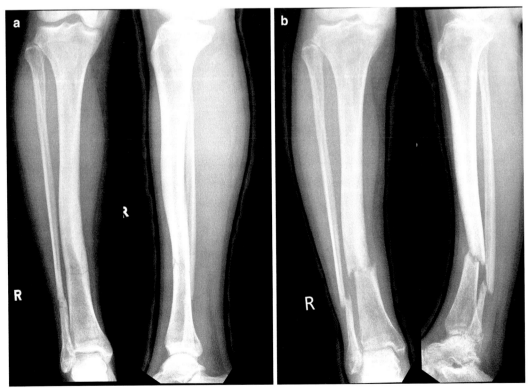

Fig. 32.2 Plain radiographs showing non-operative management, note pre-existing varus deformity of tibia and the narrow canal. (**a**) Position of the fracture immobilised in the cast. (**b**) Position following 16 weeks of treatment with non-union and displacement into varus and apex posterior

Fig. 32.3 Plain radiographs following hexapod external ring fixation

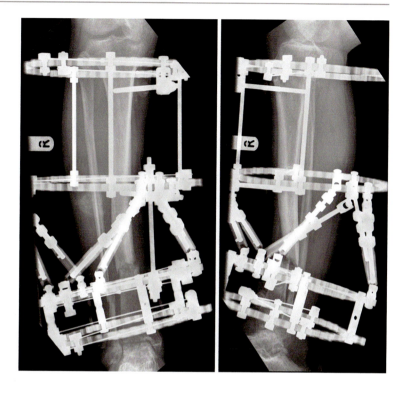

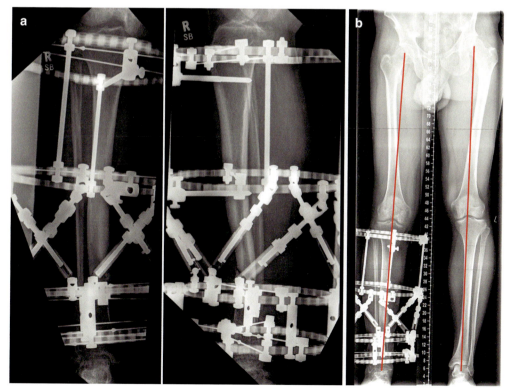

Fig. 32.4 Plain radiographs following hexapod correction. (**a**) Plain AP and lateral radiographs of the tibia showing contact and alignment restored. (**b**) Standing alignment films showing restoration of the mechanical axis. Note approximately 2.5-cm limb length discrepancy

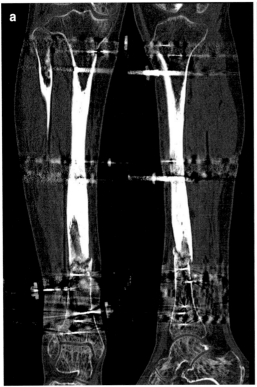

Fig. 32.5 Computed tomography following circular frame management. (**a**) After treatment in external fixation frame. (**b**) After a further 6-month treatment using LIPUS in a Sarmiento cast. Note tenuous union and adjacent cyst formation with canal occlusion

to the history of childhood injury. The fracture was monitored with expectation of progress to union. This was slow and gradual supportive distraction and compression was applied to stimulate the fracture mechanically. At 36 weeks post-injury, 20 weeks since frame application, low-intensity-pulsed ultrasound (LIPUS) (Exogen, Bioventus) treatment was commenced in a further attempt to stimulate healing. Despite these measures the fracture failed to unite, confirmed on CT scan at a year post-injury (Fig. 32.5a).

Evaluation of the Aetiology of Failure of Fixation

Clinical, Radiological and Biochemical Assessment.

A cause for the non-union was again sought. The patient confirmed that they had no relevant past or family medical history, took no medication, did not smoke or drink alcohol and ate a normal diet. A full set of laboratory blood tests were again undertaken, including a full blood count, bone profile, thyroid function tests, inflammatory markers, liver and renal function and vitamin D, which were all normal. On further questioning, the patient revealed that he has a lesion on the upper arm, which he had been due to a see specialist doctor about, though this had never happened (Fig. 32.6). On examination this was thought to represent a plexiform neurofibroma. Several small, pigmented lesions, café-au-lait spots, were also identified on the patient's back, he had previously been told these were birth marks. These cutaneous lesions alongside the deformity in the tibia, a mild anterolateral bow, and limb length discrepancy, suggested a diagnosis of neurofibromatosis type I (NF-1) with congenital pseudarthrosis of the tibia and a

Fig. 32.6 Clinical photographs showing the lesion on the patient's arm

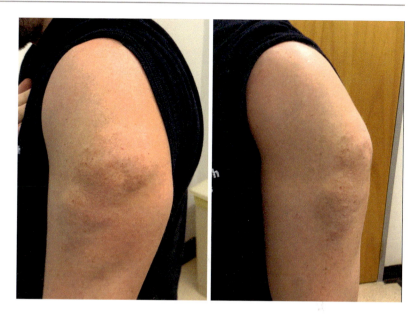

fracture. There was no spinal involvement, and the forearms and fibula were both of normal morphology. There were no axillary freckles or Lisch nodules present within the eyes. The patient was referred to a clinical geneticist for an opinion and the diagnosis confirmed on genetic testing.

Pathology of Treatment Failure

This patient was diagnosed with a late presentation of tibial pseudarthrosis and a new diagnosis of NF-1. NF-1 is caused by a single-gene mutation affecting the production of the protein neurofibromin, inherited in an autosomal dominant pattern. Historically diagnosed by clinical criteria, this has now been superseded by genetic testing [1]. Tibial pseudarthrosis is rare and is associated with NF-1 in 55% of cases. However, only 6% of those with NF-1 have a tibial pseudarthrosis [2, 3]. The pathogenesis of tibial pseudarthrosis is related to periosteal disease, causing thickening and adherence to the developing tibia. Cells with the NF-1 gene are also less responsive to biochemical mediators, namely bone morphogenetic proteins, which decreases their osteogenic potential. Specifically, osteoclasts appear to be dysfunctional and sparse, adversely affecting the balance between osteoblastic and osteoclastic activity [4]. The periosteum in tibial pseudarthrosis is inhibitory to fracture healing and invades the fracture site. Decreased cellular response to released biochemical mediators without a properly functioning periosteum means that union is rare without specific and careful surgical intervention.

In this case, though the fracture had been minimally displaced and of a relatively stable configuration, abnormalities of bone healing meant that the fracture had failed to unite by non-operative management. When this treatment failed, the fracture was realigned and stabilised by circular frame external fixation. Mechanical stimulation was applied by gradual distraction, then compression. This approach has very high success rates in aseptic non-unions, particularly following non-operative treatment [5–7]. In this case, failure to recognise the pathology again meant that the natural fracture healing mechanisms were unable to function correctly [4]. LIPUS therapy is a low-risk approach to augment fracture healing, particularly in the case of established non-unions [8]. Although no literature on the subject exists, again it is likely that the abnormalities of normal bone healing pathways present in this case led to treatment failure.

Pre-operative Planning

Treatment strategy in non-union management can be broken down into mechanical and biological considerations. Restoration of bony contact, alignment and stability provides optimal mechanics. In cases of tibial pseudarthrosis, it is necessary to excise the abnormal, inhibitory periosteum and fracture site. This alone does not guarantee success and where union does occur refracture is common. Many different treatment methods have been proposed, and to reduce refracture it is generally recommended to stabilise the fracture with combined intra- and extramedullary fixation. Biological stimulation can be provided by various means including autologous bone graft, bone morphogenetic protein (BMP) and periosteal transfer. In severe paediatric cases, generation of a cross-union to the fibula has been recommended, reducing the risk of refracture [4]. Experience and evidence of treating congenital pseudarthrosis of the tibia is based almost entirely on paediatric practice, with patients often requiring multiple surgeries and some having amputations. As most patients are treated in childhood and the condition is rare, first presentation in adults is unusual, perhaps reflected in the diagnostic difficulties seen here.

In our case this was an adult patient with relatively normal tibial morphology. Despite this there was a recalcitrant non-union with evidence of bone resorption at the fracture site. There was a pre-existing leg length discrepancy. The patient's main goal was to attain union and return to pain-free weight-bearing. Treatment options were discussed with the patient, including non-operative management in a brace, limb salvage surgery by internal or external fixation or an amputation. Though the patient carefully considered amputation, he wished a final attempt at limb salvage and did not wish further Ilizarov treatment. It was not felt that cross-union would be necessary to prevent refracture, given the amount of normal bone stock available. It was therefore agreed that we would excise the fracture site, shorten the tibia and stabilise by internal fixation. A Masquelet technique to retain length was considered but rejected on the basis that this

was likely to be a high-risk non-union and leaving a critical bone defect would increase the risk of treatment failure. It was instead planned to later restore leg length by femoral or tibial callus distraction or contralateral shortening, should union of the distal tibial fracture be attained.

Excision of the abnormal tissue at the fracture site would result in a transverse osteotomy site in the distal tibia. Its morphology along with soft tissue excision and shortening would render this site without any inherent stability. Furthermore, this site was likely to be slow to unite with a high risk of refracture. Internal fixation using a combination of an intramedullary nail and a distal tibial locking plate in compression was planned to afford maximal stability for union and reinforce the united bone to reduce the risk of refracture. A paediatric nail was to be used (GAP Nail, PEGA Medical) due to the narrow canal diameter and abnormal tibial morphology. The nature of non-union in tibial pseudoarthrosis along with removal of periosteum impairs bone healing. It was therefore planned to biologically augment the fracture site using a combination of autologous bone graft, bone marrow aspirate concentrate, platelet-rich plasma, a BMP-2 sponge and free-vascularised periosteal graft [9–11]. This combination was felt to afford a good chance of success by addressing all facets required for union [12]. It was planned to obtain bone graft by reamer-irrigator-aspirator (RIA) harvest from the contralateral femur [13]. It is noteworthy that use of the BMP-2 sponge in long bone non-union is currently off licence and the patient was counselled as such.

Revision Surgery

To allow the Ilizarov pin sites to heal and reduce the associated risk of infection on further surgical intervention, the circular frame was removed in the outpatient's clinic and the patient's limb immobilised in a cast. Whilst plans were made for surgery, the COVID-19 pandemic occurred, limiting access to healthcare. The patient remained comfortable in the cast and content for surgery to be delayed; the LIPUS treatment was therefore continued over this period. Six months later, though plain radiographs suggested some progress to union, a CT scan showed only very minor bridging at the fracture with adjacent osteolysis and cyst formation alongside canal sclerosis, consistent with the diagnosis. The patient remained symptomatic, and it was therefore agreed to proceed with surgery to correct deformity and stimulate bony healing. A pre-operative deformity correction was planned using templating software, which predicted that approximately 25 mm of further shortening would be required following excision of the non-union and adjacent abnormal bone along with a 15° closing wedge osteotomy from the current position (Fig. 32.7). This showed that intramedullary fixation should be feasible.

At surgery, RIA graft and bone marrow aspirate concentrate (BMAC) were obtained from the contralateral femur and the iliac crest, respectively. An anterior approach to the distal tibia was undertaken using the interval between the tibialis anterior and extensor hallucis longus. The anterior tibial neurovascular bundle was identified and protected as recipient vessels for later microvascular anastomosis. A transpatellar tendon approach was undertaken to allow access for the nail entry site. The non-union site was excised en bloc to healthy bleeding bone allowing angular correction of the tibial deformity by closing the wedge according to the pre-operative plan. Abnormal periosteum was excised along with this, with circumferential extension beyond the bony resection for approximately 1.5–2 cm proximally and distally, ensuring retained periosteum was morphologically normal beyond this margin. The medullary canal was occluded at the resection margin though the bone appeared vascular-

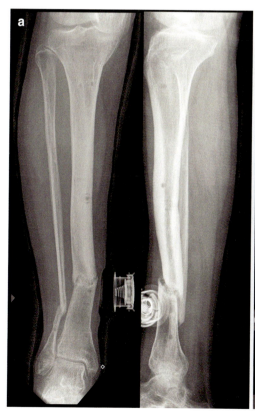
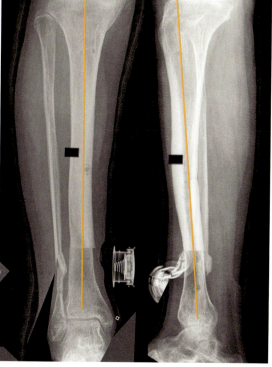

Fig. 32.7 Pre-operative planning. (**a**) Plain radiographs of non-union. (**b**) A pre-operative plan with approximately 2.5-cm shortening including closing wedge osteotomy. Orange line shows the planned course of intramedullary fixation

ised and healthy. A guidewire was used to perforate this, and further canal preparation undertaken by a combination of antegrade and retrograde techniques. A "Poller" blocking wire was placed to control reaming at the deformity site to allow nail passage according to the preoperative deformity correction plan. The guidewire was then passed to the distal segment and reaming completed to 8.5 mm and a 6.4-mm intramedullary nail passed (GAP Nail, PEGA Medical). Correction of the tibial axis was confirmed, and a long anterolateral locking plate was contoured to fit and applied with multidirectional locking screws distally around the nail (EVOS plate, Smith and Nephew). This was then applied proximally in compression and fixation completed, again with multidirectional locking screws avoiding the nail. The nail was then locked proximally and distally completing fixation. Stability was confirmed clinically. Intraoperative steps are shown in Fig. 32.8.

The medial distal femur was approached and the descending and superomedial genicular arteries dissected and followed to the medial femoral condyle. A corticoperiosteal flap was elevated from the medial femoral condyle and raised based upon a branch of the descending genicular artery. Microvascular anastomosis was undertaken end to end onto the anterior tibial artery and veins. Autologous bone graft was mixed with BMAC, platelet-rich plasma (PRP) and a small volume of graft expander (Vitoss, Stryker Medical). This was placed around the non-union site along with a BMP-2 sponge (Infuse, MedTronic). The periosteal graft was then wrapped around this and inset using bone anchors to hold it in place to the tibia and all wounds closed. The patient's limb was supported in a below-knee back slab, largely to prevent ankle movement and protect the wounds.

The patient's post-operative course was unremarkable. The limb was supported in a remov-

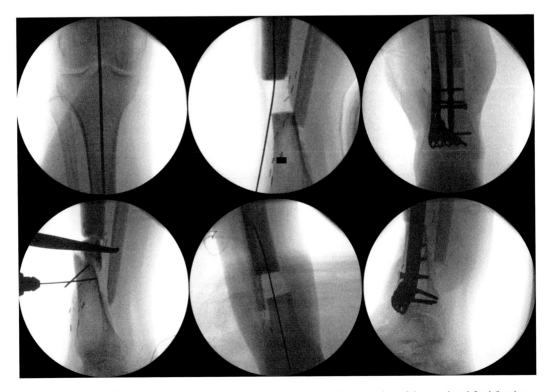

Fig. 32.8 Intraoperative fluoroscopy imaging showing planning of resection, opening of the canal and final fixation

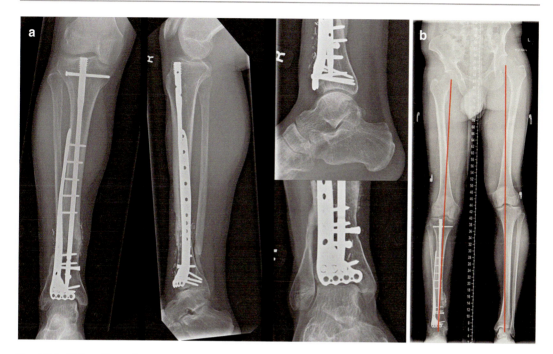

Fig. 32.9 Plain radiographs at 2 years post-surgery. (**a**) AP and lateral radiographs showing good alignment and evidence of union. (**b**) Standing alignment films showing restoration of the mechanical axis and a leg length discrepancy of around 4.5–5 cm

able walker boot from 2 weeks post-operatively, and toe-touch weight-bearing allowed with physiotherapy supervision. This was progressed to weight-bearing as tolerated at 6 weeks. The patient remained pain free on weight-bearing and at 3 months post-surgery he was allowed to remove the walker boot. Gradual return to normal activities was undertaken over the next 6 months. By 7 months post-surgery, bridging callus was visible across the non-union site and by 12 months this appeared to be remodelling and maturing. At the most recent follow-up (2 years), the patient had returned to the gym, he had pain-free mobility and good range of motion in the knee and ankle. He was aware of a 4- to 5-cm leg length discrepancy and plans were made to correct this by ipsilateral femoral lengthening or contralateral tibial shortening. The patient's function with a shoe raise at this point was good and he wished to defer this. Radiographs appeared to show solid union with no signs of hardware failure (Fig. 32.9).

Summary: Lessons Learned

This was a challenging case notwithstanding the benign appearance of the initial presentation. There were significant delays in determining the underlying pathology, despite repeated careful history taking and repeated investigation, which could have been apparent from the outset and throughout treatment. The patient did not relate the lesion on his arm to the tibial fracture and therefore did not share it. The explanation of the tibial deformity by the patient was accepted, though on discussion with his parents in hindsight, no specific injury was recalled. This highlights the need for repeated careful history taking, particularly in cases of recalcitrant non-union, which eventually secured the diagnosis. It is critical to identify the cause of non-union before treatment, the authors prefer to use the approach of considering mechanical and biological factors, the latter being local and systemic. In this case, a local biological factor significantly contributing to the non-union, resulting from a systemic condition, was not ascertained prior to the second cycle of treatment, led to its failure. This resulted in significant delays in returning the patient to function and additional treatment costs.

Once the correct diagnosis was made, careful multidisciplinary planning was undertaken including specialists from orthopaedic limb reconstruction, paediatric orthopaedics and plastic reconstructive surgery. This allowed a combined approach and successful intervention in a single stage without complication. We would recommend that all complex non-unions are treated in specialist centres where such expertise is available.

References

1. Neurofibromatosis, N. I. H. Conference statement. National Institutes of Health Consensus development conference. Arch Neurol. 1988;45:575–8.
2. O'Donnell C, Foster J, Mooney R, Beebe C, Donaldson N, Heare T. Congenital pseudarthrosis of the tibia. JBJS Rev. 2017;5:e3.
3. Wallace M. Pseudarthrosis of the tibia. In: Eltorai AEM, Eberson CP, Daniels AH, editors. Orthopedic surgery clerkship: a quick reference guide for senior medical students. Cham: Springer International Publishing; 2017. p. 635–8.
4. Paley D. Congenital pseudarthrosis of the tibia: biological and biomechanical considerations to achieve union and prevent refracture. J Children's Orthop. 2019;13:120–33.
5. Ferreira N, Marais L, Aldous C. Management of tibial non-unions: Prospective evaluation of a comprehensive treatment algorithm. SA Orthop J. 2016;15:60–6.
6. Kocaoğlu M, Eralp L, Sen C, Cakmak M, Dincyürek H, Göksan SB. Management of stiff hypertrophic nonunions by distraction osteogenesis: a report of 16 cases. J Orthop Trauma. 2003;17:543–8.
7. Szelerski Ł, Pajchert-Kozłowska A, Żarek S, Górski R, Małdyk P, Morasiewicz P. The outcomes of Ilizarov treatment in aseptic nonunions of the tibia stratified by treatment strategies and surgical techniques. Sci Rep. 2020;10:20511.
8. Zura R, Della Rocca GJ, Mehta S, Harrison A, Brodie C, Jones J, et al. Treatment of chronic (>1 year) fracture nonunion: heal rate in a cohort of 767 patients treated with low-intensity pulsed ultrasound (LIPUS). Injury. 2015;46:2036–41.
9. Chahla J, Mannava S, Cinque ME, Geeslin AG, Codina D, LaPrade RF. Bone marrow aspirate concentrate harvesting and processing technique. Arthrosc Tech. 2017;6:e441–e5.
10. Haubruck P, Tanner MC, Vlachopoulos W, Hagelskamp S, Miska M, Ober J, et al. Comparison of the clinical effectiveness of Bone Morphogenic Protein (BMP) -2 and −7 in the adjunct treatment of lower limb nonunions. Orthop Traumatol Surg Res. 2018;104:1241–8.
11. Thabet AM, Paley D, Kocaoglu M, Eralp L, Herzenberg JE, Ergin ON. Periosteal grafting for congenital pseudarthrosis of the tibia: a preliminary report. Clin Orthop Relat Res. 2008;466:2981–94.
12. Andrzejowski P, Giannoudis PV. The 'diamond concept' for long bone non-union management. J Orthop Traumatol. 2019;20:21.
13. Cox G, Jones E, McGonagle D, Giannoudis PV. Reamer-irrigator-aspirator indications and clinical results: a systematic review. Int Orthop. 2011;35:951–6.

Distal Tibial Extra-Articular Intramedullary Nail Failed Fixation

33

Michael J. Price and Peter V. Giannoudis

History of Previous Primary Failed Treatment

A 60-year-old man was admitted to a regional trauma centre after being struck by a moving vehicle. He had a medical history remarkable for schizophrenia, was independently ambulant prior to this incident and a non-smoker. Trauma primary and secondary surveys revealed an isolated left distal-third tibial and same-level fibular fracture, with the distal end of the proximal tibial fragment protruding through a 4-cm curvilinear anteromedial shin wound (Fig. 33.1). Distal pulses were intact, with preserved sensation. He was managed with wound dressing and broad-spectrum antimicrobial prophylaxis as per open fracture guidelines [1], and an above-knee plaster backslab applied following initial reduction in the emergency department.

He underwent primary surgery on a combined orthoplastic operating list within 24 h of presentation, at which the wound was debrided and the tibial fracture stabilised using a static-locked Synthes Expert intramedullary nail through a medial parapatellar approach (Fig. 33.2). His wound was primarily closed with the addition of a split skin graft harvested from the contralateral calf. Postoperative diagnosis was of a Gustilo-Anderson grade II injury [2].

The patient was placed into a below-knee plaster for 2 weeks following the index operation, and no early metalwork complications were observed on the radiographs at his first (4 weeks post-surgery) clinic review. By the eighth postoperative week there was evident callus formation at the tibial and fibular fracture sites on radiographs, but the nail had fractured at the level of the distal locking screws and the tibial fracture collapsed into flexion with valgus deformity (Fig. 33.3).

M. J. Price
Academic Department of Trauma and Orthopaedics, Leeds General Infirmary University Hospital, School of Medicine, University of Leeds, Leeds, UK
e-mail: m.j.price@doctors.org.uk

P. V. Giannoudis (✉)
Academic Department of Trauma and Orthopaedics, School of Medicine, University of Leeds, Leeds, UK

NIHR Leeds Biomedical Research Center, Chapel Allerton Hospital, Leeds, UK

© The Author(s), under exclusive license to Springer Nature Switzerland AG 2024
P. V. Giannoudis, P. Tornetta III (eds.), *Failed Fracture Fixation*,
https://doi.org/10.1007/978-3-031-39692-2_33

Fig. 33.1 Initial left tibia injury radiographs: (**a**) anteroposterior (AP) and (**b**) lateral radiographs showing the fracture sustained

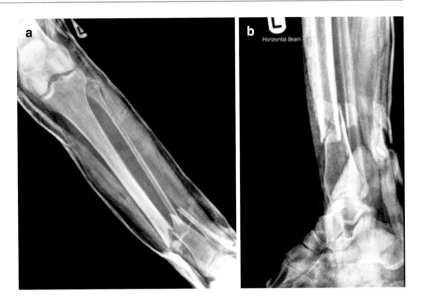

Fig. 33.2 Left tibia (lateral and AP) post-operative radiographs

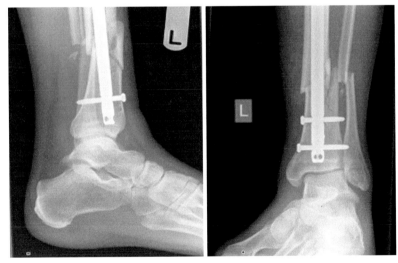

Fig. 33.3 Left tibia AP and lateral radiographs showing failure of fixation at 8 weeks post-operatively

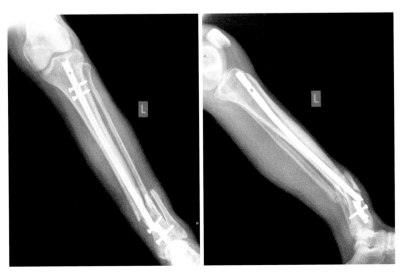

Evaluation of the Aetiology of Failure of Fixation

The post-operative radiographs (Fig. 33.2) demonstrate that the fracture was fixed into valgus, procurvatum and shortening. Moreover, the proximal distal locking screw was inserted near the original fracture line. Consequently, the abnormal biomechanical loading and inherent fracture instability led to a stress riser and failure of the nail at the level of the proximal distal locking screw level.

Clinical Examination

An 8-week post-operative review found the flexion and valgus deformity at the fracture site described above. Approximately 50% of the split-thickness skin graft had taken, particularly around the perimeter of the original defect, but there was a sizeable granuloma within the wound bed and a discharging sinus as evident in the attached clinical photographs (Fig. 33.4). The skin around the perimeter was indurated and cellulitic, with golden-coloured crusted exudate from the sinus. Distal neurovascular function remained intact, and the patient had remained systemically well.

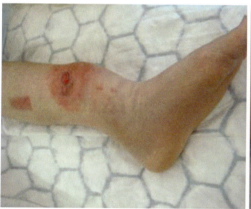
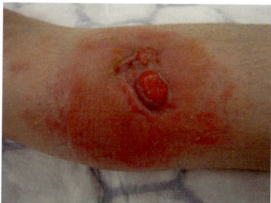

Fig. 33.4 Left tibia photographs showing redness and discharging sinus

Diagnostic-Biochemical and Radiological Investigations

Skin swabs taken from the split-thickness skin graft site between the first and second post-operative clinic reviews yielded skin commensals and a variety of enteric flora including gram-negative bacilli. Swabs taken from the discharging sinus at the third clinical review, however, yielded heavy growth of flucloxacillin-sensitive *Staphylococcus aureus*. Serial monitoring of serum inflammatory markers at the 3 post-operative reviews showed persistently elevated C-reactive protein levels of 18.7, 25 and 24, respectively. The plain radiographs taken were adequate on this occasion to allow us to evaluate the underlying problem. Computed tomography (CT) scan acquisition can help further to assess the state of the bone and the presence of sequestrum.

Preoperative Planning

Salvage options for the patient were discussed in a multidisciplinary limb reconstruction team meeting before offering revision surgery. The technique chosen was the two-stage Masquelet procedure [3].

The first stage involves radical debridement of infected tissue, and in the case of revision procedures, may require explantation of failed or infected metalwork. The resulting bone defect is then packed with polymethylmethacrylate (PMMA), enveloping both proximal and distal bone ends in order to limit fibrous ingrowth into the defect and allow the resultant endothelial membrane to span the bony zone of injury. There is fair evidence to support the addition of antibiotics to the cement for the promotion of membrane formation [4]. Internal or external bridging skeletal stabilisation should be undertaken at this stage, to render a sufficiently low-strain environment conducive to endothelial membrane formation. Any required reconstitution or reconstruction of the soft tissue envelope should also be performed at this stage, so as to minimise disruption of the fracture environment at the second stage.

Meticulous attention must then be paid to optimisation of patients' medical comorbidities, which might otherwise be deleterious to healing, such as diabetes mellitus and systemic infection.

The second stage involves approach to the fracture site between 6 and 8 weeks later, through the original incisions if possible, so as to limit disruption to the soft tissue envelope and fracture environment within. The delicate endothelial membrane is incised longitudinally and carefully elevated to facilitate extrication of the cement spacer. This leaves a defined cavity, termed a 'biological chamber', for the containment of bone graft. If there are signs of infection at this stage then repeat local debridement should be performed and tissue samples obtained to guide microbiological management, before placement of a new PMMA spacer and plan for antibiotics pending rescheduled the second stage.

Alternative surgical techniques to Masquelet may include bone transport using fine-wire circular frame fixation, vascular fibular autograft, bony allograft or cancellous bony autograft without prior membrane induction implanted in an aseptic environment.

Choices Behind Implant Selection

The presence of a wound sinus, raised inflammatory markers and positive bacterial wound swabs in this case prompted the decision to perform temporising external skeletal stabilisation with debridement at the first stage so as to facilitate adequate eradication of infection. Particular attention must then be paid to the external fixator pin sites pending the second stage, as these are a source of local infection, although consensus is yet to be reached on the optimal techniques to minimise this risk [5].

The decision to use internal fixation for definitive fracture to bridge the graft site was made in preference to prolonged ongoing treatment in an external fixation device as originally described [6]. This can take the form of the locking plate or intramedullary nail fixation, the former having the advantage in being able to more fully utilise the extensive incision required for radical debridement of infection, and advantages of the latter including a reduction in the volume of bone graft required to fill the bone defect.

Need for Bone Grafting

The Diamond Concept [7] sets out considerations for optimal healing in long bone fractures: mechanical stability must be achieved in a timely fashion to create a sufficiently low-strain environment with a competent vascular supply. A combined medical and surgical approach is required in order to eradicate infection and to optimise any comorbidities, which may be otherwise deleterious to healing.

Osteogenesis is facilitated by osteoinductive mediators such as commercially available bone morphogenetic protein 2 (BMP-2) [8] and autologous platelet-rich plasma (PRP). PRP can be obtained from 60 mL of peripheral blood, which is concentrated to 7 mL prior to implantation. This may also be supplemented by bone marrow aspirate concentrate (BMAC). The latter is especially useful for frail patients and those with otherwise impaired regenerative potential, as in this particular case.

Cancellous autograft may be obtained either from the iliac crest, or through use of the reamer-irrigation-aspirator (RIA) system as was chosen in this case. This involves antegrade reaming of the femoral shaft as for an intramedullary nail but with a suction aspirator unit to collect the cancellous reamings and marrow. Care must be taken to progress slowly, withdrawing the RIA unit in between each advance of 2–3 cm to prevent blockage of the instruments and reduce the risk of thermal osteonecrosis to the femoral shaft.

Revision Surgery

The first stage was performed 12 weeks after primary intramedullary fixation of the fracture and involved explantation of the intramedullary nail through its original medial parapatellar wound. The tibial shaft was reamed out to ensure clearance of infection, and reaming samples sent for

microbiological inspection. The sinus extending down to the site of non-union was excised and soft tissues debrided by the combined orthoplastic surgical team, and devitalised bone was removed along with invaginated fibrous tissue from the bone ends and deep tissue samples for microbiology (Fig. 33.5). Antibiotic-impregnated PMMA cement was then moulded into place at the site of the bone defect, with a surgical glove filled with cool saline used to shield the adjacent soft tissues from the exothermic reaction as the PMMA cured. Temporising skeletal fixation was achieved with the application of an external fixator spanning the ankle joint, and the wound closed primarily (Fig. 33.6).

The patient was seen in the clinic at 4, 6 and 8 weeks following the first-stage surgery, during which time they continued to take oral flucloxacillin for laboratory-proven methicillin-sensitive *Staphylococcus aureus* (MSSA) found in bone, marrow, reaming and soft tissue samples. External fixation pin sites remained clean and healthy, and no displacement of the cement spacer was seen on interim radiographs.

The second-stage procedure was performed 8 weeks after the first, in keeping with the principles set out as above. Autologous graft was harvested first, with RIA reaming to a diameter of 13 mm through the right femoral piriformis fossa and 15cc of cancellous bone and blood harvested from the right iliac crest. The external fixator was removed and the tibial wound re-incised longitudinally, beneath which the Masquelet membrane was found to have formed successfully around the surface of the PMMA spacer. This was carefully incised longitudinally, the cement explanted and further deep tissue samples sent for microbiology (Fig. 33.7). If there had been macroscopic evidence of infection at this stage, a new cement spacer would have been placed and the wounds closed to resume antimicrobial suppression therapy until such a time as the second stage could be reattempted.

The RIA-harvested autograft was supplemented with bone morphogenetic protein (BMP) and it was implanted in the defect area (Fig. 33.8) and the membrane was then closed without tension. Definitive fracture stabilisation was

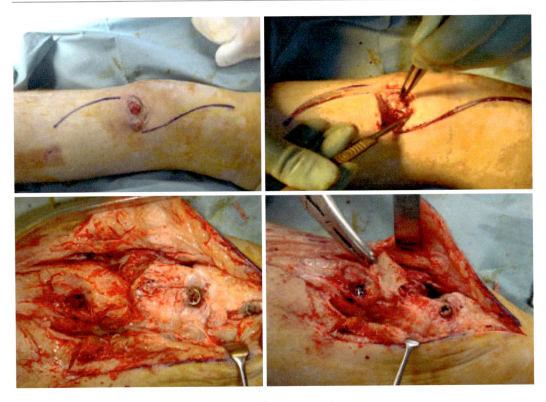

Fig. 33.5 Intraoperative debridement of soft tissue and fracture non-union

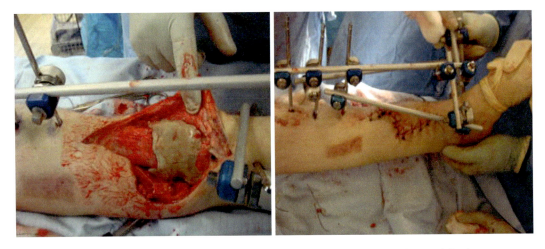

Fig. 33.6 Insertion of the PMMA spacer and after primary wound closure application of external fixation

achieved using a distally locked plate to bridge the graft site and the tibial wound was then closed in a meticulous tension-free fashion (Fig. 33.9). Intravenous flucloxacillin continued post-operatively until the second set of deep tissue samples returned clear from microbiology.

The patient was seen for wound review at 2 weeks post-operatively, and radiographs were performed, which demonstrated no early complications associated with the metalwork. He received low-molecular-weight heparin thromboprophylaxis for 12 weeks when he started mobil-

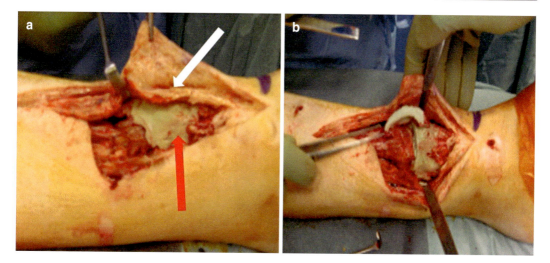

Fig. 33.7 (a) Demonstration of induced membrane (white arrow) and the PMMA spacer (red arrow); (b) excision of the PMMA spacer

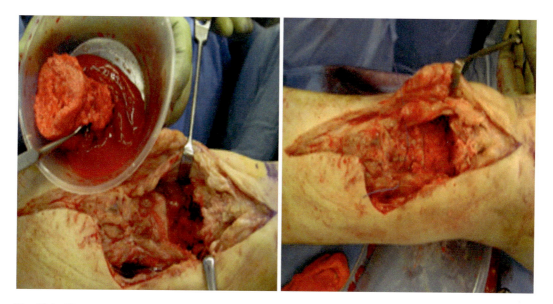

Fig. 33.8 Placement of augmented bone graft into the induced membrane cavity

ising partial weight-bearing. By 16 weeks after the second stage, the patient was able to bear weight comfortably fully with the aid of a walking frame and with satisfactory range of ankle joint movement and by 6 months no support was required. Clinical and radiological bone union was complete at 9 months of follow-up (Fig. 33.10). These findings were reflective of other reports in the literature, where authors have reported a median time to radiographic consolidation of around 218 and 232 days to full weight-bearing [6].

A separate retrospective study involving 61 tibial defects treated using the Masquelet technique found an 86% union rate with a mean time to union of 14.6 months, noting that this was independent of the size of bone defect (which were up to 230-mm length in the tibia) [9].

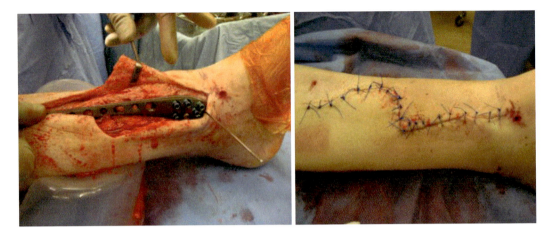

Fig. 33.9 Internal fixation with a locking plate and tension-free wound closure

Fig. 33.10 Left tibia AP and lateral radiographs demonstrating union at 12 months

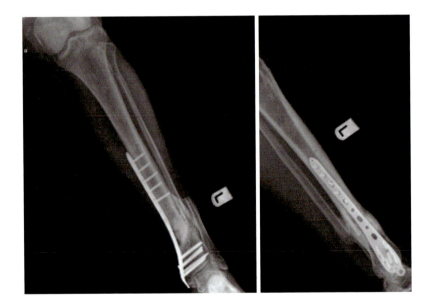

Lessons Learned

This case summarises the aetiology of failure of a distal tibia extra-articular fracture that was managed with reamed IM nailing. Due to poor reduction, malalignment (valgus) and abnormal loading, the failure of fixation was quite early. The subsequent development of infection required careful evaluation and planning. The safest approach on this occasion was felt to proceed with revision surgery using the two-stage Masquelet technique. Such a strategy can be considered by the surgeons when they are dealing with similar situations.

References

1. British Orthopaedic Association & British Association of Plastic, Reconstructive & Aesthetic Surgeons Audit Standards for Trauma: Open Fractures. https://www.boa.ac.uk/resources/boast-4-pdf.html, accessed 19.10.22.

2. Kim PH, Leopold SS. Gustilo-Anderson classification. Clin Orthop Relat Res. 2012;470(11):3270–4.
3. Masquelet AC, Giannoudis PV. The induced membrane technique for treatment of bone defects: what have I learned? Trauma Case Rep. 2021;36:100556.
4. Masquelet A, Kanakaris NK, Obert L, Stafford P, Giannoudis PV. Bone repair using the Masquelet technique. J Bone Joint Surg Am. 2019;101:1024–36.
5. Lethaby A, Temple J, Santy-Tomlinson J. Pin site care for preventing infections associated with external bone fixators and pins. Cochrane Database Syst Rev. 2013;(12):CD004551.
6. Olesen UK, Eckardt H, Bosemark P, Paulsen AW, Dahl B, Hede A. The Masquelet technique of induced membrane for healing of bone defects. A review of 8 cases. Injury. 2015;46(S8):S44–7.
7. Andrzejowski P, Giannoudis PV. The 'diamond concept' for long bone non-union management. J Orthop Traumatol. 2019;20(1):21. https://doi.org/10.1186/s10195-019-0528-0.
8. Pelissier P, Masquelet AC, Bareille R, Pelissier SM, Amedee J. Induced membranes secrete growth factors including vascular and osteoinductive factors and could stimulate bone regeneration. J Orthop Res. 2004;22(1):73–9. https://doi.org/10.1016/S0736-0266(03)00165-7.
9. Karger C, Kishi T, Schneider L, Fitoussi F, Masquelet AC, the French Society of Orthopaedic Surgery and Traumatology (SoFCOT). Treatment of posttraumatic bone defects by the induced membrane technique. Rev Chirurgie Orthop Traumatol. 2012;98(1):81–7.

Distal Tibia Extra-Articular Plating Failed Fixation

34

Zoe B. Cheung and Philip R. Wolinsky

History of Previous Primary Failed Treatment

For extra-articular distal tibia fractures, two common fixation options are plate fixation and intramedullary nailing (IMN). While an IMN is the standard for treatment of midshaft tibia fractures, its use in distal tibia fractures is challenging due to technical difficulties avoiding fracture malalignment and achieving adequate fixation in the short distal segment [1–3]. Open plate fixation of distal tibia fractures can involve extensive soft tissue dissection with the associated risks of wound complications and infection [1–3]. Minimally invasive plate osteosynthesis (MIPO) is a potential alternative, 'biologically friendly' plating technique aimed at minimizing soft tissue disruption, but soft tissue complications in the acute setting remain a concern [4]. Thus, there remains a lack of consensus regarding the optimal treatment for distal tibia fractures.

A 42-year-old man with no significant medical history sustained an isolated, Grade IIIA open injury to his left tibia after he was struck by a metal cap that burst off under high pressure from a water pipe. Examination of his left leg demonstrated a 4 × 2-cm open wound over the anteromedial aspect of the distal tibia, as well as a small open wound over his medial malleolus. He did not have any neurovascular deficits. Radiographic evaluation revealed comminuted fractures of his distal tibia and fibula without any intra-articular extension (Fig. 34.1). He received intravenous antibiotics in the emergency department and was taken urgently to the operating room.

After operative debridement of the open fracture, he had a 6-cm bone defect in his distal tibia. He underwent plate fixation of the distal tibia and fibula with placement of an antibiotic polymethylmethacrylate (PMMA) spacer in the bone defect (Fig. 34.2). Ten weeks after the index procedure, he was brought back to the operating room for removal of his antibiotic PMMA spacer and autogenous bone grafting obtained using a reamer/irrigator/aspirator (RIA) technique from the ipsilateral femur (Fig. 34.3). However, 11 months after the bone grafting procedure, he continued to have persistent pain over his fracture that was exacerbated by standing and ambulation. Radiographs demonstrated that despite some areas of interval healing, there was evidence of non-union in the distal tibia with non-circumferential healing (Fig. 34.4). There was no malalignment and no broken hardware.

Z. B. Cheung · P. R. Wolinsky (✉)
University of California, Davis,
Sacramento, CA, USA

© The Author(s), under exclusive license to Springer Nature Switzerland AG 2024
P. V. Giannoudis, P. Tornetta III (eds.), *Failed Fracture Fixation*,
https://doi.org/10.1007/978-3-031-39692-2_34

Fig. 34.1 Initial injury radiographs demonstrating comminuted fractures of the distal tibia and fibula

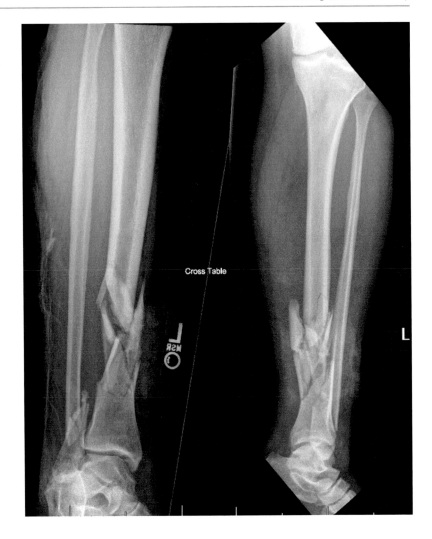

Fig. 34.2 Postoperative radiographs after the index procedure with plate fixation and placement of an antibiotic PMMA spacer in the tibial bone defect

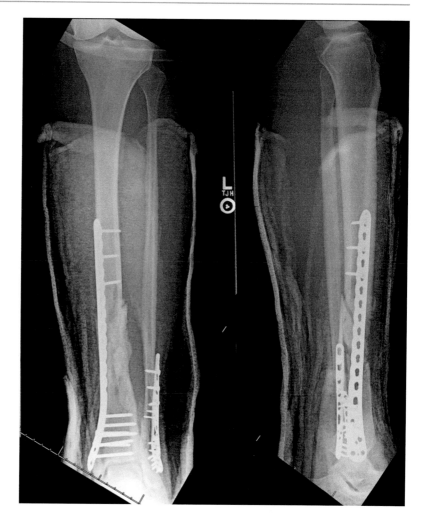

Fig. 34.3 Postoperative radiographs after removal of the antibiotic PMMA spacer and autogenous bone grafting

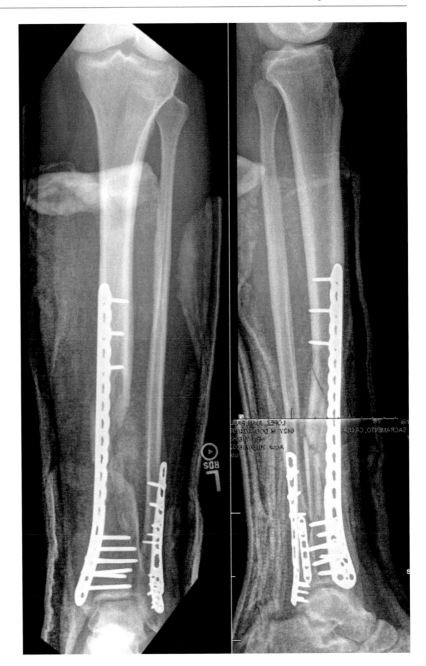

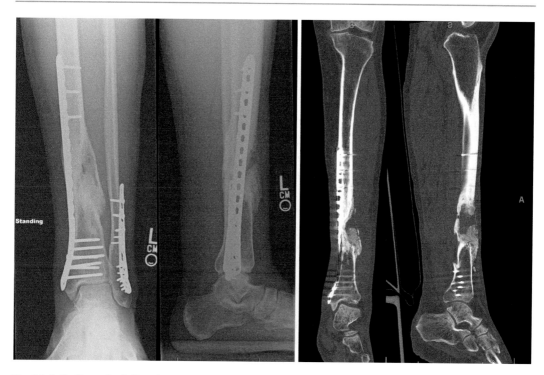

Fig. 34.4 Radiographs (left) and CT (right) obtained at 11 months after surgery illustrating an oligotrophic nonunion with non-circumferential healing with a residual bone defect

Evaluation of the Aetiology of Failure of Fixation

A variety of factors have been identified that may contribute towards impaired fracture healing and resultant non-union. Some of these factors are within the surgeon's control, while others are not. In this case, the patient sustained a high-energy, open injury that predisposed him to an impaired bone healing response. The degree of injury to bone and surrounding soft tissues has a significant influence on the potential for fracture healing. Specifically, the risk of fracture non-union has been shown to rise with increasing energy of injury [5]. The incidence of non-union has been reported to approach 15% for open fractures with an extensive soft tissue injury [5].

Mechanistically, a high-energy injury is associated with greater damage to the bone with devascularization that reduces its inherent capacity to heal and form new bone. Immediate cell death, cell death via apoptosis and bone loss from trauma or surgical debridement are other potential mechanisms that contribute to non-unions. Damage to surrounding soft tissues and periosteal stripping further reduces the ability to generate a normal bone healing response. Specifically, for diaphyseal tibia fractures, higher rates of delayed union and non-union have been observed after open fractures compared with closed fractures, regardless of fixation method [6].

This patient's high-energy, open injury was therefore a significant predisposing factor that likely contributed to subsequent non-union.

The specific location of fracture also influences the potential for bone healing. The distal diaphyseal region of the tibia is relatively hypovascular with few extraosseous blood vessels. [7] This relatively poor blood supply predisposes to delayed bone healing. MIPO plating techniques for distal tibia fractures attempt to decrease soft tissue disruption and devascularization in order to maintain a more biologically favourable environment for bone healing. [8] However, these techniques are not necessarily feasible in the setting of a high-energy, open fractures. In this patient, disruption of the extraosseous blood supply at the time of injury, as well as during subsequent plating osteosynthesis. May have contributed to impaired bone healing and the development of a distal tibia non-union.

The role of host factors as it relates to non-union is also important to consider when evaluating the aetiology of fixation failure. Specifically, major comorbidities that have been strongly associated with non-union include smoking, diabetes and vascular disease. This patient did not have any of these specific risk factors.

Clinical Examination

On examination, the anterior and medial incisions over his tibia, as well as the lateral incision over his fibula, were well healed. The percutaneous incisions that had been used for proximal fixation in the medial tibial plate were also well healed. There were no clinical signs of infection. The skin over his anterior incision was mobile. He had tenderness to palpation over the distal third of his tibia, but no detectible motion at the fracture site. He did not have any neurovascular deficits and ambulated with a slightly antalgic gait.

Diagnostic-Biochemical and Radiological investigations

Given concern for a non-union based on his clinical examination, a metal-suppression computed tomography (CT) scan with two-dimensional and three-dimensional reformats was obtained. CT imaging demonstrated healing of the posterolateral cortex, but persistence of residual gap and bone defect in the distal tibia with sclerotic bone edges (Fig. 34.4). The distal fibula fracture was healed. This is consistent with non-circumferential healing and an oligotrophic non-union of the distal tibia.

To evaluate for the possibility of infection, his diagnostic workup included inflammatory mark-

ers. An erythrocyte sedimentation rate (ESR) and C-reactive protein (CRP) were obtained, and both were within normal limits. The final results from intraoperative cultures taken at the time of his one grafting procedure 1 year prior were reviewed and confirmed to be negative. These diagnostic findings, along with his benign clinical examination, were suggestive of an aseptic non-union.

Preoperative Planning

A comprehensive treatment algorithm is needed to optimize management of distal tibia non-unions. These are challenging problems due to the short distal segment and proximity to the ankle joint. Furthermore, a healthy respect for the tenuous soft tissue envelope is required to avoid potentially catastrophic wound complications. The patient in this case had an aseptic, oligotrophic non-union of the distal tibia with a residual bone defect and no associated deformity. Preoperative planning for an oligotrophic non-union should address the deficiency in bone contact through mechanical or biological techniques, or a combination of both.

Careful preoperative planning is essential for successful treatment of non-union. Preoperative planning for removal of the existing plate fixation in this case included having the universal screw removal set readily available in the event of encountering stripped, broken or cold-welded screws. Other instruments that were available to aid in hardware removal if needed included osteotomes, needle nose pliers and a carbide drill bit or diamond-tipped burr.

New implant selection should focus on increasing and optimizing mechanical stability in order to improve the mechanical environment for bone healing. Less rigid forms of fixation, such as a bridge plate or a loose-fitting intramedullary nail in the metaphysis, provide lower mechanical stability. For reconstruction of non-unions, implants that provide more rigid fixation are preferred, such as a compression plate or a snug fitting intramedullary nail in the diaphysis. If additional mechanical stability is still deemed necessary after revision to a new implant, consideration can then be given to augmentation with a second implant.

In this case, the patient had an extra-articular distal tibia non-union after failed bridge plating with a residual bone defect and non-circumferential healing. In order to improve mechanical stability, conversion to a diaphyseal fitting intramedullary nail was selected. Reamed, locked intramedullary nailing has been shown to be effective in treating non-unions in the distal one-fourth of the tibia [9]. Furthermore, given the patient's non-circumferential healing, placement of an intramedullary nail would fill the central void such that bone healing may be able to proceed in a more napkin ring fashion without the need for central bone graft incorporation.

To address this patient's bone defect, open bone grafting was indicated. Oligotrophic non-unions are intermediate in their biological capacity for fracture healing. It is therefore prudent to improve the biological environment in conjunction with optimizing the mechanical environment.

Autogenous bone graft is considered the gold standard in the treatment of delayed union and non-union. It possesses osteoconductive, osteoinductive and osteogenic properties, while having the lowest risk of immunological rejection [10]. However, when considering autogenous bone graft harvest, it is important to recognize that there is associated donor-site morbidity [11]. An overall 8.6% rate of complications has been reported, including infection, prolonged wound drainage, large hematomas, reoperation, prolonged pain and sensory loss [11]. Furthermore, the amount of autograft available varies depending on donor site and may not be ideal for certain patient populations [12].

The medullary canal of long bones represents a potential source of cancellous autograft. The RIA technique yields autograft with osteogenic and osteoinductive properties. When compared with iliac crest bone graft (ICBG), RIA has been shown to have comparable fracture union rates, but with lower postoperative pain scores at the donor site [13, 14]. The RIA technique has the additional advantage of being able to harvest potentially larger volumes of autograft compared with anterior ICBG harvest [14]. It is therefore a good reliable option to consider for autogenous bone grafting.

In the setting of non-union, augmentation of bone grafting with growth factors such as bone morphogenetic proteins (BMPs) can also be considered. BMPs consist of cytokines within the transforming growth factor beta (TGF-β) superfamily, each of which has varying degrees of osteoinductive properties. Currently, the only BMP with FDA approval for use in a fracture setting is recombinant human BMP-2 (rhBMP-2). Specifically, rhBMP-2 is approved for use in open tibial shaft fractures in skeletally mature patients treated with intramedullary nail fixation within 14 days of the initial injury [15]. However, rhBMP-2 has been used off-label in the treatment of established non-unions [16–19]. In reconstruction of diaphyseal tibial fractures with cortical defects, use of cancellous allograft with rhBMP-2 augmentation has demonstrated similar rates of clinical union to ICBG, with less blood loss [17]. There may be an emerging role for expanded indications for rhBMP-2 use for non-union repairs, but caution should be exercised when indicating patients for this use. rhBMP-2 is contraindicated in patients who are pregnant or are planning to become pregnant within 1 year, patients with an active or a history of malignant cancer and skeletally immature patients.

The patient in this case had previously undergone autogenous bone grafting via the RIA technique from the ipsilateral femur with a 14-mm reamer. Given the size of the bone defect, autogenous bone graft harvest alone was unlikely to yield an adequate volume of graft. Therefore, the plan was to again harvest autogenous bone graft via the RIA technique, along with augmentation with cancellous bone allograft and rhBMP-2.

Revision Surgery

After completing the preoperative diagnostic workup and planning, the patient was taken to the operating room for revision surgery. The existing plate fixation in the distal tibia was removed. The prior medial incision over the distal tibia was utilized to remove the distal screws from the medial plate. Percutaneous incisions were made to remove the proximal screws and it was noted that the most proximal screw had broken. The medial distal tibia plate was then removed. The trephine from the broken screw removal set was used to remove the remaining broken screw in its entirety.

After successfully removing the primary fixation implants from the tibia, the non-union site was exposed through the prior anterolateral approach. No purulence or signs of infection were encountered during the dissection. Upon exploration of the non-union site, the cortices were noted to be healed laterally and posteriorly, but there was a residual 4- to 5-cm bone defect, and the intramedullary canals were capped off with sclerotic bone. There was also some residual bone graft from the prior procedure that had not incorporated, and curettes were used to remove this, and samples were sent for culture. The sclerotic bone on the bone ends was removed with a saline cooled drill followed by a burr in order to restore access to the intramedullary canals in the proximal and distal segments. The sclerotic bone was debrided back to bleeding bone.

After the non-union site had been prepared, the next step was autogenous bone graft harvesting. A separate incision was made over the hip in order to gain access to the piriformis fossa. After placing a guidewire into the femur and preparing a path for the reamer, a 15-mm reamer head was passed using RIA and yielded a moderate amount of autogenous bone graft (Fig. 34.5a).

Next, a suprapatellar approach was made to place the guidewire for a tibial intramedullary nail. The guidewire was advanced across the non-union site and centred in the distal segment (Fig. 34.5b). Sequential reaming was performed up to 12.5 mm, yielding additional autogenous bone graft from the tibia. An 11-mm intramedullary nail was then placed. Two proximal interlocking screws and one distal interlocking screw were placed.

The autograft obtained from the RIA and tibial reamings were combined with cancellous bone allograft to achieve an adequate volume of bone graft for the defect. After thoroughly irrigating the non-union site, the mixed bone graft was packed into the remaining defect around the intramedullary nail. Lastly, rhBMP-2 on an absorbable collagen sponge was placed over the bone graft in the open defect (Fig. 34.5c).

All the wounds were then closed in a layered fashion. The anterolateral incision was primarily closed without undue tension, but given the somewhat tenuous nature of the soft tissue envelope, incisional negative pressure wound therapy (NPWT) was applied. A well-padded postoperative splint was also applied to promote wound healing and protect the soft tissue.

Postoperatively, he was allowed to be weight-bearing as tolerated with early active and passive motion of the knee and ankle. The incisional NPWT and splint were removed on postoperative day 3 and there were no wound complications. Final intraoperative cultures were negative. His sutures were removed at 3 weeks after surgery. At his 4-month follow-up, the patient was doing well and ambulating independently with no pain at the fracture site. There was evidence of interval healing on his radiographs (Fig. 34.6). He was subsequently lost to follow-up.

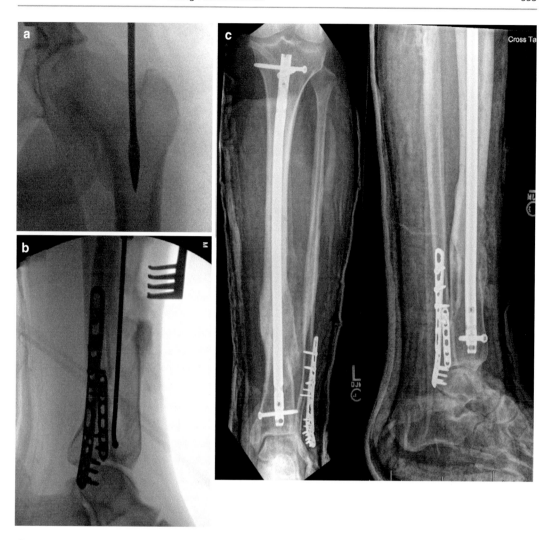

Fig. 34.5 (a) Autogenous bone graft harvest using the RIA technique. (b) Insertion of guidewire for revision osteosynthesis with an intramedullary nail. (c) Postoperative radiographs demonstrating conversion to intramedullary nail fixation with bone grafting

Fig. 34.6 Follow up radiographs at 4 months after surgery demonstrating interval healing

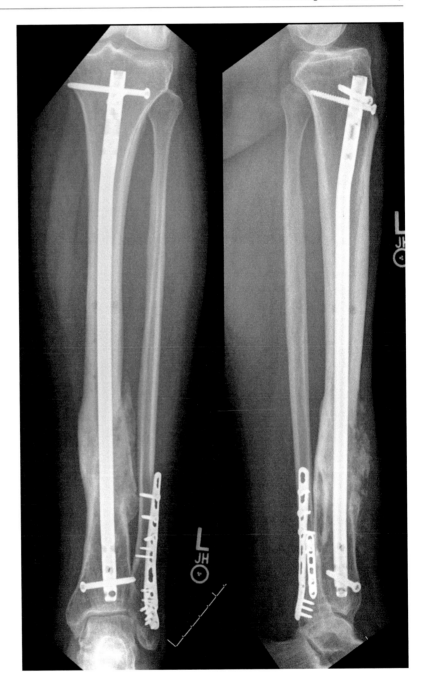

Summary: Lessons Learned

In this chapter, we presented a case of an extra-articular distal tibia non-union with a persistent bone defect after failed plating that was successfully treated with revision to an intramedullary nail with bone grafting. High-energy, open fractures of the distal tibia are at increased risk for delayed union and non-union. A comprehensive diagnostic workup and preoperative planning are essential for successful treatment of these non-unions. Reamed, locked intramedullary nailing is an excellent technique for achieving bone healing for nonunions of the distal tibia. Revision osteosynthesis with a large-diameter intramedullary nail in this case was used to achieve a snug fit in the diaphysis in order to optimize mechanical stability and change the biomechanical stresses at the non-union site. Use of an intramedullary nail in the setting of non-circumferential healing also aided in filling the central portion of the defect, such that bone healing and graft incorporation could proceed in a napkin ring fashion without the need for central healing. Judicious use of autogenous bone grafting is important for fracture healing in non-unions. Careful consideration can also be given to potential off-label use of rhBMP-2 in select patients at high risk for treatment failure.

References

1. Zelle BA, Bhandari M, Espiritu M, Koval KJ, Zlowodzki M, Evidence-Based Orthopaedic Trauma Working Group. Treatment of distal tibia fractures without articular involvement: a systematic review of 1125 fractures. J Orthop Trauma. 2006;20(1):76–9.
2. Vallier HA, Cureton BA, Patterson BM. Randomized, prospective comparison of plate versus intramedullary nail fixation for distal tibia shaft fractures. J Orthop Trauma. 2011;25(12):736–41.
3. Bleeker NJ, van de Wall BJM, IJpma FFA, Doornberg JN, Kerkhoffs GMMJ, et al. Plate vs. nail for extra-articular distal tibia fractures: how should we personalize surgical treatment? A meta-analysis of 1332 patients. Injury. 2021;52(3):345–57.
4. Barcak E, Collinge CA. Metaphyseal distal tibia fractures: a cohort, single-surgeon study comparing outcomes of patients treated with minimally invasive plating versus intramedullary nailing. J Orthop Trauma. 2016;30(5):e169–74.
5. Clancey GJ, Hansen ST Jr. Open fractures of the tibia: a review of one hundred and two cases. J Bone Joint Surg Am. 1978;60(1):118–22.
6. Vallier HA, Toan Le T, Bedi A. Radiographic and clinical comparisons of distal tibia shaft fractures (4 to 11 cm proximal to the plafond): plating versus intramedullary nailing. J Orthop Trauma. 2008;22(5):307–11.
7. Borrelli J Jr, Prickett W, Song E, Becker D, Ricci W. Extraosseous blood supply of the tibia and the effects of different plating techniques: a human cadaveric study. J Orthop Trauma. 2002;16(10):691–5.
8. Helfet DL, Shonnard PY, Levine D, Borrelli J Jr. Minimally invasive plate osteosynthesis of distal fractures of the tibia. Injury. 1997;28(Suppl. 1):A42–7.
9. Richmond J, Colleran K, Borens O, Kloen P, Helfet DL. Nonunions of the distal tibia treated by reamed intramedullary nailing. J Orthop Trauma. 2004;18(9):603–10.
10. Sen MK, Miclau T. Autologous iliac crest bone graft: should it still be the gold standard for treating nonunions? Injury. 2007;38(Suppl 1):S75–80.
11. Younger EM, Chapman MW. Morbidity at bone graft donor sites. J Orthop Trauma. 1989;3(3):192–5.
12. Baldwin P, Li DJ, Auston DA, Mir HS, Yoon RS, Koval KJ. Autograft, allograft, and bone graft substitutes: clinical evidence and indications for use in the setting of orthopaedic trauma surgery. J Orthop Trauma. 2019;33(4):203–13.
13. Belthur MV, Conway JD, Jindal G, Ranade A, Herzenberg JE. Bone graft harvest using a new intramedullary system. Clin Orthop Relat Res. 2008;466(12):2973–80.
14. Dawson J, Kiner D, Gardner W 2nd, Swafford R, Nowotarski PJ. The reamer-irrigator-aspirator as a device for harvesting bone graft compared with iliac crest bone graft: union rates and complications. J Orthop Trauma. 2014;28(10):584–90.
15. Govender S, Csimma C, Genant HK, Valentin-Opran A, Amit Y, et al. Recombinant human bone morphogenetic protein-2 for treatment of open tibial fractures: a prospective, controlled, randomized study of four hundred and fifty patients. J Bone Joint Surg Am. 2002;84(12):2123–34.
16. Johnson EE, Urist MR, Finerman GA. Repair of segmental defects of the tibia with cancellous bone grafts augmented with human bone morphogenetic protein: a preliminary report. Clin Orthop Relat Res. 1988;236:249–57.
17. Jones AL, Bucholz RW, Bosse MJ, Mirza SK, Lyon TR, et al. Recombinant human BMP-2 and allograft compared with autogenous bone graft for reconstruction of diaphyseal tibial fracturs with cortical defects: a randomized controlled trial. J Bone Joint Surg Am. 2006;88(7):1431–41.
18. Tressler MA, Richards JE, Sofianos D, Comrie FK, Kregor PJ, Obremskey WT. Bone morphogenetic protein-2 compared to autologous iliac crest bone graft in the treatment of long bone nonunion. Orthopedics. 2011;34(12):e877–84.
19. Starman JS, Bosse MJ, Cates CA, Norton HJ. Recombinant human bone morphogenetic protein-2 use in the off-label treatment of nonunions and acute fractures: a retrospective review. J Trauma Acute Care Surg. 2012;72(3):676–81.

Distal Tibial Intra-Articular Ilizarov Failed Fixation

35

Paul Nesbitt and Paul Harwood

History of Previous Primary Failed Treatment

A middle-aged female patient who was previously fit and well-sustained injuries as the result of a road traffic collision. Initial assessment in the emergency department revealed an open right total articular tibial distal tibial fracture as well as injuries to the left tibia and abdomen (Fig. 35.1a). She was taken to theatre on an urgent basis where the wound was classified as Gustilo and Anderson IIIA, debrided, washed and closed. A spanning external fixator was applied across the right ankle (Hoffmann II, Stryker) to allow the soft tissues to settle (Fig. 35.1b). Her abdominal injuries were extensive requiring a splenectomy, superior mesenteric artery angioplasty and liver packing at the same anaesthetic. The injuries to the left tibia were treated conservatively.

Following a period of resuscitation and physiological restoration in intensive care, an Ilizarov external fixator (Smith & Nephew) was applied to manage the distal tibial fracture definitively. The fracture was reduced by traction and percutaneous manipulation, the ankle was spanned to the calcaneum to protect the ankle (Fig. 35.2a, b). The patient appeared to initially progress well, mobilising in the frame. The ankle span was removed at 6 weeks post-surgery as planned. However, at the 4-month clinic visit, there was little progression toward union radiographically and the patient was struggling to walk due to pain. At 6 months post-injury, it was noted that there appeared to be an established non-union with bone resorption at the fracture site (Fig. 35.3a). This was confirmed by computed tomography (CT) (Fig. 35.3b).

P. Nesbitt
Leeds Major Trauma Center, Leeds Teaching
Hospitals, NHS, Trusts, Leeds, UK

P. Harwood (✉)
Leeds Teaching Hospitals NHS Trust, Leeds, UK

Leeds Major Trauma Centre and Limb
Reconstruction Unit, Leeds, UK
e-mail: paulharwood@nhs.net

© The Author(s), under exclusive license to Springer Nature Switzerland AG 2024
P. V. Giannoudis, P. Tornetta III (eds.), *Failed Fracture Fixation*,
https://doi.org/10.1007/978-3-031-39692-2_35

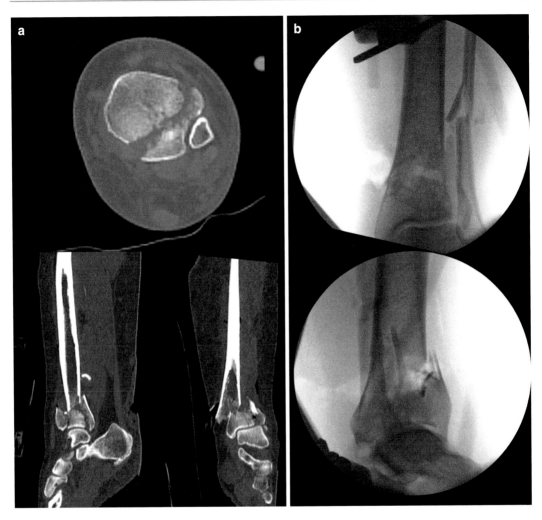

Fig. 35.1 (a) Selected CT images showing intra-articular distal tibial fracture. (b) Intra-operative images following application of spanning external fixator

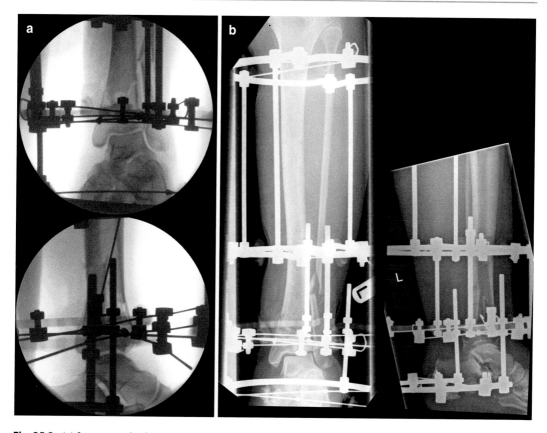

Fig. 35.2 (**a**) Intra-operative images showing fracture reduction. (**b**) Initial post-operative radiographs

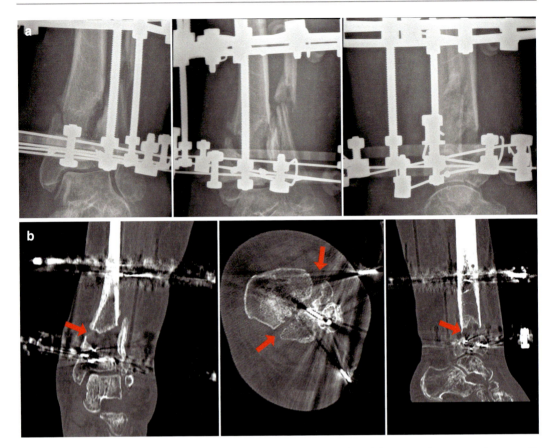

Fig. 35.3 (a) AP, oblique and lateral radiographs at 6 months post-fixation showing bone resorption at the fracture site. (b) CT scan reconstructions showing significant bone defect with apparent bony resorption, metadiaphyseal and articular non-union

Evaluation of the Aetiology of Failure of Fixation

The patient revealed she had significant weight loss, of 3 stones in 6 months, alongside palpitations and intolerance of warm environments. She had persistently loose stools since the accident. The patient had related all these symptoms to recovery from their injuries and had therefore not initially sought medical attention. She had in the last 2 weeks attended to her general practitioner who had raised the suspicion of hyperthyroid disease and referred the patient to endocrinology. Examining the limb, the Ilizarov fixator was stable and the pin sites were in good condition. The wounds from the open fracture and initial debridement were well healed with no local signs of infection. Potential causes of the non-union given the clinical assessment and radiographic findings to this point were therefore felt to be (1) infection related to the open fracture and/or (2) bone resorption due to hyper-catabolism related to thyroid disease (3) mal-reduction of the articular segment with a fracture gap evident on CT.

Clinical Examination

The patient was assessed for potential local and systemic causes of non-union. It was confirmed that she was previously fit and well, did not smoke and was an occasional drinker. The pin sites of the frame were clean. There was no obvious discharge. Active movement of the knee was associated with marked discomfort; ankle movements were limited and associated with pain. There was no ankle joint effusion. No distal neurovascular deficit was present. The frame became unstable, and it was therefore removed. The affected extremity was placed into a below knee cast.

Diagnostic-Biochemical and Radiological Investigations

Haematological investigations were undertaken in conjunction with the patient's general practitioner and subsequently an endocrinologist. These revealed grossly abnormal thyroid function with raised thyroid stimulating hormone (TSH) and free T4, a very low 25-OH vitamin D2 and elevated Calcium. Parathyroid hormone (PTH), the remainder of the bone profile and renal and liver functions were otherwise normal. White cell count and inflammatory markers were normal. Radio-labelled white cell and colloid marrow scans were undertaken which revealed no evidence of deep infection. Plasma procollagen type 1 N-terminal propeptide (P1nP) and beta-carboxy-terminal collagen crosslink (B-CTX) were both significantly elevated. These plasma markers estimate osteoblastic bone formation and osteoclastic bone resorption respectively, both being elevated suggesting a catabolic state likely related to the patient's hyperthyroidism. TSH receptor (TRAB) and thyroid peroxidase antibodies (TPO) were both elevated and a diagnosis of Graves's disease, auto-immune thyroid hyper-stimulation, was made.

The endocrine team initiated medical management of Grave's disease with carbimazole, whilst correcting the serum calcium and vitamin D. Initially the frame was maintained for a period to ascertain if correcting the patient's thyroid status might allow fracture healing to progress. However, the Grave's disease remained recalcitrant to therapy and no evidence of bone union occurred. It was advised that the risks of general anaesthesia to treat the non-union in this situation were too high without endocrine control. The endocrine team felt that thyroidectomy with replacement therapy would be required once the thyroid status was partially corrected. This was undertaken when endocrine control was finally achieved by further medical management and the patient rendered euthyroid by replacement therapy. The endocrine team advised it was then safe to proceed with non-union surgery. Further imaging was undertaken at this point to plan surgery. This revealed an intra-articular component to the non-union with a displaced anterolateral fragment potentially contributing to the aetiology (Fig. 35.4a, b).

Pathology of Treatment Failure

Grave's disease is a systemic autoimmune disorder in which thyroid antigen-specific T-cells infiltrate thyroid-stimulating hormone receptor (TSH-R) expressing tissues. The resultant autoantibodies then stimulate the TSH-R causing unregulated thyroid hormone production and secretion along with hyperplasia of the thyroid itself [1]. Thyroid hormones, triiodothyronine (T3) and thyroxine (T4), play a crucial role in the regulation of bone remodelling, which involves a balance between bone resorption by osteoclasts and bone formation by osteoblasts. Thyroid hormone enhances osteoclast activity by stimulating the expression of receptor activator of nuclear factor-kappa B ligand (RANKL) in osteoblasts, a cytokine involved in the differentiation and activation of osteoclasts. Additionally, thyroid hormone inhibits osteoblast differentiation and function by decreasing the expression of bone-specific genes, including alkaline phosphatase, osteocalcin, and collagen type I.

In hyperthyroidism, excess thyroid hormone production alters the balance of bone remodelling, by the mechanisms described above, leading to increased osteoclastic bone resorption and decreased osteoblastic bone formation. This leads to decreased bone mass, increased risk of osteoporosis and impaired bone healing. [2–4] The remodelling cycle is critically shortened, with 10% net bone loss occurring per cycle [2]. The resultant bone resorption suggests that fracture union will be difficult to achieve whilst in

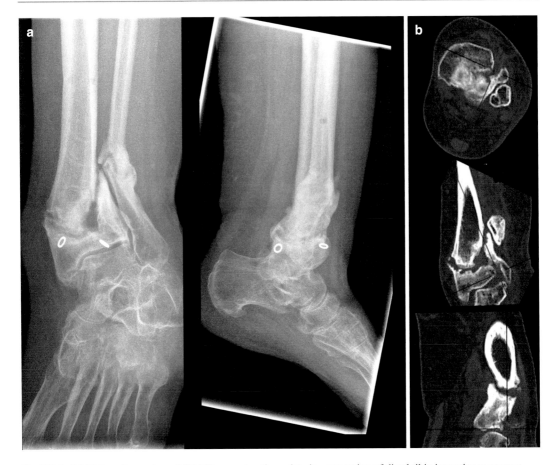

Fig. 35.4 (a) Plain radiographs and (b) CT reconstructions showing non-union of distal tibia just prior to surgery

this metabolic state, particularly where it is uncontrolled [3–6].

The treatment of tibial Pilon fractures using Ilizarov frames is well established, with union rates in excess of 96% at 12 months reported, even in open injuries [7]. This patient had suffered a high-energy open fracture with associated periosteal stripping of the bone. This results in loss of vascularity at the fracture site with an increased risk of non-union. Infection had been ruled out as far as possible by pre-operative investigation, however, in this context occult infection remains a possibility. The mal-reduction of the joint surface reduces bony contact and is also potentially contributory, as well as having implications for long-term function. It would, however, appear most likely that the undiagnosed thyroid pathology was the main determinant of outcome in this case. However, it is important to consider all these factors when planning treatment.

Pre-Operative Planning

Once rendered euthyroid, further treatment options were discussed with the patient. At 18 months post-initial injury, further imaging revealed an articular non-union with a significant bone defect at the meta-diaphysis and resultant valgus and apex posterior deformity (Fig. 35.4). The foot was in a good condition and there remained no clinical or biochemical signs of infection. The patient was only able to walk a short distance, even in a splint, and had significant pain. They were unable to weight-bear without the orthosis. Whilst amputation was considered, the patient wished a further attempt at limb salvage. The patient wished to avoid further Ilizarov treatment at this point if possible.

Treatment strategy in non-union can be broken down into mechanical and biological considerations.

Mechanically, the fracture was too unstable in an orthosis for union to occur and was malaligned with an intra-articular component to the non-union. Management requires a technique which will restore contact, alignment and appropriate stability. Biologically, the resultant normalisation of the patient's thyroid status post-thyroidectomy and hormone replacement should create an environment where a union could proceed [5]. However, the non-union continued to appear inert radiographically with little sign of biological activity. Further complexity in this case was added by the presence of a bone defect at the fracture site which was likely to be critical once alignment had been restored. An open approach was required in order to debride the non-union and reduce the articular fragments. Deep infection appeared unlikely but not impossible. It was therefore planned to manage the non-union by a two-stage induced membrane (Masquelet) technique, using internal fixation to reduce and stabilise the articular block and restore alignment. The fibula non-union would be addressed at the same time and samples sent for microbiological culture to allow treatment to be adjusted if the occult infection was identified. Bone grafting would then be undertaken at around 6 weeks.

Revision Surgery

Staged revision surgery was undertaken in two separate procedures 6 weeks apart. At the first procedure, the fracture site was exposed and the pseudarthrosis at the metadiaphysis was excised and debrided back to the bleeding bone. Multiple deep samples were sent for culture. The articular non-union was taken down and rotated back into position and compressed with a clamp. An antero-lateral distal tibial peri-articular locking plate was applied compressing this and restoring overall alignment. The fibular was realigned and plated with a locking plate. A polymethyl methacrylate cement spacer with vancomycin and gentamicin was placed in the resultant tibial defect as a first-stage induced membrane technique. This affords local antibiotics and stimulates the formation of the Masquelet membrane, which has been shown to be biologically active and enhance healing in critical bone defects and helping to address any issues with local biology. Additional cement was placed anterior to the plate to ensure good membrane formation in the surgical approach. The patient made an uneventful recovery, all of the samples were negative for pathogens on microscopy and extended culture and the wounds were healed by 6 weeks post-initial procedure. It was therefore decided to proceed to the second stage grafting as planned (Fig. 35.5).

At the second procedure, an autologous bone graft was harvested from the patient's femur using the Reamer Irrigator, Aspirator system (RIA, Depuy-Synthes UK). To enhance biological activity, this was mixed with bone marrow aspirate concentrate (BMAC) taken from the patient's iliac crest, platelet-rich plasma from peripheral blood and synthetic graft expander (Orthoss, Geistlich UK). The cement spacer was removed, preserving the Masquelet membrane, and the resultant tibial cavity was filled with bone graft mixture. The membrane was then closed around the graft (Fig. 35.6). The patient made an uneventful recovery. To reduce the risk of fatigue failure of the plate, the patient's limb was protected in an orthosis and they were asked to partially bear weight for 12 weeks post-operatively. At 20 weeks the patient's fracture had gone on to radiologic union with restoration of alignment (Fig. 35.7). Though her function was dramatically improved from that with the non-union, this did not return to normal, and she continues to receive treatment for complex regional pain syndrome.

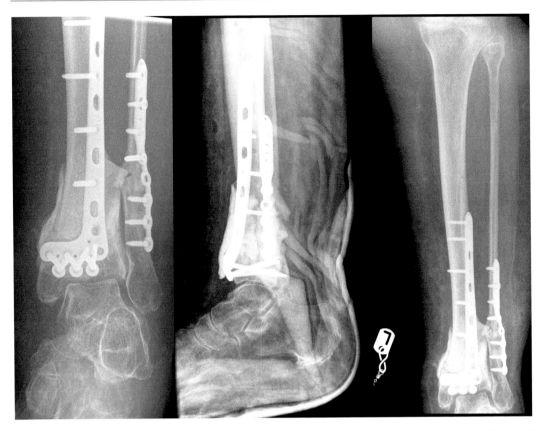

Fig. 35.5 Post-operative radiographs showing fixation, ankle joint reduction and cement spacers in the metadiaphyseal defect and anterior to the plate

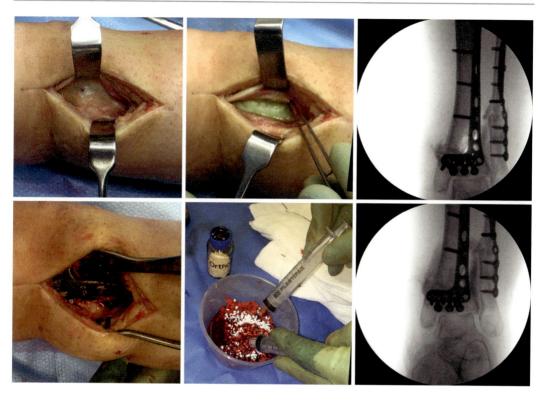

Fig. 35.6 Intra-operative photographs and image intensifier films. The membrane is identified and opened. The cement spacer is removed from the defect. RIA harvested bone graft is mixed with BMAC, PRP and graft expander and applied anterior to the plate and within the defect area

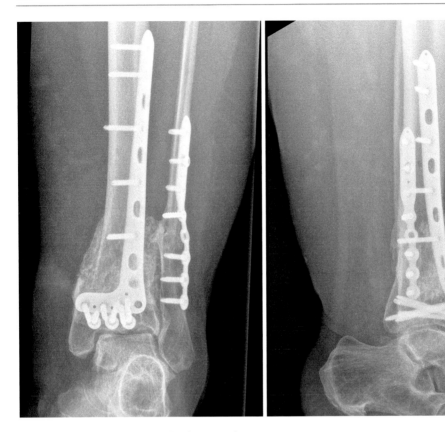

Fig. 35.7 Final radiographs showing fracture union

Summary: Lessons Learned

The aetiology of non-union is frequently multifactorial. This case highlights the need for careful assessment in all cases to identify contributory factors. It is useful to break this down into problems with the fracture mechanics and problems with the systemic and local biology. In this case following removal of the frame, stability and alignment of the non-union needed to be addressed. With regard to the local biology, the nature of the injury meant that local vascularity was likely to be sub-optimal and the possibility of infection remained. A significant issue with the patient's systemic biology was identified which needed to be addressed before non-union surgery was undertaken. The patient's thyroid disease was managed with assistance from the endocrinology team. A surgical strategy was selected which aligned with the patient's wishes to avoid further Ilizarov fixation whilst addressing the mechanical and local biological issues which had been identified and was safe should occult infection be identified. If concerns about occult infection had been greater, a spanning external fixator could have been applied at stage 1 with internal fixation being undertaken at stage 2. As this appeared unlikely, it was decided to undertake internal fixation at the first intervention to avoid potential issues with external fixator pin sites, cultures from the first stage were all negative. The non-union went on to an uneventful union following these interventions. Despite this, the patient failed to regain pre-injury function. She was nevertheless satisfied with her treatment; this does, however, highlight the need to carefully counsel patients regarding likely outcomes and consider reconstructive amputation even in situations where a limb is technically salvageable but functional outcome is likely to be very poor.

References

1. Kahaly GJ, Bartalena L, Hegedüs L, Leenhardt L, Poppe K, Pearce SH. 2018 European Thyroid Association Guideline for the management of graves' hyperthyroidism. Eur Thyroid J. 2018;7(4):167–86. Available from: https://etj.bioscientifica.com/view/journals/etj/7/4/ETJ490384.xml
2. Williams GR, Bassett JHD. Thyroid diseases and bone health. J Endocrinol Investig. 2018;41(1):99–109. Available from: https://pubmed.ncbi.nlm.nih.gov/28853052/
3. Tuchendler D, Bolanowski M. The influence of thyroid dysfunction on bone metabolism. Thyroid Res. 2014;7(1) Available from: /pmc/articles/PMC4314789/
4. Brinker MR, O'Connor DP, Monla YT, Earthman TP. Metabolic and endocrine abnormalities in patients with nonunions. J Orthop Trauma. 2007;21(8):557–70. Available from: https://journals.lww.com/jorthotrauma/Fulltext/2007/09000/Metabolic_and_Endocrine_Abnormalities_in_Patients.7.aspx
5. Vestergaard P, Mosekilde L. Fractures in patients with hyperthyroidism and hypothyroidism: a nationwide follow-up study in 16,249 patients. Thyroid. 2004;12(5):411–9. https://doi.org/10.1089/105072502760043503.
6. Daya NR, Fretz A, Martin SS, Lutsey PL, Echouffo-Tcheugui JB, Selvin E, et al. Association between subclinical thyroid dysfunction and fracture risk key points + supplemental content. JAMA Netw Open. 2022;5(11):2240823. Available from: https://jamanetwork.com/
7. Giannoudis VP, Ewins E, Taylor DM, Foster P, Harwood P. Clinical and functional outcomes in patients with distal tibial fracture treated by circular external fixation: a retrospective cohort study. Strategies Trauma Limb Reconstr. 2021;16(2):86. Available from: /pmc/articles/PMC8578245/

Distal Tibial Intra-Articular Plating Failed Fixation

36

Vincenzo Giordano, Robinson Esteves Pires, Felipe Serrão de Souza, Franco L. De Cicco, Mario Herrera-Perez, and Alexandre Godoy-Santos

History of Previous Primary Failed Treatment

A 66-year-old male patient was admitted by the emergency department after falling from a folding ladder sustaining a Gustilo type I open fracture of the right tibial pilon. The patient was conscious, haemodynamically stable, with no

---

V. Giordano (✉)
Serviço de Ortopedia e Traumatologia Prof. Nova Monteiro—Hospital Municipal Miguel Couto, Rio de Janeiro, Brazil

Ortopedia—Clínica São Vicente, Rede D'or São Luiz, Rio de Janeiro, Brazil

R. E. Pires
Departamento do Aparelho Locomotor, Universidade Federal de Minas Gerais, Belo Horizonte, Brazil

F. S. de Souza
Serviço de Ortopedia e Traumatologia Prof. Nova Monteiro—Hospital Municipal Miguel Couto, Rio de Janeiro, Brazil

F. L. De Cicco
Departamento de Ortopedia, Hospital Sotero del Río, Santiago, Chile

M. Herrera-Perez
Departamento de Ortopedia, Universidad de La Laguna, San Cristóbal de La Laguna, La Laguna, Spain

A. Godoy-Santos
Instituto de Ortopedia e Traumatologia, Hospital das Clinicas HCFMUSP, Faculdade de Medicina, Universidade de Sao Paulo, São Paulo, Brazil

other skeletal injury and normal neurovascular status on the right lower limb. Initial clinical examination revealed a small (<1 cm) wound in the distal medial region of the right leg, approximately 5.0 cm above the medial malleolus, with no apparent gross contamination. Radiographically, the fracture of the tibial pilon was displaced in the valgus, with slight comminution in the medial metaphyseal area and an associated fracture of the medial malleolus with no displacement. The fibula presented a comminuted fracture at the same level, also displaced in the valgus (Fig. 36.1).

The patient was taken to the operating room (OR) for irrigation and debridement (I&D) of the open wound. During debridement, it was noticed that the medial metaphyseal fragment was devitalised and removed. The medial wound was primarily closed with no tension and the leg was placed in a short-leg splint with the ankle in a neutral position for temporary immobilisation until definitive surgical treatment. The splint remained in place for 10 days, when the definitive surgery was performed. During this period, the wound and leg oedema were assessed daily.

Open reduction and internal fixation (ORIF) of the distal tibia and fibula were performed with the patient in a floppy lateral position with the injured limb on the top. A thigh tourniquet was applied. A posterior approach to the distal tibia

---

© The Author(s), under exclusive license to Springer Nature Switzerland AG 2024
P. V. Giannoudis, P. Tornetta III (eds.), *Failed Fracture Fixation*,
https://doi.org/10.1007/978-3-031-39692-2_36

Fig. 36.1 Initial anteroposterior (AP) (**a**) and lateral (**b**) radiographs of the right leg revealing a comminuted fracture of the distal tibia with articular extension (AO-OTA type 43C2), associated with a comminuted fracture of the fibula at the same level. Note that both fractures were displaced in valgus. Also, there was an associated fracture of the medial malleolus with no displacement

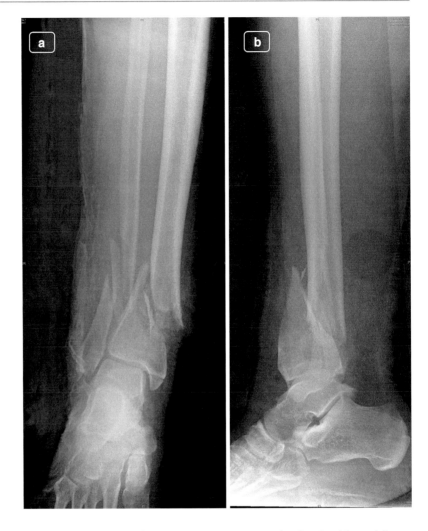

was done and the posterior malleolus was reduced and fixed with 2 straight 2.7 mm locked plates and screws [1]. Then, using the same approach, the fibula fracture was reduced and fixed with a straight 2.7 mm locked plate and screws. After the closure of the posterior surgical wound, the patient's pelvis was flopped backwards and the entire lower limb was externally rotated, so that the patient was repositioned in an oblique supine position. An anterior approach was performed to the distal tibia and the remaining component of the pilon fracture was reduced and fixed using a 3.5-mm anterolateral locked plate and screws. Finally, the non-displaced medial malleolus fracture was percutaneously fixed with a 4.0-mm cannulated cancellous screw (Fig. 36.2). No bone graft was used to fill the medial metaphyseal defect.

The patient received intravenous antibiotics for 24 h and started deep venous thrombosis prophylaxis with low molecular weight heparin. Physical therapy was started immediately after surgery, and partial weight bearing was allowed with crutches. The patient was discharged from the hospital 48 h after the definitive surgery.

The patient was followed up with regular outpatient appointments. During follow-up visits, it was observed that both the medial exposure

Fig. 36.2 Immediate post-operative AP (**a**) and lateral (**b**) radiographs of the right leg. ORIF of the fibula and the posterior component of the distal tibia were performed through a posterior approach, then anterior approach was performed to the distal tibia and the remaining component of the pilon fracture was reduced and fixed. The non-displaced medial malleolus fracture was percutaneously fixed with a 4.0 mm cannulated cancellous screw. No bone graft was used to fill the medial metaphyseal defect

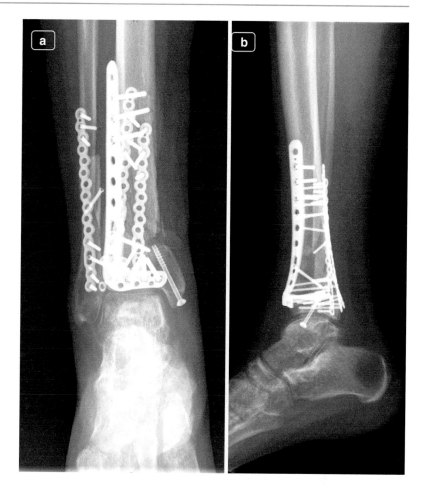

wound, and the surgical wounds healed satisfactorily, with no persistent drainage or signs of infection. The patient gradually regained ankle mobility and independence.

Two months after the operation, the patient had mild varus on the right ankle. There was no local pain or signs of infection, but the ankle was slightly swollen. X-rays taken at the time revealed that the distal fracture of the tibia had suffered a mild varus collapse, with subsidence of the medial metaphyseal wall. He was still using two crutches and performing partial weight bearing (Fig. 36.3). It was decided to stop weight-bearing.

At 3 months, the distal tibial fracture had suffered a complete varus collapse, with total subsidence of the medial metaphyseal wall (Fig. 36.4). There were radiographically signs of failure of the anteromedial plate.

Fig. 36.3 AP (**a**) and lateral (**b**) radiographs of the right leg at 2 months showing a slight displacement of the distal tibia into varus. There were no signs of implant failure

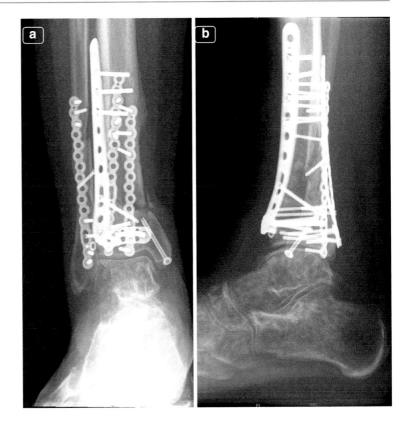

Fig. 36.4 AP (**a**) and lateral (**b**) radiographs of the right leg at 3 months revealing a complete displacement of the distal tibia into varus, with obvious signs of implant failure and some broken screws

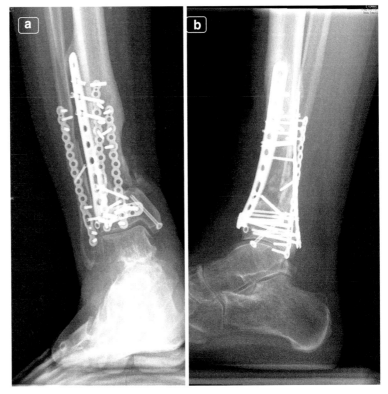

Evaluation of the Aetiology of Failure of Fixation

Radiographs showed non-union of the distal tibia. The distal tibia bone gap and the development of non-union led to abnormal loading of the distal tibia and the subsequent varus collapse.

Clinical Examination

Clinical examination revealed good local soft tissue conditions, particularly at the site of initial bone exposure. The scar tissue was elastic, with adequate wound healing. The right ankle was in varus. There was mild mobility at the tibial pilon fracture site. There was good passive plantar flexion of the ankle, with neutral dorsiflexion. There was no distal neurovascular deficit.

Diagnostic-Biochemical and Radiological Investigations

Laboratory was normal, with no significant elevation of inflammatory markers. However, infection could not be 100% excluded. For this reason, it was planned to take cultures during the re-operation. There was no callus formation in either the tibia or the fibula. The articular component of the pilon fracture healed with no step-off. The major point of concern was the posterior metaphyseal defect of the distal tibia. CT scan was planned for better evaluation of the problem.

Preoperative Planning

It was decided to remove the hardware and take cultures for infection (step 1).

Six weeks later, the patient underwent definitive reconstruction with a posterolateral tibial plate, a fibula plate, and bone graft. The preoperative planning considered not only the posterior metaphyseal defect of the distal tibia but also the varus malalignment of the right ankle.

The decision on the best source of bone graft for the posterior distal bone defect was discussed among peers, and the use of the Reamer-Irrigator-Aspirator (RIA) was preferred. RIA was basically chosen because of the possibility of harvesting a large amount of autologous bone graft from the medullary canal of the ipsilateral femur. Both antero-posterior and lateral radiographs of the femur were taken to measure the canal isthmus and the cortical thickness. In order to augment the RIA graft with inductivity, it was decided to mix it with a vial of demineralised bone matrix (DBM).

Revision Surgery

During implant removal (step 1), some screws broke and remained intraosseous. There were no major signs of infection. No bacterial growth occurred with negative results for infection. It was observed that the tibial pilon fracture did not heal (Fig. 36.5). The articular component of the pilon fracture healed with no step-off (Fig. 36.6).

Six weeks later revision surgery was performed (step 2) to manage the distal tibia non-union. The patient was initially positioned supine on a radiolucent table with a bump beneath the right gluteus region and a retrograde technique was used to harvest the graft from the ipsilateral femur with the RIA. Approximately 40 cc of autogenous bone graft was harvested. The wound was closed, and the patient was positioned prone.

In this position, a thigh tourniquet was applied. An extensive posterolateral approach to the distal tibia and fibula was done [1]. The fibula was approached first. Although there was no callus formation, there was no mobility at the fibula fracture site. Thus, an osteotomy of the fibula was performed in the original focus of the fracture, and new fibula osteosynthesis was performed using a straight 2.7-mm locked plate and screws. Through the same approach, the distal tibia was exposed, and the non-union site was debrided. Intraoperative tissue samples were collected, with no bacterial growth. The distal tibia was reduced and the posterior defect was filled with

Fig. 36.5 AP (**a**) and lateral (**b**) radiographs of the right leg after implant removal. Both fractures were fixed displaced in varus and there were no signs of bone healing

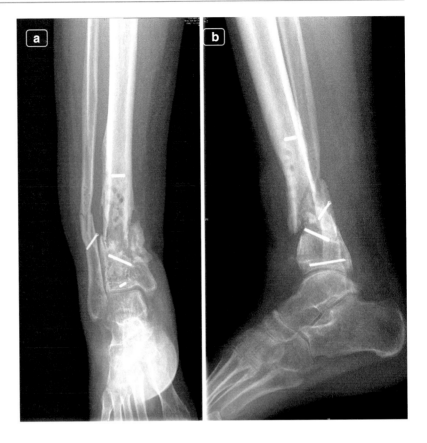

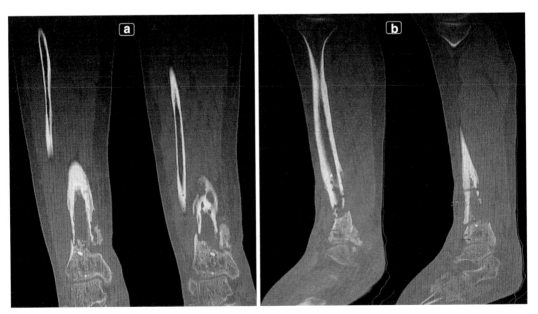

Fig. 36.6 Coronal (**a**) and sagittal (**b**) CT cuts of the right leg revealing an atrophic non-union of the distal tibia, with a major posterior defect. The articular component of the pilon fracture healed with no step-off

Fig. 36.7 AP (**a**) and lateral (**b**) radiographs of the right leg at 6 months. The pilon fracture healed uneventfully with the ankle in good position. Note the large amount of bone graft used to fill the posterior void and also the medial metaphyseal defect

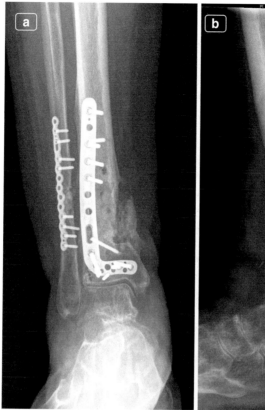
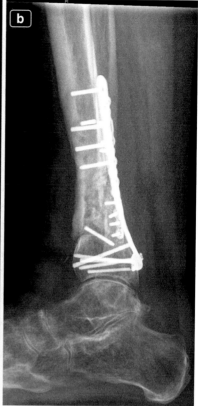

autogenous bone graft and demineralised bone matrix. Then, a 3.5-mm locked L plate and screws were used for the fixation of the distal tibia.

The patient received intravenous antibiotics for 24 h and started thromboprophylaxis with low molecular weight heparin. Again, physical therapy was started immediately after surgery, and partial weight bearing was allowed with crutches. The patient was discharged from the hospital 48 h after the definitive surgery. There were no major complaints related to either the bone graft donor site or the fixation site.

The patient was followed up with regular outpatient visits. Wounds healed satisfactorily. Ankle joint mobilisation and progressive loading were allowed. At 6 months, full weight bearing was possible without pain or limping, and X-rays showed that the fracture had healed (Fig. 36.7). Subsequently, the patient was allowed to return to his activities of daily living.

Summary: Lessons Learned

The treatment of tibial pilon fractures has evolved rapidly in recent years, mainly due to the continued understanding of the importance of surrounding soft tissues and the increasing use of a staged treatment strategy [2–4]. Despite this, the treatment of high-energy fractures still presents with a high risk of complications [5]. Fixation failure can occur due to both implant-related and soft-tissue-related problems. Therefore, non-union, malunion, wound dehiscence, skin necrosis, implant exposure, superficial infection, deep sepsis and late-onset degenerative arthritis may occur [5–7]. Pilon fracture literature has shown low quality of life due to the inability to undertake daily tasks and a late return to work [8]. Failure in foot functions has a direct effect on the quality of life in both the short and mid-term [9]. Pollak et al. [10] reported lower SF-36 scores in

103 patients after pilon fractures than after pelvic fractures or in patient groups with chronic illnesses such as AIDS and coronary artery disease at a mean of 3.2 years follow-up.

Soft tissue problems account for more than 50% of these complications, requiring additional procedures and potentially leading to implant exposure, fracture-related infection and fixation failure [7]. Open fractures and soft tissue insult in the zone of injury increase the risk of complications [6]. In addition, associated fibular fractures, metaphyseal comminution and multiple displaced articular fragments are associated with higher energy mechanisms and additional soft tissue injury [11]. In this context, it is necessary for the orthopaedic surgeon who manages these injuries to understand the reasons and avoid complications, as well as quickly recognise and manage them. Currently, it has been demonstrated that the adoption of a two-staged fixation strategy can help mitigate some concerns with soft tissue compromise while obtaining good articular alignment.

In our patient, there was an open fracture of the tibial pilon, with a medial wound in the distal region of the leg, and an associated comminuted fracture of the fibula. After initial I&D, the local soft tissues were deemed unsuitable for definitive fixation, which was delayed for 10 days. During this period, the leg was immobilised for soft tissue monitoring and preoperative planning. Temporary external bridging fixation and acute fibular fixation have been advocated to accurately restore the normal length of the fractured tibia. We chose not to use the external fixator because the use of an orthosis was sufficient to maintain the length of the tibia. Likewise, we chose not to fix the fibula, as poor reduction of the fibula fracture could lead to poor reduction of the corresponding distal tibial fragment, which would make definitive surgery more difficult.

The importance of the fibula fracture in the spectrum of the tibial pilon fracture was highlighted by several authors [12–14]. Comminuted fibular fractures are generally the result of compressive stresses occurring when the talus is displaced into the valgus. In a valgus fracture pattern, the medial tension band and soft tissues are damaged, while the lateral tension band is still intact [2, 13]. In this fracture pattern, it has been demonstrated that anterolateral plating fixation of the distal tibial plus stable fixation of the fibula assist in restoring the lateral tension band, providing better mechanical stability [2, 12, 13, 15]. In our patient, definitive fixation of the tibial pilon fracture comprised the use of anterior and posterior plates and adjuvant plate fixation of the fibula fracture. The posterior malleolus was split into two large fragments, so a staged front-back surgical planning was done with the patient in a floppy lateral position. The medial metaphyseal defect was not bone grafted nor plated, and at 3 months there was a complete varus subsidence of the pilon fracture with failed osteosynthesis. Watson [7] pointed out that the most common cause of hardware failure is the inability to achieve a stable fixation construct. Delayed union or non-union of the metaphyseal-diaphyseal junction is common and usually occurs in conjunction with hardware failure.

Recently, Haller [16] argued for and against the inclusion of a medially based plate in the fixation construct through the open wound at the time of definitive fixation. There is a complicated balance between biology and mechanics that needs to be properly defined. Thus, in some patients or situations where there is an increased risk of soft tissue complications, such as diabetes, severe vascular insufficiency, smokers and a severely damaged soft tissue envelope, the use of a medial plate should be avoided, or the risks calculated [16, 17]. Goodnough et al. [18] proposed the use of a medial column support with percutaneous large fragment fixation in pilon fractures as a viable option to provide mechanical stability while effectively managing tenuous soft tissue envelopes. Maybe this technique can be useful in certain cases; however, there is still a lack of adequate feedback to definitively adopt it on a large scale. Another possibility includes the use of circular external fixation for the definitive treatment of tibial pilon fractures, which has been shown safe and effective, with a high union and low serious complication rate [19–22]. In a systematic review and meta-analysis comparing postoperative complications and functional outcomes of open reduction and internal fixation versus circular external fixation, Malik-Tabassum et al. [21] found that both are acceptable treatment options for surgical management of tibial pilon fractures, with comparable outcomes.

When present after tibial pilon fracture fixation, complications are not infrequent and must be identified and treated early. In Duckworth et al. [23] consecutive series of tibial pilon fractures, 40.2% of patients required at least one additional operation, with removal of symptomatic metalwork being the primary indication. Adequate preoperative planning and execution are critical, as well as the choice of the fixation tactics [24, 25]. In our patient, although there was no pain or discomfort at the surgical site, and laboratory tests did not indicate active infection, the patient underwent implant removal followed by tissue culture to diagnose implant-related infection. CT scan was performed and showed a major metaphyseal-diaphyseal defect on the posterior aspect of the distal tibia. We decided to use the RIA system with an additional demineralised bone matrix to fill the defect. Although autogenous bone graft is generally harvested from the iliac crest, the adoption of alternative options such as the RIA can be considered to reduce the complications related to iliac crest graft harvest. Several authors have shown the potential of the RIA system to harvest autografts without creating a substantial secondary defect [26].

During surgery, the fibula was osteotomised to allow adequate alignment of the ankle joint, and a posterolateral 2.7-mm was used to fix it. Then, the distal tibia was fixed with a 3.5-mm locked L plate through the same approach. Posterior plate placement was chosen to avoid shortening of the posterior column of the distal tibia and to keep the bone graft in situ. Despite the satisfactory resolution of the failed fixation, the patient was followed up for 1 year and several complications can develop later after a tibial pilon fracture such as degenerative osteoarthritis. Nevertheless, this case taught us about the importance of an adequate assessment of the fracture morphology and the concept of intact periosteum. Although a valgus fracture pattern with comminuted fibular fracture and lateral tibial comminution is preferred stabilised with a laterally based plate, the existence of concomitant metaphyseal medial comminution or bone loss should be addressed [12, 13, 15, 27]. Mechanically, the use of a medial plate seems important to support the medial metaphyseal comminution when present; however, one should keep in mind that in certain patients another form of stabilisation should be used due to the high risk of complications, especially of the local soft tissues.

Disclosure Authors do not and will not have financial benefits related to the subject presented in this chapter.

References

1. Assal M, Ray A, Stern R. Strategies for surgical approaches in open reduction internal fixation of pilon fractures. J Orthop Trauma. 2015;29(2):69–79. https://doi.org/10.1097/BOT.0000000000000218.
2. Hebert-Davies J, Kleweno CP, Nork SE. Contemporary strategies in pilon fixation. J Orthop Trauma. 2020;34(Suppl. 1):S14–20. https://doi.org/10.1097/BOT.0000000000001698.
3. Patterson MJ, Cole JD. Two-staged delayed open reduction and internal fixation of severe pilon fractures. J Orthop Trauma. 1999;13(2):85–91. https://doi.org/10.1097/00005131-199902000-00003.
4. Sirkin M, Sanders R, DiPasquale T, Herscovici D Jr. A staged protocol for soft tissue management in the treatment of complex pilon fractures. J Orthop Trauma. 1999;13(2):78–84. https://doi.org/10.1097/00005131-199902000-00002.
5. Gaulke R, Krettek C. Pilon-tibiale-Frakturen: Vermeidung und Behandlung von Komplikationen. Unfallchirurg. 2017;120(8):658–66. https://doi.org/10.1007/s00113-017-0366-6.
6. Yeramosu T, Satpathy J, Perdue PW Jr, Toney CB, Torbert JT, Cinats DJ, Patel TT, Kates SL. Risk factors for infection and subsequent adverse clinical results in the setting of operatively treated pilon fractures. J Orthop Trauma. 2022;36(8):406–12. https://doi.org/10.1097/BOT.0000000000002339.
7. Watson JT. Complications in tibial pilon fractures: avoiding errors in judgment. Tech Foot Ankle Surg. 2016;15(4):175–87.
8. Bonato LJ, Edwards ER, Gosling CM, Hau R, Hofstee DJ, Shuen A, Gabbe BJ. Patient reported health related quality of life early outcomes at 12 months after surgically managed tibial plafond fracture. Injury. 2017;48:946–53. https://doi.org/10.1016/j.injury.2016.11.012.

9. Yaradılmış YU, Okkaoğlu MC, Kılıç A, Haberal B, Demirkale I, Altay M. The mid-term effects on quality of life and foot functions following pilon fracture. Ulus Travma Acil Cerrahi Derg. 2020;26(5):798–804. https://doi.org/10.14744/tjtes.2020.85601.

10. Pollak AN, McCarthy ML, Bess RS, Agel J, Swiontkowski MF. Outcomes after treatment of high-energy tibial plafond fractures. J Bone Joint Surg. 2003;85(10):1893–900. https://doi.org/10.2106/00004623-200310000-00005.

11. Olson JJ, Anand K, Esposito JG, von Keudell AG, Rodriguez EK, Smith RM, Weaver MJ. Complications and soft-tissue coverage after complete articular, open tibial plafond fractures. J Orthop Trauma. 2021;35(10):e371–6. https://doi.org/10.1097/BOT.0000000000002074.

12. Rouhani A, Elmi A, Akbari Aghdam H, Panahi F, Dokht GY. The role of fibular fixation in the treatment of tibia diaphysis distal third fractures. Orthop Traumatol Surg Res. 2012;98(8):868–72. https://doi.org/10.1016/j.otsr.2012.09.009.

13. Sameer M, Bassetty KC, Singaravadivelu V. Fixation of tibial pilon fractures based on column concept: a prospective study. Acta Orthop Belg. 2017;83(4):568–73.

14. Zelle BA, Dang KH, Ornell SS. High-energy tibial pilon fractures: an instructional review. Int Orthop. 2019;43(8):1939–50. https://doi.org/10.1007/s00264-019-04344-8.

15. Siegel J, Tornetta P III. Fracture pattern assessment of tibial pilon fractures. Tech Foot Ankle. 2016;15(4):162–8.

16. Haller J. Medial plating in open pilon fractures may be indicated in the right patient. J Orthop Trauma. 2022;36(1):e40–1. https://doi.org/10.1097/BOT.0000000000002147.

17. Oladeji LO, Platt B, Crist BD. Diabetic pilon fractures: are they as bad as we think? J Orthop Trauma. 2021;35(3):149–53. https://doi.org/10.1097/BOT.0000000000001904.

18. Goodnough LH, Tigchelaar SS, Van Rysselberghe NL, DeBaun MR, Gardner MJ, Hecht GG, Lucas JF. Medial column support in pilon fractures using percutaneous intramedullary large fragment fixation. J Orthop Trauma. 2021;35(12):e502–6. https://doi.org/10.1097/BOT.0000000000002073.

19. Giannoudis VP, Ewins E, Taylor DM, Foster P, Harwood P. Clinical and functional outcomes in patients with distal tibial fracture treated by circular external fixation: a retrospective cohort study. Strategies Trauma Limb Reconstr. 2021;16(2):86–95. https://doi.org/10.5005/jp-journals-10080-1516.

20. Jacob N, Amin A, Giotakis N, Narayan B, Nayagam S, Trompeter AJ. Management of high-energy tibial pilon fractures. Strategies Trauma Limb Reconstr. 2015;10(3):137–47. https://doi.org/10.1007/s11751-015-0231-5.

21. Malik-Tabassum K, Pillai K, Hussain Y, Bleibleh S, Babu S, Giannoudis PV, Tosounidis TH. Postoperative outcomes of open reduction and internal fixation versus circular external fixation in treatment of tibial plafond fractures: a systematic review and meta-analysis. Injury. 2020;51(7):1448–56. https://doi.org/10.1016/j.injury.2020.04.056.

22. Tornetta P 3rd, Weiner L, Bergman M, Watnik N, Steuer J, Kelley M, Yang E. Pilon fractures: treatment with combined internal and external fixation. J Orthop Trauma. 1993;7(6):489–96. https://doi.org/10.1097/00005131-199312000-00001.

23. Duckworth AD, Jefferies JG, Clement ND, White TO. Type C tibial pilon fractures: short- and long-term outcome following operative intervention. Bone Joint J. 2016;98-B(8):1106–11. https://doi.org/10.1302/0301-620X.98B8.36400.

24. Carter TH, Duckworth AD, Oliver WM, Molyneux SG, Amin AK, White TO. Open reduction and internal fixation of distal tibial pilon fractures. JBJS Essent Surg Tech. 2019;9(3):e29. https://doi.org/10.2106/JBJS.ST.18.00093.

25. Topliss CJ, Jackson M, Atkins RM. Anatomy of pilon fractures of the distal tibia. J Bone Joint Surg Br. 2005;87(5):692–7. https://doi.org/10.1302/0301-620X.87B5.15982.

26. Giannoudis PV, Tzioupis C, Green J. Surgical techniques: how I do it? The Reamer/Irrigator/Aspirator (RIA) system. Injury. 2009;40(11):1231–6. https://doi.org/10.1016/j.injury.2009.07.070.

27. Tornetta P 3rd, Gorup J. Axial computed tomography of pilon fractures. Clin Orthop Relat Res. 1996;323:273–6. https://doi.org/10.1097/00003086-199602000-00037.

Lateral Malleolus Ankle Failed Fixation

37

Georgios Kotsarinis and Peter V. Giannoudis

History of Previous Primary Failed Treatment

This is the case of a 36-year-old male, with unremarkable past medical history, who sustained an inversion injury of his left ankle whilst playing football. Subsequently, he was unable to bear weight through his left foot and he was taken to the local hospital. On examination, his left lower extremity was neurovascularly intact, but it was severely swollen around the ankle. The radiographic investigation demonstrated a left distal fibula Weber B fracture with a posterior and lateral shift of the talus creating a remarkable medial space opening (Fig. 37.1). He was manipulated under sedation; an acceptable ankle position was achieved, and he was placed in a below the knee backslab (Fig. 37.2).

Two days later, the repeat X-ray showed that the initially acceptable position was lost in the plaster of Paris (Fig. 37.3). A decision was made

for provisional closed reduction and stabilisation with an external fixator, considering the severe soft tissue swelling (Fig. 37.4).

Eleven days post-injury, the local soft tissue condition settled, and the patient was taken to the operating room for definite fixation. After administration of prophylactic antibiotics and external fixator removal, the tourniquet was inflated up to 300 mgHg, and open reduction and internal fixation, with one interfragmentary 3.5 mm screw and a 12-hole stainless steel 1/3 tubular plate, was performed (Fig. 37.5). The syndesmosis was checked with the Cotton test [1] under image intensifier and was found stable. Immediately postoperatively, the ankle was immobilised in a below knee backslab.

The patient was discharged home and advised not to weight bear until seen in the outpatient clinic. He was prescribed 4.500 IU of tinzaparin for thromboprophylaxis for a period of 4 weeks.

A week later he was seen in the clinic for a wound check and X-rays of the left ankle which demonstrated failure of fixation with lateral shift of the talus and medial space opening (Fig. 37.6).

G. Kotsarinis
Academic Department of Trauma and Orthopaedics, Leeds General Infirmary, School of Medicine, University of Leeds, Leeds, UK

P. V. Giannoudis (✉)
Academic Department of Trauma and Orthopaedics, School of Medicine, University of Leeds, Leeds, UK

NIHR Leeds Biomedical Research Center, Chapel Allerton Hospital, Leeds, UK

© The Author(s), under exclusive license to Springer Nature Switzerland AG 2024
P. V. Giannoudis, P. Tornetta III (eds.), *Failed Fracture Fixation*,
https://doi.org/10.1007/978-3-031-39692-2_37

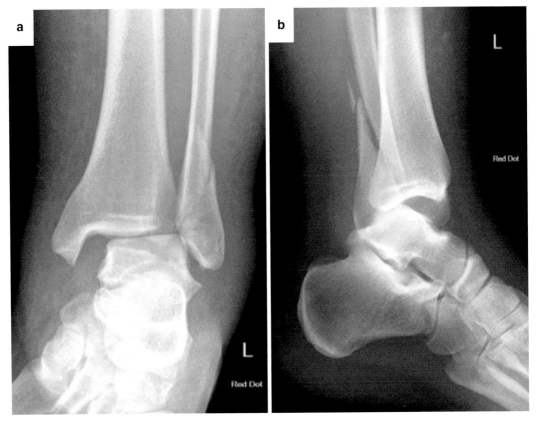

Fig. 37.1 (**a**) Anteroposterior (AP) and (**b**): lateral left ankle radiographs, demonstrating the fracture pattern and the subluxation of the ankle joint laterally and posteriorly. The significant soft tissue swelling should be noted

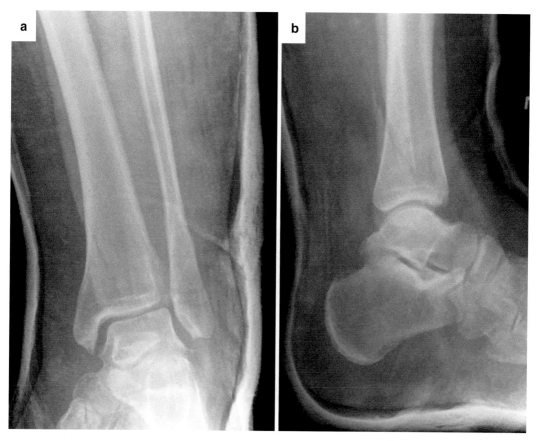

Fig. 37.2 (**a**): AP and (**b**): lateral radiographs of the left ankle after closed reduction attempt. This position was accepted to give time to the soft tissues to settle in a plaster of Paris (back slab)

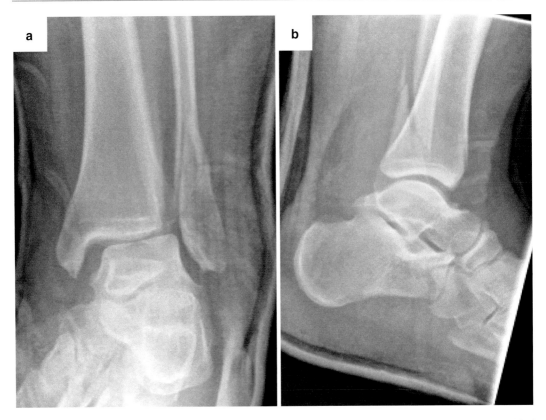

Fig. 37.3 1: AP and 2: lateral radiographs of the left ankle showing the subluxation of the ankle. The talus is shifted laterally

Fig. 37.4 Intraoperative radiographs. (**a**, **b**): Tibial, calcaneal and metatarsal pins positioning is demonstrated. (**c**, **d**): AP and lateral radiographs of the ankle after external fixator application, showing the acceptable joint position

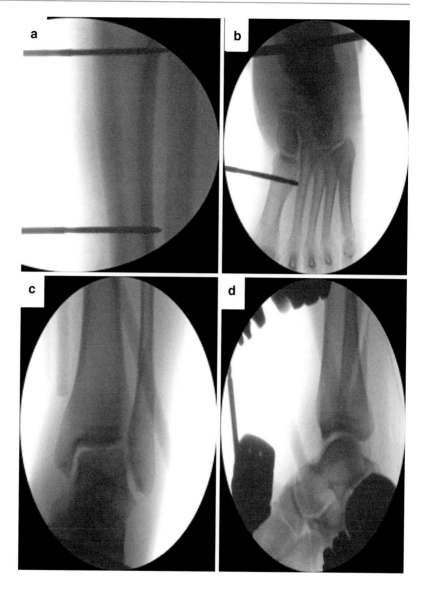

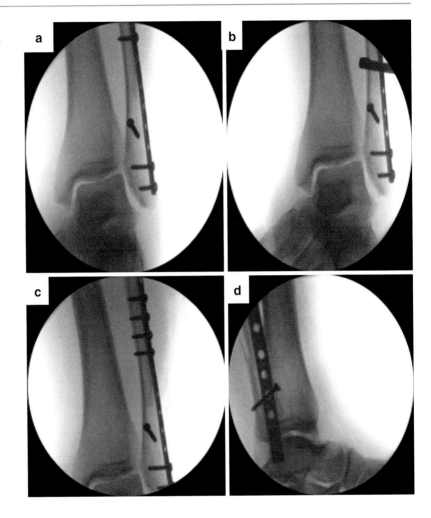

Fig. 37.5 Intraoperative radiographs. (**a**): Mortise views of the ankle under no stress. (**b**): Mortise view of the ankle applying the Cotton test. (**c, d**): AP and lateral radiographs of the ankle showing the reduction and stabilisation of the ankle with interfragmentary screw and 1/3 tubular plate

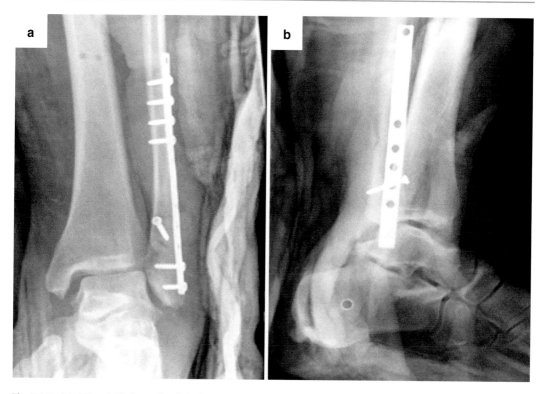

Fig. 37.6 (**a**): AP and (**b**): Lateral weight-bearing left ankle radiographs demonstrating the lateral shift of the talus and the subsequent medial space opening in the backslab

Evaluation of Aetiology of Failure of Fixation

Supination-external rotation ankle fractures are associated with a fibular fracture at the level of the joint and are also classified as Weber B. In such cases, following the biomechanics of the applied forces, significant syndesmotic disruption is not to be expected, based on the presumed integrity of the distal interosseous membrane.

The criteria for acceptable reduction of an ankle fracture on plain radiographs include articular step-off <2 mm, displacement <2 mm, medial clear space <4 mm, ball-shaped dime sign, tibiofibular overlap >5 mm on anteroposterior view, no talar shift and congruency of the ankle mortise [2–5]. These criteria were fulfilled intraoperatively, so no need for further intervention occurred at the first instance. However, plain radiographs have several limitations and lack the desired efficacy to diagnose malreduction of the fracture or malpositioning of the implant. One of these main limitations is the inability to acquire axial views and subsequently investigate any syndesmosis diastasis or subluxation [6]. According to some authors, plain radiography only reliably predicted widening at >4 mm of diastasis [7]. Moreover, measurement of medial clear space may be affected by the degree of axial rotation of the limb, image magnification, and ankle plantar flexion [8–10].

There are many tests and techniques to assess the syndesmosis intraoperatively and postoperatively: squeeze test, Cotton test, stress test, biomechanical criteria (fracture pattern), comparison with contralateral side, CT, MRI and arthroscopy [1, 11–16]. In this case, the Cotton test was utilised. However, the distal fixation of the fibula was deemed to be inadequate as there were only two screws which were rather short in length (suboptimal fixation).

Finally, it should be noted that Nielson et al. [14] found that only 42% of the unstable syndesmoses in their study were recognised intraoperatively.

Clinical Examination

Following the diagnosis of failed fixation, the patient was referred to our reconstruction unit for further management. On examination 10 days following initial fixation, the lateral malleolar wound was found to be clean, with no evidence of erythema or discharge.

There was some residual swelling over the medial malleolus. There was no distal neurovascular deficit. The function of the common and superficial peroneal nerve was intact.

Ankle movements of plantar flexion and dorsiflexion were associated with marked irritability and expressed discomfort.

Diagnostic-Biomechanical and Radiological Investigations

In this case, postoperative weight-bearing radiographs in the backslab indicated incomplete fracture fixation with syndesmosis diastasis, lateral shift of the talus and subsequent medial space opening, as shown in Fig. 37.6. Despite the clinical picture of an almost healed wound, performing baseline biochemical investigations to screen for infection is good practice (FBC, CRP, ESR). The results obtained can be considered as baseline results in case there will be issues with infection at a later stage.

The degree of malreduction and extent of syndesmosis injury can be further evaluated by the acquisition of a CT scan.

Preoperative Planning

The steps of the revision surgery consist of:

(a) Removal of the previous implant and insertion of a new implant for fixation.

(b) Confirmation of accurate distal fibula reduction.
(c) Investigation of gripping strength of the distal fragment screws.
(d) Supplementary syndesmotic screw fixation.

Implants Required:
– Small fragment set.
– ALPS distal fibula anatomical plate (Zimmer Biomet).

Revision Surgery

The previous incision was utilised, and the implant was approached through careful dissection. The reduction of the fracture with the interfragmentary screw was not anatomical as it was fixed in external rotation (fibular length was not accurate); moreover, one of the distal screws was loose with inadequate bone purchase (screw length was inaccurate). The plate and the lag screw were removed. The fibula fracture was reduced anatomically, and a lag screw was inserted (Fig. 37.7).

The fibula fracture was then stabilised with an anatomical distal fibula locking plate (Zimmer Biomet) which provided more options for distal locking screw fixation (Fig. 37.8).

After the plate application, the syndesmosis was reduced under direct visualisation, held with a reduction clamp and a four-cortices transyndesmotic screw was inserted (Fig. 37.9).

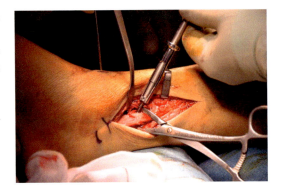

Fig. 37.7 Intraoperative picture showing insertion of lag screw

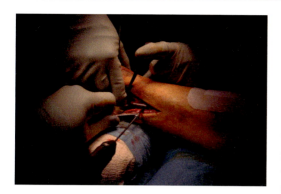

Fig. 37.8 Intraoperative picture showing insertion of proximal screws in the distal fibula anatomical locking plate

Radiographic confirmation of acceptable reduction was achieved under a stress test (application of dorsal flexion and external rotation), and the ankle was placed in a below the knee backslab (Fig. 37.10). Postoperative instructions included non-weight bearing for 6 weeks in a walker boot with immediate initiation of mild range of motion exercises. Three months postoperatively, the fracture had healed (Fig. 37.11), but the patient was experiencing some stiffness in dorsal flexion. The patient was referred to physiotherapy and 6 months postoperatively he returned to his pre-injury level of mobilisation.

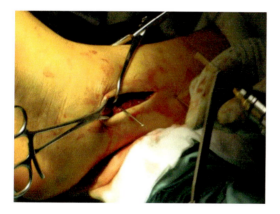

Fig. 37.9 Intraoperative image showing maintenance of syndesmosis reduction with reduction clamp

Fig. 37.10 (**a**): AP and (**b**): Lateral radiographs of the left ankle after revision surgery. There is no talar shift or medial space opening. The fracture is anatomically reduced

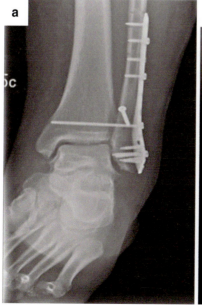
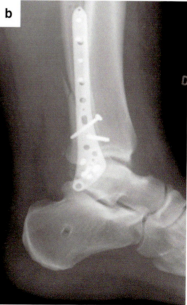

Fig. 37.11 (**a**): AP and (**b**): Lateral left ankle radiographs 3 months postoperatively. On examination, the patient could weight bear pain free, but there was some residual stiffness in dorsiflexion

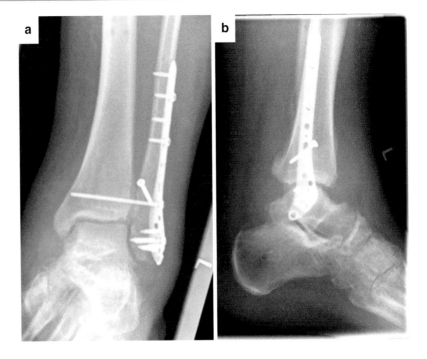

Summary: Lessons Learned

It can be challenging to confirm an anatomic ankle fracture reduction and to investigate if this needs syndesmotic fixation or not. Intraoperative image intensifier has been a significant weapon in the treatment of ankle fractures, but additional measures should be considered not to miss syndesmotic injuries. Such tips and tricks should be considered in these circumstances by the surgeon as a lateral radiograph of the contralateral uninjured ankle for comparison. This can be easily taken preoperatively in the radiology department or intraoperatively with the image intensifier and used as a reference for the accuracy of fracture's reduction.

References

1. Cotton F. Fractures and joint dislocations. Philadelphia, PA: WB Suanders; 1910.
2. Harper MC, Keller TS. A radiographic evaluation of the tibiofibular syndesmosis. Foot Ankle. 1989;10(3):156–60.
3. Leeds HC, Ehrlich MG. Instability of the distal tibiofibular syndesmosis after bimalleolar and trimalleolar ankle fractures. JBJS. 1984;66(4):490–503.
4. Pettrone FA, et al. Quantitative criteria for prediction of the results after displaced fracture of the ankle. JBJS. 1983;65(5):667–77.
5. Reckling FW, McNAMARA GR, DeSMET AA. Problems in the diagnosis and treatment of ankle injuries. J Trauma. 1981;21(11):943–50.
6. Abbasian M, et al. Reliability of postoperative radiographies in ankle fractures. Arch Bone Jt Surg. 2020;8(5):598–604.
7. Ebraheim NA, et al. Radiographic and CT evaluation of tibiofibular syndesmotic diastasis: a cadaver study. Foot & Ankle Int. 1997;18(11):693–8.
8. Goergen T, et al. Roentgenographic evaluation of the tibiotalar joint. JBJS. 1977;59(7):874–7.
9. Kragh JF Jr, Ward JA. Radiographic indicators of ankle instability: changes with plantarflexion. Foot Ankle Int. 2006;27(1):23–8.
10. Saldua NS, et al. Plantar flexion influences radiographic measurements of the ankle mortise. JBJS. 2010;92(4):911–5.

11. Boden SD, et al. Mechanical considerations for the syndesmosis screw. A cadaver study JBJS. 1989;71(10):1548–55.
12. Ebraheim NA, Elgafy H, Padanilam T. Syndesmotic disruption in low fibular fractures associated with deltoid ligament injury. Clin Orthop Relat Res. 2003;409:260–7.
13. Milz P, et al. Lateral ankle ligaments and tibiofibular syndesmosis: 13-MHz high-frequency sonography and MRI compared in 20 patients. Acta Orthop Scand. 1998;69(1):51–5.
14. Nielson JH, et al. Correlation of interosseous membrane tears to the level of the fibular fracture. J Orthop Trauma. 2004;18(2):68–74.
15. Sclafani S. Ligamentous injury of the lower tibiofibular syndesmosis: radiographic evidence. Radiology. 1985;156(1):21–7.
16. Takao M, et al. Diagnosis of a tear of the tibiofibular syndesmosis: the role of arthroscopy of the ankle. J Bone Joint Surg Br Vol. 2003;85(3):324–9.

Bimalleolar Ankle Failed Fixation

38

Jodi Siegel

History of Previous Primary Failed Treatment

This patient sustained a low-energy, bimalleolar ankle fracture after a ground-level fall. The medial malleolus is an anterior colliculus fracture and the lateral malleolus is a Weber B. He is a 60-year-old obese diabetic with peripheral neuropathy. The distal fibula fracture was fixed with a laterally based, standard one-third tubular plate and the medial malleolus was repaired with short cancellous, cannulated screws (Fig. 38.1). His weight bearing was advanced at 6 weeks. After walking without pain for a month, but with worsening ankle deformity, his care was transferred with failed fixation (Fig. 38.2).

Neuropathic diabetic ankle fracture patients require aggressive care in comparison to healthy, younger patients with the same radiographic injury [1]. Their lack of protective sensation, including pain, cannot alert patients to the loss of fracture reduction or the on-going injury to the soft tissues; additionally, the compromised mobility and potential need for medical optimization can be problematic. Rapid improvements in chronic medical conditions are obviously not possible. Neuropathy cannot be corrected; elevated haemoglobin A1c >6.5% is known to portend higher complications. Perioperative glucose control is also more difficult [2].

Radiographically, this is a routine Weber B, Lauge-Hansen supination external rotation type 4 unstable ankle fracture. In non-neuropathic patients, adequate surgical management of the distal fibula fracture can be performed as either lag screw plus neutralization plate or antiglide plate [3]. Knowing the challenges in healing for neuropathic diabetics, more aggressive surgical decision-making combined with conservative post-operative care is often necessary. This patient's ankle was repaired with a standard lateral one-third tubular plate but without a lag screw. There are multiple options available to increase the robustness of the fixation. Adding a lag screw, placing multiple screws into the tibia for additional screw purchase and using the plate to antiglide to optimize biomechanical properties are some options. In this patient, medial bicortical fixation and prolonged non-weight bearing may also have been considered.

J. Siegel (✉)
Department of Orthopaedics, University of North Carolina, Chapel Hill, NC, USA

© The Author(s), under exclusive license to Springer Nature Switzerland AG 2024
P. V. Giannoudis, P. Tornetta III (eds.), *Failed Fracture Fixation*,
https://doi.org/10.1007/978-3-031-39692-2_38

Fig. 38.1 (a, b) Post-operative AP and lateral radiographs of a rotational bimalleolar ankle fracture. (Case and figures courtesy of Paul Tornetta III, MD)

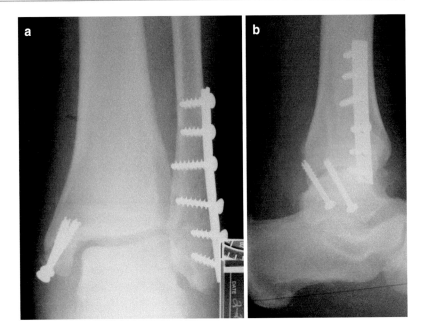

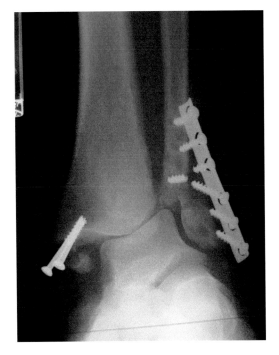

Fig. 38.2 AP radiograph at 3 months post-fixation showing failed hardware and dislocated ankle mortise

Evaluation of the Aetiology of Failure of Fixation

Neuropathic diabetic ankle fractures require a more robust surgical construction [4]. It has often been said in these patients that the conservative treatment option is surgical as without internal fixation, failure is inevitable with higher or worse complications [5, 6]. Even with planned surgical care, this patient still failed. With no evidence of infection, an inadequate hardware construct, and routine timing for weight-bearing restrictions contributed to failure. Optimizing biomechanics, with such options as antiglide plating, multiple screws into the fibula, locked plating, intramedullary implants and modifying post-operative treatment regimen is vital for success in the management of diabetic patients with ankle fractures.

Clinical Examination

As in all fracture patients, the mechanism of the injury and the patient's medical history play an important role in treatment plans and timing. Low-energy fractures in older patients with a host of medical problems and functional challenges must affect a surgeon's decision-making. Understanding the patient's mental status, current ambulatory status and functional abilities and goals is necessary for successful operative planning. Additionally, in considering the local environment of the injured area, the condition of the soft tissues surrounding the fracture can alter treatment options and decision-making. So after understanding the complexities of the patient, examining the skin is vital. Are the wounds healed? Where are the surgical scars? Are there chronic skin changes indicating advanced diabetes and/or neuropathy? Is the medial tissue comprised because of the lateral translation of the talus?

In this patient, his soft tissue envelope was relatively benign. The wounds were well healed and there was no surrounding erythema or open chronic wounds. There were no concerning chronic skin changes. The clinical alignment was valgus but not enough to cause erosive changes medially. He was able to flex and extend his toes as well as dorsi- and plantarflex the ankle with no pain. The distal sensory examination was grossly at his baseline. He had a palpable pulse as diabetes is a microvascular disease. Obtaining toe pressures is preferred by some surgeons to allow further discussion of surgical risks; that information is not available in this case.

Diagnostic-Biochemical and Radiological Investigations

Diabetes is associated with microarchitectural changes that decrease bone quality and therefore increase fracture risk [7], which is not always reflected in bone mineral density (BMD) [8]. To orthopaedic surgeons caring for diabetic patients, poor bone quality and delayed fracture healing are well-known challenges [9]. The alterations in the osteoblasts and osteoclasts, which lead to the delays in fracture healing and callus remodelling, require clinical adjustments to the robustness of the surgical construction as well as the time to weight bearing [4]. In situations where additional imaging is necessary, a CT scan examination might be helpful. In this case, it was not felt to be needed. If there is suspicion of infection, biochemical investigations including FBC, CRP and ESR can be helpful. Finally, in diabetic patients, it is essential to investigate that the blood glucose levels are well controlled with the medication taken and there is no need to revise it.

Preoperative Planning

Preoperative planning for revision cases is paramount. Restoring fracture alignment may not be simple. The fibula is short, comminuted and malaligned; the distal tibiofibular joint is dislocated. Fibular length will need to be restored. That should aid with reducing the talus under the plafond, although not always entirely. Achieving those goals could require equipment not frequently used or available in many surgery centres, which is where a lot of ankle fractures are fixed. Stabilization will require additional implants.

Pre-operative templating makes surgeons think about all of the steps and potential obstacles. It forces in-depth evaluation of the fracture. There are software packages available with many of the PACS systems that are relatively easy to learn. If that is not available, the old-school tracing paper and templates still work! Obtaining an X-ray of the contralateral side aids in planning. Figure 38.3a, b demonstrates the goal and the planned fixation strategy for this patient.

First, the hardware needs to be removed. At least one of the screws is broken. Acquiring the operative report can be helpful to know exactly what screwdriver is needed. In most PACS systems, the contrast of the image can be sharply adjusted to frequently allow visualization of the screw head. Several universal screwdriver sets are also available. Regarding broken hardware, many surgeons will leave distal hardware frag-

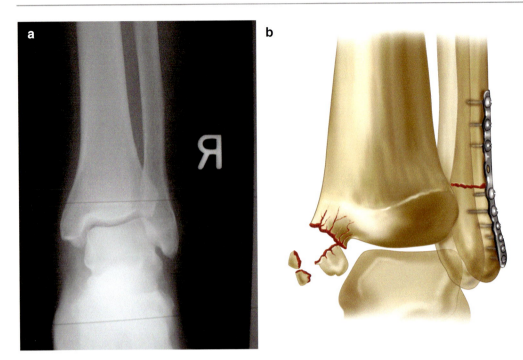

Fig. 38.3 (a, b) Contralateral ankle and pre-operative template of fixation plan

ments if they are not blocking reduction or fixation. If necessary, many companies have broken screw removal sets that include trephines and various broken screw capture systems.

Once the hardware is out, evaluate the bone and surrounding tissues. Is there any concern for infection? Consider sending bony specimens to help identify any latent infection; alternatively, abort revision surgery if there is obvious purulence. Thorough debridement and irrigation should be performed instead.

With no concerns for infection, bony healing is evaluated next. If any healing has occurred, it will require mobilization and debridement with any combination of curettes, rongeurs and osteotomes. Next fibular length will need to be restored. There are multiple techniques described for restoring fibular length. The most frequently used include employing a small fragment bone tenaculum at the fracture site to manipulate the fracture reduced or pulling on the distal segment with a small fragment lobster claw type bone holding forceps. A lamina spreader in the fracture can push the fibula out to length; care must be taken not to crush compromised bone. A Hintermann retractor placed over K-wires can distract the fibula to its normal length. Similarly, a universal distractor can be used over Steinman pins to restore length. Fixing a plate to the distal segment and then using an articulating tension/distractor device or a lamina spreader against a screw proximal to the plate can also work. Several of these options should be available. Consideration must be given to the quality of the surrounding bone when using these techniques. Poor bone quality limits the utility of the most common methods of reduction. A combination of several techniques may be necessary.

Once the fibular length is restored, the fracture needs to be reduced and provisionally held. This will coincide with reducing the talus under the mortise if restoring length has not already easily done this. Manipulation of the foot may be all that is necessary. Large peri-articular reduction forceps, with various-sized foot discs or washers to dissipate the force to a larger area of poor bone, may be necessary. This clamp can be applied to the lateral distal fibula and the medial distal tibia to medialize the talus. A lateral plate may also be used as a giant washer on the fibula.

Holding the fracture and the mortise reduced can be done with multiple smooth K-wires of various sizes (sometimes larger than what is in a small fragment type set), bone reduction forceps ± assistance from a plate, and manipulation of the foot. K-wires may be used to pin the fracture site, pin the distal fibular fragment to the tibia or pin the talus to the tibia.

Given the known struggles with diabetic neuropathic patients and their fractured bones, a robust construct is necessary. The thickness of the plate is unlikely to be the source of failure so substituting an LC-DCP plate for a standard 1/3 tubular or a location-specific, thinner, distal fibular pre-contoured locking plate is not required. The pre-contoured plates can be helpful for ease of fit, but plate position for the goals of surgery should not be sacrificed to use one of these plates. It is more important that screws can be placed through the plate, through the fibula bicortically, and into the tibia with as many screws as possible [10]. The option to lock some screws into the plate might be of value but not at the sacrifice of fixation into the tibia. Standard implants in most small fragment/location-specific type systems allow for the substitution of cortical screws for larger thread cancellous screws and the surgeon should ensure this option exists also.

Supplemental fixation could include large smooth K-wires across the tibiotalar joint left outside of the skin for ease of removal in the office [11]. External immobilization in a splint, cast or removable boot, each comes with different risks to the soft tissues.

An alternative treatment strategy to the more standard ankle fracture constructs could be to forgo the likely already damaged tibiotalar joint. Once alignment is restored, the surgeon could choose to stabilize the mortise with a tibiotalocalcaneal (TCC) nail, also frequently called a hindfoot fusion nail, with or without preparing the joint depending on the patient [12].

In terms of the need for bone grafting, given the subacute failure with known risk factors and poor fixation, it is unlikely to be advantageous. Although the potential use of allogenic non-diabetic mesenchymal stem cells in the faulty diabetic bone homeostasis and impaired fracture repair milieu is currently under investigation, there is currently no clinical knowledge of these benefits [13]. Given the known higher risk of infection in diabetic patients, the use of any type of foreign materials such as bone graft introduces more risk than any perceived benefits in the opinion of the author [14].

Revision Surgery

With all equipment options available, the surgical procedure can proceed with thoughtful decision-making based on the soft tissues, the ease or difficulty with obtaining and maintaining the reduction, the condition of the articular cartilage and the feel of the bone quality. The author prefers to operate on a radiolucent operating room table although a regular OR table would work. A large fluoroscopy unit will enter from the contralateral side. A bump was placed under the ipsilateral hip for neutral to slight internal rotation of the extremity for improved lateral access. The author prefers to use sterile bumps in the field in lieu of blankets or commercially available devices under the drapes to allow for easy intraoperative adjustments to assist with reduction. No tourniquet was used.

After sterile preparation of the skin, the entire extremity is draped to the hip to allow for easier movement of the limb; the toes are covered. A sterile bump is placed under the calf/Achilles, allowing the heel to float free; placing the heel on the bump can cause subluxation of the talus anteriorly on the plafond. Attention was first turned medially. Since the medial hardware was presumed to interfere with reduction of the mortise, and since revision medial fixation was still not guaranteed necessary, the screw heads were identified by palpation. The skin was incised through the previous scar at this level. The medial fixation was removed uneventfully.

Attention was turned laterally. There was a previous direct lateral surgical scar, which was adequate to allow for the procedure. After incising the skin and soft tissues, the plate was encountered. The soft tissues were elevated on the plate, and the non-broken screws and the plate were removed. Two distal fragments of broken screws were left as they were felt to not affect reduction and revision fixation. There was no obvious evidence of infection.

With the metal removed, the fracture deformity was easy to see. There was minimal callus. The tissues were mobilized off the bone to allow for adequate visualization. There was gross motion at the fracture but also significant stiffness of the entire ankle. The non-union was taken down and any intervening callus was removed. After adequate mobilization of the fracture site, the fracture and the mortise were reduced under direct control with bone reduction forceps at the fracture and manipulation of the foot. The fracture was reduced with smooth K-wires.

A straight plate was contoured to fit over the distal fibula while positioned in a lateral position that allowed screws to be placed into the tibia, too. Then multiple quadricortical 3.5-mm screws were placed through the plate, through the fibula and into the tibia. An additional screw was able to be placed through the plate, across the fracture. The most proximal screw was into the fibula only due to inadequate access to the tibia. The distal cluster of screws included cancellous screws. With the fracture reduced and stabilized and the talus reduced under the plafond in both the coronal and sagittal planes, two large smooth transfixion pins were placed retrograde transcalcaneal-talar-tibial to supplement the fixation [11]. Fluoroscopic images were obtained (Fig. 38.4a, b). The mortise was reduced and stable. The fibula was out to length. The medial malleolus fragment was reduced. Given that it was a small anterior colliculus fragment, offering minimal additional stability to this construct, the decision was made to avoid a larger medial incision and treat it without additional hardware (Fig. 38.5).

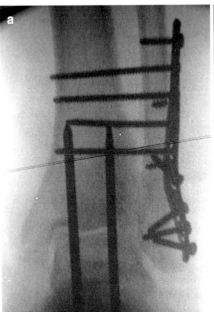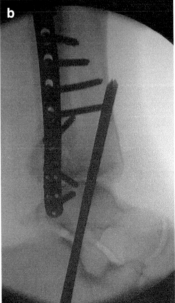

Fig. 38.4 (a, b) AP and lateral fluoroscopic images of final fixation construct

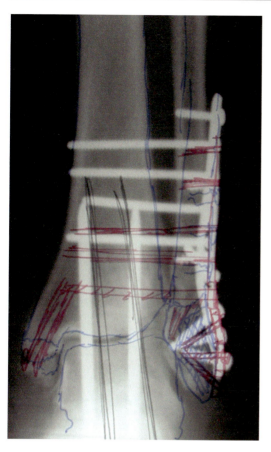

Fig. 38.5 Post-operative template overlaying fluoroscopic fixation image

The lateral tissues were able to cover all of the metal. The skin was closed with interrupted nylons with the plan to retain the sutures for a month. The transfixion pins were left outside the skin plantarly to allow for removal in the clinic. The patient was immobilized in a cast. He was made non-weight bearing. He was seen every 2 weeks for cast changes and skin checks. The pin was removed at 8 weeks; it was loose but not infected. His weight bearing was advanced at 12 weeks. At 6 months, he is walking with a painless ankle, a stable mortise and mild stiffness (Fig. 38.6a–d).

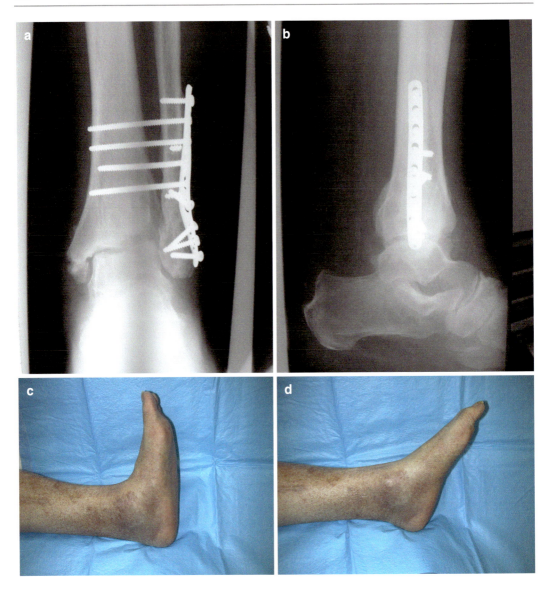

Fig. 38.6 (**a, b**) AP and lateral radiographs at 6 months showing a reduced mortise. (**c, d**): Maximal active dorsiflexion and plantarflexion at 6 months

Lessons Learned

Diabetic ankle fractures are well known to present challenges. Surgical management is considered by many to be the more conservative option and although complications are not uncommon, they are often less severe than the difficulties associated with nonsurgical treatment. Restoring anatomy, using robust fixation constructs, prescribing prolonged non-weight bearing, and employing vigilance about possible complications are mandatory for any successful attempt to salvage the extremity [15].

In this case, as with many patients who are diabetic and neuropathic, failing to adjust the treatment plan can be disastrous. The combination of the plate and screw construct, the transarticular pins, delayed weight-bearing, and the cast provided the necessary stability to hold alignment until union. Although this fixation technique was successful, the alternative approach of the tibiotalocalcaneal (TTC) intramedullary nail is an attractive option with the added benefit of immediate weight-bearing in a patient who may have already sustained irreparable damage to the articular cartilage of the ankle. Multiple studies have shown this to be a safe option to provide stable fixation that allows immediate weight bearing [16]. The patient was counselled of this option but chose an attempt to preserve his motion; therefore, a robust plate and supplementation fixation construct was chosen.

References

1. Bariteau JT, Hsu RY, Mor V, Lee Y, DiGiovanni C, Hayda R. Operative versus nonoperative treatment of geriatric ankle fractures: A Medicare Part A claims database analysis. Foot Ankle Int. 2015;36(6):648–55.
2. Lee SY, Park MS, Kwon S, Sund KH, Jung HS, Lee KN. Influence of ankle fracture surgery on glycemic control in patients with diabetes. BMC Musculoskelet Disord. 2016;17:137.
3. Kilian M, Csorgo P, Vajczikova S, Luha J, Zamborsky R. Antiglide versus lateral plate fixation for Danis-Weber type B malleolar fractures caused by supination-external rotation injury. J Clin Orthop Trauma. 2017;8(4):327–31.
4. Gougoulias N, Oshba H, Dimitroulias A, Sakellariou A, Wee A. Ankle fractures in diabetic patients. EFFORT Open Rev. 2020;5(8):457–63.
5. Flynn J, Rodriguez-del Rio F, Piza P. Closed ankle fractures in the diabetic patient. Foot Ankle Int. 2000;21(4):311–9.
6. Lovy A, Dowdell J, Keswani A, Koehler S, Kim J, Weinfeld S, Joseph D. Nonoperative versus operative treatment of displaced ankle fractures in diabetics. Foot Ankle Int. 2017;38(3):255–60.
7. Hongli J, Xiao E, Graves D. Diabetes and its effects on bone and fracture healing. Curr Osteoporos Rep. 2015;13(5):327–35.
8. Vestergaard P. Discrepancies in bone mineral density and fracture risk in patients with type 1 and type 2 diabetes—a meta-analysis. Osteop Int. 2007;18(4):427–44.
9. Ding Z, Zeng W, Rong X, Liang Z, Zhou Z. Do patients with diabetes have an increased risk of impaired fracture healing? A systematic review and meta-analysis. ANZ J Surg. 2020;90(7-8):1259–64.
10. Schon L, Marks R. The management of neuroarthropathic fracture-dislocations in the diabetic patient. Orthop Clin North Am. 1995;26(2):375–92.
11. Jani M, Ricci W, Borrelli J, Barrett S, Johnson J. A protocol for treatment of unstable ankle fractures using transarticular fixation in patients with diabetes mellitus and loss of protective sensibility. Foot Ankle Int. 2003;24(11):838–44.
12. Srinath A, Matuszewski P, Kalbac T. Geriatric ankle fracture: robust fixation versus hindfoot nail. J Orthop Trauma. 2021;35(Suppl 5):S41–4.
13. Hayes J, Coleman C. Diabetic bone fracture repair: a progenitor cell-based paradigm. Curr Stem Cell Res Ther. 2016;11(6):494–504.
14. Gortler H, Rusyn J, Godbout C, Chahal J, Schemitsch E, Nauth A. Diabetes and healing outcomes in lower extremity fractures: a systematic review. Injury. 2018;49(2):177–83.
15. Brutico A, Nasser E, Brutico J. Operative ankle fractures in complicated diabetes: outcomes of prolonged non-weightbearing. J Foot Ankle Surg. 2022;61(3):542–50.
16. Tan YY, Nambiar M, Onggo JR, Hickey BA, Babazadeh S, Tay WH, Hsuan J, Bedi H. Tibio-Talar-Calcaneal nail fixation for ankle fractures: a systematic review and meta-analysis. J Foot Ankle Surg. 2022;61(6):1325–33.

Ankle Syndesmosis Injury Failed Fixation

39

George D. Chloros, Emmanuele Santolini, Amit E. Davidson, Anastasia Vasilopoulou, and Peter V. Giannoudis

History of Previous Primary Treatment

This is the case of a 20-year-old otherwise healthy man who had fallen inside a pothole and sustained an isolated, neurovascularly intact closed left ankle injury (Fig. 39.1a, b). He was transferred to an outside regional hospital for initial management.

The fracture was immediately reduced in the emergency room, and on the same day, the patient underwent open reduction and internal fixation of his fracture. The fibula was fixed using a lateral fibular locking plate (Newclip Technics) and the syndesmosis was stabilized using a partially threaded syndesmotic screw. The medial malleolus was also reduced and fixed with two fully threaded screws (Fig. 39.2a, b).

In view of the post-operative radiographs, 5 days following the fixation, the patient was referred to the authors' tertiary centre for further management.

G. D. Chloros (✉)
Academic Department of Trauma and Orthopaedics, School of Medicine, University of Leeds, Leeds, UK

Orthopedic Surgery Working Group, Society for Junior Doctors, Athens, Greece

E. Santolini · A. E. Davidson
Academic Department of Trauma and Orthopaedics, School of Medicine, University of Leeds, Leeds, UK

A. Vasilopoulou
Orthopedic Surgery Working Group, Society for Junior Doctors, Athens, Greece

Korgialeneio Mpenakeio Hellenic Red Cross Hospital, Athens, Greece

P. V. Giannoudis
Academic Department of Trauma and Orthopaedics, School of Medicine, University of Leeds, Leeds, UK

NIHR Leeds Biomedical Research Center, Chapel Allerton Hospital, Leeds, UK

© The Author(s), under exclusive license to Springer Nature Switzerland AG 2024
P. V. Giannoudis, P. Tornetta III (eds.), *Failed Fracture Fixation*,
https://doi.org/10.1007/978-3-031-39692-2_39

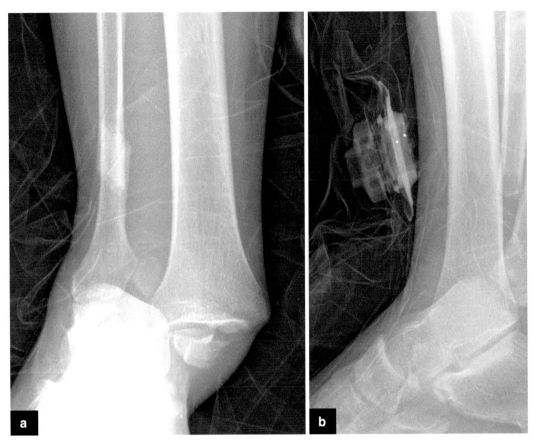

Fig. 39.1 (a) Anteroposterior and (b) lateral radiographs showing a fracture-dislocation of the right ankle on presentation

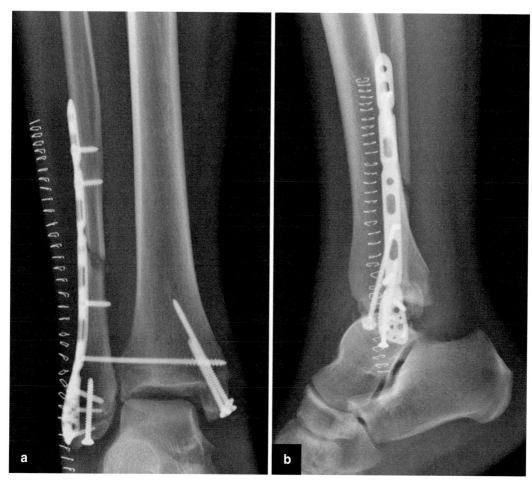

Fig. 39.2 (**a**) Mortise and (**b**) lateral post-operative radiographic views showing the initial fixation

Evaluation of the Aetiology of Failure of Fixation

At this stage, the first step is to use several plain radiographic parameters to evaluate the status of the syndesmosis (Fig. 39.3a, b): tibiofibular clear space, tibiofibular overlap and medial clear space, length of the fibula ('dime' or 'ball' sign and talocrural angle) [1, 2]. The mortise view (Fig. 39.2a) shows that all of these parameters are disrupted, and on both the mortise and lateral views (Fig. 39.2b), there appears to be a non-congruent joint line. The aetiology of failure therefore is secondary to poor technique, i.e. poor reduction of the syndesmosis.

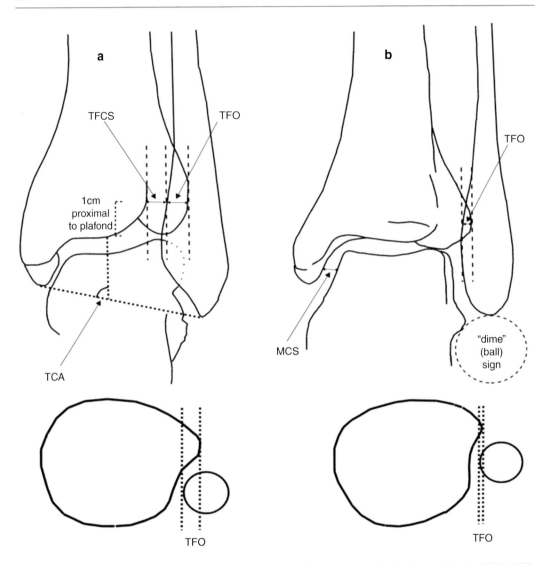

Fig. 39.3 (**a, b**) Plain radiographic parameters for evaluation of the syndesmosis on the anteroposterior (AP) radiograph (**a**) and mortise view (**b**). Measurements should be: tibiofibular clear space (TFCS): <6 mm on either view, tibiofibular overlap (TFO): <6 mm (AP view) or <1 mm (mortise view), talocrural angle (TCA): 72°–86° (AP view), medial clear space (MCS): equal to the superior clear space and < 4 mm (mortise view). 'Dime' sign: ball (or circle should not be disrupted). (Obtained with permission from George D. Chloros, MD)

Clinical Examination

On examination, 5 days post-operatively, there was moderate swelling and no wound dehiscence, drainage or any signs of early infection (Fig. 39.4). The patient was otherwise completely neurovascularly intact.

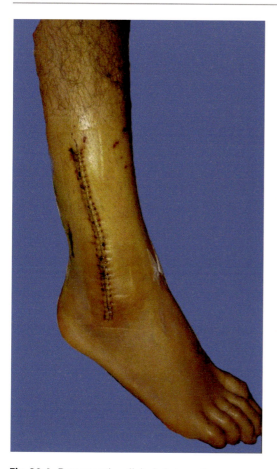

Fig. 39.4 Post-operative clinical photograph

Diagnostic-Biochemical and Radiological Investigations

In view of the radiographic evaluation, which prompted a high index of suspicion for syndesmosis malreduction, further imaging was ordered consisting of a computed tomography (CT) scan for pre-operative planning purposes (Fig. 39.5a-d).

Based on the imaging, the list of problems is as follows (Fig. 39.6):

1. Fibula malreduction – rotational defect.
2. Syndesmotic anterior dislocation.
3. Tibiotalar anterior subluxation (significant: more than 50% of the talar articular surface not articulating with the tibial plafond).
4. Medial malleolus—malreduction.
5. Posterior malfracture.

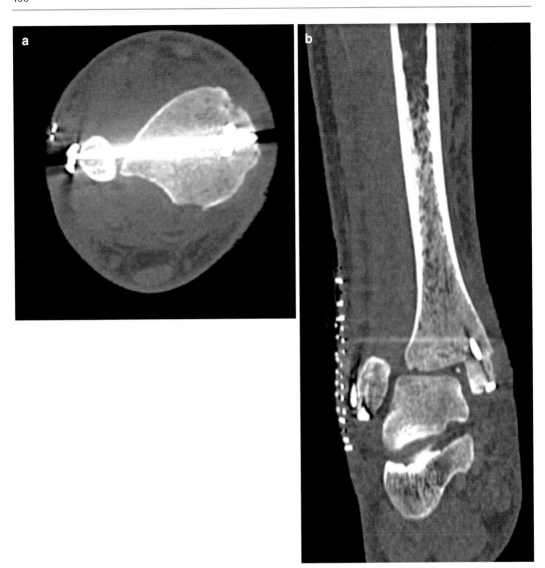

Fig. 39.5 (**a–d**) CT scan showing the status of the ankle joint and syndesmosis: (**a**) Transverse section showing that the fibula lies completely outside of the incisura. (**b**) Coronal section demonstrating significant joint incongruity. (**c**) Sagittal section showing anterior subluxation of the ankle joint. (**d**) Three-dimensional (3D) CT reconstruction showing in addition to malreduction of the medial malleolus

39 Ankle Syndesmosis Injury Failed Fixation

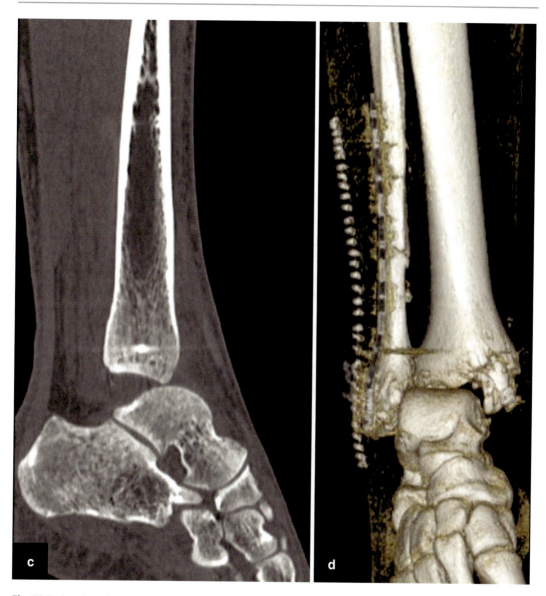

Fig. 39.5 (continued)

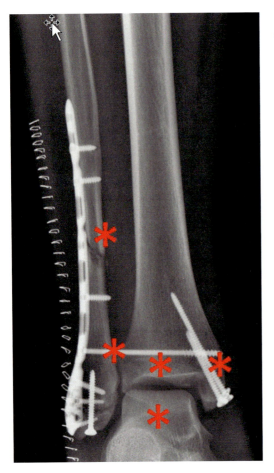

Fig. 39.6 Initial fixation issues to consider

Preoperative Planning

At this point, the goal is to restore the ankle joint anatomic congruity by addressing the aforementioned problems: removal of the hardware, revision fixation of the fibula and the medial malleolus to correct the malreduction and appropriately establish the alignment of the joint surfaces and lastly, fixation of the syndesmosis; the appropriate length, alignment and rotation of the fibula must be addressed and second the syndesmosis needs to be fixed [3–5]. It is well established that malreducing the syndesmosis, either by failing to restore the aforementioned fibular parameters or by failure to fix the fibula in the appropriate position within the incisura, leads to poor outcomes [6].

Therefore, a revision fixation is contemplated consisting of:

1. Removal of the previous screws from the medial malleolus.
   Equipment needed: small fragment set screwdriver
2. Revision reduction and fixation of the medial malleolus using partially threaded cancellous screws.
   Equipment needed: Tulloch-Brown clamp (special pointed reduction forceps); two partially threaded 4.0-mm cancellous screws
3. Removal of the fibula plate.
   Equipment needed: small fragment set screwdriver (Newclip Technics)
4. Opening of the syndesmosis and evaluation under direct vision.
   Equipment needed: dental pick, nibblers, lamina spreaders
5. Visualization, reduction and revision fixation of the fibula to make sure that anatomic alignment including length, alignment and rotation is restored.
   Equipment needed: 1.6 K-wires, one-third small fragment semi-tubular plate DepuySynthes
6. Syndesmosis reduction fixation.
   Equipment needed: fully threaded cortical 3.5-mm-long screw.

Revision Surgery

The patient was positioned supine in the operating table. Antibiotics were administered. The patient was prepped and draped in the usual sterile fashion and a thigh tourniquet was inflated to 350 mmHg. A medial incision was carried out, which was centred on the previous incision. The medial malleolus was exposed and the 4.0 screws were removed using the appropriate screwdriver. The fracture site was cleaned using a combination of dental picks and nibblers and subsequently reduced and held with a Tulloch-Brown clamp. Reduction was confirmed using biplanar fluoroscopy and was satisfactory. Two 1.6-K-wires were drilled in a parallel fashion and 4.0-mm partially threaded cannulated screws of appropriate length were inserted through the wires, which were then removed. The medial wound was closed using 3–0 subcutaneous sutures followed by 3–0 nylon skin sutures.

Attention was then drawn to the lateral side. The previous lateral incision was used and the hardware was exposed and removed using appropriate screwdrivers. The fracture site was taken down, mobilized and cleaned from the debris using a combination of instruments similar to the medial side. At this point, the lower syndesmosis was completely visualized and thoroughly debrided. The fibula was clearly posteriorly malreduced relative to the incisura, which was empty. The length, alignment and rotation of the fibula were re-established using standard reduction manoeuvre by reversing the mechanism of injury. Two crocodile reduction clamps were used to stabilize the fibula in place. A 12-hole third tubular plate was contoured to match the fibula, including distal contouring to 'hook' the lateral malleolus. Eight 3.5-mm cortical screws were subsequently inserted. Attention was turned on the syndesmosis, which was reduced under direct vision and temporarily pinned with a 1.6-mm K-wire. Fluoroscopy verified correct length, alignment and rotation of the fibula and reduction of the syndesmosis. Of note, there are mainly two methods of direct visualization and reduction of the syndesmosis, including the evaluation of the anterior incisura versus visualization of the anterior articular surface at the joint [7]. As the former method has proved less reliable (80%), the syndesmosis was reduced according the later method described by Tornetta et al., which is 93% accurate and is based on perfectly aligning the anterolateral tibial plafond cartilage and the anteromedial fibular cartilage [7]. The authors of this chapter recommend reducing the syndesmosis under direct vision as described and confirming the reduction fluoroscopically with contralateral side comparison. If the reduction is anatomic, then the projections should also be symmetrical. If this is not the case, then, re-attempt at reduction should be performed until everything 'adds-up'. Post-operatively, the patient was put in a splint, no weightbearing for 6 weeks and given deep venous thrombosis (DVT) prophylaxis. He received initial follow-up at the clinic in 2 weeks and further imaging was obtained (Fig. 39.7a, b). At this point, the splint was replaced with a cam walker boot and the patient was encouraged to actively move his ankle using Therabands. At 8 weeks, full weightbearing was permitted and the patient started formal physical therapy. The syndesmotic screw was subsequently removed at 3 months. At 6 months, radiographs show maintenance of the post-operative result (Fig. 39.8a, b). The patient had an excellent range of motion, with a pain-free, stable ankle (Fig. 39.9a, b).

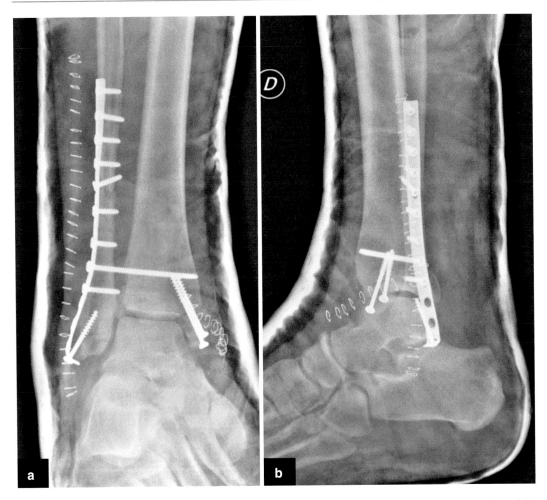

Fig. 39.7 (**a**) Anteroposterior and (**b**) lateral radiographs at 2 weeks following fixation showing restoration of the mortise

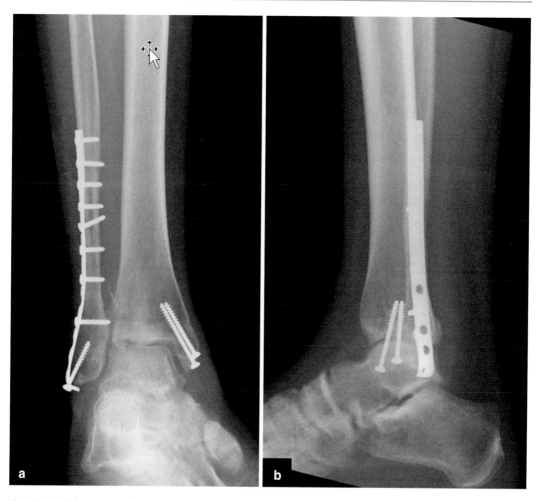

Fig. 39.8 (**a**) Anteroposterior and (**b**) lateral radiographs at 6 months showing a congruent mortise with maintenance of all the radiographic parameters. The syndesmotic screw was removed at 3 months

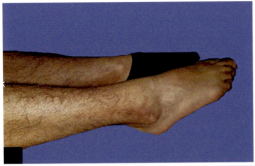

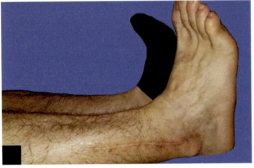

Fig. 39.9 Clinical result at 6 months showing plantarflexion and dosriflexion of the ankle joint

Discussion

There is considerable controversy in the diagnosis and detection of syndesmosis injuries, with the literature being constantly updated with new imaging for technological advances. Sufficient and updated knowledge of the currently available imaging modalities including their strengths and limitations and their appropriate application is essential and crucial in the clinical decision-making of the individual patient.

In this particular case presented, the initial syndesmosis malreduction was easily diagnosed in a straightforward manner using the usual imaging parameters, as described previously (Figs. 39.3a, b and 39.6).

However, it is important to note that nowadays, those 'classic' measurements are surrounded with significant controversy and uncertainty, and therefore should be taken with a grain of salt [2]. First and foremost, they are dependent on the magnification, rotation and position of the limb as far as plantar flexion and dorsiflexion and they have been challenged by recent CT studies [2]. Second, as outlined below,

there is significant interindividual variation, and therefore the bottom line is that x-rays should be interpreted with caution and always within the clinical context, on a case-by-case basis [2]. Frequently, stress radiographs are important in the assessment in equivocal cases [8].

Intra-Operative Imaging

As there is considerable anatomical variability among patients [9], but little intraindividual variation [10], the simple technique of templating the contralateral (uninjured) ankle with intra-operative fluoroscopy is shown to be very effective in assessing the syndesmosis, and is briefly shown in Fig. 39.10 [9, 11–13]. Furthermore, intra-operative cone beam CT may also be used

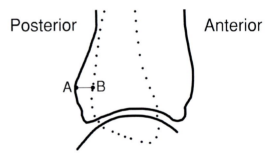

Fig. 39.10 Intra-operative reduction using the contralateral extremity as template [11]. Prior to prepping and draping, a coronal plane template is obtained by a perfect mortise view. Fibular length and rotation, by virtue of the usual radiographic parameters, as described previously, including the medial clear space, the tibiofibular clear space and the tibiofibular overlap as well as the 'ball' or 'dime' sign, is evaluated. Subsequently, for reduction in the sagittal plane, a perfect lateral of the ankle with superimposition of the medial and lateral talar domes is obtained. Posterior tibiofibular distance (A-B): The distance between the posterior aspect of the posterior malleolus of the tibia and the posterior cortex of the fibula is measured on the contralateral extremity and the image is saved for future templating. The injured limb is then reduced in both planes. The posterior tibiofibular distance should match the previously templated contralateral extremity both measured at the same level, and subsequently the surgeon may proceed with their preferred method of syndesmosis fixation. Of note, the distance between the limb and image intensifier should be kept constant to minimize magnification errors and measurements should take place at the same level for both injured and uninjured limbs. (Obtained with permission from George D. Chloros, MD)

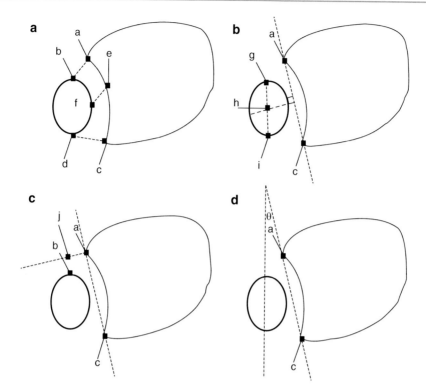

Fig. 39.11 (**a–d**): Various CT scan measurements, based on Nault et al. [1]. Note the line joining the anterior and posterior edges of the colliculi (connecting point a to point c): (**a**) Anterior tibiofibular distance (**a, b**), posterior tibiofibular distance (**c, d**), distance between tibia and fibula in the middle of the incisura (**e, f**). (**b**) Distance between the anterior part of the fibula (**g, h**) and the posterior part of the fibula (**h-i**), respectively, perpendicular to line a-c. (**c**) Distance between the anterior part of the incisura and the anterior part of the fibula (b-j). (**d**) Angle theta (θ), drawn between line a-c and a line representing the orientation of the fibula (i.e. along the longest axis of the fibula). (Obtained with permission from George D. Chloros, MD)

[1] Nault ML, Hébert-Davies J, Laflamme GY, Leduc S. CT scan assessment of the syndesmosis: A new reproducible method. Journal of Orthopaedic Trauma. 2013;27 [11]:638–641.

to accurately assess reduction [14]; however, its major current limitation is availability.

Further Advanced Imaging

Bilateral computed tomography (CT) of the ankles may be checked either pre-operatively (to diagnose syndesmosis injury) or post-operatively (to assess fixation) [10].

Pre-operative assessment is crucial in determining subtle, i.e. less than 3-mm diastases, and is superior to plain radiographs in diagnosing syndesmosis injuries [10], as about 40% of those may be overlooked based on plain radiographic evaluation even in experienced hands [15]. Figures 39.11 and 39.12 show the different parameters that can be evaluated based on the bilateral ankle CT.

Of note plain radiographs are unreliable in quantifying the status of the posterior malleolus including determining the size of the fragment and if any incarcerated fragments and in these cases a CT scan has been shown to change operative planning in 44% of cases [17]. Therefore the authors of this chapter suggest that every ankle fracture with a posterior malleolar component (unless extremely small i.e. a flake) should get a pre-operative CT scan to truly assess the injury. In the case described herein the posterior malleolus was broken but the fragment was small and fixing the syndesmosis with a screw restores the function of the posterior inferior tibiofibular ligament

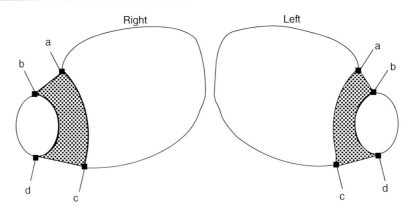

Fig. 39.12 CT for evaluation of the syndesmosis, based on Lee et al. The surface area of the syndesmosis (SAS) [16] is the surface area enclosed by the anterior colliculus (**a**), the most anterior part of the fibula (**b**), the posterior colliculus (**c**) and the most posterior aspect of the fibula (**d**). The SAS on the right side is significantly larger, compared to the left indicating disruption. (Obtained with permission from George D. Chloros, MD)
[Lee SW, Lee KJ, Park CH, Kwon HJ, Kim BS. The Valid Diagnostic Parameters in Bilateral CT scan to Predict Unstable Syndesmotic Injury with Ankle Fracture. Diagnostics (Basel). 2020;10 [10].]

Weightbearing CT

The emergence of weightbearing CT is promising, and in recent studies the diastasis in unstable ankles is significantly greater compared to conventional CT [18]. In a recent systematic review, the surface area of the syndesmosis (SAS) has been shown to be the most reliable measurement in the diagnosis of syndesmotic instability using a weightbearing CT scan [19].

MRI

Magnetic resonance imaging (MRI) has 93% specificity and 100% sensitivity for anterior inferior tibiofibular ligament (AITFL) and 100% sensitivity and specificity for posterior inferior tibiofibular ligament (PITFL) disruptions [4]; however, it is an expensive investigation and usually not required in the acute assessment of the syndesmosis.

Although this case is straightforward, in general, the decision regarding performing a revision surgery of the syndesmosis based on radiographic parameters, for example on an ankle that shows some degree of asymmetry compared to the contralateral extremity in an otherwise nonpainful patient, remains tough and controversial as it would entail a relatively important surgery with prolonged no weightbearing in an asymptomatic patient. In these tough situations, the authors of this chapter would routinely obtain a postoperative bilateral CT scan to further assess the situation, for example whether the fixation was problematic to begin with and inform the patient that they may have a higher chance of getting ankle arthritis in the future. The decision is always tough one, and recommendations are based on multiple factors, and always on a case-by-case basis. In this patient presented herein, there was obvious distortion of the radiographic parameters, and it was clearly felt that the benefit of a revision surgery to address the syndesmosis and reduce the talus back into the mortise would be the appropriate management as the risk of not having surgery would definitely lead to early-onset debilitating arthritis.

Summary: Lessons Learned

- Evaluation and treatment of 'failed' syndesmosis fixation is difficult and controversial.
- There is no unified universal approach and each case should be individualized.
- The case presented here shows successful treatment of a failed syndesmosis and mortise fixation in a patient due to obvious initial technical errors.
- However, the moto 'get it right the first time' and correctly addressing the syndesmosis is crucial in ankle fractures, but not always feasible, as unpredictable factors,

including the nature and severity of the injury, as well as patient factors may compromise outcome.
- Good knowledge of the various imaging modalities and parameters, including pre-operative, intra-operative and post-operative imaging, is critical and those should complement a thorough history and examination of the individual patient in order to lead to optimal outcomes.

References

1. Kellett JJ, Lovell GA, Eriksen DA, Sampson MJ. Diagnostic imaging of ankle syndesmosis injuries: a general review. J Med Imaging Radiat Oncol. 2018;62(2):159–68.
2. White T, Bugler K. Ankle fractures. In: Tornetta P, Ricci W, Court-Brown C, McQueen M, McKee MM, editors. Rockwood and Green's fractures in adults. 9th ed. Lippincot Williams & Wilkins; 2020. p. 2822–76.
3. Fort NM, Aiyer AA, Kaplan JR, Smyth NA, Kadakia AR. Management of acute injuries of the tibiofibular syndesmosis. Eur J Orthop Surg Traumatol. 2017;27(4):449–59.
4. Rammelt S, Obruba P. An update on the evaluation and treatment of syndesmotic injuries. Eur J Trauma Emerg Surg. 2015;41(6):601–14.
5. Walsh AS, Sinclair V, Watmough P, Henderson AA. Ankle fractures: getting it right first time. Foot (Edinb). 2018;34:48–52.
6. Kubik JF, Rollick NC, Bear J, Diamond O, Nguyen JT, Kleeblad LJ, et al. Assessment of malreduction standards for the syndesmosis in bilateral CT scans of uninjured ankles. Bone Joint J. 2021;103(1):178–83.
7. Tornetta P 3rd, Yakavonis M, Veltre D, Shah A. Reducing the syndesmosis under direct vision: where should i look? J Orthop Trauma. 2019;33(9):450–4.
8. Tornetta P 3rd, Axelrad TW, Sibai TA, Creevy WR. Treatment of the stress positive ligamentous SE4 ankle fracture: incidence of syndesmotic injury

and clinical decision making. J Orthop Trauma. 2012;26(11):659–61.
9. Chu X, Salameh M, Byun SE, Hadeed M, Stacey S, Mauffrey C, et al. The utilization of intraoperative contralateral ankle images for syndesmotic reduction. Eur J Orthop Surg Traumatol. 2022;32(2):347–51.
10. Rammelt S, Md P, Boszczyk A, Md P. Computed tomography in the diagnosis and treatment of ankle fractures: a critical analysis review. JBJS Rev. 2018;6(12):e7.
11. Harwin SF, Schreiber JJ, McLawhorn AS, Dy CJ, Goldwyn EM. Intraoperative contralateral view for assessing accurate syndesmosis reduction. Orthopedics. 2013;36(5):360–1.
12. Summers HD, Sinclair MK, Stover MD. A reliable method for intraoperative evaluation of syndesmotic reduction. J Orthop Trauma. 2013;27(4):196–200.
13. Koenig SJ, Tornetta P 3rd, Merlin G, Bogdan Y, Egol KA, Ostrum RF, et al. Can we tell if the syndesmosis is reduced using fluoroscopy? J Orthop Trauma. 2015;29(9):e326–30.
14. Vetter SY, Euler J, Beisemann N, Swartman B, Keil H, Grützner PA, et al. Validation of radiological reduction criteria with intraoperative cone beam CT in unstable syndesmotic injuries. Eur J Trauma Emerg Surg. 2021;47(4):897–903.
15. Szymański T, Zdanowicz U. Comparison of routine computed tomography and plain X-ray imaging for malleolar fractures-How much do we miss? Foot Ankle Surg. 2022;28(2):263–8.
16. Lee SW, Lee KJ, Park CH, Kwon HJ, Kim BS. The valid diagnostic parameters in bilateral CT scan to predict unstable syndesmotic injury with ankle fracture. Diagnostics (Basel). 2020;10(10):812.
17. Donohoe S, Alluri RK, Hill JR, Fleming M, Tan E, Marecek G. Impact of computed tomography on operative planning for ankle fractures involving the posterior malleolus. Foot Ankle Int. 2017;38(12):1337–42.
18. Del Rio A, Bewsher SM, Roshan-Zamir S, Tate J, Eden M, Gotmaker R, et al. Weightbearing cone-beam computed tomography of acute ankle syndesmosis injuries. J Foot Ankle Surg. 2020;59(2):258–63.
19. Raheman FJ, Rojoa DM, Hallet C, Yaghmour KM, Jeyaparam S, Ahluwalia RS, et al. Can weightbearing cone-beam CT reliably differentiate between stable and unstable syndesmotic ankle injuries? A systematic review and meta-analysis. Clin Orthop Relat Res. 2022;480(8):1547–62.

Posterior Malleolar Ankle Failed Fixation

40

Scott P. Ryan and Nicholas R. Pagani

History of Previous Primary Treatment

Posterior malleolar fractures occur in as many as half of all ankle fractures and this subset has worse outcomes [1–4]. The posterior malleolus also contributes to syndesmotic stability through its connection to the distal fibula via the posterior inferior tibiofibular ligament (PITFL). The Haraguchi classification of posterior malleolar fractures is the most commonly referenced and involves three types (Type 1, posterolateral oblique fracture of the distal tibia; Type 2, medial extension fracture involving the posterior aspect of the medial malleolus; Type 3, shell fracture of the posterior tibial cortex) (Fig. 40.1a–c) [5]. More recently, Bartonicek and Rammelt proposed a classification system with added attention to the role of incisural involvement [6]. In this classification system, Type 1 fractures are extraincisural, Type 2 are posterolateral fragments, Type 3 are two-part posteromedial fractures, and Type 4 are large posterolateral triangular fractures involving more than one-third of the fibular notch (Fig. 40.2a–d).

S. P. Ryan (✉) · N. R. Pagani
Department of Orthopaedic Surgery, Tufts Medical Center, Boston, MA, USA
e-mail: SRyan3@tuftsmedicalcenter.org;
npagani@tuftsmedicalcenter.org

In order to understand the causes of posterior malleolar fixation failure, comprehensive knowledge of the biomechanical implications of posterior malleolar fractures is necessary. Biomechanical studies analyzing the role of the posterior malleolus in ankle stability have given variable results. Harper resected 30%, 40%, and 50% of the distal tibial posterior articular surface and found no posterior talar subluxation with posterior stress [7].

Furthermore, addition of a medial malleolar fracture did not result in subluxation. Raasch removed up to 40% of the posterolateral corner of the distal tibia and reported no posterior subluxation [8]. However, when the anterior tibiofibular ligament and fibula were transected, posterior subluxation of the talus occurred when more than 30% of the distal tibia articular surface was removed. Hartford et al. reported that 25%, 33%, and 50% loss of the distal tibial posterior articular surface led to reduction of the ankle joint force-bearing area by 4%, 13%, and 22%, respectively [9]. Fitzpatrick found that talar subluxation did not occur with 50% reduction of the posterior distal tibial articular surface; however, the center of contact stress moved anteromedially following fracture [10]. Evers et al. investigated the role of posterior malleolar fragments (<25%) in trimalleolar fractures and found that contact area decreased following frac-

© The Author(s), under exclusive license to Springer Nature Switzerland AG 2024
P. V. Giannoudis, P. Tornetta III (eds.), *Failed Fracture Fixation*,
https://doi.org/10.1007/978-3-031-39692-2_40

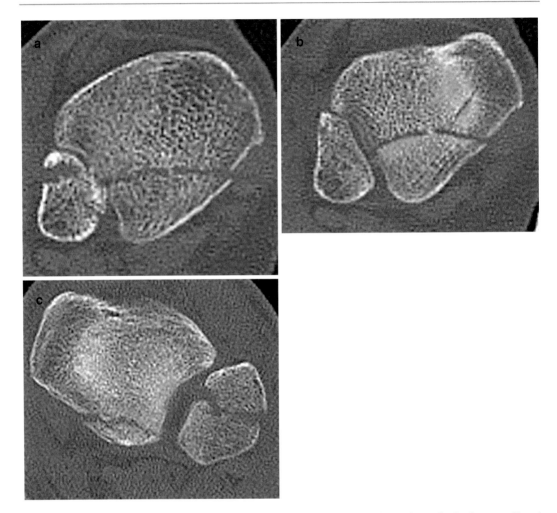

Fig. 40.1 Representative axial CT scan images of the Haraguchi classification of posterior malleolar fractures: Type 1 (**a**), Type 2 (**b**), and Type 3 (**c**)

ture while anatomic reduction and fixation of the posterior malleolar fragment restored contact pressure distribution to intact levels [11]. Finally, Gardner et al. showed that fixation of the posterior malleolar fragment in pronation external rotation fractures restored tibiofibular syndesmotic stability significantly better than a standard syndesmotic screw [12]. In summary, with the medial and lateral malleoli intact or fixed, posterior translation of the talus occurs only when posterior malleolar fragment size exceeds 40% of the articular surface. However, even relatively small posterior malleolar fragments (<25%) can lead to decreased tibiotalar contact area and increased contact pressure.

Early clinical studies demonstrated inferior results of nonoperative treatment of large posterior malleolar fractures, leading to dogma that posterior malleolar fractures involving over 25–33% of the articular surface require fixation [4, 13, 14]. However, Langenhuijsen showed that joint incongruity with posterior malleolar fragments as small as 10% of the tibial articular surface portends poor prognosis [15]. More recent studies have also highlighted the importance of incisura involvement with posterior malleolar

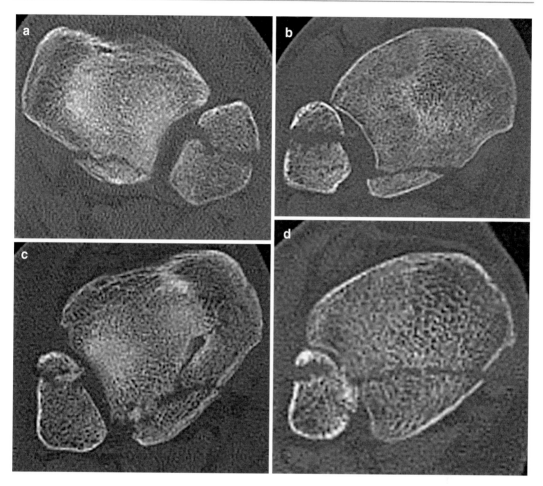

Fig. 40.2 Representative axial CT scan images of the Bartonicek and Rammelt classification of posterior malleolar fractures: Type 1 (**a**), Type 2 (**b**), Type 3 (**c**), and Type 4 (**d**)

fractures [6]. In addition to restoring the distal tibial articular surface at the posterior plafond, the objectives of posterior malleolar fixation have therefore evolved to include restoration of syndesmotic stability through anatomic reduction of the PITFL attachment and anatomic restoration of the incisura, thus facilitating accurate reduction of the distal fibula [1]. Therefore, current operative considerations have expanded beyond fracture size and displacement to also include incisura involvement, presence of intercalary fragments, plafond impaction, and syndesmotic instability.

Posterior malleolar fractures can be treated nonoperatively if the fragment is small and either extraincisural or non/minimally displaced. Operative fixation methods include indirect reduction and anterior-to-posterior screw fixation or open direct reduction and either posterior-to-anterior screw fixation or posterior plating. Larger nondisplaced fragments may be amenable to screw fixation. However, large displaced fragments or those with intercalary fragments, incisural involvement, and joint impaction typically require open reduction followed by plate or screw fixation under direct visualization.

Evaluation of the Etiology of Failure of Fixation

Failure of posterior malleolar fixation can be thought of as (1) failure to recognize a posterior malleolar fracture requiring fixation, (2) failure to achieve reduction compromising syndesmotic stability and fibular reduction, and (3) insufficient fixation method. All three can result in an incongruent tibiotalar joint.

Identification of a fracture fragment that needs fixation may not be obvious on initial or postoperative radiographs as the fibular fixation can obscure fracture lines (Fig. 40.3a, b). With the ankle externally rotated, the fibula will sit more posteriorly exposing the distal tibial fracture line (Fig. 40.3c). Therefore, external rotation lateral radiographs can improve detection and size appreciation as the X-ray beam is more in line with the obliquity of the fracture line [16]. Furthermore, numerous studies have reported that the pattern and size of posterior malleolar fractures cannot be reliably assessed with radiographs alone. Computed tomography (CT) scans are therefore indicated for suspected posterior malleolar fractures and for preoperative planning [6, 17, 18]. The authors routinely obtain preoperative CT scans on all ankle fractures with a posterior component regardless of suspected size on plain radiographs. Intraoperatively, fixation of the medial and lateral structures can lead to reduction of the posterior malleolus via ligamentotaxis when the PITFL is intact [4]. However, a gravity stress and posterior translation stress test must be performed to detect residual subluxation. Therefore, when posterior malleolar fixation is planned, most authors advocate for reduction and fixation of the posterior malleolar fracture prior to fibular fixation.

Accurate reduction and fixation of posterior malleolar fractures that involve the incisura is necessary to restore the fibular notch to allow for fibular reduction. Posterior malleolar fixation reestablishes fibular length through the PITFL and restores syndesmotic stability. Failure to anatomically reduce and stabilize the incisura can lead to rotational malalignment, shortening, and posterior displacement of the distal fibula.

Regarding fixation method, options include the use of lag screws (inserted either anterior-to-posterior or posterior-to-anterior) or a posterior buttress plate. While minimally displaced large fracture fragments with no intercalary fragments or joint impaction may be amenable to percutaneously screw fixation, posterior antiglide or buttress plating is typically recommended for fractures requiring direct open reduction. Multiple studies have shown increased biomechanical fixation strength with posterior buttress plates in comparison to both anterior-to-posterior and posterior-to-anterior screws [19, 20]. Screw fixation alone is not strong enough to support large posterior distal tibial fragments that want to displace posteriorly. This will lead to construct failure when utilized inappropriately (Fig. 40.4a, b).

Finally, there are less common instances where fractures have poor healing potential that displaced during cast treatment (i.e., poorly controlled diabetes) (Fig. 40.5a, b).

It is important to understand which posterior malleolar/posterior distal tibia fractures require direct plate fixation and why in order to prevent either postoperative subluxation with (Fig. 40.4a, b) or without (Fig. 40.3a–c) fixation failure or delayed subluxation (Fig. 40.5a, b).

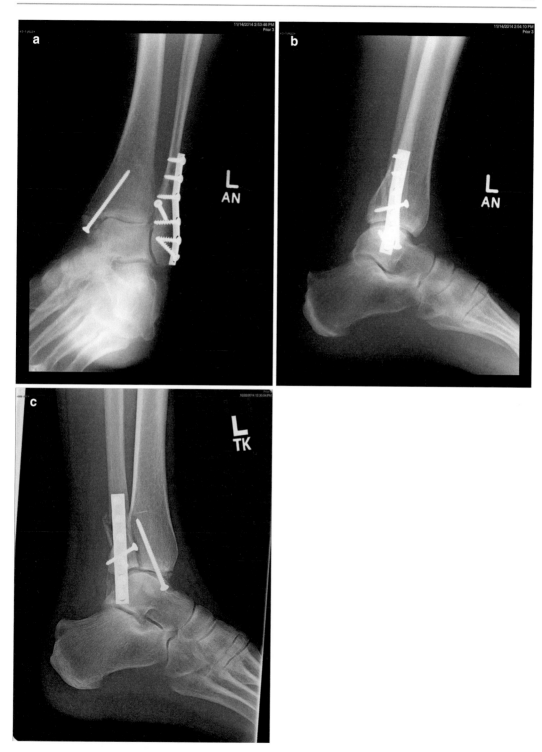

Fig. 40.3 Initial postoperative radiographs: mortise (**a**) and lateral (**b**) after lateral plating of a distal fibula fracture. A missed posterior distal tibia fracture is identified on a postoperative lateral radiograph with the ankle externally rotated to expose the primary tibial fracture line (**c**)

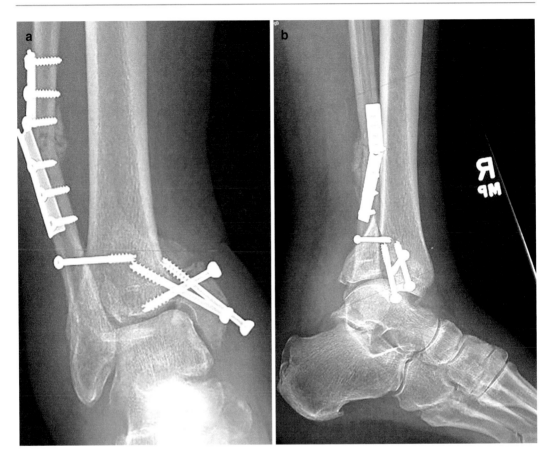

Fig. 40.4 Postoperative anteroposterior (AP) (**a**) and lateral (**b**) radiographs of a trimalleolar ankle fracture, with a large posterior malleolar fragment treated with attempted screw fixation only and syndesmotic stabilization (courtesy of Paul Tornetta III)

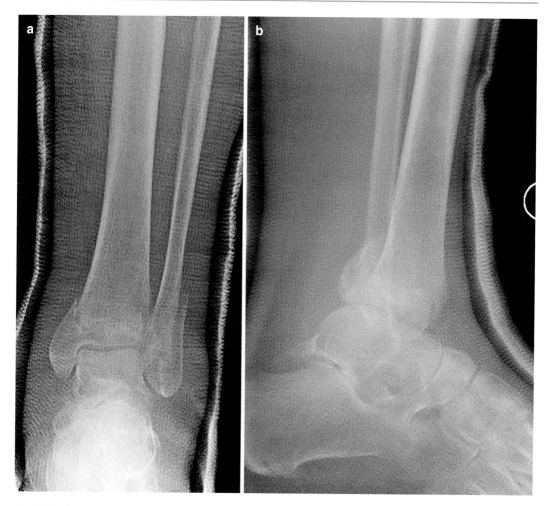

Fig. 40.5 An AP (**a**) and lateral (**b**) showing a posteriorly displaced distal tibia fracture after initial nonoperative management in a cast

Clinical Examination

The clinical examination of a patient with failed ankle fracture fixation starts with a thorough assessment of the skin and soft tissues. Depending on the interval from index fixation, surgical wounds may still be in the nascent stages of healing. Standard management principles apply to lower extremity swelling and fracture blisters. Surgeons should pay close attention to prior external fixation pin sites, open wounds or skin compromise from poorly padded splints or casts.

Detailed evaluation of prior skin incisions is critical. Bimalleolar and trimalleolar ankle fractures are commonly approached using a combination of a medial and laterally based incision to address the distal fibula. Depending on the index fixation strategy utilized, the posterior malleolus may have been addressed via percutaneous anterior incisions (for anterior-to-posterior screws), a posterolateral approach or less commonly a posteromedial approach.

In cases in which a posterolateral approach was previously used to manage the distal fibula and/or posterior malleolus, this incision can be used at the time of revision fixation to address the posterior malleolus. As described by Tornetta et al. (2011), the posterolateral approach allows for reduction and fixation of posterior malleolar fragments under direct visualization with excellent reported results [21]. If indicated, revision fixation of the distal fibula can also be performed through this approach.

If a direct lateral approach was previously used to manage the distal fibula, this will not provide adequate exposure of the posterior tibial plafond. Placement of a standard posterolateral incision is high risk in this scenario due to the close proximity and potential for skin bridge compromise. However, placing a posterolateral incision more posteriorly toward the Achilles can be done safely, as described below. In certain cases, a posteromedial approach to the posterior tibia may be necessary, but close attention should be paid regarding proximity to any existing medial incisions. Clinical and radiographic results for posterior malleolar fixation via the posteromedial approach have been reported as comparable to the posterolateral approach [22]. Furthermore, the posteromedial approach facilitates access to posterior malleolar fractures with medial extension (Haraguchi Type 2 and Bartonicek-Rammelt Type 3).

When planning incisions to a previously operated ankle, surgeons must have detailed understanding of the angiosomes of the lower leg. Historically, authors have purported that a 7-cm minimum skin bridge is necessary between surgical incisions to prevent soft tissue compromise. However, the validity of this rule has been called into question. Howard et al. (2008) reported a low soft tissue complication rate in a series of patients with multiple incisions for tibial plafond fractures with a measured skin bridge less than 7 cm [23]. Safe placement of surgical incisions within 7 cm of each other can be explained by the concept of lower leg angiosomes (defined as a composite block of tissue supplied anatomically by source vessels spanning between the skin and bone) [23–26]. The lower leg contains three angiosomes: the anterior tibial, posterior tibial, and peroneal. The standard posterolateral skin incision is located within the midportion of the peroneal angiosome and the posteromedial skin incision is within the posterior tibial angiosome. If possible, skin incisions should ideally be placed between angiosomes. However, when this is not possible, minimizing unnecessary dissection can limit trauma to source vessels feeding an overlying skin bridge. Placement of a posterolateral incision more posteriorly toward the Achilles can be done safely in the setting of a previous direct lateral incision, given the angiosome distribution described above.

In addition to the above considerations, preoperative optimization of glycemic control and nutritional status can help minimize the potential for soft tissue complications. Finally, a detailed neurovascular examination is necessary for each patient prior to surgery.

Diagnostic-Biochemical and Radiological Investigations

Initial assessment should be performed with standard radiographs. Instances of failure of initial fixation or failure of nonoperative management can be obvious (Fig. 40.4a, b). Other times it can be difficult to assess on radiographs if there is minimal displacement and subluxation of the talus as lateral fibular hardware can obscure fracture lines (Fig. 40.3c). A CT scan should be obtained to evaluate the morphology of the fracture for surgical planning. The CT scan will define the morphology of the posterior distal tibia fragment and asses for bone loss of not only the posterior malleolar fragment, but also on the talus. This can be helpful when counselling patients on expectations such as risk of posttraumatic arthritis (Figs. 40.5a, b, 40.6a, and 40.7).

Failure typically occurs within the first few months after surgery or nonoperative management and bone healing is incomplete. This is because it is typically not due to the bone quality itself but not recognizing the injury (Fig. 40.3a–c) or with an adequate stability (Fig. 40.4a, b).

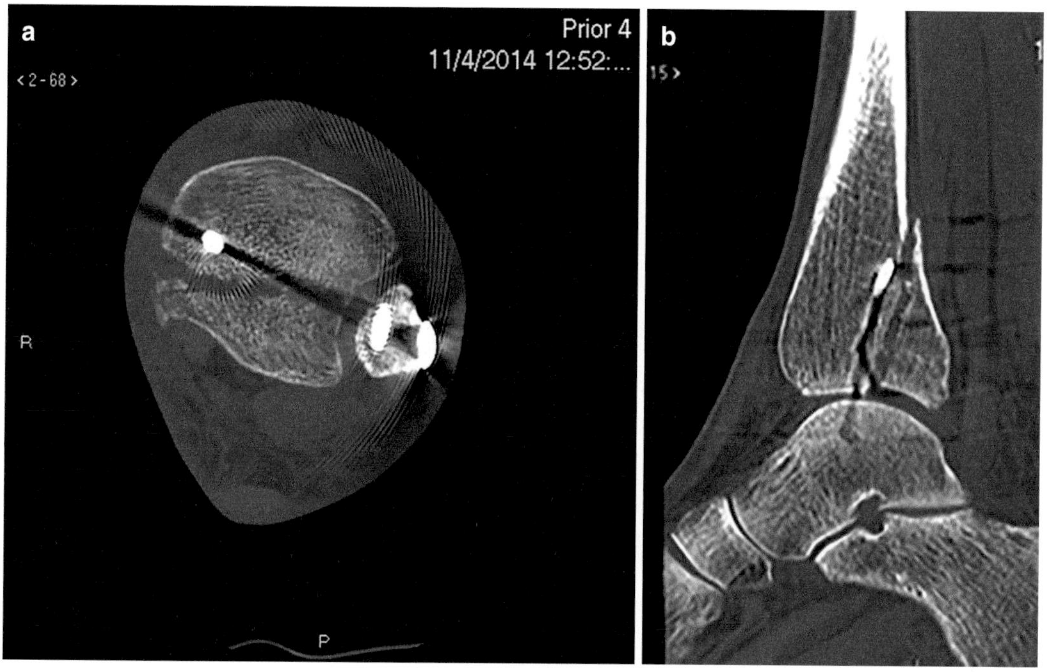

Fig. 40.6 (**a**, **b**) Respective CT cuts of the patient with the missed posterior distal tibia fracture after lateral plating of the fibula (Fig. 40.3 a–c). There is good underlying bone quality and a fracture across the entire distal tibia, which may necessitate a separate medial approach to assist in fracture mobilization. Subluxation of the talus is also appreciated with the distal tibia fragment

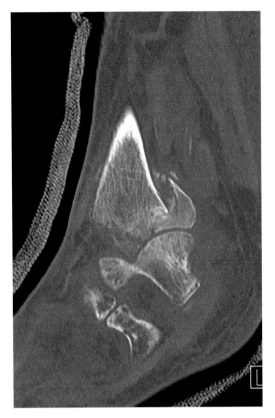

Fig. 40.7 A CT sagittal cut of the patient with attempted nonoperative management of a distal tibia and fibula fracture (Fig. 40.5b). The CT scan shows impaction of the talus on the distal tibia suggesting articular cartilage loss and loss of bone of the posterior distal tibial fragment. There is also erosion of the anterior distal tibia. Risk of posttraumatic arthritis is high

Preoperative Planning

The goal of surgery is to obtain an anatomic ankle mortise by providing resistance to posterior subluxation of the talus with stable fixation of the posterior distal tibia. Whether the fracture has failed/displaced because it was missed or inadequately stabilized, posterior plate fixation of the distal tibia is almost always required. As with all revision surgeries, preoperative templating and planning is critical to success.

The most difficult part of the preoperative plan is determining how to work around previous surgical incisions and safely approach the fracture without putting the soft tissues at risk. This is due to the fact that previous incisions for ankle fracture surgery that have not addressed the posterior malleolus directly tend to be very close to incisions required for a direct posterior approach. For example, it can be difficult or impossible to perform a posterolateral approach to the distal tibia soon after a direct lateral approach has been performed for the fibula.

The preoperative CT scan is necessary to plan the appropriate posterior surgical approach, with the most common being the posterior lateral approach to the distal tibia. However, this can be modified to a posterior medial approach if needed. The posterolateral approach is extensile and one can access almost all of the posterior distal tibia. Since most posterior malleolar fractures leading to instability have a large posterolateral fragment, this is the preferred approach for revision fixation for posterior instability.

The dogma of leaving a 7-cm skin bridge between surgical incisions has recently been questioned by Howard et al. [23]. Although they did not report a minimum distance between surgical incisions, the authors reported a low complication rate when using skin bridges averaging approximately 5 cm, with some skin bridges as small as 4 cm. What may be more relevant is limiting the portions of the incision that overlap as opposed to using an absolute number. One must be cautious however as it is necessary to have meticulous soft tissue technique and avoid excessive retraction and undermining of the soft tissue flap. Using careful soft tissue dissection and placing a posterolateral incision slightly more posteriorly toward the Achilles tendon will allow a safe approach when working around a previous direct lateral approach to the fibula. An alternative approach would be a posteromedial approach, which can be done with different deep intervals. An approach just anterior to the posterior tibial tendon is useful for more medial fractures, but it is not as extensile as the other more posterior approaches. A more posterior skin incision utilizing the interval between the flexor digitorum longus and the posterior neurovascular bundle allows a more extensile approach to the posterior and posterior lateral distal tibia. The downside of this approach is the need to identify and retract the posterior neurovascular bundle, which is not required in the posterior lateral approach. The surgeon must be prepared to need to use the previous surgical approaches at the same time if necessary for hardware removal, which is why meticulous soft tissue handling is critical.

Once the surgical approach has been determined, one must decide whether the hardware in place can remain (in the instance of a missed posterior malleolus) or removed (in the instance of failed hardware or the need to revise fibular fixation). Be prepared to remove any previous implants, which is typically standard small fragment implants and cannulated screws. A broken screw removal set may also be necessary. It is always prudent to have reviewed the previous operative note and have all necessary screw drivers available.

New Implant Selection

Surgery for failed posterior malleoli fixation or nonunion requires plate and screw stabilization on the posterior distal tibia. Screw fixation alone is not sufficient for stability and healing. Anatomic-specific posterior distal tibial plates can be useful; however, even standard one-third tubular plates under contoured to act as an antiglide or buttress plate may be sufficient. The size and type of plate needed is related to the difficulty in obtaining and maintaining the reduction and underlying bone quality. Fractures with underlying poor bone quality that have been posteriorly displaced in the subacute and chronic timeframe (i.e., >4 weeks from injury or failure) will likely require larger, more powerful plates with locking screw options as the plate may be used as the final reduction tool. Fractures with underlying good bone quality and displaced less than 4 weeks can typically be mobilized with or without the need for using the plate as a reduction tool and thus would only necessitate smaller/shorter plates. The more difficult the reduction of the posterior distal tibia (and subsequent talus), the longer and more robust the plate should be. A minimum of two screws above the fracture is required for stable fixation. Two screws can be used in cases with good bone quality and longer plates, with more screws proximal to the fracture in cases with suboptimal bone quality. Screws are typically placed across the fracture line to provide more stability to the fracture and at the level of the articular surface either outside or through the plate.

Need for Bone Grafting

Bone grafting is typically not necessary when performing revision surgery as there is bone-to-bone contact at the level of the joint and metaphysis. If there is a void in the metaphysis or at the level of the joint, allograft bone chips can be placed but autograft is typically not required.

Revision Surgery

The primary goal of revision surgery for posterior malleolar or posterior distal tibia fractures is to align the talus underneath the plafond. This is done in a two-step process. The first is to regain the length of the posterior malleolar fragment and the second is to provide posterior support to the fragment and subsequently the talus resulting in a congruent and stable joint.

The authors prefer prone positioning on a radiolucent table with the ankle at the end of the bed. This allows for surgeon positioning both on the sides of the ankle and at the foot of the bed, which can assist in reduction and instrumentation. Preoperative planning for incisions is critical to avoid soft tissue complications as previously discussed. A tourniquet can be used during this surgery, but it is not necessary with careful hemostasis. Not using a tourniquet can also preserve blood flow to previous incisions if it is in the acute postoperative period.

The work-horse incision for access to the posterior distal tibia is the posterior lateral approach in between the peroneals and the flexor halluces longus (FHL). If there is a laterally based incision, a more posterior incision closer to the Achilles can be made. The sural nerve and the lesser saphenous vein are always encountered during this approach. The deep fascia incised longitudinally in the FHL is reflected off the distal tibia for access to the fracture site. In the instance that the posterior malleolus was missed, there is typically no hardware that needs to be removed (Fig. 40.3a–c). For cases where there is failed fixation with screws (Fig. 40.4a, b), removal can be done in a percutaneous fashion by flexing the knee. If screw fixation had been placed from posterior to anterior, they can be removed at the time of approach. Any broken hardware should be removed if it is blocking reduction. A standard broken screw removal set can assist in this.

The first step in achieving reduction of the posterior distal tibia fragment and talus is to mobilize the posterior malleolar fragment. Depending on bone quality and time from initial surgery or injury, this can be difficult. There is a benefit and a detriment to having a long posterior spike of the distal tibial fragment. The benefit is obvious with improved bone stock, but the larger the fragment, the more difficult it can be to mobilize through the primary fracture line from the superior aspect. This is because the angle, which is needed to enter the fracture line, is often difficult to obtain because the calf can be in the way. In these instances, one can free up the primary fracture line from lateral to medial but be careful not to take off the tibial attachment of the posterior syndesmosis. A separate medial incision can be made to access the posterior distal tibia and help clean out the fracture line (Fig. 40.6a). Instruments useful for this can be a combination of a pituitary rongeur, small curved curettes, dental picks and small lamina spreaders. In poor bone quality it is easy to fracture off metaphyseal cortical fragments, which can make the reduction read difficult (Fig. 40.8). Carefully mobilizing through the primary fracture line in order to gain length in the reduction without losing bone stock is the most difficult aspect of the case.

The talus may need to be distracted and anteriorly translated in order to help gain length of the fracture fragment. This can be done with either temporary external fixation or a femoral distractor. The talus can then be secured in the

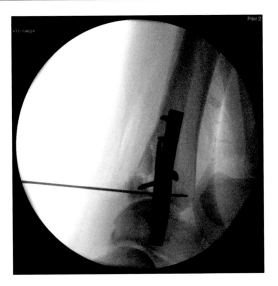

Fig. 40.8 Intraoperative image after mobilization of the posterior malleolus, which resulted in fragmentation of the cortex (compare to the CT scan in Fig. 40.6b)

reduced position using the distractor/fixator or with a Steinman pin (Fig. 40.9a–c).

The posterior tibial fragment can then be reduced to the intact tibia with a ball spike and held with K-wires (Fig. 40.8). There is often still a residual gap at the fracture site, but as long as the fragment is out to an appropriate length this gap can be compressed with either lag screws along the joint (Fig. 40.9c–e) or using an undercontoured plate as a final reduction tool (Fig. 40.10a–e). An undercontoured plate can be a powerful reduction tool. This requires an appropriate bend (or lack thereof) in the plate and acceptable bone quality in the tibial shaft to support the screw purchase during plate placement. If there is poor bone quality, the screws will not have adequate purchase to bend the plate for the final reduction maneuver. Figure 40.11a–e illustrates the case of delayed subluxation at 6 weeks (Fig. 40.5a, b), which required the use of a large plate as a reduction tool. In this instance a femoral distractor was placed to gain length, but given the time from injury, anatomic length could not be obtained while retaining bone stock. Screws were placed from proximal to distal given the bone quality and ability for the far cortex to hold the screws and maintain the anteriorly directed

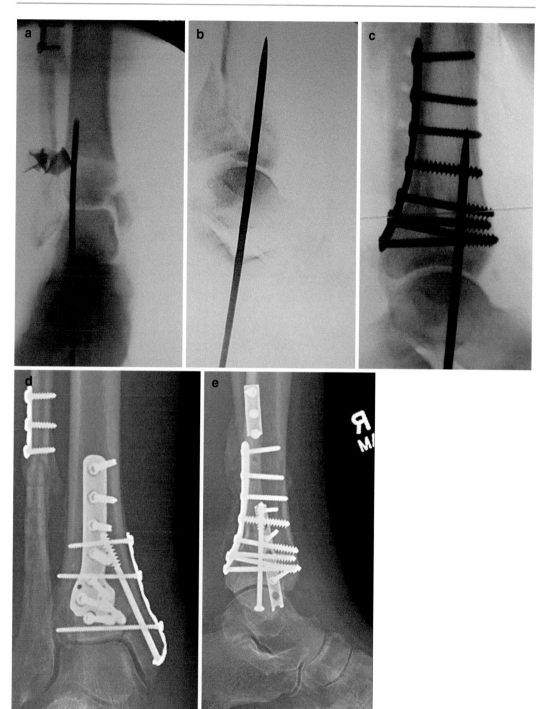

Fig. 40.9 Intraoperative image stabilizing the talus underneath the intact mortise with a Steinman pin on the AP (**a**) and lateral (**b**) radiographs. The distal tibia is then reduced to the talus and fixed (**c**). One-year postoperative mortise (**d**) and lateral (**e**) radiographs showing a healed, congruent and stable ankle mortise (courtesy of Paul Tornetta III)

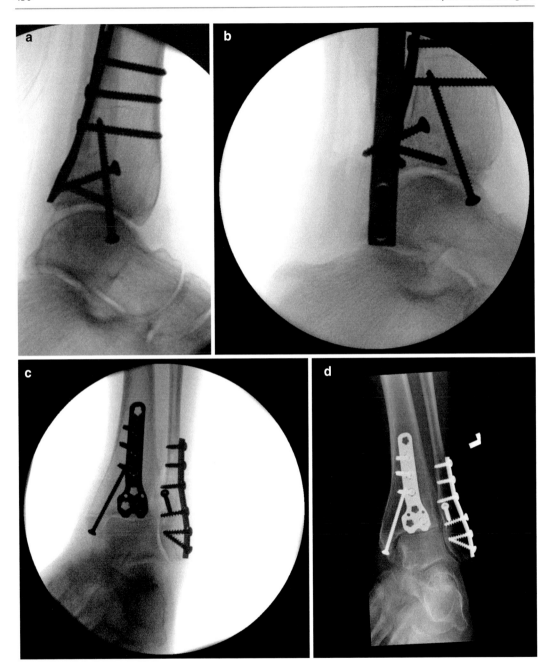

Fig. 40.10 Intraoperative imaging showing the plate being used as the final reduction tool with the posterior malleolus out to length. Lateral (**a**), externally rotated lateral showing the fracture line out to length, reduced with the unicortical screw extra-articular (**b**) and mortise (**c**). One year postoperatively the ankle is in anatomic alignment on the mortise (**d**) and lateral (**e**) radiographs. The patient requested lateral plate removal, which was done at 1 year postoperatively, and the postoperative lateral (**f**) radiograph shows a congruent ankle joint and healed fracture line

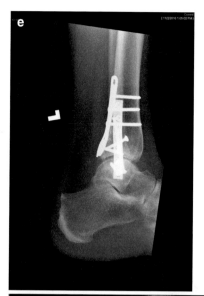

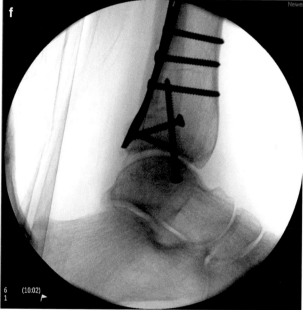

Fig. 40.10 (continued)

reduction force of the plate. The plate was still able to function by providing posterior stability to the talus during healing. Although the talus healed slightly in a slightly posterior translation, functional outcome was not impacted.

A standard layered closure is then performed with vertical mattress nylon sutures for the skin. A deep drain is left at the surgeon's discretion. The ankle is then immobilized in a short leg AO splint. Patients are typically admitted to the hospital overnight and discharged within 1–2 days after adequate pain control and drain removal. Patients are then seen at 1–2 weeks of follow-up for a wound check and placement of a short leg cast. Immobilization of the ankle is performed until the wound is healed, which can be between

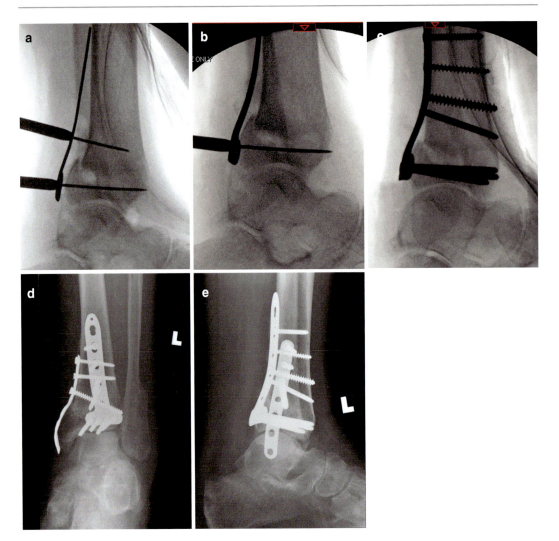

Fig. 40.11 Intraoperative imaging using the plate as a reduction tool with plate placement and provisional stabilization (**a**), proximal screw placement (**b**) and final construct (**c**). Sequential screw placement will bend the plate and provide the anteriorly directed force on the distal tibia, which stabilizes the talus. The patient is healed at 6 months on the mortise (**d**) and lateral (**e**) radiographs

2 and 6 weeks as the posterior skin incision can take longer to heal, especially with other incisions nearby. After the incision is healed, physical therapy for range of motion and strengthening is performed. Radiographs are obtained at 2, 6, 12, 26 and 52 weeks postoperatively. Weight-bearing is typically begun at 10–12 weeks postoperatively depending on how patients are doing clinically and whether there are comorbidities that would delay healing (i.e., diabetes). Weight-bearing is being as tolerated with assisted device and in the boot is discontinued by 4 months in noncomplicated patients and as late as 6 months in patients with diabetes.

Lessons Learned

The goal of treating any fracture around the ankle is to provide stability such that the talus can heal in an anatomic alignment within the mortise. Posterior malleoli fractures that are large enough to result in posterior subluxation of the talus are typically treated with a direct approach and plate and screw fixation. In the instances where this fracture is missed, inadequately fixed or failed nonoperative management, surgery can be challenging. Identifying which posterior malleolar fractures require a direct approach and plate fixation during the initial surgery is critical in preventing failure and complications. The two main obstacles for successful revision surgery include safely working around previous incisions and obtaining length and anterior translation of the talus in order to reduce the distal tibial fragment. Stable fixation will prevent posterior translation of the distal tibia fragment and subsequently the talus, which will result in a stable ankle mortise and improved outcome.

References

1. Rammelt S, Bartoníček J. Posterior malleolar fractures. JBJS Rev. 2020;8(8):e19.00207.
2. Jaskulka RA, Ittner G, Schedl R. Fractures of the posterior tibial margin: their role in the prognosis of malleolar fractures. J Trauma Inj Infect Crit Care. 1989;29(11):1565–70.
3. Tejwani NC, Pahk B, Egol KA. Effect of posterior malleolus fracture on outcome after unstable ankle fracture. J Trauma Inj Infect Crit Care. 2010;69(3):666–9.
4. Odak S, Ahluwalia R, Unnikrishnan P, et al. Management of posterior malleolar fractures: a systematic review. J Foot Ankle Surg. 2016;55(1):140–5.
5. Haraguchi N, Haruyama H, Toga H, et al. Pathoanatomy of posterior malleolar fractures of the ankle. J Bone Jt Surg Ser A. 2006;88(5):1085–92.
6. Bartoníček J, Rammelt S, Kostlivý K, et al. Anatomy and classification of the posterior tibial fragment in ankle fractures. Arch Orthop Trauma Surg. 2015;135(4):505–16.
7. Harper MC. Posterior instability of the Talus: an anatomic evaluation. Foot Ankle Int. 1989;10(1):36–9.
8. Raasch WG, Larkin JJ, Draganich LE. Assessment of the posterior malleolus as a restraint to posterior subluxation of the ankle. J Bone Jt Surg Ser A. 1992;74(8):1201–6.
9. Hartford JM, Gorczyca JT, McNamara JL, et al. Tibiotalar contact area: contribution of posterior malleolus and deltoid ligament. Clin Orthop Relat Res. 1995;320:182–7.
10. Fitzpatrick DC, Otto JK, McKinley TO, et al. Kinematic and contact stress analysis of posterior

malleolus fractures of the ankle. J Orthop Trauma. 2004;18(5):271–8.
11. Evers J, Fischer M, Zderic I, et al. The role of a small posterior malleolar fragment in trimalleolar fractures: a biomechanical study. Bone Jt J. 2018;100-B(1):95–100.
12. Gardner MJ, Brodsky A, Briggs SM, et al. Fixation of posterior malleolar fractures provides greater syndesmotic stability. Clin Orthop Relat Res. 2006;447:165–71.
13. Heim D, Niederhauser K, Simbrey N. The Volkmann dogma: a retrospective, long-term, single-center study. Eur J Trauma Emerg Surg. 2010;36(6):515–9.
14. Rammelt S, Bartoníček J. Posterior malleolar fractures: a critical analysis review. JBJS Rev. 2020;8(8):e19.00207.
15. Langenhuijsen JF, Heetveld MJ, Ultee JM, et al. Results of ankle fractures with involvement of the posterior tibial margin. J Trauma. 2002;53(1):55–60.
16. Ebraheim NA, Mekhail AO, Haman SP. External rotation-lateral view of the ankle in the assessment of the posterior malleolus. Foot Ankle Int. 1999;20(6):379–83.
17. Yao L, Zhang W, Yang G, et al. Morphologic characteristics of the posterior malleolus fragment: a 3-D computer tomography based study. Arch Orthop Trauma Surg. 2014;134(3):389–94.
18. Donohoe S, Alluri RK, Hill JR, et al. Impact of computed tomography on operative planning for ankle fractures involving the posterior malleolus. Foot Ankle Int. 2017;38(12):1337–42.
19. Hartwich K, Lorente Gomez A, Pyrc J, et al. Biomechanical analysis of stability of posterior antiglide plating in osteoporotic pronation abduction ankle fracture model with posterior tibial fragment. Foot Ankle Int. 2017;38(1):58–65.
20. De Vries JS, Wijgman AJ, Sierevelt IN, et al. Long-term results of ankle fractures with a posterior malleolar fragment. J Foot Ankle Surg. 2005;44(3):211–7.
21. Tornetta P, Ricci W, Nork S, et al. The posterolateral approach to the tibia for displaced posterior malleolar injuries. J Orthop Trauma. 2011;25(2):123–6.
22. Zhong S, Shen L, Zhao JG, et al. Comparison of posteromedial versus posterolateral approach for posterior malleolus fixation in trimalleolar ankle fractures. Orthop Surg. 2017;9(1):69–76.
23. Howard JL, Agel J, Barei DP, et al. A prospective study evaluating incision placement and wound healing for tibial plafond fractures. J Orthop Trauma. 2008;22(5):299–305.
24. Taylor GI, Pan WR. Angiosomes of the leg: anatomic study and clinical implications. Plast Reconstr Surg. 1998;102(3):599–616.
25. Taylor GI. The angiosomes of the body and their supply to perforator flaps. Clin Plast Surg. 2003;30(3):331–42.
26. Taylor GI, Palmer JH. The vascular territories (angiosomes) of the body: experimental study and clinical applications. Br J Plast Surg. 1987;40(2):113–41.

Talar Fracture Failed Fixation

41

Xinbao Wu, Xiaofeng Gong,
and Peter V. Giannoudis

History of Previous Failed Treatment

This is the case of a 32-year-old otherwise healthy woman who was involved in a traffic accident and sustained an isolated, neurovascularly intact closed right talar fracture (Fig. 41.1a, b). She was transferred to an outside regional hospital for initial management.

The patient underwent surgical reconstruction at the regional hospital a week after the original injury. An anteromedial approach with medial malleolar osteotomy was performed, followed by open reduction and internal fixation (ORIF) of the talar neck fracture and deltoid ligament repair. The fracture was fixed using a medial locking plate with two cannulated screws for an antero-posterior fixation (Fig. 41.2a, b). The injured lower limb was then immobilized by a plaster for 3 months, after which the case mobilized with aids for 9 months.

The case experienced medial ankle pain after the initial operative treatment and had a maximum walking distance of around 3000 m. Simultaneously, it was difficult for the patient in doing squatting, going upstairs and uphill. She was referred to our unit for further management.

X. Wu (✉)
Department of Orthopaedics and Traumatology, Beijing Jishuitan Hospital, Capital Medical University, Beijing, China

Laboratory of Bone Tissue Engineering, Beijing Laboratory of Biomedical Materials, Beijing Research Institute of Orthopaedics and Traumatology, Beijing Jishuitan Hospital, Beijing, China

National Centre for Orthopaedics, Beijing, China

X. Gong
National Centre for Orthopaedics, Beijing, China

Department of Foot and Ankle Surgery, Beijing Jishuitan Hospital, Capital Medical University, Beijing, China

P. V. Giannoudis
Academic Department of Trauma and Orthopaedics, School of Medicine, University of Leeds, Leeds, UK

NIHR Leeds Biomedical Research Center, Chapel Allerton Hospital, Leeds, UK
e-mail: peter.giannoudis@nhs.net

© The Author(s), under exclusive license to Springer Nature Switzerland AG 2024
P. V. Giannoudis, P. Tornetta III (eds.), *Failed Fracture Fixation*,
https://doi.org/10.1007/978-3-031-39692-2_41

Fig. 41.1 (**a**, **b**): The anteroposterior (AP) and lateral radiographs of the right ankle showing a displaced talar neck fracture with a medial subtalar subluxation

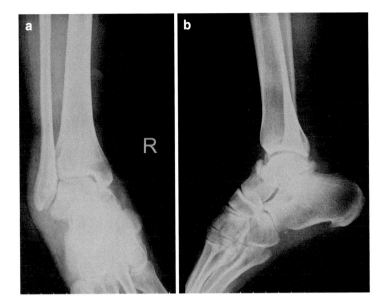

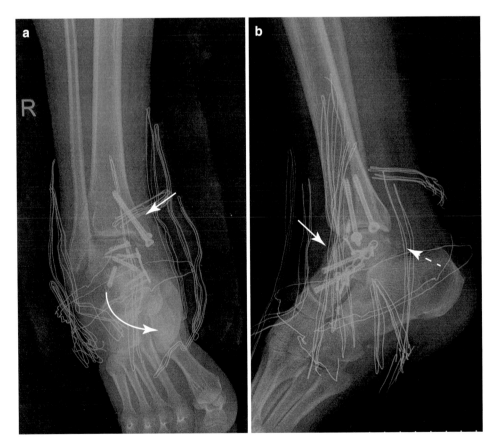

Fig. 41.2 (**a**, **b**): Post-operative anteroposterior (AP) (**a**) and lateral (**b**) radiographs demonstrating the initial fixation. With a careful observation, malreduction of the medial malleolar osteotomy (arrow) with residual medial subtalar subluxation (curve arrow) (**a**) and the malreduction of the talar neck fracture (arrow) with overlap of the subtalar joint (dotted arrow) (**b**) can be identified

Evaluation of the Aetiology of Failure of Fixation

Following talar neck fracture fixation, failure of the original objective of the reconstruction is realized several months down the line as it was the situation in the case presented here.

For displaced talar neck fractures, it is necessary to use a combined medial and lateral approach to expose both sides of the fracture, otherwise poor reduction may occur. A single medial approach to expose the talar neck fracture was the important risk factor that led to the poor reduction and malunion during the initial surgery. The poor reduction was not identified due to the angle of the X-ray projection from the postoperative ankle joint lateral radiographs, but the abnormal hindfoot varus would be found if carefully checking the anteroposterior radiograph. Subsequently, this hindfoot varus deformity obviously appeared while the patient started mobilizing with full weight-bearing. In general terms, malreduction of the talar neck fracture and the hindfoot varus deformity can be recognized by checking the weight-bearing lateral radiograph of the ankle joint (Fig. 41.3a–e).

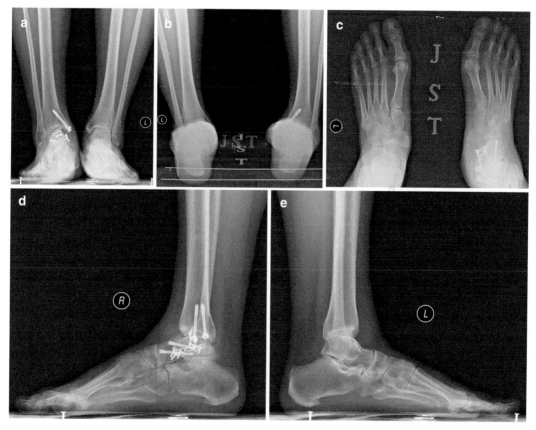

Fig. 41.3 (**a–e**): Standard weight-bearing radiographs of the foot and ankle illustrating the medial tibiotalar arthrosis (**a**), hindfoot varus (**b**) and forefoot supination (**c** and **d**) compared to the contralateral side (**e**), and malreduction of the talar neck fracture

Clinical Examination

The physical examination showed that the anteromedial incision has healed well, with obvious hindfoot varus (Fig. 41.4). The gait was antalgic with weight-bearing over the lateral border of the foot. The right ankle joint had 0° of dorsiflexion and 20° of plantar flexion, accompanying with the contracture of the Achilles tendon. The inversion and eversion strength were normal and neurovascular condition was intact. The American Orthopaedic Foot and Ankle Society (AOFAS) score was 47 points, and the Foot Function Index (FFI) score was 46 points.

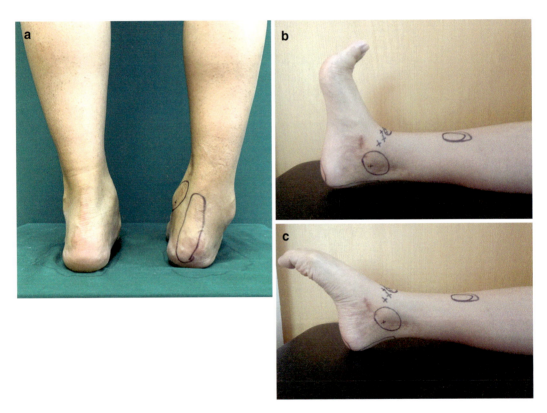

Fig. 41.4 (a–c) One-year post-operative clinical photographs suggesting the hindfoot varus (a) with decreased dorsiflexion (b) and plantarflexion (c)

Diagnostic-Biochemical and Radiological Investigations

Weight-bearing foot and ankle radiographs showed a malunion of the talar neck with hindfoot varus. For the preoperative planning, given the radiographic evaluation for the malunion of talar neck fracture, a computed tomography (CT) scan (Fig. 41.5a–c) and weight-bearing CT (WBCT) (Fig. 41.6a–c) were used to rule out the avascular necrosis (AVN), and further to determine the tibiotalar and subtalar joint arthrosis.

Based on the imaging, issues to address are as follows (Fig. 41.6):

1. Talar neck malreduction with hindfoot varus malunion.
2. Medial subtalar subluxation.
3. Tibiotalar and subtalar arthrosis.
4. No extensile AVN of the talus.

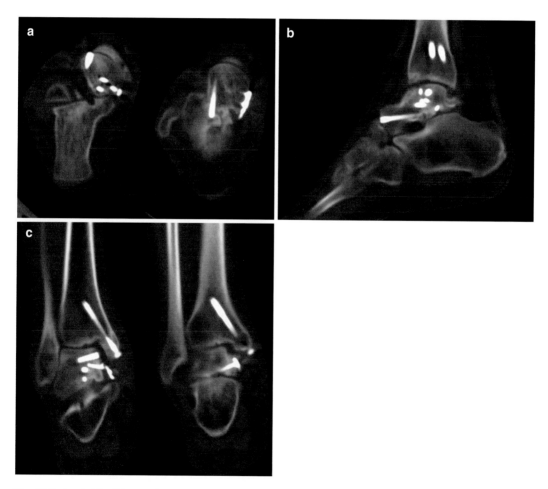

Fig. 41.5 (**a–c**): The CT scan showing the malreduction of the talar neck fracture and hindfoot varus: (**a**) Transverse section showing the abnormal lateral talar neck curve and medial subtalar subluxation. (**b**) Sagittal section demonstrating the subtalar arthrosis. (**c**) Coronal section illustrating the medial tibiotalar arthrosis and medial subtalar subluxation with arthrosis

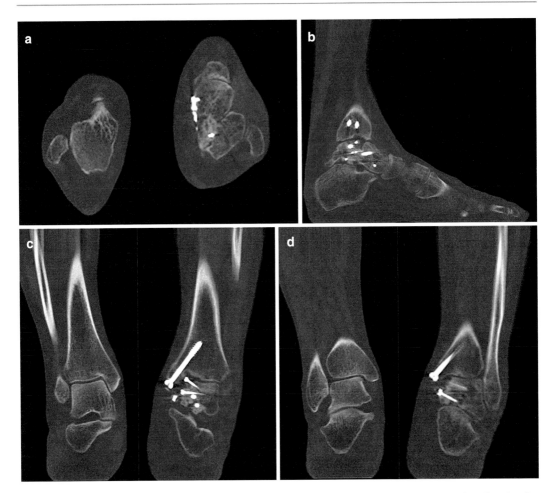

Fig. 41.6 (a–d): WBCT demonstrating the malreduction of the talar neck fracture and hindfoot varus: (**a**) Transverse section showing the malreduction of the talar neck with a clear lateral fracture line, which should be found during the surgery. (**b**) Sagittal section demonstrating subtalar arthrosis. (**c** and **d**) Coronal section showing medial tibiotalar arthrosis and medial subtalar subluxation with more obvious arthrosis, against the opposite side

Preoperative Planning

Poor reduction of the talar neck fracture usually results in hindfoot varus, which has a significant impact on standing and walking, so surgical correction is necessary.

Therefore, the goal of the revision surgery is to correct the malreduction of the talar neck fracture to ensure the anatomic congruity with the three surrounding joints. First, all hardware should be removed; then, along with the fracture line of malunion, dual-incision approaches will be needed to implement an osteotomy to correct the deformity of hindfoot varus and restore the alignment of the subtalar joint; finally, miniplates and screws will be used for a combined medial and lateral fixation to maintain the normal length of talus with bone grafting followed. K-wire application would allow temporarily fixation of the subtalar joint. Restoration of lack of dorsiflexion would require Achilles tendon lengthening.

Having discussed the surgery plan with the patient, it was decided not to address the tibiofibular joint arthrosis and subtalar joint arthrosis. It was felt that if the patient's condition deteriorates at a later stage, either a supramalleolar osteotomy or a subtalar arthrodesis could be conducted.

A summary of the preoperative planning is shown below:

1. Removing the previous hardware from the medial side of the talus through the previous anteromedial approach.
   Equipment needed: small fragment set screwdriver
2. Using the anterolateral approach to expose the lateral talar neck.
3. Talar neck osteotomy.
   Equipment needed: K-wire, mini-osteotome and chisel
4. Reduction of the subtalar joint.
   Equipment needed: rongeur, curette
5. Revision fixation of the talar neck fracture to restore the medial and lateral length, alignment and rotation.
   Equipment needed: 1.5, 2.0 K-wires, mini-fragment locking plate system
6. Maintenance of the subtalar joint reduction.
   Equipment needed: 2.0 K-wires
7. Bone grafting from the proximal tibia.
   Equipment needed: mini-osteotome, chisel
8. Hoke Achilles tendon lengthening.

Revision Surgery

The patient was positioned supine on the operating table. Prophylactic antibiotics (Cefuroxime 1.5 g) were administered. The patient was prepped and draped in the usual sterile fashion and a thigh tourniquet was inflated to 280 mmHg. An anteromedial incision was carried out, which was centred on the previous incision. The medial malleolus and the medial talar neck were exposed and the previous plate and screws were removed using the appropriate screwdriver. The lateral talar neck and the subtalar joint were exposed through the anterolateral ankle approach (Fig. 41.7).

Since the lateral side of the talus was not exposed during the initial surgery, there was no scar, where it was easy to identify the fracture line (Fig. 41.7a). The fracture line on the medial side was also difficult to be recognized and needed to be confirmed from the dorsal side of the neck (Fig. 41.7b). With the C-arm fluoroscopy, the original fracture was identified using a K-wire, and then an osteotome was used to implement an osteotomy and completely open the original fracture surface. Two K-wires are then placed on both sides of the talar neck osteotomy, and a K-Wire distractor is mounted over these two K wires not only to control the distraction but also the rotation of the talar neck. The fracture end was pulled apart and was cleaned with a scraper. Loosening

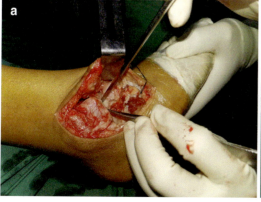 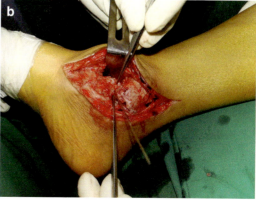

Fig. 41.7 (**a, b**): (**a**) Anterolateral and (**b**) anteromedial approaches were used to expose the talar neck malunion. It is easier to identify the fracture site from the lateral side at first (**a**) and then followed to the medial side (Please insert in the pictures letters A and B to differentiate)

the scar tissue adhered to the lateral side of the subtalar joint can improve the subtalar joint valgus, while the hindfoot varus was corrected with the aid of a distractor mounted in the medial side.

A locking plate was fixed on the lateral side of the fracture after reduction, while two fully threaded screws were used to fix the medial side to avoid the medial column shortening. The subtalar joint was maintained in slight eversion and fixed by two K-wires. A series of fluoroscopic images of the ankle joint was taken to verify the correction of the fracture deformity and the hindfoot varus.

A small incision was made at the tibial tuberosity. Using a 2.5-mm drill to make a square cortical window, cancellous bone was harvested and grafted around the talar neck fracture. A Hoke percutaneous Achilles tendon lengthening by triple semisection was employed after checking the ankle dorsiflexion, which could not reach the neutral position. Post-operative radiographs are shown in Fig. 41.8a, b.

The wounds were closed using 3-0 subcutaneous sutures followed by 4-0 nylon skin sutures.

At 22 months of post-operative follow-up, the patient was very satisfied with the clinical outcome with the AOFAS score was improved from 47 preoperatively to 82 points, and the Foot Function Index (FFI) score was improved from 46 to 12 points. The pain was almost relieved, and the range of motion of the ankle joint was significantly improved, but the range of motion of the subtalar joint was slightly improved (Fig. 41.9a–c). The anteroposterior and lateral radiographs are shown in Fig. 41.10a, b.

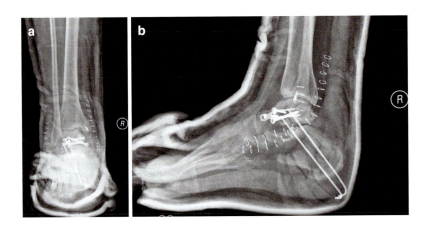

Fig. 41.8 (a, b): (a) Anteroposterior and (b) lateral radiographs after surgery after the revision fixation showing reduction of the talar neck fracture and maintenance of the subtalar joint with 2 K-wires

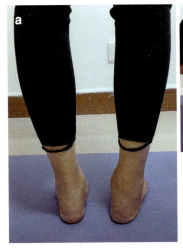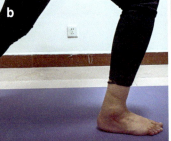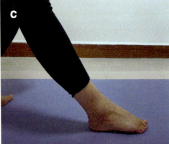

Fig. 41.9 (a–c): Clinical outcomes at 22 months post-operatively showing slight hindfoot varus and improved ankle range of motion

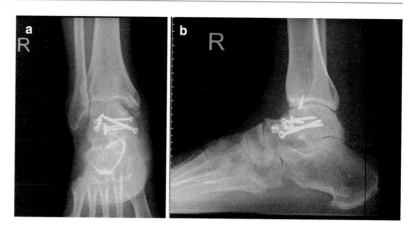

Fig. 41.10 (**a**) Anteroposterior and (**b**) lateral radiographs 22 months postoperatively showing maintenance of the medial tibiotalar joint space (**a**), improved hindfoot varus (**a**) and forefoot supination (**b**) with narrowed subtalar joint space

Discussion

Talar neck fractures are well addressed by dual-incision approaches to improve the accuracy of reduction, which ensures an optimal alignment of fracture to avoid malrotation at the talar neck. Intraoperatively, the reduction should be checked with the C-arm, using the anteroposterior and lateral views, and the Canale and Kelly view, which facilitates the visualization of the talus neck [1]. Failure to follow the principles mentioned above would increase the risk of malreduction of the talar neck fractures.

Two primary types of malunion deformity can be recognized, the dorsal and the varus malunion. Both can be identified with lateral and hindfoot radiographs, respectively. Patients with dorsal malunion sustain pain and restricted dorsiflexion of the ankle caused by impingement on the anterior tibia. It can be treated successfully with resection of the dorsal beak [2].

Patients with union of hindfoot varus deformity often experience painful and rigid feet varus during walking. Canale identified that patients with union of hindfoot varus deformity had a higher incidence of developing degenerative arthritis in the subtalar joint [3]. Some case reports with a small sample size described various revision surgeries for union of talar neck deformity after surgery, including ankle arthrodesis, fusion of the subtalar and/or calcaneocuboid joint, triple arthrodesis, tibiocalcaneal arthrodesis or total ankle replacement. For patients with remaining cartilage in the peritalar joints, but without talar collapse or AVN, revision surgery to anatomically reconstruct talar neck fractures with union of deformity has advantages in the recovery of foot function. Some retrospective case studies demonstrated a satisfactory clinical and radiographic outcome.

Considering the risk of damage to the vascular supply associated with the talar neck osteotomy, Monroe [4] and Barg [5] used a single anteromedial approach to expose the talar neck. In the case illustrated herein, the preoperative WBCT (Fig. 41.6a) showed that there were no comminuted fractures at the lateral talar neck fracture line, which enables to accurately locate the original fracture. In order to accurately perform osteotomy based on the original fracture line, the author used a dual-incision approach to expose both sides of the talar neck.

In the author's experience, the hindfoot varus is usually uncorrected after the osteotomy. At this time, it is necessary to release the adhesion of subtalar joint completely, and it will be very useful to correct the hindfoot varus with the K-Wire distractor from the medial side. For this patient, taking the relatively intact lateral cortex and dorsal contour of the talar neck as a reference, the rotation and length of the talar neck can be accurately reduced with the control of K-Wire distractor.

Once the underlying deformity of the talar neck is completely corrected, there will always be a gap in the medial side, which makes bone grafting necessary. Some authors advocated that insertion of a tricortical iliac crest bone graft is necessary to restore the medial length and screw fixation to maintain the reduction [5, 6]. For this patient, using a lateral plate is stable and much easier to match the relatively intact lateral talar contour, whereas leaving the void in the medial talar neck can be sufficiently filled with cancellous bone graft from the proximal tibia.

Additional surgeries are usually combined with the osteotomy and revision fixation, including Achilles tendon lengthening, medial and/or posterior release, subtalar joint arthroscopy and subtalar arthrodesis. During the revision surgery of this patient, percutaneous Hoke lengthening was needed to improve the ankle joint dorsiflexion. Subtalar fixation with two K-wires was the preferred method used, which were removed 6 weeks after surgery. Over the 2-year follow-up, the patient had no obvious pain in the subtalar joint, which suggested the hindfoot alignment was more important than the subtalar joint movement.

Summary: Lessons Learned

– Talar neck fractures are well exposed by dual-incision approaches to improve the reduction and to avoid malrotation of the talar neck.
– Treatment of "failed" talar neck fracture fixation is difficult and the prognosis is uncertain.
– For patients who are chosen to undergo osteotomy and revision surgery, the indications should be strictly and carefully controlled.

Generally, it is suitable for patients with well-preserved cartilage, no AVN, or collapse, and individualized treatment plans should be developed.
– The case presented herein ended up having improved clinical outcome with mild hindfoot varus, without necessitating further surgical treatment at 22 months after surgery.
– The remaining hindfoot varus also pointed out the importance of the anatomical reduction in the initial fracture fixation; otherwise, the results of the secondary reconstruction will be unpredictable.
– Additional surgeries are usually combined with the osteotomy and revision fixation, including Achilles tendon lengthening and subtalar arthrodesis, although the timing of subtalar arthrodesis remains controversial.

References

1. Rammelt S, Swords M, Dhillon MS, Sands AK. Manual of fracture management-foot and ankle. Georg Thieme Verlag; 2019. p. 310–1.
2. Canale ST, Kelly FB Jr. Fractures of the neck of the talus. J Bone Joint Surg. 1978;60A:143–56.
3. Canale ST. Fractures of the neck of the talus. Orthopedics. 1990;13:1105–15.
4. Monroe MT, Manoli A 2nd. Osteotomy for malunion 20 of a talar neck fracture: a case report. Foot Ankle Int. 1999;20(3):192–5.
5. Barg A, Suter T, Nickisch F, et al. Osteotomies of the talar neck for posttraumatic malalignment. Foot Ankle Clin. 2016;21(1):77–93.
6. Rammelt S, Winkler J, Heineck J, et al. Anatomical reconstruction of malunited talus fractures: a prospective study of 10 patients followed for 4 years. Acta Orthop. 2005;76(4):588–96.

Fifth Metatarsal Fracture Failed Fixation

42

George D. Chloros, Adam Lomax, and Peter V. Giannoudis

History of Previous Primary Failed Treatment

This is the case of a 34-year-old male smoker with poorly controlled type 2 diabetes who fell from a step and sustained a zone 3 fracture of the right fifth metatarsal (Fig. 42.1). The patient was treated conservatively in a non-weightbearing cast for 6 weeks, and then he was put in a boot to partially weightbear. Temporarily, the symptoms improved; however, 10 months following conservative treatment, the patient represented himself with persistent symptoms with increased tenderness and swelling compatible with a non-union (Fig. 42.2). At this point, the patient was clinically noted to have a cavus foot with a slight plantar flexion of the first metatarsal. At that point, a bone scan was undertaken which confirmed fracture non-union. Therefore, at 13 months post-injury a decision was made to address the symptomatic non-union with open reduction and internal fixation using a 5 mm intramedullary screw. There were no complications, and the patient was put non-weightbearing for 6 weeks, then progressive weightbearing over the course of another 4 weeks to full weightbearing thereafter. However, he was still symptomatic now almost 2 years after the original injury and 1 year after his surgery, with evidence of non-union on radiographs and computed tomography (CT) (Fig. 42.3). Therefore, a decision to proceed with revision surgery was undertaken. The non-union was taken down, the old screw was removed and revised with a new screw and bone graft. Of note, the screw was again a 5 mm screw as it was felt at the time that it had already reached the maximum capacity of the metatarsal. The postoperative regimen included a 6-week interval of non-weightbearing, followed by another 4 weeks of progressive weightbearing until fully weightbearing. The patient's symptoms on the lateral side of the foot were temporarily alleviated however, at 8 months after the revision surgery, he still ended up with painful non-union (Fig. 42.4). It was, therefore, referred to our institution for further management.

G. D. Chloros (✉)
Academic Department of Trauma and Orthopaedics, School of Medicine, University of Leeds, Leeds, UK

Orthopedic Surgery Working Group, Society for Junior Doctors, Athens, Greece

A. Lomax
Academic Department of Trauma and Orthopaedics, Leeds General Infirmary, School of Medicine, University of Leeds, Leeds, UK
e-mail: adam.lomax1@nhs.net

P. V. Giannoudis
Academic Department of Trauma and Orthopaedics, School of Medicine, University of Leeds, Leeds, UK

NIHR Leeds Biomedical Research Center, Chapel Allerton Hospital, Leeds, UK

© The Author(s), under exclusive license to Springer Nature Switzerland AG 2024
P. V. Giannoudis, P. Tornetta III (eds.), *Failed Fracture Fixation*,
https://doi.org/10.1007/978-3-031-39692-2_42

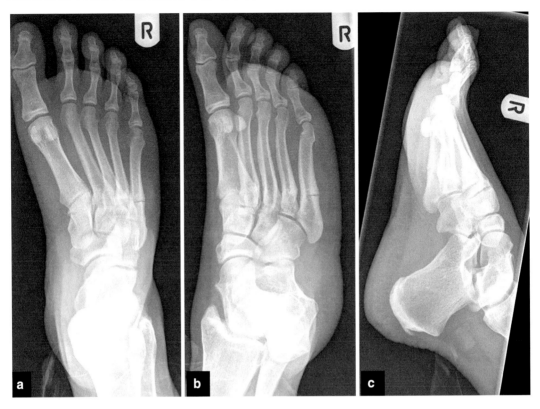

Fig. 42.1 Corresponding anteroposterior (AP) (**a**), oblique (**b**) and lateral (**c**) injury films of the patient showing a zone 3 fifth metatarsal fracture. (Obtained with permission from George. D. Chloros, MD)

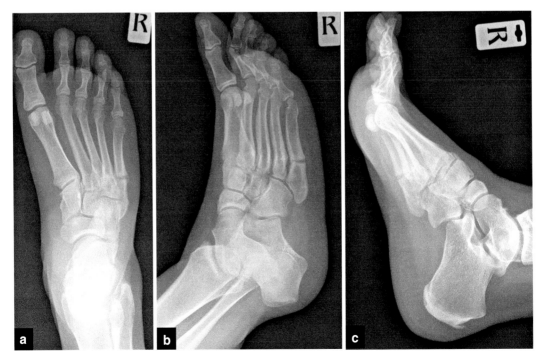

Fig. 42.2 Corresponding AP (**a**), oblique (**b**) and lateral (**c**) films showing persistence of the fracture line at 10 months. (Obtained with permission from George. D. Chloros, MD)

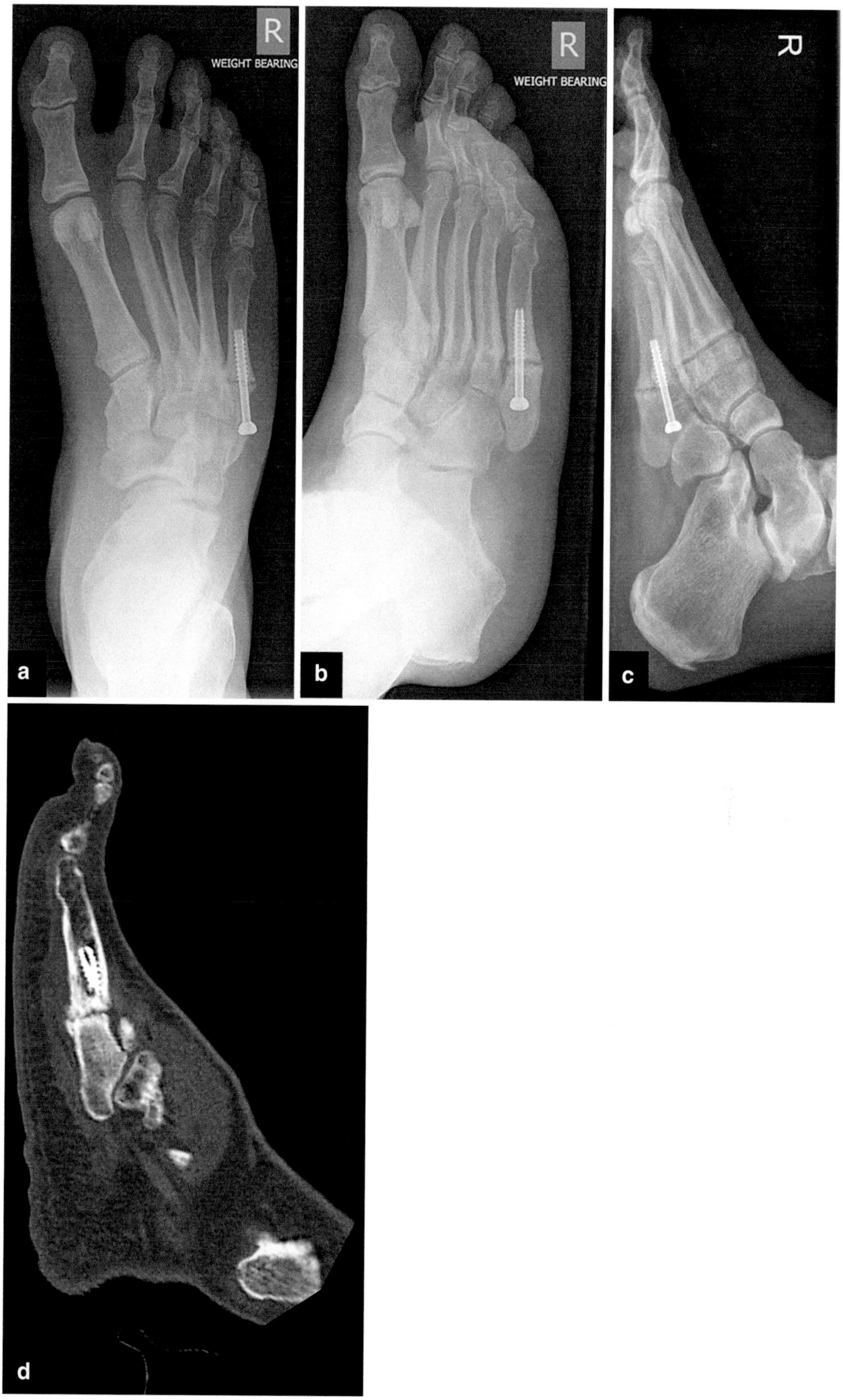

Fig. 42.3 Corresponding AP (**a**), oblique (**b**) and lateral (**c**) films as well as CT (**d**), showing persistent non-union, 1 year after original fixation (2 years post original injury). (Obtained with permission from George. D. Chloros, MD)

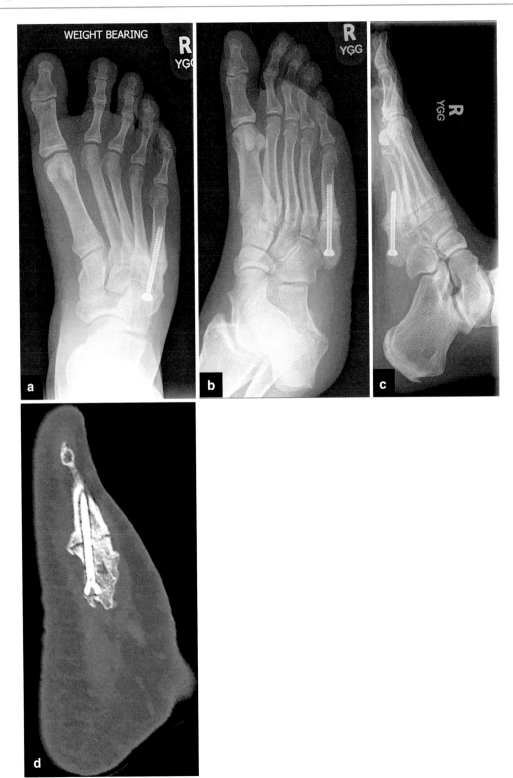

Fig. 42.4 Corresponding AP (**a**), oblique (**b**) and lateral (**c**) films as well as CT (**d**) showing persistent non-union, 8 months post-revision surgery. Of note, there is a stress reaction at the base of the fourth metatarsal further indicating overloading of the lateral column. (Obtained with permission from George. D. Chloros, MD)

Evaluation of the Aetiology of Failure of Fixation

The patient has already undergone two surgical procedures to address his persistent non-union, which haven't been able to solve the problem. In this particular case, several factors which may predispose to failure of treatment have to be considered, including diabetes, smoking, vitamin D deficiency, using a screw of the same diameter during the revision surgery as well as not offloading the lateral column by failing to address the concomitant cavovarus deformity [1–8].

Clinical Examination

Upon standing he has varus hindfoot mal alignment (Fig. 42.5). There is an obvious wear pattern on the lateral aspect of his footwear. He has a non-correctable heal varus with a positive Silfverskiold test. On a talar neutral foot he has planter flexion of the first metatarsal. He has a healed scar from his previous surgery and there is tenderness in this area. There is no pain on moving any of the joints in the foot.

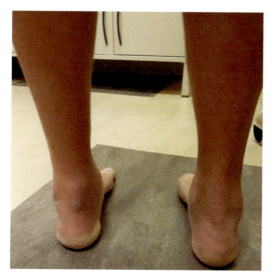

Fig. 42.5 Clinical picture of the patient demonstrating a Bilateral cavovarus deformity. (Obtained with permission from George. D. Chloros, MD)

Diagnostic-Biochemical and Radiological Investigations

Addressing all the aforementioned predisposing factors in the setting of hypertrophic non-union is essential [1, 4]. Although the patient claimed that he has been in control of his diabetes, his latest HbA1c was 54 (range 20–41). He has now stopped smoking as he used to smoke about 4–5 cigarettes per day at the time of his injury and during his first surgery. The rest of his metabolic panel, including vitamin D levels and calcium metabolism, was within normal limits. At that point, an increased calcaneal pitch is noted, as well as a stress reaction to his fourth metatarsal base as well (Fig. 42.4), which clearly indicates that the patient is overloading his lateral column [1, 2, 8].

Preoperative Planning

At this point, a revision fixation needs to be undertaken consisting of: (1) Achilles tendon lengthening, (2) lateralizing calcaneal osteotomy, (3) first metatarsal dorsiflexion osteotomy and (4) fifth metatarsal non-union takedown, with revision of intramedullary fixation and application of autograft to be harvested from the calcaneal osteotomy.

The following implants are selected:

- 6.5 mm solid intramedullary screw—higher diameter to exchange the previous one (5 mm).
- Cortical 3.5 screw to secure the first metatarsal dorsiflexion osteotomy.
- 4-hole plate (Calcaneus Step-plate, Arthrex®, Naples, FL) to secure the lateralizing calcaneal osteotomy.

In less complicated cases, in which there is an associated failure of hardware (either a screw or a plate) (Fig. 42.6a, b), the fragments of the broken metalwork need to be removed prior to implementing the appropriate treatment plan including revision of fixation for example, intramedullary screw, plating, tension-band wiring (Fig. 42.7a–c).

Fig. 42.6 (a) Oblique foot radiograph showing failure of fixation secondary to insertion of a smaller than ideal diameter screw. (b) Oblique radiograph showing failure of plate fixation. (Obtained with permission from George. D. Chloros, MD)

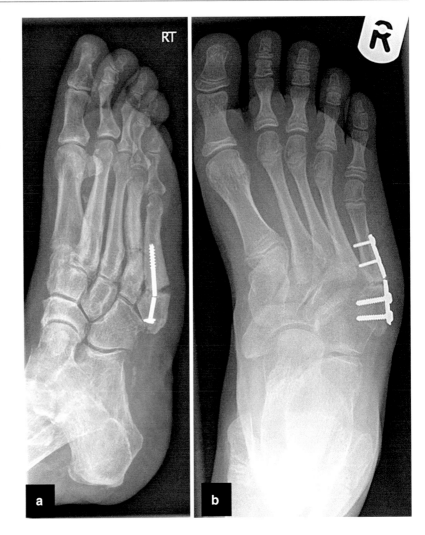

42 Fifth Metatarsal Fracture Failed Fixation

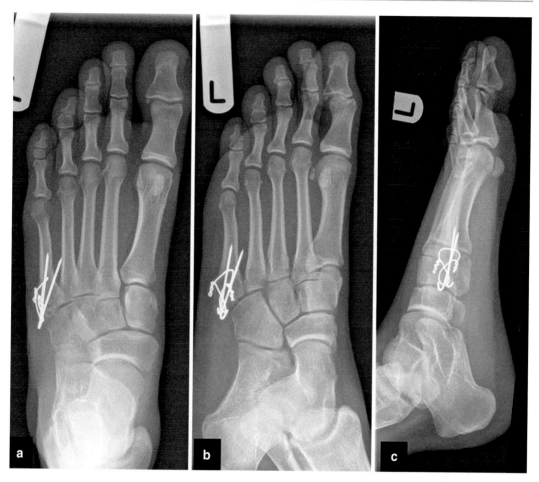

Fig. 42.7 (**a**) Anteroposterior, (**b**) oblique and (**c**) lateral radiograph showing tension band wire fixation of a fifth metatarsal fracture. (Obtained with permission from George. D. Chloros, MD)

Revision Surgery

The patient is positioned supine in the operating table with a sandbag under the ipsilateral hip. A marking pen is used to outline an incision beginning at the tip of the fibula and extending down to the fifth metatarsal base and a second incision just medial to the Extensor Hallucis Longus (EHL) tendon and distal to the first tarsometatarsal (TMT) joint. A tourniquet is inflated to 300 mmHg.

Initially, the Hoke percutaneous tendo-Achilles lengthening was carried out and with manual dorsiflexion pressure, approximately 15 degrees of dorsiflexion was now possible and finger palpation confirmed continuity of the tendon.

Subsequently, attention is drawn to the lateral calcaneus, and subperiosteal dissection is carried out anteriorly and posteriorly. Under fluoroscopy, a guidewire is used to mark directly onto the calcaneus the level of the proposed osteotomy which is carried out using a microsagittal saw. A second angle osteotomy is performed in order to remove a 3 mm wedge from the lateral aspect of the calcaneus allowing to perform a slide along with a closing lateral wedge osteotomy. After completion of the osteotomy, the weightbearing tuberosity of the calcaneus was slid laterally approximately 5 mm. The osteotomy is temporarily secured with 2x 2.0 mm K-wires and the plate is applied to secure it in place (Fig. 42.8a).

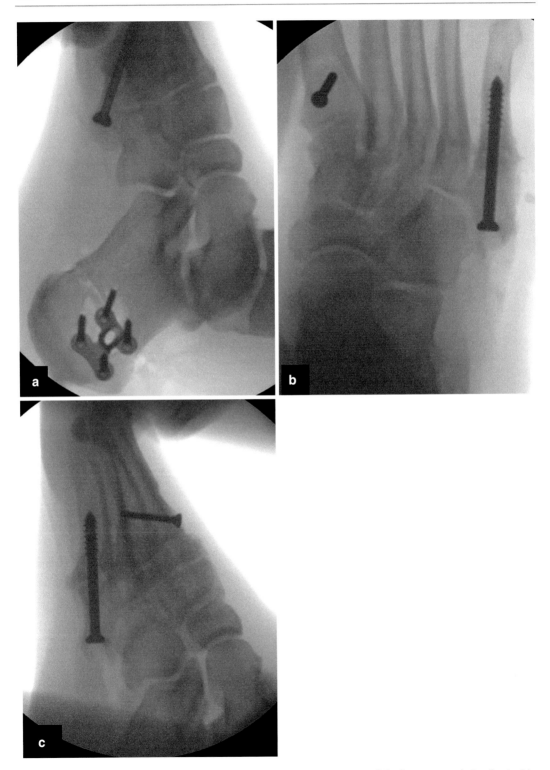

Fig. 42.8 (a–c): Intraoperative fluoroscopic images: (**a**) Lateral image showing the calcaneal slide osteotomy; (**b**) anteroposterior and (**c**) lateral images showing the fixation of the fifth metatarsal with a screw, along with the dorsiflexion osteotomy of the first metatarsal also fixed with a screw. (Obtained with permission from George. D. Chloros, MD)

Then, attention is directed to the first metatarsal incision. The EHL tendon is identified and retracted laterally. The underlying first metatarsal is subperiosteally dissected medially and laterally exposing its base and a marking pen and fluoroscopy are now used to mark the location of the first metatarsal base osteotomy. A microsagittal saw is then used to perform the osteotomy from dorsal to plantar taking care not to violate the plantar cortex. The first pass with the saw blade is made parallel to the first TMT joint, whereas the second was made 2 mm distal to this but towards the same apex plantarly. A small wedge of bone is removed from between the 2 saw cuts and a greenstick manoeuvre with dorsiflexion of the osteotomy site is closed with slight dorsiflexion of the first metatarsal. A push-up test now confirms that the first metatarsal is now only slightly plantar to the fifth. A 3.5 mm cortical screw is used to secure the osteotomy in place as shown in Fig. 42.8b, c.

Finally, attention is drawn to the fifth metatarsal through the former incision. The interval between the peroneus brevis and the lateral band of the plantar fascia was identified, and blunt dissection was carried down to the fifth metatarsal base. The screw is removed easily using a screwdriver. Another incision is made at the level of the non-union following the previous incision. The non-union site is taken down, and the bone ends freshened-up using curettes. A guidewire was placed at the fifth metatarsal base, past the non-union. The cannulated drill was then used over the guidewire to beyond the fracture site, and it was passed several times at the fracture site in an attempt to try to break up the intramedullary sclerosis. The 5.5 cannulated tap was initially used over the guidewire, and based upon fluoroscopy was felt that the 6.5 cannulated tap would still have clearance. Therefore, the 6.5 cannulated tap was now passed over the guidewire to be on the fracture site. The guidewire was then removed. Using the standard measurements, a 6.5 mm x 45 mm solid partially threaded screw was used and advanced into the intramedullary canal. A solid screw is chosen to increase the bending stiffness of the construct. The autograft was placed at the level of the non-union. Final fluoroscopic X-rays were obtained in multiple planes. Closure was obtained using a 2.0 Vicryl interrupted sutures for the subcutaneous tissue and 3.0 Vicryl rapide for the skin in a non-interrupted fashion. A modified Jones dressing was applied and the tourniquet was deflated.

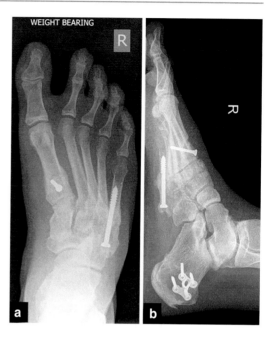

Fig. 42.9 AP (**a**) and lateral (**b**) films at 8 months after the last procedure showing complete healing of his previous recalcitrant non-union, as well as of the osteotomies. (Obtained with permission from George. D. Chloros, MD)

Postoperatively, the patient was put in a below-knee cast, non-weightbearing for 6 weeks total, then progression to full weightbearing by 10 weeks. An Exogen bone stimulator was also prescribed to accelerate the healing. At 8 months postoperatively, the patient had no complaints and had healed completely as shown in Fig. 42.9.

Summary: Lessons Learned

This case summarizes a young patient with known risk factors for non-union including smoking and type 2 diabetes who underwent two failed fixations with intramedullary screw. Unfortunately, the presence of a cavovarus deformity clinically and secondary sclerosis of the base of the fourth metatarsal was initially not taken into account leading to failure of treatment. The third and final surgery included correcting the cavovarus deformity at the same time of revision screw intramedullary fixation of the fifth metatarsal provided resolution of the symptoms. This case teaches us that addressing all the possible factors and having in mind that in cavovarus feet overloading of the lateral column may lead to recalcitrant non-union and needs to be addressed simultaneously.

References

1. Chloros GD, Kakos CD, Tastsidis IK, Giannoudis VP, Panteli M, Giannoudis PV. Fifth metatarsal fractures: an update on management, complications, and outcomes. EFORT Open Rev. 2022;7(1):13–25.
2. Fleischer AE, Stack R, Klein EE, Baker JR, Weil L Jr, Weil LS Sr. Forefoot adduction is a risk factor for jones fracture. J Foot Ankle Surg. 2017;56(5):917–21.
3. O'Malley M, DeSandis B, Allen A, Levitsky M, O'Malley Q, Williams R. Operative treatment of fifth metatarsal jones fractures (Zones II and III) in the NBA. Foot Ankle Int. 2016;37(5):488–500.
4. Miller JR, Dunn KW, Ciliberti LJ Jr, Patel RD, Swanson BA. Association of vitamin D with stress fractures: a retrospective cohort study. J Foot Ankle Surg. 2016;55(1):117–20.
5. Kane JM, Sandrowski K, Saffel H, Albanese A, Raikin SM, Pedowitz DI. The epidemiology of fifth metatarsal fracture. Foot Ankle Spec. 2015;8(5):354–9.
6. Carreira DS, Sandilands SM. Radiographic factors and effect of fifth metatarsal Jones and diaphyseal stress fractures on participation in the NFL. Foot Ankle Int. 2013;34(4):518–22.
7. Smith TO, Clark A, Hing CB. Interventions for treating proximal fifth metatarsal fractures in adults: a meta-analysis of the current evidence-base. Foot Ankle Surg. 2011;17(4):300–7.
8. Raikin SM, Slenker N, Ratigan B. The association of a varus hindfoot and fracture of the fifth metatarsal metaphyseal-diaphyseal junction: the Jones fracture. Am J Sports Med. 2008;36(7):1367–72.

Calcaneus Fracture Failed Fixation

43

Mandeep S. Dhillon and Ankit Khurana

History of Previous Primary Failed Treatment

A 39-year-old male sustained 7 months previously an isolated closed Sanders type IV calcaneal fracture following a fall from a height. There was no neurovascular deficit at presentation to his local hospital besides some surrounding soft tissue swelling. Ten days later, when the swelling had subsided, he was taken to the operating theatre and underwent fixation via a lateral approach. His postoperative course was uncomplicated and was discharged home 4 days after fixation. Subsequently, he was followed up at the local hospital in the outpatient clinic and after 3 months he was advised to start mobilising full weight bearing. Nonetheless, as he was experiencing a lot of heel pain and difficulty in walking by 6 months he was referred to our institution for further management (Fig. 43.1).

M. S. Dhillon (✉)
Department of Orthopaedics, Postgraduate Institute of Medical Education and Research, Chandigarh, India

Department of Physical Medicine, Postgraduate Institute of Medical Education and Research, Chandigarh, India

A. Khurana
Department of Orthopaedic Surgery, Dr. BSA Medical College and Hospital, Govt of NCT Delhi, Rohini, Delhi, India

© The Author(s), under exclusive license to Springer Nature Switzerland AG 2024
P. V. Giannoudis, P. Tornetta III (eds.), *Failed Fracture Fixation*,
https://doi.org/10.1007/978-3-031-39692-2_43

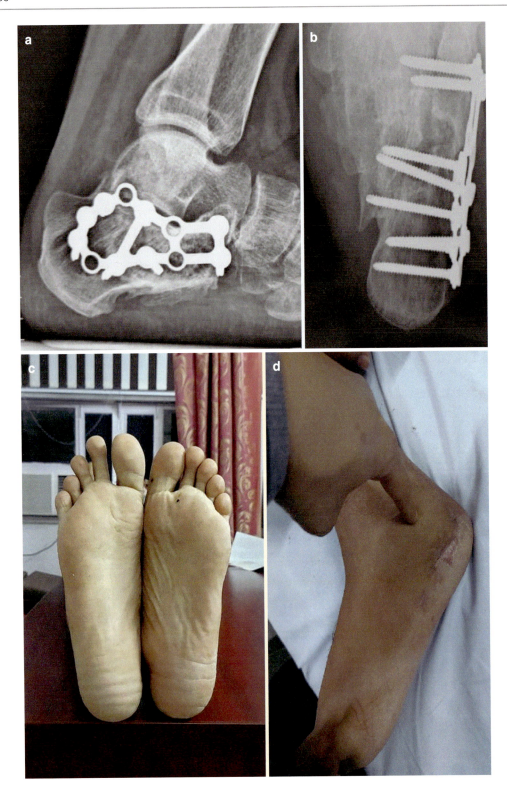

Fig. 43.1 (**a, b**) Lateral and axial view of an inadequately fixed calcaneus fracture seen after 7 months of surgery. (**c, d**) Clinical picture showing deformed heel with widening when seen from below; lateral aspect shows the scar of previous surgery and point of tenderness. (**e, f**) CT scan showing the deformed calcaneus and the lateral impingement. Note the metal artifact seen in CT due to plate in position

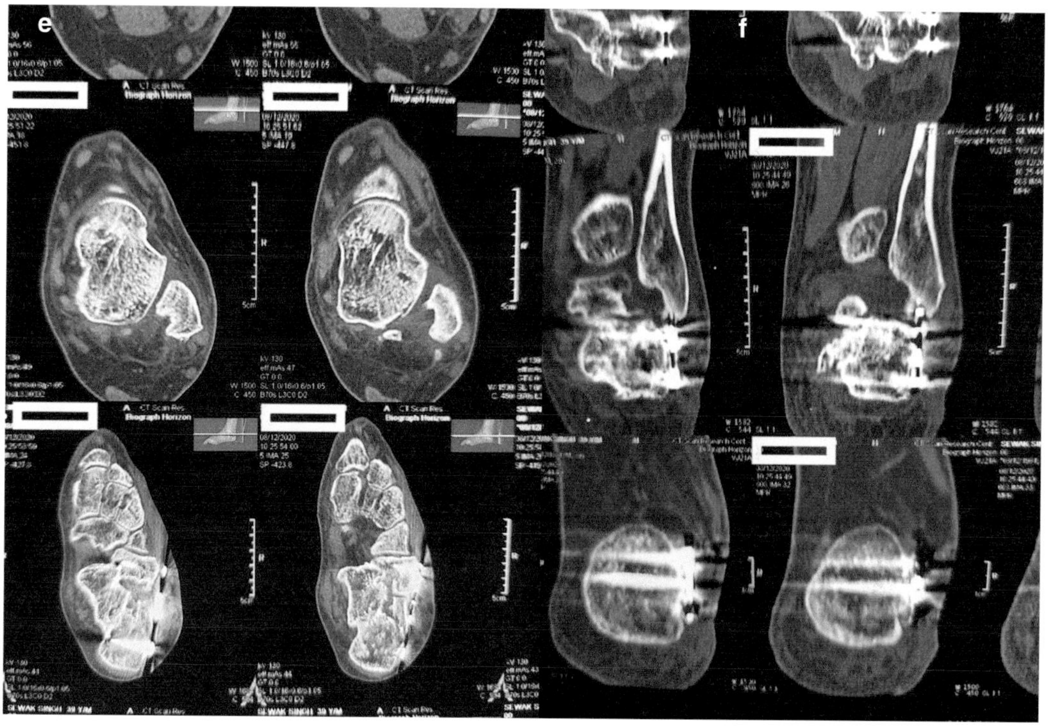

Fig. 43.1 (continued)

Evaluation of the Aetiology of Failure of Fixation

Due to malreduction, the calcaneal wall was displaced laterally against the tip of the lateral malleolus, producing symptoms of peroneal tendon impingement. This was aggravated somewhat by the heel varus. Secondly, the incongruity of the subtalar joint surface led to subtalar joint pain, and the initiation of secondary arthritis. Another cause for pain was anterior tibiotalar impingement following loss in hindfoot height.

Clinical Examination

On examining the involved foot, there was limitation of ankle dorsiflexion with limitation of subtalar motion; tenderness over the subtalar joint was elicited. Subtalar movements were painful, and there was tenderness over the peroneal tendons. There was evident heel widening, oedema and loss of heel height. The surgical scars of the previous extensile lateral approach had healed with primary intention.

Diagnostic-Biochemical and Radiological Investigations

With the clinical picture of pain with implant in situ, it was prudent to rule out infection even though the clinical picture did not suggest any evidence of the same. A routine total leucocyte count (TLC), erythrocyte sedimentation rate (ESR) and C-reactive protein (CRP) was done and was found to be within normal limits. A non-contrast computed tomography (CT) scan was done to further assess the cause of the patients' symptoms.

Role of X-rays: AP, lateral and Harris axial views of the foot are necessary to assess the degree of loss in hindfoot height, loss of Bohler and pitch angles and also to check for any varus or valgus deformity of the foot (Fig. 43.2).

The changes seen on X rays can be used as a tool to aid in surgical planning. A loss of calcaneal height > 8 mm compared to the contralateral foot and a reduction in talar declination angle more than 20° as an indication to perform subtalar distraction bone block arthrodesis [1].

However, X-rays are limited by their inability to provide detailed information regarding degree and location of arthritic changes as well as status of soft tissue structures around the foot [2].

Role of CT scan: A computerised tomographic (CT) scan of the calcaneus is always preferred since it offers a more detailed view of the altered calcaneal morphology as well as gives us a three-dimensional (3D) picture of the deformity (Fig. 43.3).

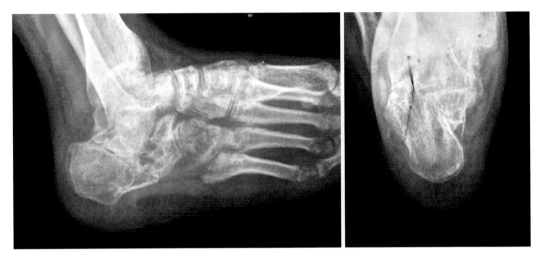

Fig. 43.2 Lateral and axial view of a different case showing residual malunion of calcaneus with deformity, after removal of K-wires used for fixation

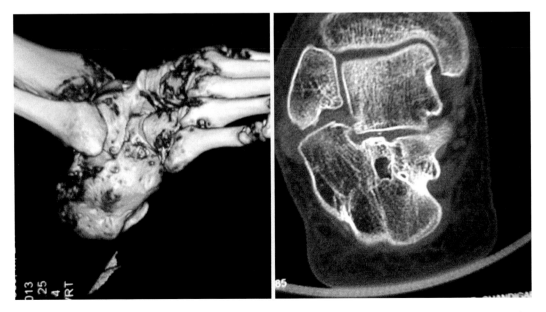

Fig. 43.3 3D reconstruction of another calcaneus malunion showing deformity and impingement; Axial cuts showing tuberosity varus, heel height shortening and lateral shift of calcaneus fragment with impingement under fibula

Stephen and Sanders [3] proposed a CT-based classification to define the problems which could arise after a calcaneus fracture, which has been fixed or not [4].

Type 1: is when the principal problem is due to a lateral wall impingement and the overall anatomy of the bone has been adequately reconstituted and there is no problem in the subtalar joint. This is the least common presentation, and is most easily rectified.

Type 2: is when there is lateral deformity and some degree of arthritis in the subtalar joint, but the heel height is by and large maintained. This would require implant removal and subtalar in situ arthrodesis, along with lateral wall excision.

Type 3: is the worst type where in addition to the above two, there is a loss of heel height and shift of the tuberosity into Varus mostly, but occasionally valgus is encountered. Here there may be need for the above two procedures plus interposition grafting of subtalar joint along with a calcaneus displacement or corrective osteotomy.

Since the advent of the classification, CT scans have had a role to play in the management of calcaneus malunions too. The main disadvantage with CT scan is that it is unable to correctly visualise the soft tissue and tendons around the hindfoot.

Role of magnetic resonance imaging (MRI): The role of MRI though limited is useful for diagnosing peroneus longus and peroneus brevis tears. MRI is the most sensitive imaging modality to detect plantar and heel pad abnormalities. Thus, MRI definitely is useful in long-term fractures with persistent pain. In the latter setting, it is able to diagnose peroneal tendon impingement and dislocations, evaluate the tarsal tunnel and the integrity of the heel pad. Although MRI is a useful imaging modality, yet its drawbacks are that it is unable to differentiate small osteophytes, spurs and bony fragments from the surrounding tendons [5].

Preoperative Planning

In the described case, the issues were chronic pain due to subtalar arthrosis, incongruous subtalar joint, loss of heel height and mechanical block to dorsiflexion (due to talar declination less than 10°). The goal of the planned procedure was thus to restore hindfoot height, correct ankle impingement, eliminate subfibular impingement and decrease pain due to subtalar arthritis.

To address these issues, a plan was formulated to remove the implant as well as the lateral exostosis in order to decrease peroneal impingement, restore heel height by distracting the sub-talar joint and finally fusing the joint in distraction to eliminate pain due to subtalar arthritis.

Revision Surgery

Patient was laid in a lateral decubitus position with the affected side facing upwards. The bone graft site was also painted and draped. A standard posterolateral approach to the subtalar joint was used. After creating full-thickness skin flaps, the prominent hardware was seen and plate was exposed (Fig. 43.4a, b); this was removed using a combination of a curved osteotome and gouges and peroneal tendons were decompressed.

Since this was a type 2 malunion, subtalar arthrodesis was warranted along with the lateral wall excision. Through the same incision, the subtalar joint was exposed and a laminar spreader was used for distracting the subtalar joint. After adequate exposure, the articular surfaces were freshened and denuded (Fig. 43.4c). The subtalar joint gap was measured and an appropriately sized graft was harvested and placed in position. The rest of the joint was filled with cancellous shavings and bone from excised lateral wall. The fusion was fixed with 2 partially threaded cancellous screws (Fig. 43.4d, e), and incisions were closed over a drain (Fig. 43.4f). Fusion was achieved 6 months later and at 12 months the screws were removed.

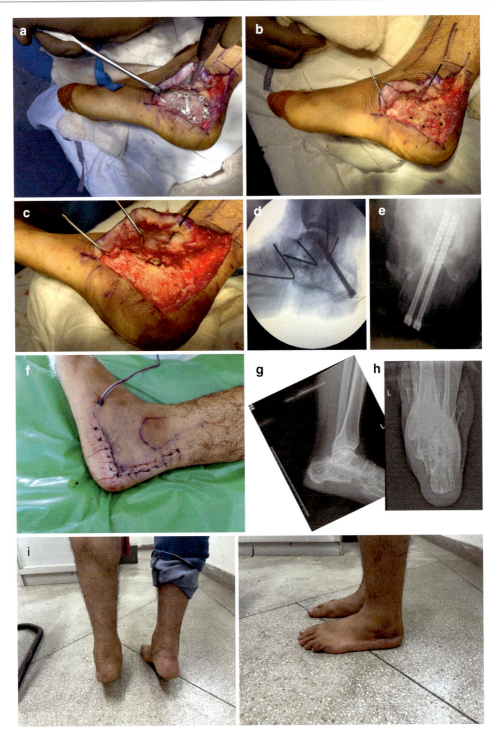

Fig. 43.4 (**a, b**) Same case after extensile approach; note the prominent plate. The lateral wall prominence stays even after removal of the plate. (**c**) After lateral wall exostectomy, the next step was subtalar debridement and subtalar fusion. (**d, e**) After subtalar fusion using bone graft and 2 partially threaded cancellous screws. (**f**) Closure of the wound over a drain. (**g**) **lateral;** (**h**) **axial view:** Three years follow-up of the case after fusion. (**i, j**) Clinical function at follow-up

At 3-year follow-up patient had good radiological union, with minimal deformity seen on axial views (Fig. 43.4g, h). Clinically he had minimal deformity and good function (Fig. 43.4i, j).

Discussion

The calcaneus is an irregular, roughly box-shaped bone sitting below the talus. Its long axis is orientated along the mid-line of the foot, but it deviates lateral to the mid-line anteriorly. Due to its unique and unparalleled anatomy, fixing calcaneal fractures requires expertise and has a steep learning curve [6–8].

The second issue causing complications after fixation is the tenuous soft tissue sleeve over the calcaneus and the close association of the Sural nerve and peroneal tendons on the lateral side. In central fractures that are displaced, not only is the shape of the bone deformed but the facet fragments are pushed down into the centre of the cancellous bone, and the lateral wall 'bursts out' laterally, along with a superior and varus tilt of the tuberosity fragment; this is often like a broken egg, making it very difficult to reform the 3D anatomy exactly [9, 10].

Modern methods of treatment now also include indirect methods of reduction and MIS interventions; thus, it is important to correctly evaluate the case and diagnose the factors responsible for failure, and appropriate identification of causes of pain and disability [9, 11].

When fixing displaced intra-articular calcaneus fractures (DIACFs), there are multiple problems even in the early stages. These may range from improper reduction, inadequate stabilisation, impending soft tissue breakdown and hindfoot deformity. Attempt at fixation with K-wires alone is no longer done, as the hold in comminuted fractures is minimal and the bone tends to collapse (Fig. 43.5a–d).

Screw fixation also has to be done with care, as the key point is obtaining a good reduction, and proper placement of screws should be to maintain this reduction till bony healing. (Fig. 43.6a, b). Even fixations with plates are often done badly, and early collapse of the bone maybe seen in comminuted fractures, with poor reduction and poor stabilisation (Fig. 43.7).

Conventional thought processes label lateral impingement as the commonest midterm issue, and sub-talar arthritis as the commonest cause for pain in the long term, when the bone anatomy is inadequately reconstructed. There is now a better understanding of the patho-anatomy of calcaneus malunion and hindfoot biomechanics and other factors causing pain are also being identified [12, 13]. Very rarely is early revision of a bad implant done, as repeated surgery in this area has soft tissue consequences due to already compromised skin (Fig. 43.8).

The primary fracture line (in most cases) separates the calcaneal tuberosity from the sustentaculum tali, whereas the secondary fracture line progresses in the sagittal plane anywhere along the length of the bone. As a result the tuberosity fragment gets displaced laterally, while the sustentaculum remains attached to the Talus by the inter-osseous ligaments (hence known as the 'constant fragment') [14, 15]. This results in deformity characteristic of most calcaneal malunions. However, when attempts at fixation are done, many structures maybe disrupted and a malunion after fixation maybe very different from a malunion in an untreated case (Fig. 43.3).

Patients may also present with a painful heel following surgery. An additional cause of pain in surgically managed calcaneus is prominent hardware, which could threaten the skin.

When trying to treat a case of failed fixation for calcaneus fractures, many things have to be taken into consideration [16–19]. The case may present early with bone collapse and poor soft tissues or they present late with problems associated with calcaneus malunion. The three main things which have to be evaluated in any particular case are the restoration of the anatomy in all three dimensions, the congruity of the joints, especially the subtalar joints, and whether there is any bulge of the lateral wall, causing impingement of the soft tissues between this and the fibula.

In fact, when a revision surgery is contemplated for a failed fixation, it is actually the treatment of a calcaneus malunion and ideally

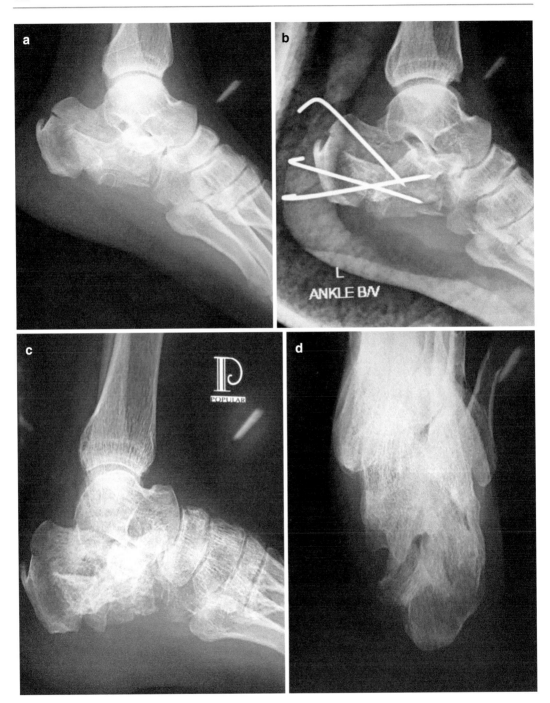

Fig. 43.5 (**a, b**) Comminuted calcaneus fracture after attempted fixation by percutaneous K-wire; there is almost no reduction of either the tuberosity or the subtalar joint. (**c, d**) Deformed calcaneus after K-wire removal at 3 months; this bone is not reconstructable and will need a corrective osteotomy and subtalar fusion

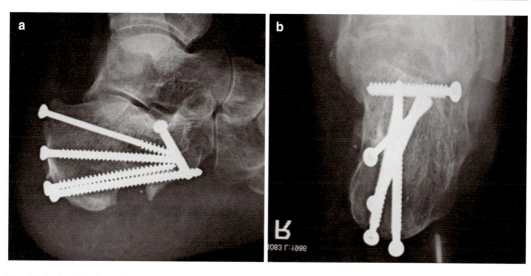

Fig. 43.6 (**a, b**) Deformed calcaneus after attempted indirect reduction and screw fixation, at 5 months; this bone will need a corrective osteotomy and subtalar fusion

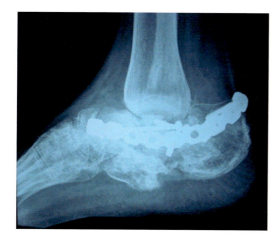

Fig. 43.7 Lateral view of another malunion despite an attempt at reduction and fixation, with plate in situ. These cases do not fit into the standard cases of malunion defined in the literature, with the patterns of displacement and deformities being different. (Adapted from Dhillon, MS: Fractures of the Calcaneus, Edition 2, 2023, Jaypee Bros N Delhi, with permission)

should be deferred to a period when the bone has already united and osteotomies could be successful.

The alterations associated with malunion or inadequately treated calcaneal fractures are as follows:

1. Loss of heel height: Loss of height in malunited calcaneal fractures leads to a reduction in talocalcaneal angle, calcaneal pitch as well as Bohler angle. As a result, the talus becomes somewhat horizontal and comes to lie in a relatively dorsiflexed position. This leads to impingement between the talar dome and the anterior tibial plafond. Symptoms manifest as pain on the dorsal aspect of the foot which are exacerbated on dorsiflexion of the ankle. This condition could eventually lead to ankle arthritis. Loss of calcaneal height also leads to a reduction in the mechanical leverage of the gastrocnemius muscle which causes gait alterations (especially in the stance phase). Shoe wear becomes difficult as the lateral malleolus rubs against the shoe counter due to the lowered heel. All the above have the potential to be a cause of pain [2].

2. Varus and valgus deformity of heel: Varus malunions are seen mostly in calcaneal fractures managed non-operatively or due to improper reduction in the tuberosity fragment during surgery, whereas valgus malunions are less often seen. Since the movements of the subtalar joint are coupled to the transverse tarsal joint, the new position of the hindfoot

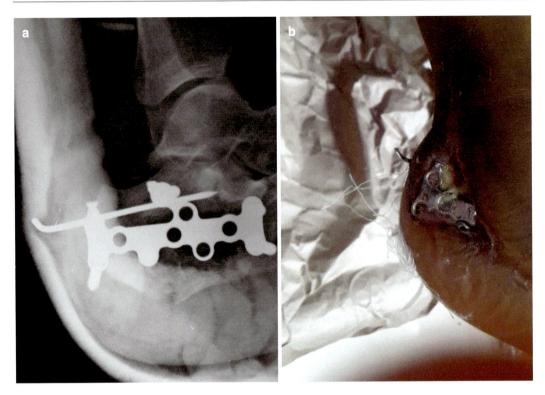

Fig. 43.8 (a, b) Lateral view showing a badly fixed calcaneus fracture with the plate exposed through the skin incision

locks the transverse tarsal joint thereby reducing its flexibility. This reduces the shock absorbing capacity of the hindfoot and may lead to accelerated degeneration of the subtalar and transverse talar joints.
3. Heel widening: There is significant heel widening in malunited calcaneus fractures which is a result of lateral wall blowout; if not addressed this leads to bony impingement on the peroneal tendons and sub-fibular abutment.
4. Post-traumatic arthrosis: Malreduction of fracture fragments in either operatively or non- operatively cases managed can lead to post traumatic arthritis of the subtalar joint. Many times the high energy nature of the injury causes irreversible damage to the articular cartilage [15]. In such cases, patient will still have a higher probability of developing arthritis regardless of the reduction attempts. Besides the sub-talar joint, the transverse tarsus and ankle joint may also be involved secondary to torsional force transmission to these joints, particularly during the stance phase of gait. Poeze et al. have shown that there is an inverse relationship between the rate of post operative subtalar arthritis and the magnitude of patient load, which proves that a learning curve for operative treatment of these fractures exists [20].
5. Soft tissue problems and other pain causative factors.

Pain aetiology may be due to a single or multiple causative factors, and thus it is important to correctly identify the cause of pain. In a study evaluating the various complications of intra-articular calcaneus fractures, Lim and Leung have stated that the causes of pain in non-operatively managed fractures are different from those which had been treated surgically [21]. In non-operatively treated calcaneal fractures, heel pain arises chiefly due to post-traumatic arthritis of the subtalar joint and malunion. In those cases, however, where the fracture has been managed primarily by either open or minimally invasive surgery (MIS), the cause of pain is usually the prominent hardware since malunion is often minimal [22]. Various nerve injuries can also take place during calcaneal fracture surgery either due to direct injury, traction injury or even due to idiopathic mechanisms such as complex regional pain syndrome (CRPS).

In the case presented above, problems like heel width, heel height and heel alignment were restored. Peroneal impingement was sorted by lateral exostectomy and in addition, subtalar pain was eliminated by arthrodesing the joint. Thus, identification of pain generators and causes of discomfort is essential so that same can be addressed in all the procedures planned.

Summary: Lessons Learned

Despite fixation, several calcaneus fractures end up with poor outcomes. Fixation failure is usually the result of either inadequate reduction or inadequate stabilisation, usually with the minimally invasive methods like K-wires or screw fixation. Even improper plating of a malreduced fracture will lead to problems in the foot.

The three most common causes of residual heel pain (when evaluated in isolation) are subtalar arthritis, peroneal tendon impingement and pain due to prominent hardware. While subtalar arthritis and lateral wall problems are seen more frequently in fractures managed non-operatively, hardware-related pain was the predominant cause in patients who had been primarily treated operatively either via open reduction internal fixation (ORIF) or MIS.

Poorer functional outcome is also associated with loss of hindfoot height and varus deformity, which may persist despite internal fixation. This usually requires subtalar fusion in the corrected position along with hardware removal, which gives satisfactory outcomes.

References

1. Jackson JB, Jacobson L, Banerjee R, Nickisch F. Distraction subtalar arthrodesis. Foot Ankle Clin. 2015;20(2):335–51.
2. Dhillon MS, Bali K, Prabhakar S. Controversies in calcaneus fracture management: a systematic review of the literature. Musculoskelet Surg. 2011;95:171–81.
3. Stephens HM, Sanders R. Calcaneal malunions: results of a prognostic computed tomography classification system. Foot Ankle Int. 1996;17(7):395–401.
4. Stapleton JJ, Belczyk R, Zgonis T. Surgical treatment of calcaneal fracture malunions and post-traumatic deformities. Clin Podiatr Med Surg. 2009;26(1):79–90.
5. Poeze M, Verbruggen JPAM, Brink PRG. The relationship between the outcome of operatively treated calcaneal fractures and institutional fracture load: a systematic review of the literature. J Bone Joint Surg Am Vol. 2008;90(5):1013–21.
6. Dhillon MS, Aggarwal S, Dhatt S, Jain M. Epidemiological pattern of foot injuries in India: preliminary assessment of data from a tertiary hospital. J Postgrad Med Edu Res. 2012;46(3):144–7.
7. Dhillon MS, editor. Fractures of the calcaneus. 1st ed. New Delhi: Jaypee Brothers Medical Publishers; 2013. https://doi.org/10.5005/jp/books/11781. https://www.jaypeedigital.com/book/9789350903438
8. Coughlin MJ. Calcaneal fractures in the industrial patient. Foot Ankle Int. 2000;21(11):896–905.
9. Buckley RE, Meek RN. Comparison of open versus closed reduction of intraarticular calcaneal fractures: a matched cohort in workmen. J Orthop Trauma. 1992;6(2):216–22.
10. Chen W, Li X, Su Y, Zhang Q, Smith WR, Zhang X, et al. Peroneal tenography to evaluate lateral hindfoot pain after calcaneal fracture. Foot Ankle Int. 2011;32(8):789–95.
11. Zwipp H, Rammelt S. Posttraumatische Korrekturoperationen am Fuß. Zentralbl Chir. 2003;128(3):218–26.
12. Chandler JT, Bonar SK, Anderson RB, Davis WH. Results of in situ subtalar arthrodesis for late sequelae of calcaneus fractures. Foot Ankle Int. 1999;20(1):18–24.
13. Banerjee R, Saltzman C, Anderson RB, Nickisch F. Management of calcaneal malunion. Am Acad Orthop Surg. 2011;19(1):27–36.
14. Lim EVA, Leung JPF. Complications of intraarticular calcaneal fractures. Clin Orthop Relat Res. 2001;391:7–16.
15. Clare MP, Crawford WS. Managing complications of calcaneus fractures. Foot Ankle Clin. 2017;22(1):105–16.
16. Shah R. Malunion calcaneus: understanding it, classification and treatment planning. In: Dhillon

MS, editor. Fractures of the calcaneus. Jaypee Brothers Medical Publishers (P) Ltd.; 2013. p. 109. Available from: https://www.jaypeedigital.com/book/9789350903438/chapter/ch14.

17. Carr JB, Hansen ST, Benirschke SK. Subtalar distraction bone block fusion for late complications of Os Calcis fractures. Foot Ankle. 1988;9(2):81–6.

18. Romash MM. Reconstructive osteotomy of the calcaneus with subtalar arthrodesis for malunited calcaneal fractures. Clin Orthop Relat Res. 1993;290:157–67.

19. Huang P-J, Fu Y-C, Cheng Y-M, Lin S-Y. Subtalar arthrodesis for late sequelae of calcaneal fractures: fusion in situ versus fusion with sliding corrective osteotomy. Foot Ankle Int. 1999;20(3):166–70.

20. Gotha HE, Zide JR. Current controversies in management of calcaneus fractures. Orthop Clin N Am. 2017;48(1):91–103.

21. Dhillon MS, Prabhakar S. Treatment of displaced intra-articular calcaneus fractures: a current concepts review. SICOT J. 2017;3:59.

22. Braly WG, Bishop JO, Tullos HS. Lateral decompression for malunited Os calcis fractures. Foot Ankle. 1985;6(2):90–6.

Lisfranc Fracture Failed Fixation

44

Mark Yakavonis and Gregory Wayresz

History of Previous Primary Failed Treatment

A 40-year-old diabetic male who had a mechanical fall from a height of 6 feet at work was found to have a ligamentous Lisfranc injury with subluxation of his second metatarsal laterally on the tarsal metatarsal articulation (Fig. 44.1).

He was treated at an outside facility with an open reduction internal fixation (ORIF) with two cannulated 3.5 mm screws immediately after the injury (Fig. 44.2).

Due to continued pain thought to be symptomatic hardware, the hardware was removed 1 year post-op by outside surgeon (Fig. 44.3).

M. Yakavonis (✉)
Department of Orthopaedics, Boston University
Medical Center, Boston, MA, USA

G. Wayresz
Department of Orthopaedics, Massachusetts General
Hospital, Boston, MA, USA
e-mail: gwaryasz@mgb.org

© The Author(s), under exclusive license to Springer Nature Switzerland AG 2024
P. V. Giannoudis, P. Tornetta III (eds.), *Failed Fracture Fixation*,
https://doi.org/10.1007/978-3-031-39692-2_44

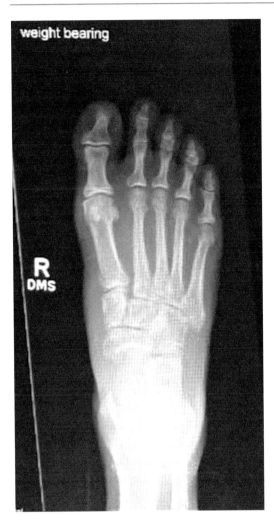

Fig. 44.1 Initial Injury radiograph

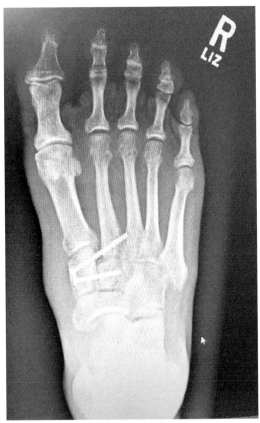

Fig. 44.2 Postoperative imaging from his index procedure

(Fig. 44.2). Additionally, the subluxation of the first Tarsometatarsal joint (TMT) joint was missed. Medial column stability is required for successful outcomes and the support for the arch of the foot. Omitting stable medial column fixation will in most cases lead to continued instability and flattening of the foot or planovalgus deformity with some pronation. While the author does not routinely fuse ligamentous injuries, this is also an option.

Clinical Examination

Patient presented for a second opinion with ongoing dorsal mid foot pain with ambulation despite hardware removal. Clinically his pain was worse over the second tarsal metatarsal joint with palpation. The foot had a planovalgus position when walking.

Diagnostic-Biochemical and Radiological Investigations

There were no signs or history of infection so no further infection workup was undertaken in this case. The most important element of the evaluation in these cases are weightbearing radiographs. In this case, they showed persistent lateral subluxation of his second metatarsal at the tarsal metatarsal joint but a congruent first TMT joint (Fig. 44.4).

Weightbearing computed tomography (CT) scan confirmed the subluxation of his second metatarsal at the tarsal metatarsal joint (Fig. 44.5).

In this patient, bone quality did not appear to be an issue. The impaired healing was ligamentous in nature. His hemoglobin A1C was found to be less than 8.

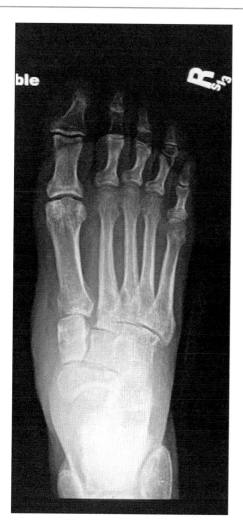

Fig. 44.3 Imaging after removal of hardware

Evaluation of the Etiology of Failure of Fixation

The fixation failed due to malreduction of the index procedure. Note persistent lateral subluxation of the second metatarsal on the middle cuneiform

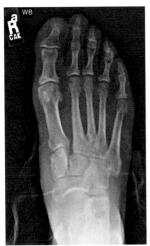

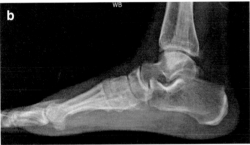

Fig. 44.4 (**a** and **b**) AP and lateral Foot radiographs on presentation

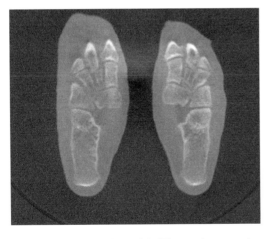

Fig. 44.5 Weightbearing axial CT scan demonstrating incongruity of the second TMT joint with excellent alignment fi the first TMT joint

Preoperative Planning

Since hardware had already been removed, additional hardware removal was not necessary. The consideration was for type of surgery.

Given that the malunion is ligamentous in nature as well as the timing between original injury and timing of second surgery, the decision was made to proceed further with arthrodesis. This is further supported as the patient was diabetic.

Implant Selection: Implant selection was guided by the desire for compression across the arthrodesis sites. A 3.5 mm screw was selected due to increased strength as well as nitinol staples to provide compression cross the fusion site. The screw was placed in a lag by technique fashion across the second metatarsal. Alternatively, a dorsal plate can be used if bone quality is an issue, or the reduction is highly unstable after debridement.

Need for Bone Grafting: In the setting of fusion of the second tarsal metatarsal joint as well as the intercuneiform, joint sometimes a small amount of bone graft will be necessary. If needed, we would proceed with harvesting of calcaneal bone graft through small incision laterally. In this case, there was no need for graft.

Revision Surgery

The prior dorsal incision of about 3–4 cm was centered over the second tarsal metatarsal joint. Dissection was carried down to expose the extensor hallucis longus. The extensor hallucis longus was retracted medially and the extensor hallucis brevis as well as the neuromuscular bundle were retracted laterally. Subperiosteal dissection was carried out over the second tarsal metatarsal joint as well as the medial intercuneiform joint. The first TMT joint was evaluated and found to be stable. A curette, rongeur, and pituitary were used to denude the second tarsal metatarsal joint of all cartilage. Care was taken to remove cartilage from the plantar aspect of the joint so as not to dorsiflex the second metatarsal at the time of fusion. In a similar fashion, the medial intercuneiform joint was denuded of all cartilage. Next, all fibrous tissues in the space between the first and second metatarsal were cleared using a pituitary and curette. Using a 2.0 mm drill, holes were made at both fusion sites to encourage subchondral bleeding. The medial inter cuneiform joint was compressed using a pointed reduction clamp. A nitinol staple was placed dorsally to stabilize and compress the fusion site. The pointed reduction clamp was removed and placed on the second metatarsal to the medial cuneiform to both close down the first and second metatarsal space as well as compress the second tarsal metatarsal joint. We then drilled through the dorsal second metatarsal with a 3.5 mm drill over 1 cm distal to the tarsal meta tarsal joint, careful to overdrill only through the second metatarsal. A 2.7 mm drill was used to drill through the middle cuneiform. A burr was used to create a slight rivet distal to the entrance of the screw in the second metatarsal to create room for the head of the screw to compress and not translate the fusion site. At this point, to provide extra stability, particularly in rotation, another nitinol staple was placed across the second tarsal metatarsal joint. Periosteum was closed over the fusion sites. The skin was closed with a nylon suture.

Patient was placed into a splint and made nonweightbearing and was discharged home the same day of the surgery with adequate pain control from a preoperative peripheral nerve block.

At 2 weeks, the sutures were removed, and the patient was placed into a Cam boot to allow for ankle range of motion. Progressive weightbearing was allowed at 6 weeks in the boot. Patient transitioned to stiff soled shoe at 3 months and maintained their reduction with relief of the majority of their pain (Fig. 44.6).

Fig. 44.6 (a–c) Final radiographs after arthrodesis

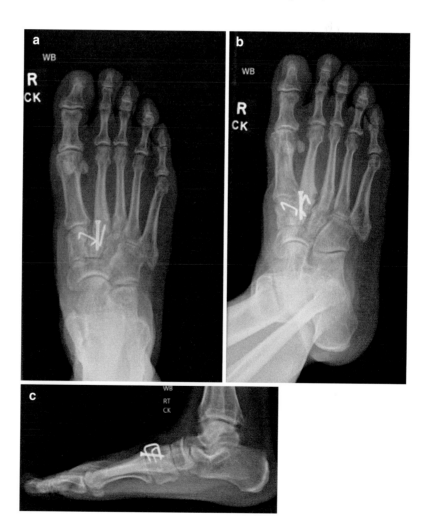

Lessons Learned

The treatment of ligamentous Lisfranc injuries has been greatly debated, with some advocating for primary fusion and some arguing for ORIF.

Proponents for primary fusion argue for better outcomes and less complications and reoperations [1]. However, a recent study refutes this outside of planned hardware removal [2]. In this case, the original Lisfranc injury was subtle in which a strong argument can be made for ORIF. However, to execute this perfectly, an anatomic reduction must be achieved [3, 4].

Fixation options for subtle Lisfranc injuries range from cannulated screws to cortical screws to bridge plates and more recently suture button devices. Arguments can be made for each of these devices provided there is an anatomic reduction.

In the case of this particular patient, while the Lisfranc injury was subtle, a strong consideration could be made for fusion given that the patient was diabetic.

When fusing the tarsal metatarsal joints, it is important to focus on denuding the cartilage particularly in the plantar aspect of the joint and if graft is needed, it can often be taken from the calcareous as the amount of graft needed is small. On option to enhance a repair which was not performed in this case is to create a dorsal spot weld by using a burr to connect the second metatarsal with the medial and middle cuneiforms. The slight divot is then filled with bone graft [5].

References

1. Coetzee JC, Ly TV. Treatment of primarily ligamentous Lisfranc joint injuries: primary arthrodesis compared with open reduction and internal fixation. Surgical technique. J Bone Joint Surg Am. 2007;89:122–7.
2. Buda M, Kink S, Stavenuiter R, et al. Reoperation rate differences between open reduction internal fixation and primary arthrodesis of Lisfranc injuries. Foot Ankle Int. 2018;39(9):1086–96.
3. Kuo R, Tejwani N, DiGiovanni C, et al. Outcome after open reduction and internal fixation of Lisfranc joint injuries. JBJS Am. 2000;82A:1609–18.
4. Demirkale I, Tecimel O, Celik I, et al. The effect of the Tscherne injury pattern on the outcome of operatively treated Lisfranc fracture dislocations. Foot Ankle Surg. 2013;19(3):188–93.
5. Hansen S. Arthrodesis of the tarsometatarsal. In: Functional reconstruction of the foot and ankle. Philadelpha: Lippincott Williams and Wilkins; 2000. p. 332–4.

Index

A
Achilles tendon allograft, 264
Acromioclavicular (ACJ) dislocation
  aetiology of, 57
  biochemical and radiological investigations, 58–59
  clinical examination, 57
  first stage revision surgery, 59–60
  history of, 55
  pre-operative planning, 59
  radiographs of, 56
  second stage revision surgery, 60–61
AIDS, 376
Altered plate, 170
American Orthopaedic Foot and Ankle Society Score
    (AOFAS), 438
Anaesthesia, 82
Angiosomes, 424
Ankle fracture, 393, 395, 417
  biomechanical and radiological investigation, 386
  clinical examination, 386
  evaluation of etiology of fixation failure, 385, 386
  history of failed primary treatment, 379–383, 385
  intraoperative image intensifier, 388
  preoperative planning, 386
  revision surgery, 386–388
Ankle syndesmosis injuries
  biochemical and radiological investigation, 405, 406
  clinical examination, 404
  evaluation of aetiology of fixation failure, 403, 404
  history of previous primary treatment, 401
  intraoperative imaging, 412
  preoperative planning, 408
  revision surgery, 408, 409, 411, 412
Anterior inferior tibio-fibular ligament (AITFL), 414
Anterior ring injury, 184
Anteromedial approach, 435
Anteroposterior, 151, 152
AOFAS score, 442
Arthrodesis, 471
Aseptic non-unions, 30
Atrophic non-unions, 30
Autogenous bone graft, 373, 377
Autograft, 449

Autologous bone graft, 363
Avascular necrosis (AVN), 88

B
Bending fractures, 168
Beta-carboxy-terminal collagen crosslink (B-CTX), 361
Bimalleolar and trimalleolar ankle fractures, 423
Bimalleolar ankle fracture, 392.
    See also Ankle fractures
Biomechanical criteria, 385
Bone grafting, 427
Bone healing, 23
  anatomic reduction, 45
  concept of, 37
  contact healing, 24
  direct fracture healing, 24
  direct healing, 41
  fixation construct failure, 44
  fracture fragments, 42
  fracture healing, 43
  gap healing, 24
  indirect fracture healing, 23, 41
  intramedullary nailing, 47
  length of the plate, 46
  locking bolts/screws, 48
  nail diameter, 48
  nail length, 48
  non-compliance, 50
  osteoinductive and osteogenic, 40
  plate-screw density, 46
  plating, 45
  plating techniques, 45
  post-operative protocols, 49
  principles of, 39–40
  reamed *vs.* unreamed nails, 47–48
  rigid plate fixation, 43
  single *vs.* double plating, 46
  stepwise approach, 51–52
  types of, 40
Bone mineral density (BMD), 393
Bone quality, 394
Buttress plate, 196, 197

© The Editor(s) (if applicable) and The Author(s), under exclusive license to Springer Nature
Switzerland AG 2024
P. V. Giannoudis, P. Tornetta III (eds.), *Failed Fracture Fixation*,
https://doi.org/10.1007/978-3-031-39692-2

C

Calcaneus fracture
  biochemical and radiological investigations, 457–459
  clinical examination, 456, 457
  complications after fixation, 461
  DIACFs, 461
  evaluation of aetiology of fixation failure, 457
  failed fixation for, 461
  fracture line, 461
  functional outcome, 465
  history of previous primary treatment, 455
  inadequately treated alteration, 463
  methods of treatment, 461
  nerve injuries, 465
  patho-anatomy, 461
  postoperative course, 455
  preoperative planning, 459
  revision surgery, 459, 461
Capitellum, 137–141
  clinical examination, 140
  preoperative planning, 141
  previous primary failed treatment, 137
  radiological investigations, 140
  revision surgery, 141, 142
C-arm fluoroscopy, 441
Chronic hepatitis B infection, 201
Clavicle fractures
  aetiology of, 68
  anatomy, 65
  bone grafting, 72
  clinical examination, 69
  extrinsic factors, 68
  failure of fixation, 66
  intrinsic factors, 68
  mid-shaft region, 66
  operative indications, 67
  orthogonal plating, 71
  plain X-ray images, 70
  preoperative planning, 71
  reconstruction plates, 67
  revision surgery, 72–73
Complex Regional Pain Syndrome (CRPS), 465
Compression fractures, 168
A computerised tomographic (CT) scan, 377, 406, 413,
       419, 420, 424, 426, 456, 458
"Constant fragment", 461
Coronary artery disease, 376
Cotton test, 379, 385
C-reactive protein (CRP), 457
CT scan. See A computerised tomographic (CT) scan

D

Deformity, 184, 187
Deltotrapezial fascia, 61
Demineralised bone matrix (DBM), 373
Diabetic ankle fractures, 398
Displaced intra-articular calcaneus fractures
       (DIACFs), 461
Distal femoral periprosthetic fractures

biochemical and radiological investigations, 252
clinical examination, 252
etiology of, 252
failed treatment, 249
preoperative planning, 252–253
revision surgery, 253–255
Distal femur fracture, 10
Distal fibula, 424
Distal fibula fracture, 391
Distal humerus fractures, 117
  anatomical combi plate, 124
  biochemical and haematological investigations, 122
  Chevron olecranon osteotomy, 124
  clinical examination, 122
  etiology of, 122
  general anaesthesia, 124
  intercondylar fracture, 124
  left iliac crest, 126
  medial and lateral wounds, 117
  medial distal plate screw, 117
  neurovascular deficit, 117
  olecranon osteotomy, 127
  post-operative course, 126
  pre-operative planning, 123
  3-D anterior view, 128
Distal locking volar plate, 162
Distal radius, 157, 163, 165, 168–171
Distal radius fractures, 159, 162
  biochemical and radiological investigations, 160
  clinical examination, 160
  failure of fixation, 159
  preoperative planning, 160
  revision surgery, 160
Distal tibia, 425
Distal tibia fractures
  autogenous bone graft, 351
  bone morphogenetic proteins (BMPs), 351
  clinical examination, 350
  etiology of, 349–350
  MIPO plating techniques, 349
  preoperative planning, 350
  reamer/irrigator/aspirator (RIA) technique, 345
  revision surgery, 351
  RIA and tibial reamings, 352
  suprapatellar approach, 352
Distal tibia intraarticular fracture fixation failure
  biochemical and radiological investigation, 373
  clinical examination, 373
  evaluation of aetiology of fixation failure, 373
  history of previous primary failed
       treatment, 369–372
  ilizarov fixation, 357, 360–363, 366
  ORIF, 369
  preoperative planning, 373
  revision surgery, 373–375
Distal tibial meta-diaphysis, 325
  anteroposterior (AP) and lateral radiographs, 326
  clinical, radiological, and biochemical
       assessment, 328
  hexapod external ring fixation, 327

Index

475

hexapod ring fixator, 325
initial presentation, 333
intraoperative fluoroscopy imaging, 332
medial distal femur, 332
multidisciplinary planning, 334
post-operative course, 332
pre-operative planning, 330, 331
revision surgery, 330–333
tibial pseudarthrosis, 329
Dorsal distraction plate, 170
Dorsal intercarpal segment instability (DISI), 176
Dorsal radio-carpal (DRC), 176

E
Elbow, 131, 134, 136, 137, 140, 141
Elbow instability, 146
Erythrocyte sedimentation rate (ESR), 350, 457
Extracapsular proximal femoral fractures
biochemical and radiological investigations, 213
clinical examination, 213
etiology of, 213
flexion/extension deformity, 215
intramedullary nail, 212
osteotome osteoclasis, 214
post-operative radiographs, 216
pre-operative planning, 213–214
primary treatment, 211–213
proximal locking screws, 212
revision surgery, 214–217
3D reconstruction, 212

F
Failed fixation, 167
Failed hardware, 185
Failed pelvic fracture fixation, 182, 189
anterior ring injury, 184, 185
clinical examination, 182
diagnostic, 183
evaluation, failure of fixation, 182
history, previous treatment, 181
posterior injury, 185, 186
revision surgery, 186–189
Fibula fracture, 376, 386
Fibula osteosynthesis, 373
Fibular fixation, 420
Fifth metatarsal fractures
biochemical and radiological investigations, 449
cavovarus foot deformity, 449, 453, 454
clinical examination, 449
Exogen bone stimulator, 453
failure of treatment, 449
hardware failure, 449
history of previous primary treatment, 445, 448
hypertrophic nonunion, 449
intraoperative fluoroscopic images, 452
non-union, 445, 449, 453, 454
preoperative planning, 449
revision surgery, 451, 453
Fixation construct failures, 45

Flexor halluces longus (FHL), 427, 428
Foot Function Index (FFI) score, 438, 442
Foot, 469
Forearm
clinical examination, 153
diaphyseal radius, 151
instability, 147–149
malalignment, 152
preoperative planning, 153, 154
radiological investigations, 153
ulna fracture, 151
Fracture fixation
acetabular fractures, 6
ankle fractures, 10
calcaneal fractures, 11
distal femur, 8
distal humeral fractures, 2
distal radius fractures, 3
distal tibia fractures, 9
distal ulna fractures, 4
femoral shaft fractures, 7
forearm fractures, 3
humeral shaft, 2
incidence and rates of, 12–14
Lisfranc fractures, 11
olecranon fractures, 2
overview, 1
pelvic ring fractures, 5
proximal femoral fractures, 6
proximal humeral fractures, 1
radial head fractures, 3
tibial plateau fractures, 8
tibial shaft fractures, 9
Fracture healing, mechanics of, 25
Fragment-specific fixation, 170

G
Grave's disease, 361
Gustilo type I open fracture, 369

H
Haversian remodeling, 41
Heel pain, 465
Hindfoot fusion nail, 395
Hindfoot varus, 437–440, 442–444
Humeral midshaft fracture, 44
Humeral neck
anatomy of, 87
bone grafting, 93
clinical examination, 90
displaced fracture, 88
extension deformity, 89
implant selection, 92–93
intramedullary strut graft, 94
mechanisms of failure, 88
medullary canal, 93
modes of failure, 92
preoperative planning, 91–92
revision fixation, 91, 93

Humeral shaft fractures, 97
  AP and lateral views, 115
  autogenous bone grafting, 101
  biochemical and radiological investigations,
          99–100
  cerclage wires, 112
  clinical evaluation, 98
  clinical examination, 113
  C-reactive protein levels, 113
  dual plating, 107
  entry and exit ballistic wounds, 102
  etiology of, 98, 111–113
  exchange nailing, 101
  femoral canal, 105
  fixation failure, 104
  fluoroscopic and intraoperative images, 114
  implant selection, 100
  initial management, 102–104
  intramedullary (IM) nailing, 97
  Masquelet technique, 103
  oligotrophic nonunion, 106
  plate augmentation, 101
  preoperative planning, 100, 113
  primary treatment, 109–111
  removal and plate osteosynthesis, 100
  revision surgery, 102–105, 113
Hyperthyroidism, 34, 361

I
Ilizarov fixation
  biochemical and radiological investigations, 361
  clinical examination, 360
  evaluation of etiology of fixation failure, 360
  history of previous primary failed
          treatment, 357
  pathology of treatment failure, 361, 362
  pre-operative planning, 362, 363
  revision surgery, 363
Infection, 373
Intra-articular calcaneus fractures, 464
Intracapsular neck of femur fracture, 201
  aetiology, 204–205
  biochemical and radiological investigations, 205
  clinical examination, 205
  osteotomy, 207
  preoperative planning, 205
  review his wounds, 201
  revision surgery, 205–208
Intramedullary nail (IM)
  anteroposterior (AP) and lateral radiographs, 342
  biochemical and radiological investigations, 338
  bone grafting, 339
  clinical examination, 337–338
  etiology of, 337
  implant selection, 338–339
  preoperative planning, 338–339
  revision surgery, 339–341
  tibia injury radiographs, 336
  valgus deformity, 335

Intramedullary nailing (IMN), 345
Intravenous antibiotics, 370, 375

K
Kapandji, 157, 160
K-wires, 394, 395

L
LARS™ ligament, 60
Lateral malleolus failed fracture
  clinical examination, 393
  diagnostic-biochemical and radiological
          investigations, 393
  evaluation of etiology of fixation failure, 392
  history of previous primary failed
          treatment, 391
  preoperative planning, 393–395
  revision surgery, 395–397
Limited compression dynamic compression plate
          (LC-DCP), 153–155
Lisfranc fracture dislocation
  AP and lateral foot radiograph, 470
  biochemical and radiological investigation, 469
  bone grafting, 470
  clinical examination, 469
  evaluation of aetiology of fixation failure, 469
  fusion, 470, 472
  history of previous primary treatment, 467
  implant selection, 470
  medial column stability, 469
  ORIF, 472
  postoperative imaging, 468
  preoperative planning, 470
  revision surgery, 470, 471
  treatment, 472
Low energy fracture, 393
Low molecular weight heparin, 370, 375

M
Magnetic resonance imaging (MRI), 414, 459
Medial extension fracture, 417
Metaphyseal-diaphyseal defect, 377
Metaphysis, 427
Methicillin-sensitive staphylococcus aureus
          (MSSA), 339
Midshaft femoral fracture, 8
  biochemical and radiological investigations, 232
  clinical examination, 232
  etiology of, 232
  lag screw sheath assembly, 233
  NCB plate and lag screws, 231
  polyaxial distal femoral plate, 230
  pre-operative planning, 232
  previous primary treatment, 227–232
  radiographs of left femur, 234
  revision surgery, 232–234
  sagittal plane, 233

Index 477

Minimally invasive plate osteosynthesis (MIPO), 345
MRI. *See* Magnetic resonance imaging

N
Negative pressure wound therapy (NPWT), 352
Neuropathic diabetic ankle fracture, 391, 392
Non-union, 357, 360–363, 366
  aseptic, 30–31
  definition of, 27–28
  metabolic workup, 33–34
  radiographic and mechanical workup, 32–33
  septic, 28–30

O
Olecranon, 131–133, 136
  clinical examination, 133
  fixation failure, 131
  haematological investigations, 133
  preoperative planning, 134
  revision surgery, 134
  tension band wiring, 131
Oligotrophic non-unions, 30
Open reduction and internal fixation (ORIF), 131, 145,
      369, 371, 379, 467, 469–472
  biochemical and radiological investigations, 240–241
  biologic considerations, 242
  clinical examination, 240
  dual incision approach, 242
  etiology of, 239–240
  implant selection, 241
  post-operative course, 243–246
  pre-operative planning, 241
  previous primary treatment, 237
Osteoblasts/osteoclasts, 393
Osteotomy, 373, 444, 451

P
PACS systems, 393
Pain, 464
Palpable pulse, 393
Parathyroid hormone (PTH), 361
Patella alta, 275
Patella baja, 261
Patella fracture fixation failure
  biochemical and radiological investigations, 284–285
  clinical examination, 284
  etiology of, 284
  patella bridges, 281
  post-revision surgery radiographs, 287
  preoperative planning, 285
  revision surgery, 285–288
  right patella fracture, 283
  right patella preoperative radiographs, 282
Patellar tendon (PT) ruptures
  biochemical and radiological Investigations, 273–274
  clinical examination, 272–273
  etiology of, 272
  graft jacket, 277

Nylon sutures, 278
  preoperative planning, 274
  previous failed primary treatment, 271
  revision surgery, 274–276
  tibial tubercle, 275
  transosseous (TO) techniques, 272
Pelvic ring, 181, 184–187
Perilunate injury, 173, 176
  biochemical and radiological investigations, 176
  clinical examination, 176
  evaluation failure fixation, 176
  preoperative planning, 176
  previous primary treatment, 173
  revision surgery, 177
Physical therapy, 370, 375
Physiotherapy, 387
Pilon fracture, 370, 371, 373, 375
PITFL, 419, 420
Plate fixation, 47
Polymethylmethacrylate (PMMA), 338
Polymethylmethacrylate (PMMA) spacer, 345
Post traumatic arthrosis, 464
Posterior inferior tibio-fibular ligament (PITFL),
      414, 417
Posterior injury, 185
Posterior malleolar fracture
  clinical examination, 423, 424
  diagnostic-biochemical and radiological
        investigations, 421, 422, 424
  evaluation of aetiology of fixation failure, 420
  Haraguchi classification, 417, 418
  history of previous primary treatment, 417–419
  implant selection, 427
  incisura involvement, 418
  posterior antiglide or buttress plating, 420
  preoperative planning, 426, 427
  revision surgery, 427, 428, 430, 432
Posterior subluxation of talus, 417, 426, 433
Posterior tibial cortex, 417
Posterior wall acetabular fractures
  clinical examination, 197
  failure of fixation, 196, 197
  history, previous primary treatment, 193
  preoperative planning, 197
  radiological investigations, 197
  revision surgery, 197, 198
Posterolateral approach, 373, 423, 426, 459
Posterolateral oblique fracture, 417
Posteromedial approach, 424, 426
Pre-operative assessment, 413
Procollagen type 1 N-terminal propeptide
      (P1nP), 361
Prophylactic antibiotics, 379, 441
Proximal humerus
  aetiology of, 77
  clinical examination, 78–79
  implant selection, 81
  investigations, 79–80
  postoperative management, 83–84
  preoperative planning, 81
  surgery, 81–83

Proximal tibia fractures
  anteroposterior and lateral views, 316
  atrophic non-unions, 319
  clinical examination, 317
  erythrocyte sedimentation rate (ESR), 317
  etiology, 317
  hypertrophic nonunion, 318
  interfragmentary compression, 319
  intraoperative fluoroscopic views, 313
  overview of, 311
  preoperative planning, 318
  revision surgery, 319–323
Proximal tibial fractures, 305
  adequate reduction and fixation, 310
  AP and lateral radiographs, 309
  biomechanical and radiological investigations, 306
  clinical examination, 306
  etiology of, 305–306
  fracture displacement, 308
  implants required, 308
  preoperative planning, 306–308, 310
  proper implant placement, 310
  revision surgery, 308
  supplemental fixation, 310
  trans-patellar approach, 305
Pseudoarthrosis, 31

Q

Quadriceps tendon (QT)
  Achilles allograft, 268
  biochemical and radiological investigations, 261–262
  clinical examination, 260–261
  etiology of, 260
  preoperative planning, 262–263
  previous failed treatment, 259
  revision surgery, 263–265

R

Radial head fractures
  assessment, 145–147
  failed fixation, 145, 146, 148
  fixation failure incidence, 145
  preoperative planning, 147–149
  revision surgery, 149, 150
Radius, 152
Reamer-Irrigator-Aspirator (RIA), 373, 377
Receptor activator of nuclear factor-kappa B ligand (RANKL), 361
Rehabilitation, 143
Revision, 169
RIA. *See* Reamer-Irrigator-Aspirator
RIA-harvested autograft, 339
Road traffic collision (RTC), 173

S

Scapho-lunate (SL), 173, 174
Shearing fractures, 168

SHUKLA Nail Extraction System device, 100
Soft-tissue, 375, 376, 395, 461, 464
Squeeze test, 385
Stability and strain theory, 25–27
  external fixators mechanics, 27
  intramedullary device mechanics, 27
  plate fixation mechanics, 26–27
Stepwise approach, 52
Stress test, 385, 387
Subcutaneous tissue, 453
Subluxation, 385
Subtalar arthrodesis, 459
Subtalar joint, 442
Subtrochanteric femoral fracture, 42
  biochemical and radiological investigations, 221
  clinical examination, 221
  etiology of, 221
  preoperative planning, 222
  previous treatment history, 219, 221
  revision surgery, 222–224
Subtrochanteric proximal femoral fracture, 7
Supination-external rotation ankle fractures, 385
Surface area of syndesmosis (SAS), 414
Syndesmosis, 379, 385–387, 408, 409, 412, 414
Synthes Screw Removal Set, 100
Systemic autoimmune disorder, 361

T

Talar fracture
  anteromedial approach, 443
  anteroposterior (AP) and lateral radiographs, 436
  biochemical and radiological investigation, 439
  clinical examination, 438
  evaluation of aetiology of fixation failure, 437
  hindfoot varus, 437–440, 442–444
  incision approach, 443
  medial and lateral approach, 437
  ORIF, 435
  post-fracture fixation, 443
  post-operative AP and lateral radiographs, 436
  preoperative planning, 440, 441
  revision surgery, 441
Tarsal metatarsal joint, 469, 472
Technical error, 199
Tension band wiring, 131, 133
Thyroid stimulating hormone (TSH), 361
Tibial pilon fracture, 362, 369, 373, 375–377
Tibial plateau
  biochemical and radiological investigations, 295–296
  bone grafts, 296
  clinical assessment, 294
  etiology of, 293
  implant selection, 296
  preoperative planning, 296
  previous primary treatment, 289–293
  revision surgery, 296–302
Tibiotalocalcaneal (TTC), 399
Tinzaparin, 379
Toe pressure, 393

Index

Total Leucocyte Count (TLC), 457
Tricortical iliac crest bone graft, 444
Trimalleolar fractures, 417

U
Ulna fracture, 157

V
Vascular endothelial growth factor (VEGF), 24

W
Wedge lateral cortex osteotomy, 206

Weight bearing, 432, 437
Weight-bearing CT (WBCT), 414, 439
Weightbearing CT scan, 469
Wound, 393
Wrist denervation, 4

X
X-ray, 420, 457, 458

Z
Z-plasty, 264

Printed in the United States
by Baker & Taylor Publisher Services